Mechanism and Clinical Management of Cardiac Arrhythmias

Mechanism and Clinical Management of Cardiac Arrhythmias

Editor: Joe Tyler

hayle medical
New York

Hayle Medical,
750 Third Avenue, 9th Floor,
New York, NY 10017, USA

Visit us on the World Wide Web at:
www.haylemedical.com

ISBN 978-1-64647-555-1 (Hardback)

Cataloging-in-Publication Data

Mechanism and clinical management of cardiac arrhythmias / edited by Joe Tyler.
p. cm.
Includes bibliographical references and index.
ISBN 978-1-64647-555-1
1. Arrhythmia. 2. Arrhythmia--Treatment. 3. Arrhythmia--Diagnosis.
4. Heart--Diseases. 5. Heart beat. 6. Cardiology. I. Tyler, Joe.
RC685.A65 M43 2023
616.128--dc23

Contents

Preface

Cardiac arrhythmias are conditions that involve irregularities in the heart beat. It can be generally classified based on the speed of the heart rate as tachycardia and bradycardia. Tachycardia is a condition in which the heart beats more than 100 times per minute. There are several types of tachycardia such as atrial fibrillation, atrial flutter, supraventricular tachycardia, ventricular fibrillation, and ventricular tachycardia. Bradycardia involves a heart rate less than 60 beats per minute. It can be categorized into sick sinus syndrome and conduction block. Some common symptoms of cardiac arrhythmia are chest pain, palpitations, anxiety, etc. Clinical management of cardiac arrhythmias includes different types of medications and invasive therapies. Electrical cardioversion is a type of treatment in which an electrical impulse is conveyed through the chest wall. It is used to synchronize the heart and allow the normal rhythm to restart. This book provides significant information of cardiac arrhythmias to help develop a good understanding of their mechanism and clinical management. It is a vital tool for all researching and studying these medical conditions.

This book unites the global concepts and researches in an organized manner for a comprehensive understanding of the subject. It is a ripe text for all researchers, students, scientists or anyone else who is interested in acquiring a better knowledge of this dynamic field.

I extend my sincere thanks to the contributors for such eloquent research chapters. Finally, I thank my family for being a source of support and help.

Editor

1

Development of a High-Throughput Flow Cytometry Assay to Monitor Defective Trafficking and Rescue of Long QT2 Mutant hERG Channels

Scott A. Kanner[1], Ananya Jain[2] and Henry M. Colecraft[1,2,3]*

[1] Doctoral Program in Neurobiology and Behavior, Columbia University College of Physicians and Surgeons, New York, NY, United States, [2] Department of Physiology and Cellular Biophysics, Columbia University College of Physicians and Surgeons, New York, NY, United States, [3] Department of Pharmacology, Columbia University College of Physicians and Surgeons, New York, NY, United States

***Correspondence:**
Henry M. Colecraft
hc2405@cumc.columbia.edu

Long QT Syndrome (LQTS) is an acquired or inherited disorder characterized by prolonged QT interval, exertion-triggered arrhythmias, and sudden cardiac death. One of the most prevalent hereditary LQTS subtypes, LQT2, results from loss-of-function mutations in the hERG channel, which conducts I_{Kr}, the rapid component of the delayed rectifier K^+ current, critical for cardiac repolarization. The majority of LQT2 mutations result in Class 2 deficits characterized by impaired maturation and trafficking of hERG channels. Here, we have developed a high-throughput flow cytometric assay to analyze the surface and total expression of wild-type (WT) and mutant hERG channels with single-cell resolution. To test our method, we focused on 16 LQT2 mutations in the hERG Per-Arnt-Sim (PAS) domain that were previously studied via a widely used biochemical approach that compares levels of 135-kDa immature and 155-kDa fully glycosylated hERG protein to infer surface expression. We confirmed that LQT2 mutants expressed in HEK293 cells displayed a decreased surface density compared to WT hERG, and were differentially rescued by low temperature. However, we also uncovered some notable differences from the findings obtained via the biochemical approach. In particular, three mutations (N33T, R56Q, and A57P) with apparent WT-like hERG glycosylation patterns displayed up to 50% decreased surface expression. Furthermore, despite WT-like levels of complex glycosylation, these mutants have impaired forward trafficking, and exhibit varying half-lives at the cell surface. The results highlight utility of the surface labeling/flow cytometry approach to quantitatively assess trafficking deficiencies associated with LQT2 mutations, to discern underlying mechanisms, and to report on interventions that rescue deficits in hERG surface expression.

Keywords: long QT syndrome type 2, HERG channels (Kv11), ion channel trafficking, flow cytometry, cardiac arrhythmias

INTRODUCTION

Long QT Syndrome (LQTS) is an inherited or acquired disorder characterized by delayed cardiac action potential repolarization, which predisposes to polymorphic ventricular tachycardias (torsade de pointes), syncope, and sudden cardiac death (SCD) (Moss and Kass, 2005; Bohnen et al., 2016). Congenital LQTS occurs in approximately 1 in 2000 live births (Schwartz et al., 2009), and accounts for a significant portion of ~400,000 cases of SCD in the United States each year (Tester and Ackerman, 2009; George, 2013). Loss-of-function mutations in several genes have been linked to LQTS (LQT1-LQT13), with around 70% occurring in genes encoding pore-forming subunits for the primary repolarizing K^+ currents in ventricular cardiomyocytes – KCNQ1 (LQT1) and hERG (LQT2) (Bohnen et al., 2016).

The hERG potassium channels assemble as a tetramer of four Kv11.1 α_1 pore-forming subunits, and conduct I_{Kr}, the rapid component of the delayed rectifier K^+ current (Trudeau et al., 1995). I_{Kr} is critical for proper cardiac repolarization, as well as the suppression of arrhythmic events caused by premature stimuli (Sanguinetti et al., 1995; Vandenberg et al., 2012). Over 500 LQT2 mutations in hERG have been described to date, with ~40% consisting of non-sense mutations and ~60% being missense mutations (Schwartz et al., 2009; Smith et al., 2016). Four classes of mutations have been described: Class 1 mutations affect channel synthesis or translation; Class 2 mutations affect channel trafficking and intracellular transportation; Class 3 mutations alter channel gating; and Class 4 affect ion permeability (Smith et al., 2016). It has become apparent that the vast majority (~88%) of LQT2 mutations are Class 2 type, featuring compromised channel trafficking to the plasma membrane (Anderson et al., 2006, 2014; Smith et al., 2016). Understanding the mechanisms regulating hERG trafficking and how these may be dysregulated in disease is important for molecular insights into the pathophysiology of LQT2.

The hERG channels undergo several levels of post-translational processing and maturation before the functional channel reaches the cell surface (**Figure 1**). They are synthesized in the endoplasmic reticulum (ER), which provides an environment for optimum folding and assembly. In the ER, the 132-kDa protein undergoes N-linked core glycosylation of the protein, generating a 135-kDa immature protein (Zhou et al., 1998b; Petrecca et al., 1999; Gong et al., 2002) (**Figure 1**, left – step 1). From the ER, hERG that is properly folded and assembled is exported via COPII vesicles (Delisle et al., 2009) to the Golgi where it is matured through N-linked complex glycosylation to generate a 155-kDa protein that is biochemically distinguishable from the immature form (**Figure 1**, left – step 2). Most studies investigating hERG trafficking defects in inherited or acquired LQT2 have taken advantage of these biochemical signatures, utilizing immunoblot assays to distinguish relative expression of 135-kDa immature and 155-kDa mature bands and, thereby, infer surface expression (**Figure 1**, left – step 3) (Zhou et al., 1998b, 1999; Gong et al., 2002, 2005; Guo et al., 2009; Dennis et al., 2011; Apaja et al., 2013; Ke et al., 2013).

The conclusion that a majority of LQT2 mutations are of the Class 2 type (i.e., trafficking-deficient) come from observations that there is either a relative or a complete loss of the 155-kDa mature hERG protein in most of these instances (Anderson et al., 2006, 2014; Ke et al., 2013). An important feature of many trafficking-deficient LQT2 mutants is that they are not irretrievably lost, but can be rescued by incubation at low temperature or with chemical chaperones such as the Kv11.1 channel blocker, E-4031 (Zhou et al., 1999; Ficker et al., 2002; Anderson et al., 2006). Such correction typically results in the re-emergence of the mature 155-kDa band, thereby providing a signature that can be monitored to evaluate rescue efficacy (**Figure 1**, right).

Despite the evident efficacy of the biochemical assay to probe hERG protein trafficking, there are some potential limitations to this approach. First, it does not provide a direct measure of surface channels. This is pertinent giving findings that glycosylation may not be absolutely required for surface trafficking (Gong et al., 2002), and the possibility that some fully glycosylated channels may still be compromised in their ability to reach the cell surface (Dennis et al., 2011; Smith et al., 2011). Second, the method may lack subcellular discrimination since glycosylated channels could potentially reside in the Golgi as well as post-Golgi compartments including the cell surface and endosomes. Finally, the biochemical approach is relatively labor-intensive which limits opportunities for rapid high throughput screening strategies to identify novel trafficking correctors as potential therapeutics. Here, we sought to develop an optical high-throughput assay to monitor surface and total hERG protein expression that would be useful to discern mechanisms underlying LQT2 trafficking deficiencies and also amenable as an assay for identifying new hERG protein trafficking correctors.

RESULTS

Design and Implementation of a Flow Cytometric Assay to Analyze WT and Mutant hERG Surface Expression

Previous studies from our laboratory and others have shown the utility of a 13-residue high-affinity bungarotoxin binding site (BBS) introduced as an extracellular epitope tag to faithfully label surface population of distinct ion channels and membrane proteins (Sekine-Aizawa and Huganir, 2004; Wilkins et al., 2008; Yang et al., 2010; Aromolaran et al., 2014; Cassidy et al., 2014). Building on previous work that utilized an extracellular HA epitope for surface detection of hERG (Ficker et al., 2003; Wible et al., 2005), we introduced the BBS tag into the extracellular S1-S2 loop of hERG to enable efficient detection of surface channels in non-permeabilized cells with Alexa Fluor 647-conjugated bungarotoxin (BTX_{647}) (**Figure 2A**). We also fused YFP to the C-terminus of hERG to enable simultaneous fluorescence detection of total hERG expression (**Figure 2A**). Human embryonic kidney (HEK293) cells transiently transfected with wild-type (WT) BBS-hERG-YFP displayed robust fluorescence signals for total (yellow; YFP) and surface (red; BTX_{647}) channel pools when imaged by confocal microscopy (**Figure 2B**). We used flow cytometry to quantify total and surface BBS-hERG-YFP channel pools in an unbiased and high-throughput manner, all with single cell resolution (**Figure 2C**). Consistent with the confocal microscopy results, cells expressing WT BBS-hERG-YFP (i.e., YFP-positive cells) displayed robust surface expression, with red fluorescence signals up to a 100-fold higher than a threshold level established with single color controls (**Figures 2C,D**).

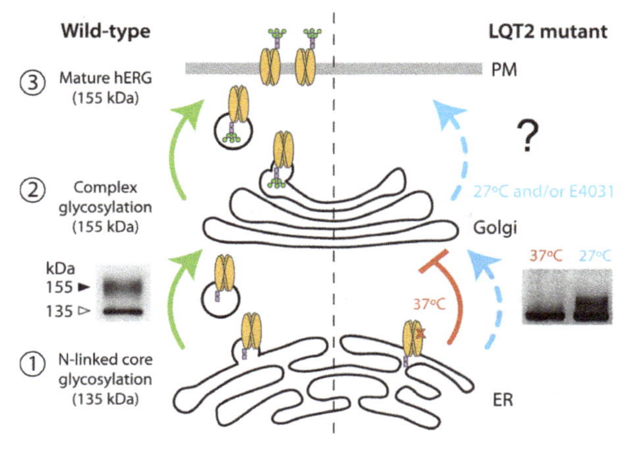

FIGURE 1 | hERG maturation, glycosylation, and surface trafficking. (Left) Forward trafficking of WT hERG (green) is represented. WT hERG undergoes assembly and post-translational N-linked core glycosylation (purple squares) in the endoplasmic reticulum (step 1) and complex glycosylation (green circles) in the Golgi (step 2). Functional channels on the cell surface contain the fully glycosylated 155-kDa mature form of hERG (step 3). Immunoblot (inset, Left) adapted from Gong et al. (2002) represents core glycosylated (135-kDa) and complex glycosylated (155-kDa) hERG bands. (Right) Correctable LQT2 mutant (i.e., Class 2 trafficking defect) is represented at 37°C (red) and incubation with low temperature/chemical chaperone (blue). Immunoblot (inset, Right) adapted from Zhou et al. (1999) demonstrates temperature-dependent rescue of complex glycosylation.

As an initial test of the robustness of this assay to report on trafficking-deficient LQT2 mutants, we examined the impact of introducing an LQT2-causing point mutation in hERG, C44F, which is known to be trafficking-deficient as it is not post-translationally processed to the 155-kDa mature form of the protein (Lupoglazoff et al., 2001; Anderson et al., 2014). Consistent with this view, mutant BBS-hERG$_{C44F}$-YFP displayed no surface BTX$_{647}$ red fluorescence in YFP-positive cells (**Figures 2E–G**).

Surface Labeling Assay Reveals Distinct Subtypes of LQT2-Causing Mutations in the PAS Domain

The hERG1a protein contains two major intracellular domains – the N-terminal Per-Arnt-Sim (PAS) domain and C-terminal cyclic nucleotide binding domain (CNBD) – which interact and require proper folding for effective channel trafficking and gating (Muskett et al., 2011; Gianulis et al., 2013; Ng et al., 2014; Wang and MacKinnon, 2017) (**Figure 3A**). In a recent comprehensive study, Anderson et al. (2014) conducted a large-scale analyses of hERG channel mutations to better understand and characterize trafficking properties of the channel resulting from mutations in distinct domains. They expressed mutant hERG channels in a heterologous expression system, under two corrective conditions – incubation at decreased temperature (27°C) or with the drug E-4031, a potassium channel blocker and pharmacological chaperone. Utilizing the immunoblot assay, they confirmed the predominance of impaired trafficking as the mechanism underlying loss-of-function of LQT2 mutant channels, and further demonstrated five distinct subclasses of mutations: (1) WT-like, (2) correctable by low temperature alone, (3) corrected by E4031 alone, (4) corrected by both low temperature and

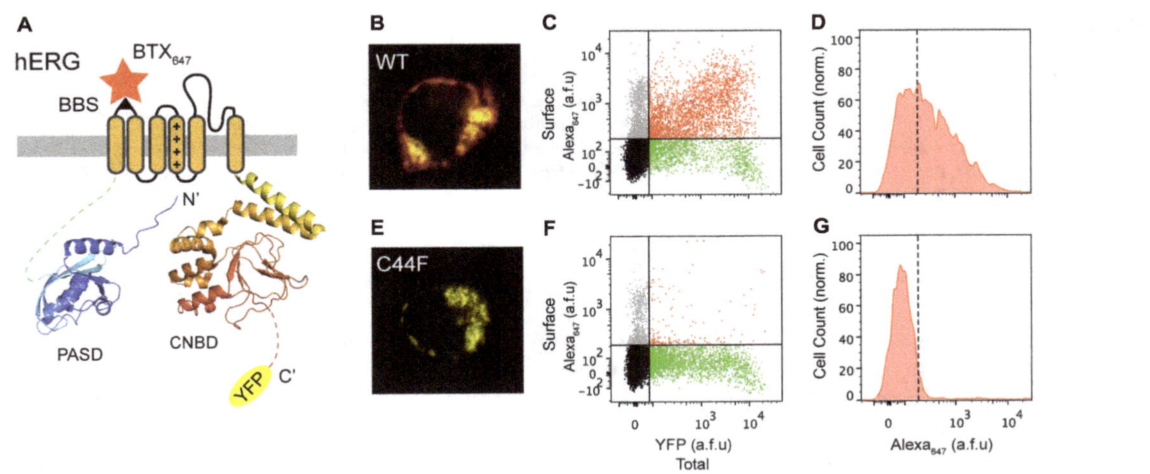

FIGURE 2 | Surface labeling of hERG channels. **(A)** Cartoon of BBS-hERG-YFP subunit. PASD (blue) and CNBD (red) structures adapted from Wang and MacKinnon (2017) (PDB: 5VA2). The bungarotoxin binding site (BBS) epitope (S1-S2) allows for selective labeling of surface hERG channels while YFP signal represents total hERG protein expression. **(B)** Confocal image of a live cell expressing BBS-hERG-YFP and stained with BTX$_{647}$. **(C)** Flow cytometry dot plot showing surface (BTX$_{647}$ fluorescence) and total (YFP fluorescence) hERG expression in cells expressing BBS-hERG-YFP. Vertical and horizontal lines represent thresholds for YFP and BTX$_{647}$-positive cells, respectively, based on the analyses of single color controls. Represented are YFP-positive cells with BTX$_{647}$ signal above (red dots) or below threshold (green dots); BTX$_{647}$-positive cells with YFP signal below threshold (gray dots); and untransfected cells (black dots). **(D)** Histogram of BTX$_{647}$ fluorescence in cells expressing WT BBS-hERG-YFP, generated from population of YFP-positive cells. Dotted line is threshold value for BTX$_{647}$ signal. **(E–G)** Data for cells expressing LQT2 mutant BBS-hERG$_{C44F}$-YFP channels; same format as **B–D**.

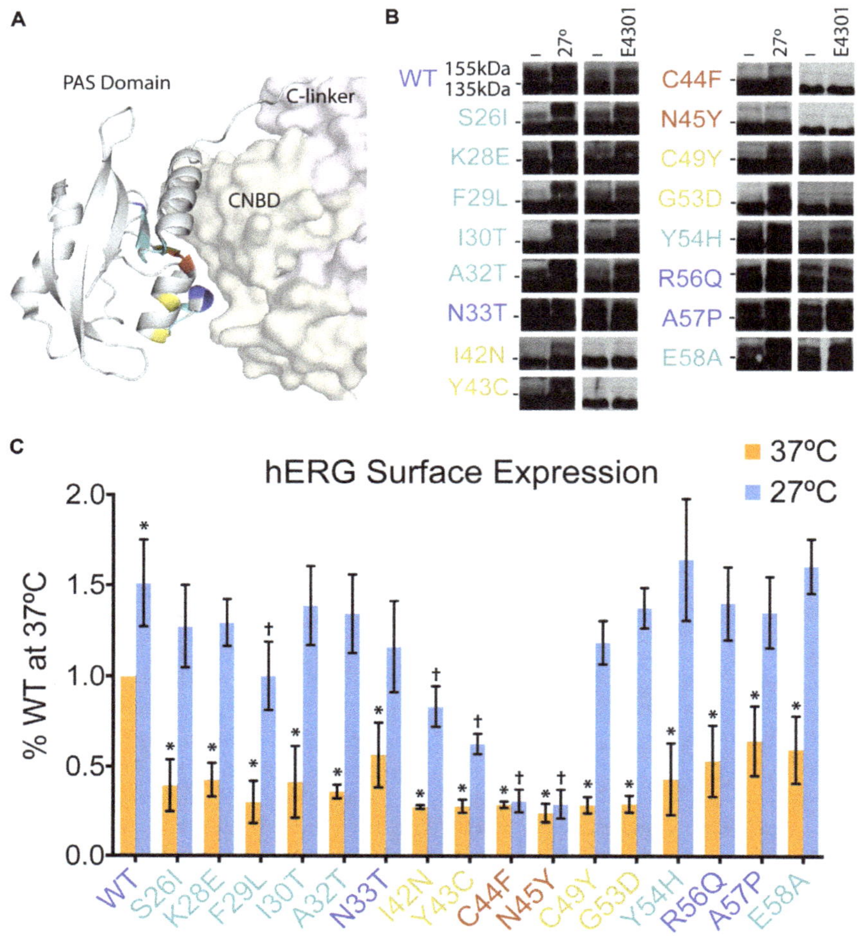

FIGURE 3 | Low temperature rescue of defective surface trafficking in 16 LQT2 hERG channels with mutations in the PAS domain. **(A)** Structure of the hERG PAS domain in complex with CNBD, adapted from Wang and MacKinnon (2017) (PDB: 5VA2). Positions of 16 LQT2 mutations highlighted according to their reported impact on hERG trafficking as assessed by the prevalence of the 155-kDa mature protein and the rescue of this band by low temperature and/or E4031–WT glycosylation (blue), uncorrectable (red), temperature correctable only (yellow), and temperature and E4031 correctable (teal). **(B)** Western blot analyses of PAS domain LQT2 mutants reproduced from Anderson et al. (2014) (with permission from Nature Communications). Horizontal dashes at the sides of the blots represent 140 kDa. **(C)** Quantification of surface hERG channels ($Alexa_{647}$ fluorescence) from flow cytometry experiments (n = 8878–30497 cells; N = 4) for WT and LQT2 mutant hERG channels at 37 and 27°C. Data are normalized to WT hERG surface expression at 37°C. *p < 0.02 versus WT 37°C, †p < 0.02 versus WT 27°C, two-way ANOVA followed by Dunnett's test.

E4031, and (5) uncorrectable by either low temperature or E4031.

The comprehensive study by Anderson et al. (2014), in combination with previous studies looking at PAS domain mutations (Gianulis and Trudeau, 2011; Harley et al., 2012; Ke et al., 2013; Perry et al., 2016), provided a valuable resource and opportunity to test the robustness of the flow cytometry approach and its potential utility in providing mechanistic information beyond that provided by the biochemical method. To accomplish this, we focused on 16 mutations clustered in the PAS domain that based on the relative prevalence of 155-kDa fully glycosylated band were previously classified as: (1) WT-like (N33T, R56Q, A57P; blue), (2) uncorrectable (C44F, N45Y; red), (3) temperature correctable only (I42N, Y43C, C49Y, G53D; yellow), and (4) both low temperature and E4031 correctable (S26I, K28E, F29L, I30T, A32T, Y54H, E58A; teal) (**Figure 3B**; Western blots reproduced from Anderson et al., 2014).

We expressed WT and mutant BBS- and YFP-tagged hERG channels in HEK293 cells, under both 37°C and low temperature (27°C) conditions. Quantification of surface intensity from four independent experiments are shown, normalized to WT surface expression at 37°C (**Figure 3C**). Reassuringly, comparison of the surface density data to the immunoblotting study shows areas of concordance. First, we observed that all the LQT2 mutant channels displayed significant deficits in surface density compared to WT when cells were incubated at 37°C. Second, incubation at 27°C resulted in rescued surface density for all mutants except C44F and N45Y. However, there were some notable differences from the previous study. We observed a significant reduction in surface density of N33T, R56Q, and A57P channels that were previously classified as WT-like based on their glycosylation pattern at 37°C (**Figure 3C**). Moreover, the low temperature rescue of I42N and Y43C channels was only partial, which was not evident by the biochemical assay (**Figures 3B,C**) (Anderson et al., 2014).

Overall, these results validate the utility of the flow cytometry approach to quantify surface expression of WT and LQT2 hERG channels in a robust and sensitive manner, and to quantitatively evaluate correction of trafficking deficiencies.

LQT2 Mutations With WT-Like Glycosylation Patterns Demonstrate Reduced Surface Expression, Impaired Forward Trafficking, and Distinct Half-Lives at the Cell Surface

The discrepancy between the biochemical and flow cytometry approaches in the assignment of WT-like properties to N33T, R56Q, and A57P channels was interesting as it suggested that the presence of a WT-like abundance of the 155-kDa mature protein does not necessarily translate to normal channel surface density. On the basis of the flow cytometry approach, these mutants would be more appropriately characterized as temperature correctable, rather than WT-like (**Figures 4A–D**).

It was instructive to consider the potential mechanisms contributing to the deficits in surface expression of these mutant channels despite their WT glycosylation patterns. In principle, these could be mediated by impaired forward trafficking, decreased stability of the channel at the surface, or a combination of both mechanisms. An advantage of the flow cytometry approach is it can be adapted to probe these possibilities utilizing two complementary, optical pulse-chase assays (Kanner et al., 2017). To test differences in forward trafficking, we utilized a live-cell assay to analyze the delivery of new channels to the surface over time (**Figure 4E**). Live, non-permeabilized cells expressing WT or mutant BBS-hERG-YFP channels at 37°C for 24 h were moved to 4°C to halt all trafficking processes and subsequently exposed to unconjugated BTX to block all extracellular BBS epitopes initially present at the plasma membrane (pulse). Cells were then incubated at 37°C for varying time periods (chase), after which cells were returned to 4°C and the newly delivered surface channels labeled with BTX_{647} and quantified by flow cytometry. Control cells expressing WT BBS-hERG-YFP demonstrated a steady delivery of new channels to the surface (**Figure 4F**). In contrast, all three mutants demonstrated impaired delivery of new channels to the surface as evident by a significantly reduced plateau in BTX_{647} fluorescence (**Figure 4F**).

To determine the residence time of channels at the cell surface, we utilized a second optical, pulse-chase assay to measure removal of channels from the plasma membrane (**Figure 4G**). Live, non-permeabilized cells expressing WT and mutant BBS-hERG-YFP channels incubated at 27°C for 24 h (to ensure a comparable number of channels initially at the cell surface) were moved to 4°C and labeled with biotinylated bungarotoxin (BTX-biotin) at 4°C (pulse). Cells were then incubated at 37°C for varying time periods to resume trafficking (chase), and subsequently labeled with streptavidin-conjugated Alexa Fluor 647 (SA-647) at 4°C. In this paradigm, SA-647 labeling would only occur on channels that were initially present at the surface and labeled with BTX-biotin during the pulse period. As expected, WT hERG channels demonstrated an exponential decrease in surface labeling over time (**Figure 4H**). Interestingly, the three mutants demonstrated different rates of decline in surface labeling (**Figure 4H**), implying different rates of internalization, with R56Q displaying the most rapid removal from the cell surface.

DISCUSSION

In this study, we sought to develop a high-throughput optical flow cytometric assay that enables quantitative assessment of WT and LQT2 hERG channel trafficking, and rescue of trafficking-deficient mutants by low temperature or pharmacological chaperones. The method is complementary to other previously described approaches to monitor hERG channel trafficking, including a biochemical assay that assesses relative abundance of immature 135-kDa and fully glycosylated 155-kDa forms of the protein. By comparing results from the flow cytometric analyses of 16 PAS domain mutant hERG channels to published data of the same mutations assessed by the biochemical approach, we find not only areas of concordance that validates the assay, but also some discrepancies that highlight advantages of the flow cytometry method. We discuss the flow cytometry assay and our results in the context of established methods to monitor hERG channel trafficking and some of the results obtained with these approaches.

Complex Glycosylation as a Marker for hERG Maturation and Surface Trafficking

The first studies elucidating glycosylation as a critical player in the maturation of WT hERG channels were reported almost two decades ago (Zhou et al., 1998b, 1999; Petrecca et al., 1999). It was further shown that while certain LQT2 mutations displayed post-translational processing similar to WT, others exhibited an impaired maturation evident as an absence of the 155-kDa fully processed protein band (Zhou et al., 1998a; Anderson et al., 2006, 2014). Moreover, treatment of cells with protease led to the digestion and disappearance of the mature 155-kDa band, with no effect on the immature 135-kDa band, consistent with the mature protein being predominantly at the cell surface (Zhou et al., 1998b; Rajamani et al., 2006). Consequently, biochemical analyses of the relative abundance of 135- and 155-kDa hERG bands has been a standard widely adopted tool to analyze trafficking of WT and mutant hERG channels under different conditions. Nevertheless, it is noteworthy that Gong et al. (2002) demonstrated that while N-linked glycosylation of hERG occurs at residue N598, mutating this site did not abolish hERG channel surface expression despite the disappearance of the 155-kDa form of the protein. Hence, while glycosylation is important for hERG maturation, it is not absolutely required for assembly and expression of functional hERG channels at the cell surface. This suggests the possibility that a sole reliance on the biochemical assay to categorize mechanisms underlying LQT2

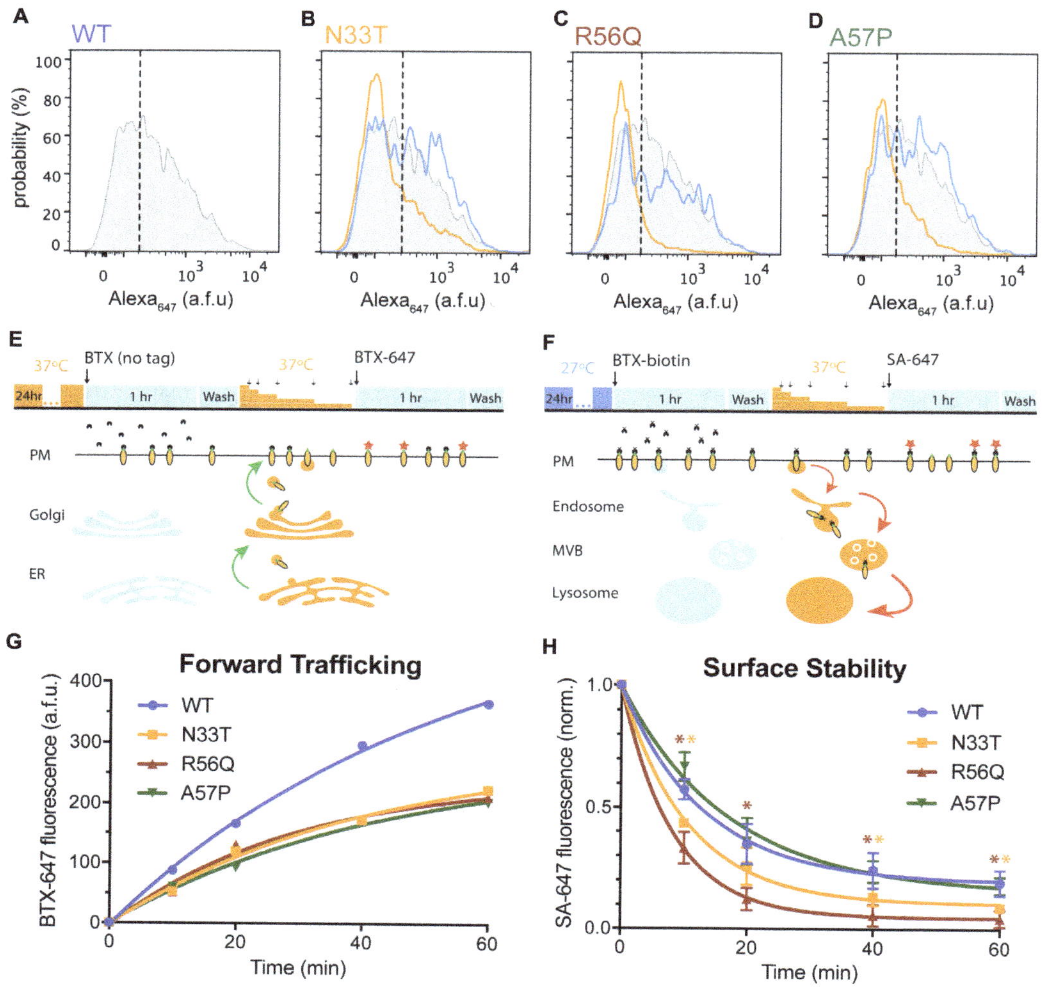

FIGURE 4 | LQT2 hERG channels with WT glycosylation patterns show reduced surface expression. **(A–D)** Representative histograms representing surface intensity from HEK293 cells expressing BBS- and YFP-tagged **(A)** WT HERG (gray) at 37°C, and LQT2 mutants **(B)** N33T, **(C)** R56Q, and **(D)** A57P incubated at 37°C (orange) and 27°C (blue). **(E)** Schematic adapted from Kanner et al. (2017), showing optical pulse-chase assay for measuring BBS-hERG-YFP forward trafficking. Cells expressing BBS-hERG-YFP were incubated at 37°C for 24 h prior to the experiment. BBS-tag on channels initially at the cell surface was blocked by incubation with untagged α-bungarotoxin (BTX) at 4°C. Cells were washed and placed back at 37°C for varying time intervals (10, 20, 40, 60 min) to resume delivery of new channels to the surface membrane. Newly delivered channels were labeled with Alexa Fluor 647 conjugated BTX (BTX_{647}) at 4°C and analyzed using flow cytometry. **(F)** Time evolution of BBS-hERG-YFP delivery to the surface for WT (•, n = 7312–8016 cells; N = 2), N33T (■, n = 6886–7533 cells; N = 2), R56Q (▲, n = 7756–9248 cells; N = 2), A57P (▼, n = 9159–10139 cells; N = 2). Smooth curves are fits of an exponential growth function to the data: $y=A(1-e^{-t/\tau})$. For WT (•), $A = 560.7 \pm 47.5$, $\tau = 53.6 \pm 9.5$ min; N33T (■), $A = 293.1 \pm 42.2$, $\tau = 42.2 \pm 12.3$ min; R56Q (▲), $A = 248.6 \pm 35.5$, $\tau = 30.4 \pm 10.4$ min; A57P (▼), $A = 276.2 \pm 40.0$, $\tau = 44.5 \pm 12.6$ min. **(G)** Schematic adapted from Kanner et al. (2017), showing optical assay for measuring BBS-hERG-YFP stability at the cell surface. Cells expressing BBS-hERG-YFP were incubated at 27°C for 24 h prior to the experiment. Channels initially at the cell surface were labeled with biotin-conjugated BTX (BTX-biotin) at 4°C. Cells were washed and incubated at 37°C for varying time intervals (10, 20, 40, 60 min) to allow for internalization of surface channels. The remaining surface channels were labeled with Alexa Fluor 647-conjugated streptavidin (SA-647) at 4°C. **(H)** Time evolution of loss of surface BBS-hERG-YFP channels WT (•, n = 8184–10128 cells; N = 3), N33T (■, n = 8499–10175 cells; N = 3), R56Q (▲, n = 9460–12338 cells; N = 3), A57P (▼, n = 7123–8911 cells; N = 3). Smooth curves are fits of an exponential decay function to the data: $y=(1-A)e^{-t/\tau}+A$. For WT (•), $A = 0.19 \pm 0.02$, $\tau = 12.9 \pm 0.9$ min; N33T (■), $A = 0.10 \pm 0.02$, $\tau = 10.6 \pm 0.8$ min; R56Q (▲), $A = 0.05 \pm 0.004$, $\tau = 8.2 \pm 0.2$ min; A57P (▼), $A = 0.15 \pm 0.05$, $\tau = 16.5 \pm 3.2$ min. * and *, $p < 0.05$ for N33T and R56Q, respectively, compared to WT; two-way ANOVA followed by Dunnett's test.

mutations could potentially misclassify some as being in the Class 2 trafficking-deficient category.

There has been relatively scant research on the prevalence of the opposite phenomenon: Does a WT-like glycosylation pattern guarantee channel surface density similar to WT hERG? Previous studies found that despite rescue of the mature 155-kDa band in antidepressant-induced and inherited G601S LQT2 by lysosomal inhibitors and microtubule depolymerization, respectively, there was no subsequent rescue in functional hERG expression at the surface membrane (Dennis et al., 2011; Smith et al., 2011). Of the 16 PAS domain LQT2 mutations we studied, three had been previously classified as WT-like on the basis of their glycosylation patterns (Anderson et al., 2014). Remarkably, we found that all three exhibited significantly reduced surface expression compared to WT hERG, demonstrating lack of an absolute correlation between relative abundance of the 155-kDa mature protein form and its level of expression at the cell surface. We further found that the putative WT-like LQT2 mutant channels displayed impaired forward trafficking. Given that these mutants have WT glycosylation patterns, they have presumably reached or passed through the Golgi compartment. We cannot distinguish from our results whether the impaired forward trafficking arises from deficits in transport from the Golgi to the cell surface, or whether it mostly reflects shortfalls in some post-Golgi recycling compartments. This is pertinent as robust Rab11-mediated recycling of hERG channels has been observed (Lamothe and Zhang, 2013; Chen et al., 2015).

Differential Plasma Membrane Stability of LQT2-Causing Mutants

Our flow cytometry method indicated that the residence time of WT hERG channels at the cell surface was short, with an apparent half-life of ~9 min. The measured half-life was even shorter with the LQT2 mutations R56Q (~5.7 min), and to a lesser extent N33T (7.3 min), but not A57P (~11.7 min). Overall, the flow cytometry approach suggests a more rapid removal of surface hERG channels than has been previously reported. There have been several approaches applied to analyze the turnover or stability of hERG channels at the cell surface. One method uses the biochemical approach to follow the loss of the fully glycosylated hERG protein band in cells treated with brefeldin A. The half-life for the disappearance of the fully glycosylated hERG protein from this approach is on the order of ~10 h. This biochemical method measures the turnover of mature hERG proteins, and is distinguished from our approach which directly measures the removal of surface channels. Notably, it has been demonstrated using the biochemical approach that some LQT2 mutations, including R56Q, display a decreased protein stability compared to WT hERG (Ke et al., 2013). Our finding that R56Q is more rapidly removed from the cell surface is in broad agreement with this previous report.

Another approach similar in principle to the method described here utilizes a hemagglutinin (HA) tag engineered into the extracellular S1-S2 loop of hERG. The labeling and fate of surface channels are then detected either by confocal microscopy in single cells, or cell surface ELISA in a population of cells (Wible et al., 2005; Apaja et al., 2013; Karnik et al., 2013). Apaja et al. (2013) utilized the cell surface ELISA approach to measure the plasma membrane residence time of WT and LQT2 hERG proteins. They measured a plasma membrane half-life of the WT protein of ~ 9 and 3 h in HeLa and H9C2i cells, respectively. It is not clear why the two methods, which seem similar in principle, give rise to such disparate values for the residence time of hERG channels in the plasma membrane. One possibility is that the different cell types used in the studies could have an impact. To this point, Apaja et al. (2013) observe a threefold difference in the hERG plasma membrane residence time between HeLa and H9C2i cells. Another factor could be the stable versus transient expression of hERG channels in heterologous systems. As demonstrated in several studies with cystic fibrosis transmembrane conductance regulator (CFTR) trafficking, differences among absolute half-lives of channels at the cell surface may appear in heterologous systems and primary cells (albeit with similar relative changes of mutant relative to WT) (Sharma et al., 2004; Swiatecka-Urban et al., 2005; Cholon et al., 2010). Thus, future studies applying the BTX_{647} labeling method in the native cellular context of primary adult rodent cardiomyocytes will be important for distinguishing among these different possibilities.

A caveat for approaches that utilize epitope and fluorescent protein tags is the potential for unanticipated effects on hERG channel trafficking. This concern is mitigated by our findings that: (1) the tagged WT hERG trafficks robustly to the cell surface, and (2) the impact of PAS domain mutations on hERG surface density is largely consistent with expectations based on previous analyses of glycosylation patterns and low temperature rescue.

Flow Cytometry as a Versatile Assay to Classify Trafficking-Deficient hERG Mutants and Elucidate New Therapeutic Strategies

Beyond the enhanced sensitivity and capacity to increase mechanistic insights, an important advantage of the flow cytometry method is its versatility compared to existing approaches. Existing ELISA-based assays rely on total fluorescence/chemiluminescence from cell populations. The lack of single cell resolution limits comparisons to homogeneous populations and potentially overlooks critical points in quality control (i.e., punctate/apoptotic cells, variable protein expression). Confocal studies allow for cellular/subcellular visualization, but do not provide the ability to easily quantify a large number of cells in an unbiased fashion. The flow cytometry method combines benefits of both approaches, enabling rapid analyses of a large population of cells with single-cell resolution, accounting for variations in transfection efficiency, and permitting normalization of channel surface expression to total protein expression levels. As such, there is no need to make stable cell lines for different mutations, and the capability to simultaneously analyze many colors at a time allows for potential applications that require multiplexing. Lastly, recent development and availability of 96-well flow cytometry protocols allow this approach to be adapted for medium- to high-throughput formats to identify novel correctors of hERG channel trafficking in a mutation-specific manner (Krutzik and Nolan, 2006; Duensing and Watson, 2018).

Although we have not conducted functional studies on these LQT2 mutants, it is important to note that previous studies observed changes in gating kinetics in certain PAS domain mutations (Chen et al., 1999; Gianulis and Trudeau, 2011). As such, the mere rescue of trafficking deficiencies may not be sufficient for therapeutic rescue of hERG function in the complex electrical milieu of the cardiac action potential (Perry et al., 2016). This highlights the need for combinatorial approaches for treating LQT2 pathology at both the cell biological (i.e., impaired forward trafficking, reduced residency time at the cell surface), and biophysical (i.e. conductance, gating kinetics) level. As there is no single mutation that is dominant in LQTS (with more variants being continually discovered), the use of new methods, such as flow cytometry, to further hone existing classifications of mutations and elucidate therapeutic subclasses will be critical in the pursuit of precision medicine for inherited arrhythmias and other ion channelopathies.

MATERIALS AND METHODS

Molecular Biology and Cloning of Plasmid Vectors

The BBS-hERG-YFP constructs were engineered on the previously described hERG1a-YFP template (Puckerin et al., 2016), which utilized overlap extension PCR to fuse enhanced yellow fluorescent protein (EYFP) in frame to the C-terminus of hERG1a. A 13-residue bungarotoxin-binding site (BBS; TGGCGGTACTACGAGAGCAGCCTGGAGCCCTACC CCGAC) (Sekine-Aizawa and Huganir, 2004; Yang et al., 2010) was then introduced between residues T436/E437 in the extracellular S1–S2 loop of hERG using the Quik-Change Lightning Site-Directed Mutagenesis Kit (Stratagene) according to the manufacturer's instructions. 16 LQT2 mutations were introduced in the PAS domain of BBS-hERG-YFP via site-directed mutagenesis.

Cell Culture and Transfections

Low passage human embryonic kidney (HEK293) cells were cultured at 37°C in Dulbecco's Modified Eagle's Medium (DMEM) supplemented with 8% fetal bovine serum (FBS) and 100 mg/mL of penicillin–streptomycin. HEK293 cell transfection was accomplished using the calcium phosphate precipitation method. Briefly, plasmid DNA was mixed with 7.75 μL of 2M $CaCl_2$ and sterile deionized water (to a final volume of 62.5 μL). The mixture was added dropwise, with constant tapping to 62.5 μL of 2x Hepes buffered saline containing (in mM): HEPES 50, NaCl 280, Na_2HPO_4 1.5, pH 7.09. The resulting DNA-calcium phosphate mixture was incubated for 20 min at room temperature and then added dropwise to HEK293 cells (60–80% confluent). Cells were washed with Ca^{2+}-free phosphate buffered saline after 4–6 h and maintained in supplemented DMEM.

Flow Cytometry Assay of Total and Surface Q1 Channels

Cell surface and total ion channel pools were assayed by flow cytometry in live, transfected HEK293 cells as previously described (Yang et al., 2010; Aromolaran et al., 2014). Briefly, 48 h post-transfection, cells cultured in 12-well plates gently washed with ice cold PBS containing Ca^{2+} and Mg^{2+} (in mM: 0.9 $CaCl_2$, 0.49 $MgCl_2$, pH 7.4), and then incubated for 30 min in blocking medium (DMEM with 3% BSA) at 4°C. HEK293 cells were then incubated with 1 μM Alexa Fluor 647 conjugated α-bungarotoxin (BTX-647; Life Technologies) in DMEM/3% BSA on a rocker at 4°C for 1 h, followed by washing three times with PBS (containing Ca^{2+} and Mg^{2+}). Cells were gently harvested in Ca^{2+}-free PBS, and assayed by flow cytometry using a BD LSRII Cell Analyzer (BD Biosciences, San Jose, CA, United States). CFP- and YFP-tagged proteins were excited at 407 and 488 nm, respectively, and Alexa Fluor 647 was excited at 633 nm.

Optical pulse chase assays to monitor rates of channel forward trafficking and internalization were conducted on live, transfected HEK293 cells as previously described (Kanner et al., 2017). For the forward trafficking studies, cells were incubated at 37°C for 24 h prior to the experiments. Cells were placed on 4°C to halt trafficking processes and washed twice with PBS containing Ca^{2+} and Mg^{2+}. For forward trafficking experiments, cells were incubated with 3 μM untagged BTX in DMEM/3% BSA at 4°C for 1 h to block surface channels, and then washed three times with PBS containing Ca^{2+} and Mg^{2+}. Cells were incubated with DMEM/3% BSA and placed at 37°C to resume trafficking for different time intervals (0, 10, 20, 40, 60 min). Cells were then returned to 4°C and newly delivered channels were labeled with 1 μM BTX-647 in DMEM/3% BSA for 1 h. Finally, cells were washed three times with PBS containing Ca^{2+} and Mg^{2+}, gently harvested in Ca^{2+}-free PBS, and assayed by flow cytometry. For surface stability/internalization experiments, cells were incubated at 27°C for 24 h prior to the experiments. Cells were placed on ice (4°C) to halt trafficking processes and washed twice with PBS containing Ca^{2+} and Mg^{2+}. Cells were then incubated in DMEM/3% BSA blocking medium for 30 min at 4°C followed by a 1 h incubation at 4°C (pulse) with 1 μM biotinylated α-bungarotoxin (BTX-biotin; Life Technologies), with gentle rocking. Cells were washed three times in PBS containing Ca^{2+} and Mg^{2+} and placed in DMEM/3% BSA at 37°C for different time intervals (0, 10, 20, 40, 60 min) to resume trafficking (chase). Cells were returned to 4°C, washed once with PBS, and channels remaining at the surface were labeled with streptavidin-conjugated Alexa Fluor 647 (Life Technologies). Finally, cells were washed three more times with PBS with Ca^{2+} and Mg^{2+}, harvested in Ca^{2+}-free PBS, and assayed by flow cytometry.

Data and Statistical Analyses

Data were analyzed off-line using FlowJo, Microsoft Excel, Origin and GraphPad Prism software. Statistical analyses were performed in Origin or GraphPad Prism using built-in functions. Statistically significant differences between means ($p < 0.05$) were determined using two-way ANOVA, followed by Dunnett's correction for multiple comparisons. Data are presented as means ± SD.

AUTHOR CONTRIBUTIONS

SK designed and conducted the experiments, analyzed and interpreted the data, and wrote the manuscript. AJ conducted the experiments and analyzed the data. HC designed the experiments, analyzed and interpreted the data, and wrote the manuscript.

ACKNOWLEDGMENTS

We thank Dr. Gail Robertson (University of Wisconsin) for providing hERG cDNA; Dr. Ademuyiwa Armolaran for constructing BBS-hERG-YFP; and Ming Chen for the excellent technical support.

REFERENCES

Anderson, C. L., Delisle, B. P., Anson, B. D., Kilby, J. A., Will, M. L., Tester, D. J., et al. (2006). Most LQT2 mutations reduce Kv11.1 (hERG) current by a class 2 (trafficking-deficient) mechanism. *Circulation* 113, 365–373. doi: 10.1161/CIRCULATIONAHA.105.570200

Anderson, C. L., Kuzmicki, C. E., Childs, R. R., Hintz, C. J., Delisle, B. P., and January, C. T. (2014). Large-scale mutational analysis of Kv11.1 reveals molecular insights into type 2 long QT syndrome. *Nat. Commun.* 5:5535. doi: 10.1038/ncomms6535

Apaja, P. M., Foo, B., Okiyoneda, T., Valinsky, W. C., Barriere, H., Atanasiu, R., et al. (2013). Ubiquitination-dependent quality control of hERG K+ channel with acquired and inherited conformational defect at the plasma membrane. *Mol. Biol. Cell* 24, 3787–3804. doi: 10.1091/mbc.E13-07-0417

Aromolaran, A. S., Subramanyam, P., Chang, D. D., Kobertz, W. R., and Colecraft, H. M. (2014). LQT1 mutations in KCNQ1 C-terminus assembly domain suppress IKs using different mechanisms. *Cardiovasc. Res.* 104, 501–511. doi: 10.1093/cvr/cvu231

Bohnen, M. S., Peng, G., Robey, S. H., Terrenoire, C., Iyer, V., Sampson, K. J., et al. (2016). Molecular pathophysiology of congenital long QT syndrome. *Physiol. Rev.* 97, 89–134. doi: 10.1152/physrev.00008.2016

Cassidy, J. S., Ferron, L., Kadurin, I., Pratt, W. S., and Dolphin, A. C. (2014). Functional exofacially tagged N-type calcium channels elucidate the interaction with auxiliary alpha2delta-1 subunits. *Proc. Natl. Acad. Sci. U.S.A.* 111, 8979–8984. doi: 10.1073/pnas.1403731111

Chen, J., Guo, J., Yang, T., Li, W., Lamothe, S. M., Kang, Y., et al. (2015). Rab11-dependent recycling of the human ether-a-go-go-related gene (hERG) channel. *J. Biol. Chem.* 290, 21101–21113. doi: 10.1074/jbc.M115.636324

Chen, J., Zou, A., Splawski, I., Keating, M. T., and Sanguinetti, M. C. (1999). Long QT syndrome-associated mutations in the Per-Arnt-Sim (PAS) domain of HERG potassium channels accelerate channel deactivation. *J. Biol. Chem.* 274, 10113–10118. doi: 10.1074/jbc.274.15.10113

Cholon, D. M., O'Neal, W. K., Randell, S. H., Riordan, J. R., and Gentzsch, M. (2010). Modulation of endocytic trafficking and apical stability of CFTR in primary human airway epithelial cultures. *Am. J. Physiol. Lung Cell. Mol. Physiol.* 298, L304–L314. doi: 10.1152/ajplung.00016.2009

Delisle, B. P., Underkofler, H. A., Moungey, B. M., Slind, J. K., Kilby, J. A., Best, J. M., et al. (2009). Small GTPase determinants for the Golgi processing and plasmalemmal expression of human ether-a-go-go related (hERG) K+ channels. *J. Biol. Chem.* 284, 2844–2853. doi: 10.1074/jbc.M807289200

Dennis, A. T., Nassal, D., Deschenes, I., Thomas, D., and Ficker, E. (2011). Antidepressant-induced ubiquitination and degradation of the cardiac potassium channel hERG. *J. Biol. Chem.* 286, 34413–34425. doi: 10.1074/jbc.M111.254367

Duensing, T. D., and Watson, S. R. (2018). Antibody screening using high-throughput flow cytometry. *Cold Spring Harb. Protoc.* 2018:dbto093773. doi: 10.1101/pdb.top093773

Ficker, E., Dennis, A. T., Wang, L., and Brown, A. M. (2003). Role of the cytosolic chaperones Hsp70 and Hsp90 in maturation of the cardiac potassium channel HERG. *Circ. Res.* 92, e87–e100. doi: 10.1161/01.RES.0000079028.31393.15

Ficker, E., Obejero-Paz, C. A., Zhao, S., and Brown, A. M. (2002). The binding site for channel blockers that rescue misprocessed human long QT syndrome type 2 ether-a-gogo-related gene (HERG) mutations. *J. Biol. Chem.* 277, 4989–4998. doi: 10.1074/jbc.M107345200

George, A. L. Jr. (2013). Molecular and genetic basis of sudden cardiac death. *J. Clin. Invest.* 123, 75–83. doi: 10.1172/JCI62928

Gianulis, E. C., Liu, Q., and Trudeau, M. C. (2013). Direct interaction of eag domains and cyclic nucleotide-binding homology domains regulate deactivation gating in hERG channels. *J. Gen. Physiol.* 142, 351–366. doi: 10.1085/jgp.201310995

Gianulis, E. C., and Trudeau, M. C. (2011). Rescue of aberrant gating by a genetically encoded PAS (Per-Arnt-Sim) domain in several long QT syndrome mutant human ether-á-go-go-related gene potassium channels. *J. Biol. Chem.* 286, 22160–22169. doi: 10.1074/jbc.M110.205948

Gong, Q., Anderson, C. L., January, C. T., and Zhou, Z. (2002). Role of glycosylation in cell surface expression and stability of HERG potassium channels. *Am. J. Physiol. Heart Circ. Physiol.* 283, H77–H84. doi: 10.1152/ajpheart.00008.2002

Gong, Q., Keeney, D. R., Molinari, M., and Zhou, Z. (2005). Degradation of trafficking-defective long QT syndrome type II mutant channels by the ubiquitin-proteasome pathway. *J. Biol. Chem.* 280, 19419–19425. doi: 10.1074/jbc.M502327200

Guo, J., Massaeli, H., Xu, J., Jia, Z., Wigle, J. T., Mesaeli, N., et al. (2009). Extracellular K+ concentration controls cell surface density of IKr in rabbit hearts and of the HERG channel in human cell lines. *J. Clin. Invest.* 119, 2745–2757. doi: 10.1172/JCI39027

Harley, C. A., Jesus, C. S., Carvalho, R., Brito, R. M., and Morais-Cabral, J. H. (2012). Changes in channel trafficking and protein stability caused by LQT2 mutations in the PAS domain of the HERG channel. *PLoS One* 7:e32654. doi: 10.1371/journal.pone.0032654

Kanner, S. A., Morgenstern, T., and Colecraft, H. M. (2017). Sculpting ion channel functional expression with engineered ubiquitin ligases. *eLife* 6:e29744. doi: 10.7554/eLife.29744

Karnik, R., Ludlow, M. J., Abuarab, N., Smith, A. J., Hardy, M. E., Elliott, D. J., et al. (2013). Endocytosis of HERG is clathrin-independent and involves arf6. *PLoS One* 8:e85630. doi: 10.1371/journal.pone.0085630

Ke, Y., Ng, C., Hunter, M. J., Mann, S. A., Heide, J., Hill, A. P., et al. (2013). Trafficking defects in PAS domain mutant Kv11. 1 channels: roles of reduced domain stability and altered domain–domain interactions. *Biochem. J.* 454, 69–77. doi: 10.1042/BJ20130328

Krutzik, P. O., and Nolan, G. P. (2006). Fluorescent cell barcoding in flow cytometry allows high-throughput drug screening and signaling profiling. *Nat. Methods* 3, 361–368. doi: 10.1038/nmeth872

Lamothe, S. M., and Zhang, S. (2013). The serum- and glucocorticoid-inducible kinases SGK1 and SGK3 regulate hERG channel expression via ubiquitin ligase Nedd4-2 and GTPase Rab11. *J. Biol. Chem.* 288, 15075–15084. doi: 10.1074/jbc.M113.453670

Lupoglazoff, J. M., Denjoy, I., Berthet, M., Neyroud, N., Demay, L., Richard, P., et al. (2001). Notched T waves on Holter recordings enhance detection of patients with LQt2 (HERG) mutations. *Circulation* 103, 1095–1101. doi: 10.1161/01.CIR.103.8.1095

Moss, A. J., and Kass, R. S. (2005). Long QT syndrome: from channels to cardiac arrhythmias. *J. Clin. Invest.* 115, 2018–2024. doi: 10.1172/JCI25537

Muskett, F. W., Thouta, S., Thomson, S. J., Bowen, A., Stansfeld, P. J., and Mitcheson, J. S. (2011). Mechanistic insight into human ether-a-go-go-related gene (hERG) K+ channel deactivation gating from the solution structure of the EAG domain. *J. Biol. Chem.* 286, 6184–6191. doi: 10.1074/jbc.M110.199364

Ng, C. A., Phan, K., Hill, A. P., Vandenberg, J. I., and Perry, M. D. (2014). Multiple interactions between cytoplasmic domains regulate slow deactivation of Kv11.1 channels. *J. Biol. Chem.* 289, 25822–25832. doi: 10.1074/jbc.M114.558379

Perry, M. D., Ng, C. A., Phan, K., David, E., Steer, K., Hunter, M. J., et al. (2016). Rescue of protein expression defects may not be enough to abolish the pro-arrhythmic phenotype of long QT type 2 mutations. *J. Physiol.* 594, 4031–4049. doi: 10.1113/JP271805

Petrecca, K., Atanasiu, R., Akhavan, A., and Shrier, A. (1999). N-linked glycosylation sites determine HERG channel surface membrane expression. *J. Physiol.* 515, 41–48. doi: 10.1111/j.1469-7793.1999.041ad.x

Puckerin, A., Aromolaran, K. A., Chang, D. D., Zukin, R. S., Colecraft, H. M., Boutjdir, M., et al. (2016). hERG 1a LQT2 C-terminus truncation mutants display hERG 1b-dependent dominant negative mechanisms. *Heart Rhythm* 13, 1121–1130. doi: 10.1016/j.hrthm.2016.01.012

Rajamani, S., Anderson, C. L., Valdivia, C. R., Eckhardt, L. L., Foell, J. D., Robertson, G. A., et al. (2006). Specific serine proteases selectively damage KCNH2 (hERG1) potassium channels and I(Kr). *Am. J. Physiol. Heart Circ. Physiol.* 290, H1278–H1288. doi: 10.1152/ajpheart.00777.2005

Sanguinetti, M. C., Jiang, C., Curran, M. E., and Keating, M. T. (1995). A mechanistic link between an inherited and an acquired cardiac arrhythmia:

HERG encodes the IKr potassium channel. *Cell* 81, 299–307. doi: 10.1016/0092-8674(95)90340-2

Schwartz, P. J., Stramba-Badiale, M., Crotti, L., Pedrazzini, M., Besana, A., Bosi, G., et al. (2009). Prevalence of the congenital long-QT syndrome. *Circulation* 120, 1761–1767. doi: 10.1161/CIRCULATIONAHA.109.863209

Sekine-Aizawa, Y., and Huganir, R. L. (2004). Imaging of receptor trafficking by using alpha-bungarotoxin-binding-site-tagged receptors. *Proc. Natl. Acad. Sci. U.S.A.* 101, 17114–17119. doi: 10.1073/pnas.0407563101

Sharma, M., Pampinella, F., Nemes, C., Benharouga, M., So, J., Du, K., et al. (2004). Misfolding diverts CFTR from recycling to degradation: quality control at early endosomes. *J. Cell Biol.* 164, 923–933. doi: 10.1083/jcb.200312018

Smith, J. L., Anderson, C. L., Burgess, D. E., Elayi, C. S., January, C. T., and Delisle, B. P. (2016). Molecular pathogenesis of long QT syndrome type 2. *J. Arrhythm.* 32, 373–380. doi: 10.1016/j.joa.2015.11.009

Smith, J. L., McBride, C. M., Nataraj, P. S., Bartos, D. C., January, C. T., and Delisle, B. P. (2011). Trafficking-deficient hERG K(+) channels linked to long QT syndrome are regulated by a microtubule-dependent quality control compartment in the ER. *Am. J. Physiol. Cell Physiol.* 301, C75–C85. doi: 10.1152/ajpcell.00494.2010

Swiatecka-Urban, A., Brown, A., Moreau-Marquis, S., Renuka, J., Coutermarsh, B., Barnaby, R., et al. (2005). The short apical membrane half-life of rescued {Delta}F508-cystic fibrosis transmembrane conductance regulator (CFTR) results from accelerated endocytosis of {Delta}F508-CFTR in polarized human airway epithelial cells. *J. Biol. Chem.* 280, 36762–36772. doi: 10.1074/jbc.M508944200

Tester, D. J., and Ackerman, M. J. (2009). Cardiomyopathic and channelopathic causes of sudden unexplained death in infants and children. *Annu. Rev. Med.* 60, 69–84. doi: 10.1146/annurev.med.60.052907.103838

Trudeau, M. C., Warmke, J. W., Ganetzky, B., and Robertson, G. A. (1995). HERG, a human inward rectifier in the voltage-gated potassium channel family. *Science* 269, 92–95. doi: 10.1126/science.7604285

Vandenberg, J. I., Perry, M. D., Perrin, M. J., Mann, S. A., Ke, Y., and Hill, A. P. (2012). hERG K(+) channels: structure, function, and clinical significance. *Physiol. Rev.* 92, 1393–1478. doi: 10.1152/physrev.00036.2011

Wang, W., and MacKinnon, R. (2017). Cryo-EM structure of the open human Ether-a-go-go-Related K(+) channel hERG. *Cell* 169, 422.e10–430.e10. doi: 10.1016/j.cell.2017.03.048

Wible, B. A., Hawryluk, P., Ficker, E., Kuryshev, Y. A., Kirsch, G., and Brown, A. M. (2005). HERG-Lite: a novel comprehensive high-throughput screen for drug-induced hERG risk. *J. Pharmacol. Toxicol. Methods* 52, 136–145. doi: 10.1016/j.vascn.2005.03.008

Wilkins, M. E., Li, X., and Smart, T. G. (2008). Tracking cell surface GABAB receptors using an alpha-bungarotoxin tag. *J. Biol. Chem.* 283, 34745–34752. doi: 10.1074/jbc.M803197200

Yang, T., Xu, X., Kernan, T., Wu, V., and Colecraft, H. M. (2010). Rem, a member of the RGK GTPases, inhibits recombinant CaV1.2 channels using multiple mechanisms that require distinct conformations of the GTPase. *J. Physiol.* 588, 1665–1681. doi: 10.1113/jphysiol.2010.187203

Zhou, Z., Gong, Q., Epstein, M. L., and January, C. T. (1998a). HERG channel dysfunction in human long QT syndrome. Intracellular transport and functional defects. *J. Biol. Chem.* 273, 21061–21066.

Zhou, Z., Gong, Q., and January, C. T. (1999). Correction of defective protein trafficking of a mutant HERG potassium channel in human long QT syndrome. Pharmacological and temperature effects. *J. Biol. Chem.* 274, 31123–31126. doi: 10.1074/jbc.274.44.31123

Zhou, Z., Gong, Q. M., Ye, B., Fan, Z., Makielski, J. C., Robertson, G. A., et al. (1998b). Properties of HERG channels stably expressed in HEK 293 cells studied at physiological temperature. *Biophys. J.* 74, 230–241. doi: 10.1016/S0006-3495(98)77782-3

2

Complex Interaction Between Low-Frequency APD Oscillations and Beat-to-Beat APD Variability in Humans is Governed by the Sympathetic Nervous System

Stefan Van Duijvenboden[1†], Bradley Porter[2†], Esther Pueyo[3,4], David Adolfo Sampedro-Puente[3], Jesus Fernandez-Bes[3], Baldeep Sidhu[2], Justin Gould[2], Michele Orini[5], Martin J. Bishop[2], Ben Hanson[6], Pier Lambiase[1], Reza Razavi[2], Christopher A. Rinaldi[7], Jaswinder S. Gill[7] and Peter Taggart[1]*

[1] Institute of Cardiovascular Science, University College London, London, United Kingdom, [2] School of Imaging Sciences and Biomedical Engineering, King's College London, London, United Kingdom, [3] BSICOS Group, I3A, IIS Aragón, University of Zaragoza, Zaragoza, Spain, [4] CIBER-BBN, Madrid, Spain, [5] Department of Clinical Pharmacology, Queen Mary University of London, London, United Kingdom, [6] Department of Mechanical Engineering, University College London, London, United Kingdom, [7] Guy's and St Thomas' NHS Foundation Trust, London, United Kingdom

***Correspondence:**
Peter Taggart
p.taggart@ucl.ac.uk

† These authors share first authorship

Background: Recent clinical, experimental and modeling studies link oscillations of ventricular repolarization in the low frequency (LF) (approx. 0.1 Hz) to arrhythmogenesis. Sympathetic provocation has been shown to enhance both LF oscillations of action potential duration (APD) and beat-to-beat variability (BVR) in humans. We hypothesized that beta-adrenergic blockade would reduce LF oscillations of APD and BVR of APD in humans and that the two processes might be linked.

Methods and Results: Twelve patients with normal ventricles were studied during routine electrophysiological procedures. Activation-recovery intervals (ARI) as a conventional surrogate for APD were recorded from 10 left and 10 right ventricular endocardial sites before and after acute beta-adrenergic adrenergic blockade. Cycle length was maintained constant with right ventricular pacing. Oscillatory behavior of ARI was quantified by spectral analysis and BVR as the short-term variability. Beta-adrenergic blockade reduced LF ARI oscillations (8.6 ± 4.5 ms^2 vs. 5.5 ± 3.5 ms^2, $p = 0.027$). A significant correlation was present between the initial control values and reduction seen following beta-adrenergic blockade in LF ARI ($r_S = 0.62$, $p = 0.037$) such that when initial values are high the effect is greater. A similar relationship was also seen in the beat-to beat variability of ARI ($r_S = 0.74$, $p = 0.008$). There was a significant correlation between the beta-adrenergic blockade induced reduction in LF power of ARI and the witnessed reduction of beat-to-beat variability of ARI ($r_S = 0.74$, $p = 0.01$). These clinical results accord with recent computational modeling studies which provide mechanistic insight into the interactions of LF oscillations and beat-to-beat variability of APD at the cellular level.

Conclusion: Beta-adrenergic blockade reduces LF oscillatory behavior of APD (ARI) in humans *in vivo*. Our results support the importance of LF oscillations in modulating the response of BVR to beta-adrenergic blockers, suggesting that LF oscillations may play role in modulating beta-adrenergic mechanisms underlying BVR.

Keywords: action potential duration, beat-to-beat variability, oscillations, human heart, sympathetic, beta-adrenergic blockade

INTRODUCTION

Factors which influence the stability of ventricular repolarization are important in arrhythmogenesis. Enhanced oscillation of ventricular repolarization in the low frequency range and increased beat-to-beat variability (BVR) of ventricular repolarization are two of the strongest predictors of arrhythmia and sudden cardiac death (Atiga et al., 1998; Haigney et al., 2004; Thomsen et al., 2004; Gallacher et al., 2007; Tereshchenko et al., 2009; Abi-Gerges et al., 2010; Hinterseer et al., 2010; Jacobson et al., 2011; Średniawa et al., 2012; Rizas et al., 2014, 2016, 2017; Baumert et al., 2016; Bauer et al., 2019). Both are enhanced by sympathetic stimulation and recent studies suggest a possible interactive mechanism (Porter et al., 2018). However, the mechanisms underlying the effect of beta-adrenergic stimulation on LF oscillations of repolarization and beat-to-beat variability of repolarization remain unclear.

Oscillations of ventricular repolarization measured from the ECG T-wave vector referred to as periodic repolarisation dynamics (PRD) have been attributed to oscillations in APD at the frequency of the sympathetic nerves (approx. 0.05–0.1 Hz). Ventricular action potential duration (APD) measured as activation-recovery intervals (ARI) has recently been shown to oscillate in this frequency range (Hanson et al., 2014). The LF power of APD has been shown to be increased by sympathetic provocation (Porter et al., 2018). The recent finding of LF oscillations in short term variability of ventricular APD (Porter et al., 2018) raises the possibility of an association between LF oscillations of APD and BVR.

Computational modeling has provided early insight into the mechanisms underlying these oscillations of APD, the effect of beta-adrenergic stimulation and their relationship to the initiation of ventricular arrhythmias (Pueyo et al., 2016a,b). More recent studies on the effect of beta-adrenergic blockade suggest that the cellular mechanisms underlying modulation of LF APD and BVR of APD are strongly influenced by the initial conditions of APD (Sampedro-Puente et al., 2019). One of the objectives of the present study was to examine this hypothesis in humans *in vivo*.

We have studied 12 patients during cardiac catheterization allowing us to measure ARIs as an approximation for APD at 10 right ventricular (RV) and 10 left ventricular (LV) endocardial sites in order to investigate the effect of acute beta-adrenergic blockade on LF oscillations of ventricular APD and on BVR of APD, and the possible interaction between the two. Cycle length was held constant with RV pacing to avoid confounding effects due to the cycle length dependency of APD.

MATERIALS AND METHODS

Ethical Approval

The study was approved by the Ethics Committee of Guy's and Thomas' Hospitals and conformed to the standards set by the Declaration of Helsinki (latest revision: 59th World Medical Association General Assembly). All patients gave written, informed consent.

Subjects

Studies were performed in 12 patients (10 males, 2 females, aged 41–69, median 61) during the course of routine clinical radiofrequency ablation procedures for atrial fibrillation. Four patients had paroxysmal atrial fibrillation, and eight patients had persistent atrial fibrillation. All subjects had normal biventricular systolic function. **Table 1** demonstrates further patient characteristics. Studies were performed in the un-sedated state and cardio-active medications (beta-blockers, non-dihydropyridine calcium channel blockers, digoxin, and flecainide) were discontinued for 5 days before the study.

Protocol

Utilizsing the routine transseptal puncture of an AF ablation, a decapolar catheter was placed in the left ventricle via the left atrium and mitral valve. The pacing catheter and second decapolar catheter were placed in the right ventricle. Routine AF ablation femoral venous access was utilized for placement of all catheters. The transseptal puncture was conducted under radiographic guidance. **Figure 1A** shows the set-up of both recording decapolar catheters and the pacing catheter. Subjects were paced from the right ventricular apex using a Biotronik (Berlin, Germany) stimulator (model UHS 3000) at 2x diastolic

TABLE 1 | Patient characteristics.

Diabetes	2 (17%)
Sleep apnoea	0 (0%)
Hypertension	5 (42%)
Left atrial diameter	4.2±0.4 cm
Presence of left ventricular hypertrophy	2 (17%)
Presence of diastolic dysfunction	2 (17%)
Beta-blocker	7 (60%)
Non-dihydropyridine calcium channel blocker	1 (8%)
Amiodarone	0 (0%)
Digoxin	1 (8%)
Flecainide	1 (8%)

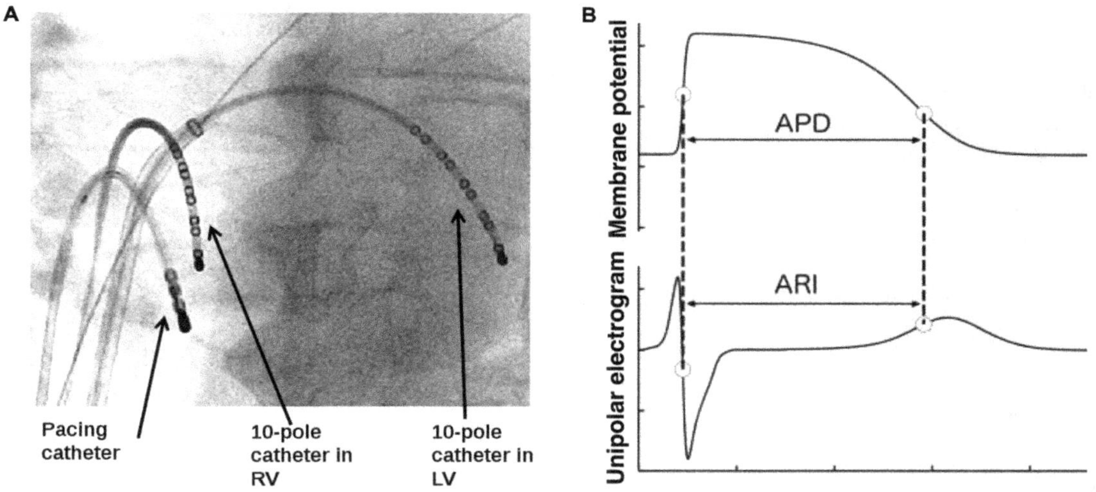

FIGURE 1 | Diagram of **(A)** decapolar catheter electrodes in RV and LV and pacing wire and **(B)** the schematic illustration of relation between the activation recovery interval (ARI) in the unipolar EGM and the ventricular action potential duration (APD).

threshold and 2 ms pulse width, at a cycle length >20 beats/min faster than the intrinsic AF rate (median: 500 ms; range: 360–500 ms) to avoid breakthrough of intrinsic beats. A 2-min period of adaptation to the paced cycle length was applied before starting a controlled breathing protocol. Breathing was controlled throughout the protocol at 0.25 and 0.5 Hz. Recordings took place for 90s during each controlled breathing cycle. First, a control period was established with the breathing protocol performed in absence of any autonomic blocking agents. Pacing was then stopped and the subject received metoprolol at a dose sufficient to reduce the intrinsic heart rate by 10 beats/min (iv; dose range, 2–10 mg), and after a further 10 min for equilibration the pacing (at the same paced cycle length as the control) and breathing protocol was repeated as above. The entire study protocol was completed prior to conducting the AF ablation.

Measurements

Continuous synchronous recordings of femoral arterial blood pressure and unipolar electrograms (UEGs) at 10 endocardial RV and 10 endocardial LV sites (**Figure 1A**) were obtained before routine clinical radiofrequency ablation procedures for atrial fibrillation in the cardiac catheterization lab at St Thomas' Hospital in London, as described previously (Hanson et al., 2012; van Duijvenboden et al., 2015). UEGs and blood pressure recordings were digitized at 1,200 Hz (Ensite 3000; Endocardial Solutions) and analyzed offline.

Data Analysis

UEGs were analyzed for ventricular APDs at each recording site by measuring activation-recovery intervals (ARIs) using the Wyatt method (Wyatt et al., 1981). This method has been validated in theoretical, computational, and experimental studies (Wyatt et al., 1981; Haws and Lux, 1990; Coronel et al., 2006; Potse et al., 2009). According to this method, activation is measured at the moment of minimum dV/dt of the QRS complex of the UEG and repolarization at the moment of maximum dV/dt of the T-wave (**Figure 1B**). ARIs were measured automatically using in house developed algorithms. Heuristic-based screening was used to identify and discount any cases where the T-wave was indistinct or corrupt. Blood pressure recordings were analyzed for systolic blood pressure (SBP) and the maximum rate of systolic pressure increase (dP/dt_{max}) as a measure of myocardial contractility. Measurement of dP/dt_{max} from the femoral artery has been shown to provide good tracking of left ventricular contractility (Monge Garcia et al., 2018).

To establish evenly sampled series, any beats for which ARI, SBP or dP/dt_{max} measurements could not be determined were replaced by linear interpolation between the surrounding beats. Recordings were rejected from the analysis if these surrogate beats constituted more than 10% of any series.

The low frequency (LF) power in each ARI series was estimated by calculating the bandpower in the low-frequency band (0.04–0.15 Hz) using the Thomson's multitaper method with three Slepian tapers, which is known to be robust against noise (Thomson, 1982). The same analysis was applied to the calculate the high frequency (HF) power in in a frequency band of the breathing frequency (either 0.25 or 0.5 Hz) ± 10%. The LF and HF powers were then averaged for RV and LV poles.

Beat-to-beat variability of ARI was assessed by computing the short term variability (STV) of ARIs for each endocardial recording site over the entire recording as per established STV measures (Johnson et al., 2013; Baumert et al., 2016). The STV ARI (STV-ARI) was computed using a moving window of 10 consecutive beats:

$$STV = \frac{\sum |ARI_{i-1} - ARI_i|}{N\sqrt{2}}$$

where ARI_i is the ARI at the ith beat and N is the number of beats. For each pole, we computed the mean STV in time and then averaged these values across poles. The STV of SBP (STV-SBP) and dP/dt_{max} (STV-dP/dt_{max}) were computed using the same formula and number of beats as for ARI.

Statistical Analysis

Results were averaged across the two separate breathing cycles for both control recordings and following introduction of beta-adrenergic blockade. Results are presented as mean ± standard deviation for normally distributed variables and as median and interquartile range (IQR) for non-normally distributed variables. The effect of beta-adrenergic blockade on LF power for ARI, SBP and dP/dt_{max} was tested for statistical significance using the two-tailed paired Wilcoxon signed-rank test. To evaluate whether there were different responses in ARI STV between individual electrodes ($n = 20$), we used the non-parametric Kruskal–Wallis test. Results were considered significant at $p < 0.05$.

RESULTS

Effect of Beta-Adrenergic Blockade on Combined Group Data

Example ARI, SBP and dP/dt_{max} time series of one patient breathing at 15 breaths/min (0.25 Hz) during control and following beta-adrenergic blockade are shown in **Figure 2**. In this example, clear LF oscillations are visible in all traces during control. which are attenuated following beta-adrenergic blockade. At the same time, there is a clear reduction in the STV.

In the group data, beta-adrenergic blockade resulted in a significant reduction of LF power of ARI (8.6 ± 4.5 ms^2 vs. 5.5 ± 3.5 ms^2, $p = 0.027$) (**Figure 3A**) and the LF power of SBP ($1.4 \times 10^{-3} \pm 1.2 \times 10^{-3}$ $mmHg^2$ vs. $0.4 \times 10^{-3} \pm 0.5 \times 10^{-3}$ $mmHg^2$, $p = 0.027$) (**Figure 3B**). A trend to reduction was observed for the LF power of dP/dt_{max} ($0.7 \times 10^{-6} \pm 1 \times 10^{-6}$ vs. $0.1 \times 10^{-6} \pm 0.2 \times 10^{-6}$ $mmHg^2/s^2$, $p = 0.129$) (**Figure 3C**).

No effect of beta-adrenergic blockade was seen on the HF power of ARI ($6.5 \times 10^{-3} \pm 3 \times 10^{-3}$ ms^2 vs. $6.1 \times 10^{-3} \pm 3.4 \times 10^{-3}$ ms^2, $p = 0.91$), SBP ($1.9 \times 10^{-3} \pm 1 \times 10^{-3}$ $mmHg^2$ vs. $1.7 \times 10^{-3} \pm 1 \times 10^{-3}$ $mmHg^2$, $p = 0.424$), nor dP/dt_{max} ($7.6 \times 10^{-7} \pm 7.4 \times 10^{-7}$ $mmHg^2/s^2$ vs. 3.2 ± 3.9 $mmHg^2/s^2$, $p = 0.052$).

No immediate effect of beta-adrenergic blockade was seen on mean ARI for group data (186.9 ± 22.8 vs. 186.5 ± 20.5 ms, $p = 0.4$) or the beat-to-beat variability (STV-ARI: 4.26 ± 1.3 vs. 4.03 ± 0.96 ms, $p = 0.97$). We also did not observe an effect on the beat-to-beat variability of SBP (STV-SBP: 5.52 ± 2.25 vs. 4.75 ± 2.68 mmHg, $p = 0.380$), but the STV dP/dt_{max} was significantly reduced (STV-dP/dt_{max} 166 ± 102 vs. 102 ± 80 mmHg/s, $p = 0.005$).

The ARI STV response to beta-adrenergic blockade was not different across breathing frequencies: mean ARI STV reduction −0.1 (±0.7) for 15 breaths/min versus 0.2 (±1.4) ms for 30 breaths/min, $p = 0.8$. Furthermore, as shown in **Figure 4**, there were no significant differences in ARI STV reduction between electrode sites in the RV and LV ($p = 0.87$ and $p = 0.56$ for RV and LV, respectively). We also tested the differences in STV baseline and reduction between RV and LV. Mean values of STV baseline and reduction were slightly higher in the LV, but the differences were not

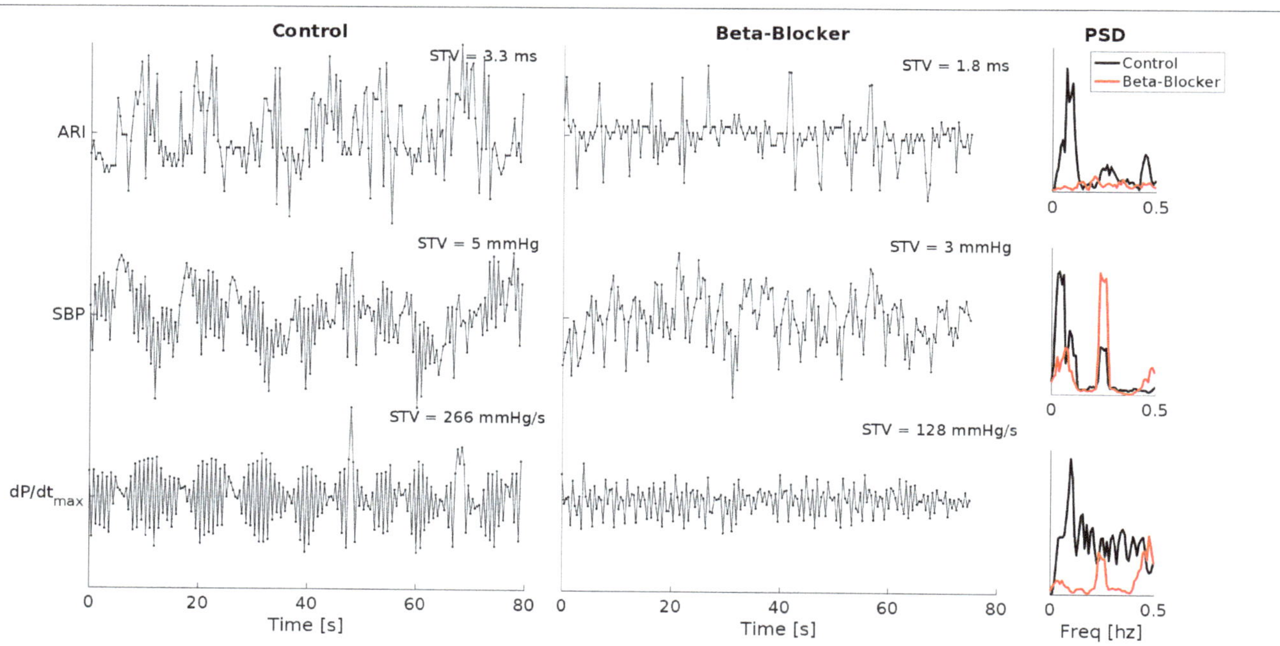

FIGURE 2 | Example ARI, SBP and dP/dt_{max} time series of one patient breathing at 15 breaths/min (0.25 Hz) during control and following beta-adrenergic blockade. Clear low-frequency oscillations are visible in all traces during control, which are attenuated following beta-adrenergic blockade. Also note the reduction in the short time variability (STV) measures. PSD, power spectral density.

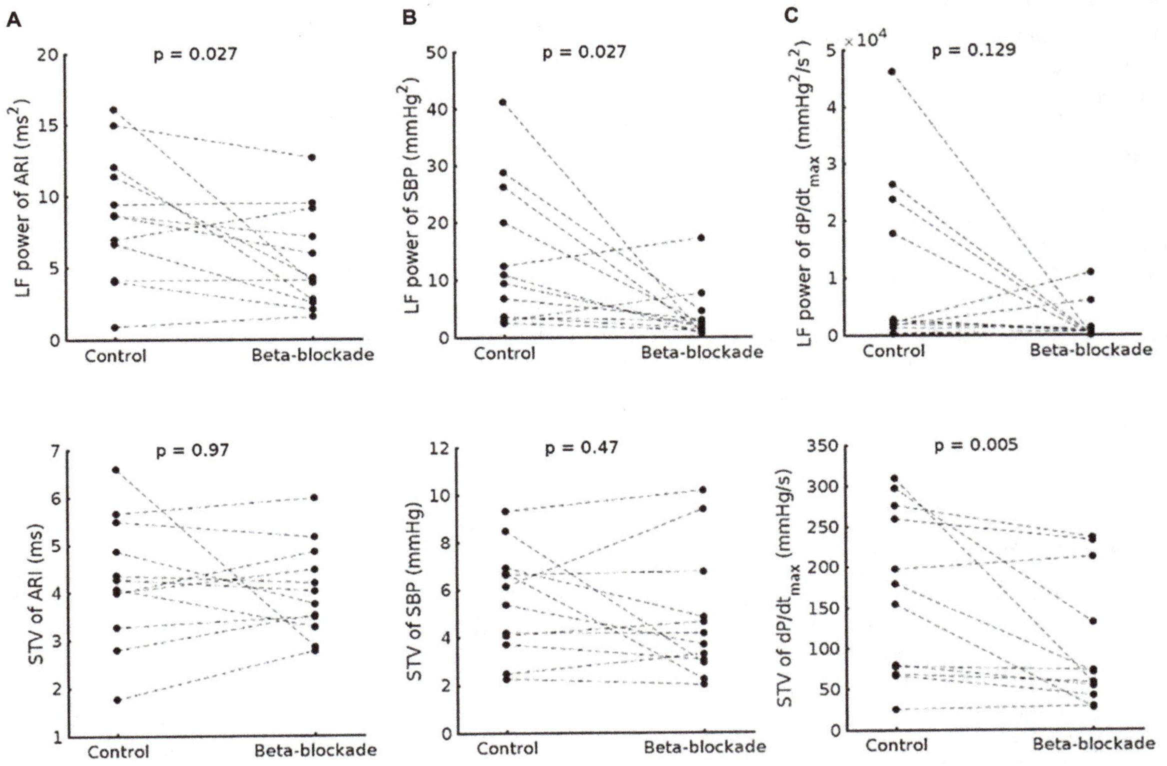

FIGURE 3 | Effect of beta-adrenergic blockade on the low frequency (LF) power (top) and short-term variability (STV) (bottom) of **(A)** activation-recovery intervals (ARIs), **(B)** systolic blood pressure (SBP) and **(C)** the maximum rate of systolic pressure increase (dP/dt$_{max}$).

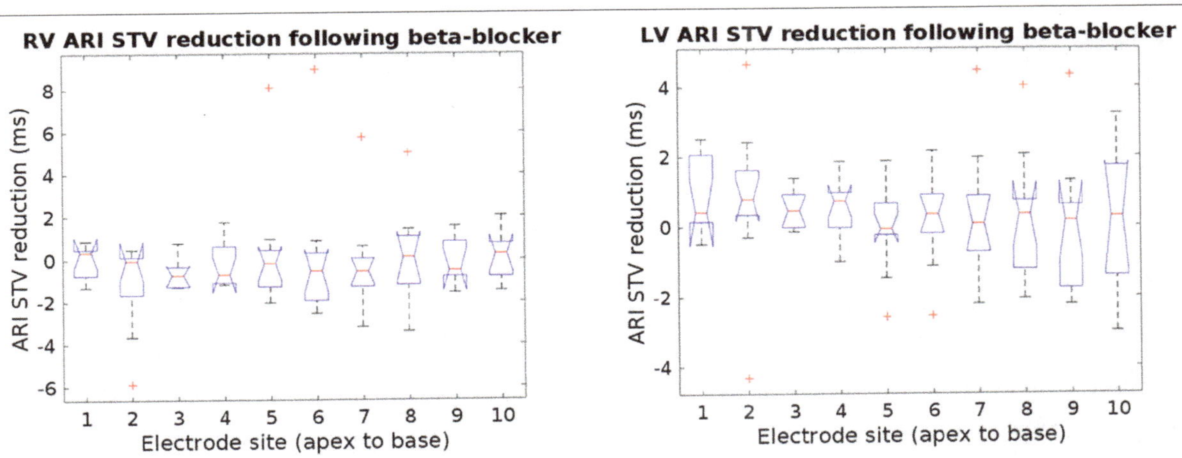

FIGURE 4 | Reduction of ARI short-time variability (STV) following beta-blocker from individual electrodes in the right and left ventricle (RV and LV). No significant changes in STV reduction were found across electrode sites. Outliers are marked by crosses.

statistically significant: mean ARI STV baseline: 8.7 ± 8.1 vs. 9.3 ± 5.0 ms, $p = 0.4$; mean ARI STV reduction: −0.1 ± 1.8 vs. 0.3 ± 1.0, $p = 0.1$, for RV and LV, respectively. Finally, we also investigated whether the LF power and STV response to beta-adrenergic blockade was different in patients who had previously been treated with beta-blocker ($n = 7$, **Table 1**) compared to those who had not ($n = 5$). Although medication was discontinued for 5 days before the study in all patients, we found that the average response in both ARI LF power and ARI STV was slightly higher in patients treated with beta-blockers, but the numbers were too small to allow robust statistical analysis (mean reduction in LF power: 4.3 ± 5.3 vs. 1.5 ± 1.3 ms^2; mean reduction in ARI STV reduction: 0.7 ± 1.5 vs. −0.4 ± 0.5 ms).

Influence of Initial Values on the Response to Beta-Adrenergic Blockade

The effect of beta-adrenergic blockade on the group data was small. However, a wide range of control values was evident and when our results were expressed in relation to control values a highly significant effect of beta-adrenergic blockade was apparent. Subjects in whom the initial control values of LF of ARI were large showed a greater change in the magnitude of the oscillations following beta-adrenergic blockade compared to subjects in whom the initial values were low. When control oscillations of ARI were large beta-adrenergic blockade reduced their magnitude. When control oscillations were small the response to beta-adrenergic blockade was minimal or variable ($r_s = 0.62$, $p = 0.037$) (**Figure 5A**). A similar relationship was observed for ARI-STV (rs = 0.74, $p = 0.008$) (**Figure 5B**), and the LF power of SBP and dP/dt_{max} ($r_s = 0.78$, $p = 0.004$ and $r_s = 0.84$, $p = 0.001$, respectively) (**Figures 5C,D**).

Relationship Between Low Frequency Power and Beat-to-Beat Variability of ARI

There was a strong relationship between the reduction in LF power of ARI and the reduction of STV-ARI in response to beta-adrenergic blockade (rs = 0.72, $p = 0.01$) (**Figure 6**). No significant relationships were found between the reduction of LF power and SBP-STV (rs = 0.42, $p = 0.2$) or dP/dt_{max}-STV (rs = 0.36, $p = 0.3$). There was also no significant relationships between the reduction in HF power and STV for ARI, SBP, and dP/dt_{max}: (ARI-STV: rs = 0.48, $p = 0.1$. SBP-STV: rs = 0.38, $p = 0.3$; dP/dt_{max} –STV: rs = 0.56, $p = 0.06$).

DISCUSSION

We studied the effect of acute beta-adrenergic blockade on LF oscillations of ventricular APD (approximated by ARI) and on beat-to-beat APD variability. LF power and STV ARI measurements were made from 10 RV and 10 LV sites and then averaged in patients with normal ventricles. Cycle length was maintained constant with right ventricular pacing to eliminate confounding effects of cycle length dependency and breathing was controlled throughout the protocol at 0.25 and 0.5 Hz. Our main findings were: (1) we observed a wide variation of control values of LF power and beat-to-beat variability of ARI, SBP and dP/dt_{max}; (2) beta-adrenergic blockade was associated with a significant reduction of LF power of ARI and SBP, (3) individually no clear impact of beta-adrenergic blockade on the beat-to-beat variability of ARI, SBP and dP/dt_{max} was demonstrated, however, (4) there was a strong correlation between the reduction seen in the LF power of ARI, SBP, and dP/dt_{max} following beta-adrenergic blockade, and the reduction in beat-to-beat variability.

Whereas oscillations in heart rate variability have long been recognized and the underlying mechanisms the subject of much debate (Parati et al., 2006), oscillations of ventricular APD at the low frequency have only relatively recently been identified (Hanson et al., 2014). These LF APD oscillations identified in

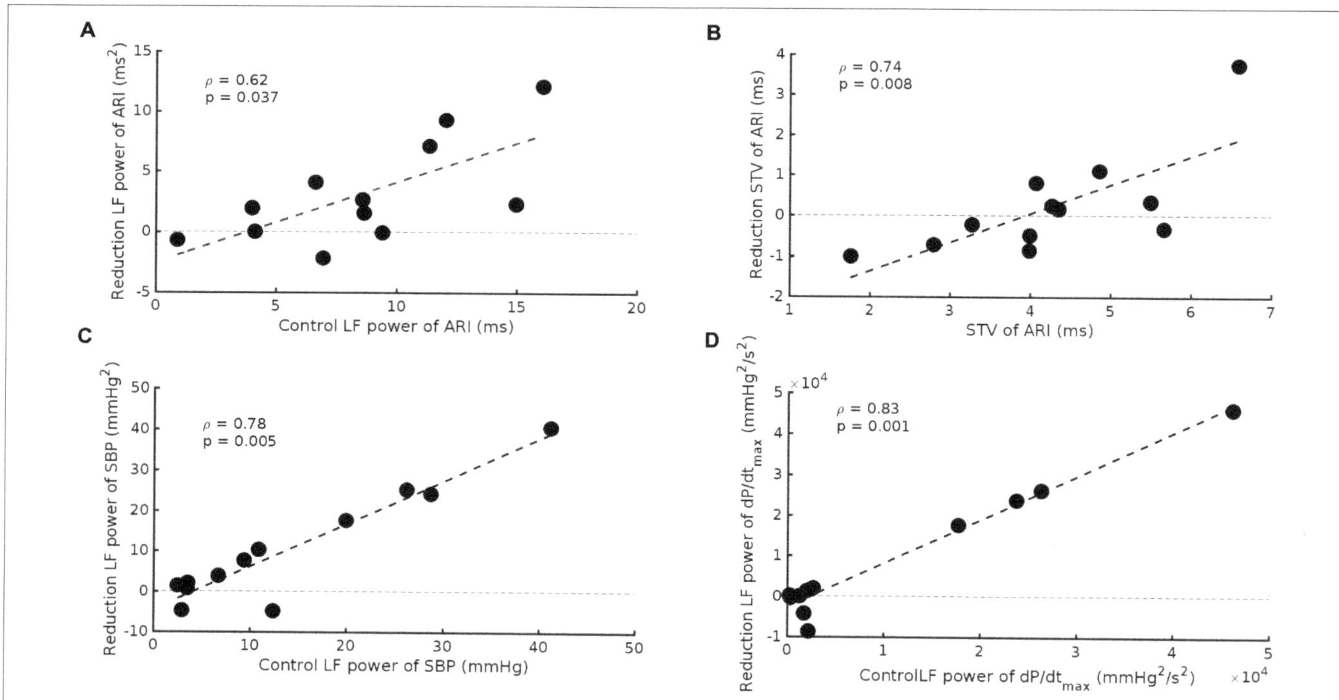

FIGURE 5 | Scatterplots demonstrating the significant relationship between baseline values and the reduction seen following beta-adrenergic blockade in: **(A)** LF power of ARI, **(B)** beat-to-beat variability of ARI (STV ARI), **(C)** LF power of systolic blood pressure (SBP), and **(D)** the LF power of the maximum rate of systolic pressure increase (dP/dt_{max}).

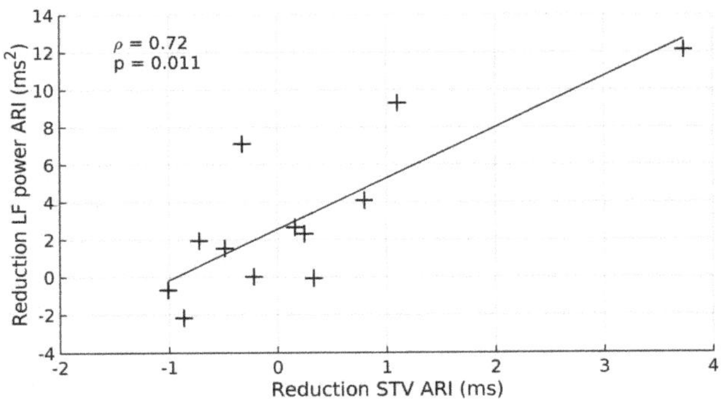

FIGURE 6 | Scatterplot demonstrating the significant relationship between the beta-adrenergic blockade induced reduction in the LF power ARI and the witnessed reduction in beat-to-beat variability of ARI (STV ARI). +, data point.

humans using ARI recordings from the ventricular myocardium, are independent of variation in R-R interval and independent of respiration (Hanson et al., 2014). They frequently occur in association with LF oscillations in blood pressure (Mayer waves) (Julien, 2006). Oscillation of ventricular repolarization at the low frequency has recently been identified from the body surface ECG T-wave vector and these are also independent of R-R interval variability and respiration and are attributed to LF oscillation of ventricular APD (Rizas et al., 2014). When enhanced these oscillations are strongly predictive of arrhythmia and sudden cardiac death (Rizas et al., 2014, 2016, 2017, 2019; Hamm et al., 2017). The magnitude of both ARI and T-wave vector oscillations is increased during sympathetic stimulation (Rizas et al., 2014; Porter et al., 2017, 2018) and it has been suggested they may be related to the intrinsic low frequency oscillation of sympathetic nerve activity.

Enhanced beat-to-beat variability of repolarization, measured clinically as QT variability or experimentally as APD variability, is well known to predispose to malignant ventricular arrhythmias (Atiga et al., 1998; Haigney et al., 2004; Thomsen et al., 2004; Gallacher et al., 2007; Tereshchenko et al., 2009; Abi-Gerges et al., 2010; Hinterseer et al., 2010; Jacobson et al., 2011; Średniawa et al., 2012; Baumert et al., 2016). BVR has been shown to be enhanced by beta-adrenergic stimulation (Johnson et al., 2010, 2013; Porter et al., 2017). Paradoxically studies using beta-adrenergic blockade have shown a mixed response of BVR in QT interval measurements with either no change or an increase or decrease (Baumert et al., 2016). In this work we demonstrate firstly a strong dependence of the effect of beta blockade on initial conditions, and secondly a possible interaction between LF power and beat-to-beat variability of ARI. Importantly, we observed that changes in beat-to-beat variability were more enhanced following beta-adrenergic blockade when LF power was reduced. In contrary, small or no changes were observed in beat-to-beat variability in individuals for which the LF power was not modulated. Although these findings may have important mechanistic implications in this context, it should be noted that beat-to-beat variability and low frequency power are both measures of variability, hence the observed relationship between LF power and beat-to-beat variability could also be a mathematical consequence. Nevertheless, the results could provide an explanation on the conflicting results reported on the effect of beta-adrenergic blockade on beat-to-beat variability. Recently it has also been observed that the intrinsic beat-to-beat variation in APD also exhibits phasic variation at the low frequency, which is enhanced during increased sympathetic stimulation (Porter et al., 2018), which may further support a possible interaction between LF ARI and intrinsic beat-to-beat variation in ARI. Interestingly, preliminary data from this study shows that the response of LF ARI power and beat-to-beat variability following beta-adrenergic blockade were more pronounced in individuals that had previously been treated with beta-blockers. While the number were too small to draw any final conclusions, it might highlight a role of the dynamic nature of beta-adrenergic receptors, but it is also possible that these patients had a higher sympathetic tone during control. Future work will further investigate this finding.

The present work was conducted in patients with normal hearts and we cannot exclude the possibility that the relationships we observed may have been different in patients with arrhythmias. However, in this context the following observations in patients with arrhythmias are worth mention. In a recent study in heart failure patients ARI recordings as a measure of local action potential duration were obtained from the left ventricular epicardial lead of an implanted cardiac defibrillator device. 11 of 43 patients received appropriate shock treatment for sustained ventricular tachycardia or fibrillation, and ARI variability was significantly higher in these patients compared to patients who did not develop arrhythmia (Porter et al., 2019). In the present paper we observed a relationship between the initial BVR and the corresponding reduction following beta blockade. Consequently beta-adrenergic blockade may have a greater effect on BVR in individuals at increased arrhythmic risk compared to those at low risk.

Clinical conditions associated with high arrhythmia risk are commonly accompanied by adverse ventricular remodeling with downregulation of ionic currents and dysregulation of Ca2+handling and reduced repolarization reserve (Armoundas et al., 2001). Beta-adrenergic stimulation in the presence of reduced repolarization reserve (Iks block) has been shown to dramatically increase BVR and be proarrhythmic (Johnson et al., 2010). The importance of downregulation of IKs in promoting excess BVR during beta-adrenergic stimulation was further demonstrated in a study identifying a role of calcium mediated mechanisms in the generation of arrhythmias (Johnson et al., 2013). In a recent study in the chronic AV block dog model using monophasic action potential recordings, remodeling resulted in an increase of low frequency oscillations of ventricular MAP duration. Furthermore, low frequency BVR measured as beat to beat differences of MAP duration, also increased. Increased low frequency power was positively related to Torsades de Pointes inducibility (Sprenkeler et al., 2019). These results suggest an interaction between the remodeling process, low frequency oscillation and beat to beat variability of ventricular repolarization as playing an important role in arrhythmogenesis. The findings are in keeping with recent computational modeling studies involving phasic low frequency beta-adrenergic and mechanical stimulation. When remodeling was simulated by reducing repolarization reserve (reduced Ikr) and incorporating calcium overload early after depolarizations and triggered activity were readily induced (Pueyo et al., 2016b; Sampedro-Puente et al., 2019).

While a number of studies have investigated the cellular mechanisms underlying modulation of BVR by beta-adrenergic stimulation and the consequent effect on arrhythmia initiation (Johnson et al., 2010, 2013; Szentandrássy et al., 2015), only a few have so far examined mechanisms underlying low frequency oscillation of ventricular APD (Pueyo et al., 2016b; Sampedro-Puente et al., 2019). Regarding BVR ion channel stochasticity and calcium cyclical variation have both been identified as major contributors. Regarding low frequency oscillations of ventricular APD a direct action of beta-adrenergic stimulation and mechano-electric feedback has been suggested.

Recent computational research has shown that the major ionic contributors to inter-individual differences in LF oscillations of APD and beat-to-beat APD variability are I_{Kr}, I_{CaL}, and I_{K1} (Sampedro-Puente et al., 2019). In this study, a set of stochastic human ventricular action potential models was developed by individually varying the ionic conductances of I_{Kr}, I_{CaL}, and I_{K1} from their nominal values in the O'Hara-Virág-Varró-Rudy (ORd) action potential model (O'Hara et al., 2011). Beta-adrenergic and mechanical stretch effects were included in the models to simulate sympathetic modulation of ventricular electrophysiology at the cell level (Pueyo et al., 2016b; Sampedro-Puente et al., 2019). For each of the simulated models, normalized measures of LF oscillation magnitude of APD (nmLF) and beat-to-beat APD variability (STV-APD) were computed before and after beta-adrenergic blockade. In accordance with the clinical observations of this study, beta-adrenergic blockade in these simulated cells led to a remarkable reduction in nmLF and also in STV-APD. Importantly, these simulations showed a wide range of nmLF and STV-APD initial values as well as of their changes in response to beta-adrenergic blockade. In line with the presented clinical data, higher nmLF and STV-APD initial values were associated with larger beta-adrenergic blockade-induced decreases in the magnitudes of both markers. A strong correlation was observed between the effects of beta-adrenergic blockade on nmLF and STV-APD.

The reduction in nmLF in response to beta-adrenergic blockade, which could be observed to a greater or lesser extent in all the virtual cells, can be explained on the basis of beta-adrenergic stimulation enhancing LF oscillations of APD via differential phosphorylation and dephosphorylation kinetics of cellular PKA targets (mainly I_{CaL} and I_{Ks}) (Pueyo et al., 2016b; Sampedro-Puente et al., 2019). For STV-APD, the reduction induced by beta-adrenergic blockade is justified by the fact that beta-adrenergic stimulation modulates, on the one hand, the LF oscillations of APD and, on the other hand, the stochastic gating of ionic currents active during the repolarization phase (Sampedro-Puente et al., 2019).

Mechanoelectric feedback (MEF) has been suggested to contribute to the development of LF oscillations and BVR of APD in humans *in vivo* (Hanson et al., 2014) and by computational simulation, these adrenergic and mechanical actions have been shown to synergistically potentiate the oscillatory behavior and temporal variability of cellular ventricular repolarization (Pueyo et al., 2016b; Sampedro-Puente et al., 2019), in accord with the well-known potentiation of MEF effects by beta-adrenergic stimulation (Horner et al., 1996; Puglisi et al., 2013). The role of MEF, possibly through stretch-activated channels, in contributing to BVR is supported by experimental evidence in the chronic atrioventricular-block dog model, where beat-to-beat preload changes have been shown to increase short-term variability of monophasic APD (Stams et al., 2016). The timing of electro-mechanical coupling may also be important. In a canine model IKs block prolonged APD altering the timing of ventricular repolarization in relation to the ventricular pressure curve. Under these conditions the addition of left stellate stimulation induced Torsades de Points (ter Bekke et al., 2019).

The importance of risk stratification for arrhythmia and sudden death to guide patient selection for ICD implantation has already been stressed. A number of non-invasive markers of risk have been proposed including amongst others heart rate variability, baroreflex sensitivity, microvolt T-wave alternans, heart rate turbulence, Tpeak-Tend as an index of dispersion of repolarization and QT interval variability, all of which are modulated by autonomic activity (Baumert et al., 2016; Priori et al., 2016; Tse et al., 2017). However, despite showing promise none of these has so far influenced clinical practice. Numerous studies have examined the predictive power of BVR estimated in humans as QT variability or intracardiac QT interval as have been comprehensively summarized by Baumert et al. (2016). While many studies showed encouraging results a significant number were less so. It was concluded by these authors that analysis of joint RR and QT dynamics seems to allow detecting repolarization stability preceding malignant ventricular arrhythmias in patients post MI, and prospective studies are needed on the predictive value of QTV as part of a multivariate risk stratification procedure in different well-defined populations. The variable that has shown the most consistent association with sudden cardiac death is reduced left ventricular ejection fraction and remains the gold standard for risk stratification of patients with ischemic heart disease and primary prevention (Priori et al., 2016). A conceptually attractive aspect of the application of BVR is that experimental work in a canine complete AV block model indicates that the strong association with inducible TdP/VF reflects ventricular remodeling which is a characteristic feature of at-risk patients (Smoczynska et al., 2019). A recent multicenter prospective clinical trial involving 44 centers in 15 EU countries now provides convincing evidence for enhanced low frequency oscillations of ventricular repolarization, measured from the ECG T-wave vector referred to as Periodic Repolarization Dynamics (PRD), to be one of the strongest predictors of ventricular arrhythmia and sudden death in post MI patients (Bauer et al., 2019). Comparison of the potential clinical value of each of these various biomarkers is hindered by the fact that most studies have focused on just one or a small number of these parameters and the lack of any standardization of methodology and study population. Future research should focus on evaluating the prognostic value of possible combinations of these biomarkers in prospective multivariate analysis in specific patient populations.

Limitations

The study population were patients with ostensibly normal ventricles undergoing routine ablation procedures for supraventricular arrhythmias. Eight of the 12 patients had persistent atrial fibrillation and therefore the possibility of some ventricular remodeling cannot be excluded. However, the routine procedure for atrial fibrillation ablation involves transseptal puncture to allow access to the left atrium from the right atrium. This enables placement of an LV decapolar catheter for the research procedure (right atrium to left atrium to left ventricle via the mitral valve) without the need for arterial puncture for retrograde access to the left ventricle. In many years experience of acquiring basic electrophysiological data from the *in vivo* human heart in order to complement laboratory studies, we have always considered it a priority to integrate the research protocol with the clinical protocol avoiding additional invasive procedures. We recognize that it would be ideal to have longer recordings when studying LF related parameters, but to comply with clinical studies we designed the study with view to limiting the duration of the study as much as possible.

Recordings were made from 20 localized right and left ventricular endocardial sites and then averaged. It is possible that other regions may have yielded different results. Furthermore, averaging may confound local beat-to-beat variabilities, although we did not find evidence for this when comparing the STV reduction across electrode sites and between left and right ventricle. In addition, breathing frequency may also play a role. In this work we report averaged data from two different breathing frequencies (15 and 30 breaths/min), but the reduction in ARI STV between the two breathing frequencies was not found to be significantly different.

Clinical Implications

Understanding the mechanisms underlying the interaction between beta-adrenergic stimulation, the LF oscillatory behavior of APD and beat-to-beat APD variability is important for the development of therapeutic strategies for the prevention of arrhythmia and sudden cardiac death. Enhanced oscillations of ventricular repolarization in the LF range measured from the ECG T-wave vector and referred to as periodic repolarization dynamics (PRD) have emerged as one of the strongest predictors of arrhythmia and sudden cardiac death in cardiac patients and are the subject of ongoing clinical trials (Rizas et al., 2014, 2016, 2017, 2019; Hamm et al., 2017; Bauer et al., 2019). The present work identifies several specific features of the interaction between beta-adrenergic stimulation, the LF oscillatory behavior of APD and beat-to-beat APD variability that are reproducible by computational modeling which enables mechanistic insight to be gained at the cellular level.

CONCLUSION

In patients with normal ventricles acute beta-adrenergic blockade modulated LF oscillatory behavior of ventricular APD (measured as ARIs) and beat-to-beat variability of APD in a manner that was dependent on baseline APD variability. A strong correlation was present between the effect of beta-adrenergic blockade on LF oscillation of APD and beat-to-beat variability of APD. These findings are discussed in relation to computational modeling which reproduced the clinical findings and investigated cellular mechanisms. These observations provide valuable insight into the strong association of LF oscillations of ventricular repolarization and arrhythmic and sudden cardiac death. Further work is warranted to improve our understanding in order to develop therapeutic strategies.

AUTHOR CONTRIBUTIONS

BP, SV, JG, and PT conceived and designed the experiments. All authors took responsibility in analyzing and interpreting the data, contributed to drafting or revising the manuscript, and approved the final version of the manuscript.

REFERENCES

Abi-Gerges, N., Valentin, J. P., and Pollard, C. E. (2010). Dog left ventricular midmyocardial myocytes for assessment of drug-induced delayed repolarization: short-term variability and proarrhythmic potential. *Br. J. Pharmacol.* 159, 77–92. doi: 10.1111/j.1476-5381.2009.00338.x

Armoundas, A. A., Wu, R., Juang, G., Marbán, E., and Tomaselli, G. F. (2001). Electrical and structural remodeling of the failing ventricle. *Pharmacol. Ther.* 92, 213–230. doi: 10.1016/S0163-7258(01)00171-171

Atiga, W. L., Calkins, H., Lawrence, J. H., Tomaselli, G. F., Smith, J. M., and Berger, R. D. (1998). Beat-to-beat repolarization lability identifies patients at risk for sudden cardiac death. *J. Cardiovasc. Electrophysiol.* 9, 899–908. doi: 10.1111/j.1540-8167.1998.tb00130.x

Bauer, A., Klemm, M., Rizas, K. D., Hamm, W., von Stülpnagel, L., Dommasch, M., et al. (2019). Prediction of mortality benefit based on periodic repolarisation dynamics in patients undergoing prophylactic implantation of a defibrillator: a prospective, controlled, multicentre cohort study. *Lancet* 394, 1344–1351. doi: 10.1016/S0140-6736(19)31996-8

Baumert, M., Porta, A., Vos, M. A., Malik, M., Couderc, J. P., Laguna, P., et al. (2016). QT interval variability in body surface ECG: measurement, physiological basis, and clinical value: position statement and consensus guidance endorsed by the European heart rhythm association jointly with the ESC working group on cardiac cellular electroph. *Europace* 18, 925–944. doi: 10.1093/europace/euv405

Coronel, R., de Bakker, J. M. T., Wilms-Schopman, F. J. G., Opthof, T., Linnenbank, A. C., Belterman, C. N., et al. (2006). Monophasic action potentials and activation recovery intervals as measures of ventricular action potential duration: experimental evidence to resolve some controversies. *Hear. Rhythm* 3, 1043–1050. doi: 10.1016/j.hrthm.2006.05.027

Gallacher, D. J., Van de Water, A., van der Linde, H., Hermans, A. N., Lu, H. R., Towart, R., et al. (2007). In vivo mechanisms precipitating torsades de pointes in a canine model of drug-induced long-QT1 syndrome. *Cardiovasc. Res.* 76, 247–256. doi: 10.1016/j.cardiores.2007.06.019

Haigney, M. C., Zareba, W., Gentlesk, P. J., Goldstein, R. E., Illovsky, M., McNitt, S., et al. (2004). QT interval variability and spontaneous ventricular tachycardia or fibrillation in the Multicenter Automatic Defibrillator Implantation Trial (MADUT) II patients. *J. Am. Coll. Cardiol.* 44, 1481–1487. doi: 10.1016/j.jacc.2004.06.063

Hamm, W., Rizas, K. D., Stülpnagel, L. V., Vdovin, N., Massberg, S., Kääb, S., et al. (2017). Implantable cardiac monitors in high-risk post-infarction patients with cardiac autonomic dysfunction and moderately reduced left ventricular ejection fraction: design and rationale of the SMART-MI trial. *Am. Heart J.* 190, 34–39. doi: 10.1016/j.ahj.2017.05.006

Hanson, B., Child, N., Van Duijvenboden, S., Orini, M., Chen, Z., Coronel, R., et al. (2014). Oscillatory behavior of ventricular action potential duration in heart failure patients at respiratory rate and low frequency. *Front. Physiol.* 5:414. doi: 10.3389/fphys.2014.00414

Hanson, B., Gill, J., Western, D., Gilbey, M. P., Bostock, J., Boyett, M. R., et al. (2012). Cyclical modulation of human ventricular repolarization by respiration. *Front. Physiol.* 3:379. doi: 10.3389/fphys.2012.00379

Haws, C. W., and Lux, R. L. (1990). Correlation between in vivo transmembrane action potential durations and activation-recovery intervals from electrograms. Effects of interventions that alter repolarization time. *Circulation* 81, 281–288. doi: 10.1161/01.CIR.81.1.281

Hinterseer, M., Beckmann, B. M., Thomsen, M. B., Pfeufer, A., Ulbrich, M., Sinner, M. F., et al. (2010). Usefulness of short-term variability of QT intervals as a predictor for electrical remodeling and proarrhythmia in patients with nonischemic heart failure. *Am. J. Cardiol.* 106, 216–220. doi: 10.1016/j.amjcard.2010.02.033

Horner, S. M., Murphy, C. F., Coen, B., Dick, D. J., and Lab, M. J. (1996). Sympathomimetic modulation of load-dependent changes in the action potential duration in the in situ porcine heart. *Cardiovasc. Res.* 32, 148–157. doi: 10.1016/0008-6363(96)00087-9

Jacobson, I., Carlsson, L., and Duker, G. (2011). Beat-by-beat QT interval variability, but not QT prolongation per se, predicts drug-induced torsades de pointes in the anaesthetised methoxamine-sensitized rabbit. *J. Pharmacol. Toxicol. Methods* 63, 40–46. doi: 10.1016/j.vascn.2010.04.010

Johnson, D. M., Heijman, J., Bode, E. F., Greensmith, D. J., Van Der Linde, H., Abi-Gerges, N., et al. (2013). Diastolic spontaneous calcium release from the sarcoplasmic reticulum increases beat-to-beat variability of repolarization in canine ventricular myocytes after β-adrenergic stimulation. *Circ. Res.* 112, 246–256. doi: 10.1161/CIRCRESAHA.112.275735

Johnson, D. M., Heijman, J., Pollard, C. E., Valentin, J. P., Crijns, H. J. G. M., Abi-Gerges, N., et al. (2010). IKs restricts excessive beat-to-beat variability of repolarization during beta-adrenergic receptor stimulation. *J. Mol. Cell. Cardiol.* 48, 122–130. doi: 10.1016/j.yjmcc.2009.08.033

Julien, C. (2006). The enigma of mayer waves: facts and models. *Cardiovasc. Res.* 70, 12–21. doi: 10.1016/j.cardiores.2005.11.008

Monge Garcia, M. I., Jian, Z., Settels, J. J., Hunley, C., Cecconi, M., Hatib, F., et al. (2018). Performance comparison of ventricular and arterial dP/dtmax for assessing left ventricular systolic function during different experimental loading and contractile conditions. *Crit. Care* 22:325. doi: 10.1186/s13054-018-2260-1

O'Hara, T., Virág, L., Varró, A., and Rudy, Y. (2011). Simulation of the undiseased human cardiac ventricular action potential: model formulation and experimental validation. *PLoS Comput. Biol.* 7:e1002061. doi: 10.1371/journal.pcbi.1002061

Parati, G., Mancia, G., Di Rienzo, M., Castiglioni, P., Taylor, J., and Studinger, P. (2006). Point: counterpoint point: counterpoint: cardiovascular variability is / is not an index of autonomic control of circulation. *J. Appl. Physiol.* 101, 676–688. doi: 10.1152/japplphysiol.00446.2006.Point

Porter, B., Bishop, M. J., Claridge, S., Behar, J., Sieniewicz, B. J., Webb, J., et al. (2017). Autonomic modulation in patients with heart failure increases beat-to-beat variability of ventricular action potential duration. *Front. Physiol.* 8:328. doi: 10.3389/fphys.2017.00328

Porter, B., Bishop, M. J., Claridge, S., Child, N., Van Duijvenboden, S., Bostock, J., et al. (2019). Left ventricular activation-recovery interval variability predicts spontaneous ventricular tachyarrhythmia in patients with heart failure. *Hear. Rhythm* 16, 702–709. doi: 10.1016/j.hrthm.2018.11.013

Porter, B., Van Duijvenboden, S., Bishop, M. J., Orini, M., Claridge, S., Gould, J., et al. (2018). Beat-to-Beat variability of ventricular action potential duration oscillates at low frequency during sympathetic provocation in humans. *Front. Physiol.* 9:147. doi: 10.3389/fphys.2018.00147

Potse, M., Vinet, A., Opthof, T., and Coronel, R. (2009). Validation of a simple model for the morphology of the T wave in unipolar electrograms. *Am. J. Physiol. Heart Circ. Physiol.* 297, H792–H801. doi: 10.1152/ajpheart.00064.2009

Priori, S. G., Blomström-Lundqvist, C., Mazzanti, A., Blom, N., Borggrefe, M., Camm, J., et al. (2016). 2015 ESC guidelines for the management of patients with ventricular arrhythmias and the prevention of sudden cardiac death. *Russ. J. Cardiol.* 7, 5–86.

Pueyo, E., Dangerfield, C. E., Britton, O. J., Virág, L., Kistamás, K., Szentandrássy, N., et al. (2016a). Experimentally-based computational investigation into beat-to-beat variability in ventricular repolarization and its response to ionic current inhibition. *PLoS One* 11:e0151461. doi: 10.1371/journal.pone.0151461

Pueyo, E., Orini, M., Rodríguez, J. F., and Taggart, P. (2016b). Interactive effect of beta-adrenergic stimulation and mechanical stretch on low-frequency oscillations of ventricular action potential duration in humans. *J. Mol. Cell. Cardiol.* 97, 93–105. doi: 10.1016/j.yjmcc.2016.05.003

Puglisi, J. L., Negroni, J. A., Chen-Izu, Y., and Bers, D. M. (2013). The force-frequency relationship: insights from mathematical modeling. *Adv. Physiol. Educ.* 37, 28–34. doi: 10.1152/advan.00072.2011

Rizas, K. D., Doller, A. J., Hamm, W., Vdovin, N., von Stuelpnagel, L., Zuern, C. S., et al. (2019). Periodic repolarization dynamics as risk predictor after myocardial infarction: prospective validation study. *Hear. Rhythm* 16, 1223–1231. doi: 10.1016/j.hrthm.2019.02.024

Rizas, K. D., Hamm, W., Kääb, S., Schmidt, G., and Bauer, A. (2016). Periodic repolarisation dynamics: a natural probe of the ventricular response to sympathetic activation. *Arrhythmia Electrophysiol. Rev.* 5, 31–36. doi: 10.15420/aer.2015

Rizas, K. D., McNitt, S., Hamm, W., Massberg, S., Kääb, S., Zareba, W., et al. (2017). Prediction of sudden and non-sudden cardiac death in post-infarction patients with reduced left ventricular ejection fraction by periodic repolarization dynamics: MADIT-II substudy. *Eur. Heart J.* 38, 2110–2118. doi: 10.1093/eurheartj/ehx161

Rizas, K. D., Nieminen, T., Barthel, P., Zürn, C. S., Kähönen, M., Viik, J., et al. (2014). Clinical medicine Sympathetic activity – associated periodic repolarization dynamics predict mortality following myocardial infarction. *J. Clin. Invest.* 124, 1770–1780. doi: 10.1172/JCI70085DS1

Sampedro-Puente, D. A., Fernandez-Bes, J., Porter, B., van Duijvenboden, S., Taggart, P., and Pueyo, E. (2019). Mechanisms underlying interactions between low-frequency oscillations and beat-to-beat variability of celullar ventricular repolarization in response to sympathetic stimulation: implications for arrhythmogenesis. *Front. Physiol.* 10:916. doi: 10.3389/fphys.2019.00916

Smoczynska, A., Beekman, H. D., and Vos, M. A. (2019). The increment of short-term variability of repolarisation determines the severity of the imminent arrhythmic outcome. *Arrhythmia Electrophysiol. Rev.* 8, 166–172. doi: 10.15420/aer.2019.16.2

Sprenkeler, D. J., Beekman, J. D. M., Bossu, A., Dunnink, A., and Vos, M. A. (2019). Pro-Arrhythmic ventricular remodeling is associated with increased respiratory and low-frequency oscillations of monophasic action potential duration in the chronic atrioventricular block dog model. *Front. Physiol.* 10:1095. doi: 10.3389/fphys.2019.01095

Średniawa, B., Kowalczyk, J., Lenarczyk, R., Kowalski, O., Sędkowska, A., Cebula, S., et al. (2012). Microvolt T-wave alternans and other noninvasive predictors of serious arrhythmic events in patients with an implanted cardioverter-defibrillator. *Kardiol. Pol.* 70, 447–455.

Stams, T. R. G., Oosterhoff, P., Heijdel, A., Dunnink, A., Beekman, J. D. M., van der Nagel, R., et al. (2016). Beat-to-beat variability in preload unmasks latent risk of Torsade de Pointes in anesthetized chronic atrioventricular block dogs. *Circ. J.* 80, 1336–1345. doi: 10.1253/circj.CJ-15-1335

Szentandrássy, N., Kistamás, K., Hegyi, B., Horváth, B., Ruzsnavszky, F., Váczi, K., et al. (2015). Contribution of ion currents to beat-to-beat variability of action potential duration in canine ventricular myocytes. *Pflugers Arch. Eur. J. Physiol.* 467, 1431–1443. doi: 10.1007/s00424-014-1581-4 ter Bekke, R. M. A., Moers, A. M. E., de Jong, M. M. J., Johnson, D. M., Schwartz, P. J., Vanoli, E., et al. (2019). Proarrhythmic proclivity of left-stellate ganglion stimulation in a canine model of drug-induced long-QT syndrome type 1. *Int. J. Cardiol.* 286, 66–72. doi: 10.1016/j.ijcard.2019.01.098

Tereshchenko, L. G., Fetics, B. J., and Berger, R. D. (2009). Intracardiac QT variability in patients with structural heart disease on class III antiarrhythmic drugs. *J. Electrocardiol.* 42, 505–510. doi: 10.1016/j.jelectrocard.2009.07.011

Thomsen, M. B., Verduyn, S. C., Stengl, M., Beekman, J. D. M., De Pater, G., Van Opstal, J., et al. (2004). Increased short-term variability of repolarization predicts d-sotalol-induced torsades de pointes in dogs. *Circulation* 110, 2453–2459. doi: 10.1161/01.CIR.0000145162.64183.C8

Thomson, D. J. (1982). Spectrum estimation and harmonic analysis. *Proc. IEEE* 70, 1055–1096. doi: 10.1109/PROC.1982.12433

Tse, G., Gong, M., Wong, W. T., Georgopoulos, S., Letsas, K. P., Vassiliou, V. S., et al. (2017). The tpeak - tend interval as an electrocardiographic risk marker of arrhythmic and mortality outcomes: a systematic review and meta-analysis. *Hear. Rhythm* 14, 1131–1137. doi: 10.1016/j.hrthm.2017.05.031

van Duijvenboden, S., Hanson, B., Child, N., Orini, M., Rinaldi, C. A., Gill, J. S., et al. (2015). Effect of autonomic blocking agents on the respiratory-related oscillations of ventricular action potential duration in humans. *Am. J. Physiol. Heart Circ. Physiol.* 309, H2108–H2117. doi: 10.1152/ajpheart.00560.2015

Wyatt, R. F., Burgess, M. J., Evans, A. K., Lux, R. L., Abildskov, J. A., and Tsutsumi, T. (1981). Estimation of ventricular transmembrane action potential durations and repolarization times from unipolar electrograms. *Am. J. Cardiol.* 47:488. doi: 10.1016/0002-9149(81)91028-6

3

Golgin-97 Targets Ectopically Expressed Inward Rectifying Potassium Channel, Kir2.1, to the *trans*-Golgi Network in COS-7 Cells

*Tarvinder K. Taneja†, Donghui Ma†, Bo Y. Kim and Paul A. Welling**

Department of Physiology, Maryland Center for Kidney Discovery, School of Medicine, University of Maryland, Baltimore, Baltimore, MD, United States

***Correspondence:**
Paul A. Welling
pwelling@umaryland.edu

† These authors have contributed equally to this work.

The inward rectifying potassium channel, Kir2.1, is selected as cargo at the *trans*-Golgi network (TGN) for export to the cell surface through a unique signal-dependent interaction with the AP1 clathrin-adaptor, but it is unknown how the channel is targeted at earlier stages in the secretory pathway for traffic to the TGN. Here we explore a mechanism. A systematic screen of Golgi tethers identified Golgin-97 as a Kir2.1 binding partner. *In vitro* protein-interaction studies revealed the interaction is direct, occurring between the GRIP domain of Golgin-97 and the cytoplasmic domain of Kir2.1. Imaging and interaction studies in COS-7 cells suggest that Golgi-97 binds to the channel en route through the Golgi. RNA interference-mediated knockdown of Golgin-97 prevented exit of Kir2.1 from the Golgi. These observations identify Golgin-97 as a Kir2.1 binding partner that is required for targeting the channel to the TGN. Based on our studies in COS-7 cells, we propose Golgi-97 facilitates formation of AP1-dependent export carriers for Kir2.1 by coupling anterograde delivery of Kir2.1 with retrograde recycling of AP-1 containing endosomes to the TGN.

Keywords: potassium channel, golgi apparatus, clathrin, inward rectifying K channel, membrane trafficking

INTRODUCTION

Highly orchestrated trafficking processes ensure that cardiac ion channels are expressed on appropriate membrane domains at suitable densities to maintain the electrical rhythm of the heart. Targeting of the inward rectifying potassium channel, Kir2.1, to the t-tubule and sarcolemma in ventricular myocytes (Ma et al., 2011), for example, is made possible by a series of sequential processes that deliver newly synthesized channels from the endoplasmic reticulum to the Golgi (Ma et al., 2001), control *trans*-Golgi network (TGN) to the cell surface (Ma et al., 2011), and drive association with appropriate lipid domains (Vaidyanathan et al., 2013, 2018; Han et al., 2014) and scaffolding complexes (Leonoudakis et al., 2004a,b; Rubi et al., 2017). The importance of membrane trafficking is underscored by human disease; mutations in Kir2.1 that disrupt proper trafficking (Bendahhou et al., 2003; Ballester et al., 2006; Ma et al., 2011) cause Andersen–Tawil syndrome (Plaster et al., 2001), which predisposes affected patients to cardiac arrhythmias.

Although great progress has been made in unraveling many of the mechanisms that control the transport of Kir2.1 in the secretory pathway, it still remains poorly understood how the channel is sorted in the Golgi from resident Golgi-proteins for transport to the TGN. Differences in transmembrane spans and lipid partitioning (Patterson et al., 2008) are generally believed to provide a universal mechanism. In the present study, we consider a new Golgi segregation process, involving Golgin molecules.

Members of the Golgin protein family are well appreciated to act as specific tethers that selectively capture transport vesicles for SNARE-mediated fusion with distinct membrane compartments of the Golgi (Munro, 2011; Witkos and Lowe, 2015; Gillingham and Munro, 2016). Different Golgins associate with different Golgi regions and have distinct capture activities toward vesicles of different origins (Wong and Munro, 2014). Additionally, anterograde trafficking of several proteins through the Golgi, including the HERG cardiac potassium channel (Bundis et al., 2006), require specific Golgin molecules.

In the course of defining the TGN export mechanism in Kir2.1 (Ma et al., 2011) and related channels (Li et al., 2016), we made a serendipitous observation that implicated Golgin-97 in intra Golgi trafficking. We found mutations in the TGN export signal caused marked accumulation of the channel throughout the entire Golgi apparatus, suggesting export from the TGN might be closely coupled to anterograde transport through the Golgi. Remarkably, the Golgi-export mutants in the *cis*-Golgi tightly co-localized with Golgi-97, a golgin molecule that is usually confined to the TGN, making us wonder if a Golgin-97 interaction mechanism might explain how channels are selected in the Golgi for delivery to the TGN. Here, we test this idea.

MATERIALS AND METHODS

Antibodies

Antibodies used in this study were: anti-HA mouse monoclonal antibody (Covance Inc., Princeton, NJ, United States), anti-HA rabbit monoclonal (Upstate Cell Signaling Solutions, Waltham, MA, United States), anti-myc rabbit polyclonal, (Santa Cruz Biotechnology, Inc., Santa Cruz, CA, United States), anti-Golgin-97 (Invitrogen, #A21270), anti-p230 (BD Transduction Laboratories, Lexington, KY, United States #611230), anti-GM130 (BD Transduction Laboratories, #51-9001978), horseradish peroxidase (HRP)-conjugated goat anti-mouse or anti-rabbit (Jackson Laboratory, Bar Harbor, ME, United States), Goat anti-GST-HRP (Amersham Biosciences, Piscataway, NJ, United States), Alexa Fluor-conjugated secondary antibodies (Invitrogen Molecular Probes, Eugene, OR, United States).

Molecular Biology

All Kir2.1 constructs are derived from the mouse Kir2.1 channel cDNA (NM_008425). As described before (Ma et al., 2001), an external hemagglutinin (HA) epitope tag was engineered into the channel at a location that does not affect that the physiological function or biochemical properties of the channel (Ma et al., 2007). For some interaction studies, a myc-tag was incorporated in frame on to the N-terminus of Kir2.1 cytoplasmic C-terminal domain fragments. cDNAs for human Golgin-97 (MGC 22154), ARL1 (MGC 12286), and Golgi Matrix Protein 130 (Golga2, MGC 78452) were acquired from distributors of the IMAGE collection, and mouse p230/Golgin 245 was purchased from ATCC (10089301), and tagged in frame to the ORFs at the N or C-termini with HA or myc-epitopes. Site-directed mutagenesis was carried out using a PCR based strategy with PfuTurbo DNA polymerase (QuikChange, Stratagene). The pcDNA3.1 mammalian expression vector (Invitrogene, Inc.) was used to express the cloned channel genes in COS7 cells. For GST pull-down analyses, recombinant DNA fragments were subcloned into pGEX-5X-2. All sequences were confirmed by dye termination DNA sequencing analysis (University of Maryland School of Medicine Biopolymer Core).

Cell Culture and Transfection

COS7 cells were cultured in high glucose DMEM medium (Invitrogene, Inc., Carlsbad, CA, United States) supplemented with 10% Fetal Bovine Serum, 100 U/ml penicillin and 100 μg/ml streptomycin in a humidified atmosphere at 37°C in 5% CO2. Cells were transfected using Fugene 6 or X-tremeGENE 9 transfection reagent (Roche Ltd., Basel, Switzerland).

RNA Interference

The double-stranded siRNA to target human form of Golgin-97 and non-targeting siRNA were purchased from Thermo/Dharmacon Inc. (Lafayette, CO, United States). The Golgi-97 probe corresponded to sense sequence 5′-GAUCACAGCCCUGGAACAAUU-3′. Cells were transfected with ~160 pmole of either probe, and transfected on the subsequent day with Kir2.1 and/or non-targeting Golgin cDNAs, and then assayed after an additional ~36 h.

Immunoprecipitation

COS-7 cells were lysed in ice-cold detergent buffer (1% Triton X-100, 1× PBS, with protease inhibitors) and the clarified supernatant (15,000 g spin, 15 min) was incubated with Protein A + G beads (Cal Biochem, cat IP05), and 1 μg of immunoprecipitating antibody for 4 h rotating at 4°C. Beads were washed for 5 min with 1× PBS for three times; bound proteins were eluted with 2× Laemmli sample buffer for 30 min at room temperature; and the entire immunoprecipitate was run on a SDS-gel, and transferred to nitrocellulose for immunoblot analysis.

Quantitative Chemiluminescence Detection of Surface Proteins

To quantify cell surface expression of Kir2.1 in mammalian cells, 36 h after transfection COS7 were fixed with 3% paraformaldehyde (PFA) for 15 min on ice, blocked on ice with blocking buffer (5% Fetal Bovine Serum in 1× PBS, 30 min), incubated with mouse monoclonal anti-HA (Covance Inc.; 1:300 dilution in blocking buffer, 1 h at room temperature), washed (with 1× PBS, three times for 5 min), incubated with goat anti-mouse IgG HRP-conjugated secondary antibody (1:1000 dilution, Jackson) (in blocking buffer, 30 min), and then extensively washed (1× PBS, 5 min/time for four times in total). After washing, the cells were scraped off from the plates and resuspended well into 500 μl 1× PBS. From the cell suspension, 10 μl of cell suspension was withdrawn and incubated with 100 μl of mixed SuperSignal ELISA Pico solution (Pierce Biotechnology, Inc., Rockford, IL, United States), and subsequently chemiluminescence signal was measured as previously described (Ma et al., 2007). To normalize the data for total protein expression level, western-blot analyses were carried out in parallel with anti-HA, or anti-Kir2.1 (Chemicon Inc.), and then quantified by densitometry analysis. Reported values are the average of triplicate transfections from three different experiments.

Production of Recombinant GST Fusion Proteins and Pull-Down Analysis

The GST fusion proteins were purified on glutathione-agarose beads according to the standard protocol supplied from Amersham Biosciences, except using two times more lysis buffer than the original volume suggested in the protocol to maximize the yield. To purify the recombinant protein to high homogeneity, the GST beads were further washed with high salt buffer (0.5 M NaCl, 25 mM HEPES, and 2.5 mM $MgCl_2$, pH7.0) twice before balancing with 1× KOAc buffer (115 mM KOAc, 25 mM HEPES, and 2.5 mM $MgCl_2$, pH7.0) for pull-down analysis. The relative amount of fusion protein was quantitated by SDS-PAGE electrophoresis and then stained with coomassie blue in parallel with serial diluted BSA standard. For pull-down assays, 10 μg of purified GST beads were incubated with 100 μg of cellular lysates. After overnight incubation at 4°C, the GST beads were extensively washed with 1× PBS buffer containing 0.1% Triton X-100 to remove any non-specific binding (4 times for 10 min each time). Proteins bound on the beads were eluted by SDS-loading dye, fractionated by SDS-PAGE gel electrophoresis, blotted onto nitrocellulose membrane, and then probed with the relevant antibody.

RESULTS

Kir2.1 Interacts Specifically With Golgin-97

We considered the possibility that Kir2.1 might be pre-selected as secretory cargo in the Golgi for export at the TGN by interaction with specific Golgin tethering molecules. To explore this hypothesis, we first surveyed members of the two main classes of Golgi tethers (GM130 and the GRIP domain containing Golgins, Golgin-245/p230, and Golgin-97) for interaction with Kir2.1. As measured by co-immunoprecipitation from COS7 cells that were transfected with Kir2.1, we found that the wild-type channel Kir2.1 (WT) and the TGN-export mutant (Δ314–315) channel but not the ER-export mutant (ΔFCY) interact with Golgin-97, as expected for an interaction that is initiated within the Golgi (**Figure 1A**). Consistent with this idea, we found more of the TGN-export mutant (Δ314–15) channel co-immunoprecipitated with Golgin-97 than the WT channel

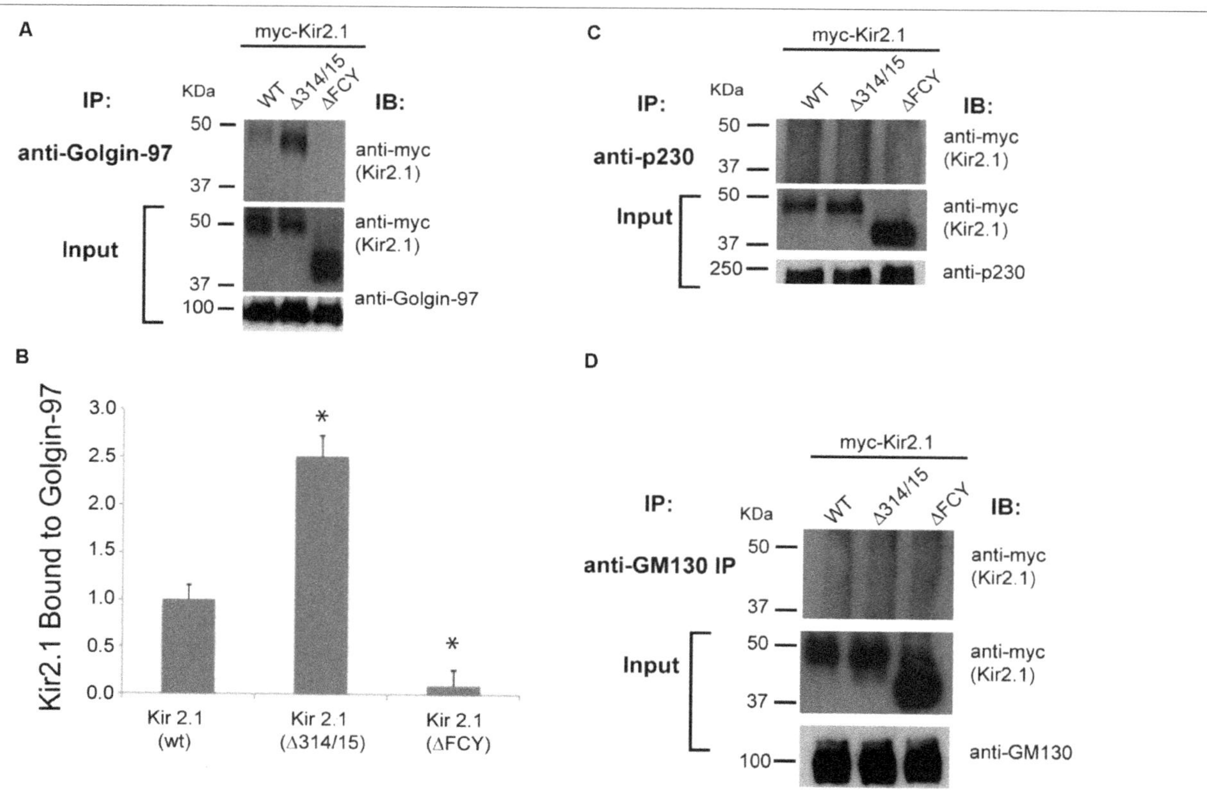

FIGURE 1 | Kir2.1 specifically binds to Golgin-97. Immunoprecipitation (IP) performed with **(A)** anti-Golgin-97; **(C)** anti-p230; **(D)** anti-GM130 antibodies from COS cells transfected with myc-Kir2.1 wild type (WT), the TGN-export mutant (Δ314–315), and the ER-export mutant (ΔFCY) and then immunoblotted (IB) with myc-antibodies to detect Kir2.1 in the Golgin immunoprecipitates. 5% input is shown below; **(B)** Quantification of the relative amounts of Kir2.1 immunoprecipatated with Golgin-97. *$P < 0.05$.

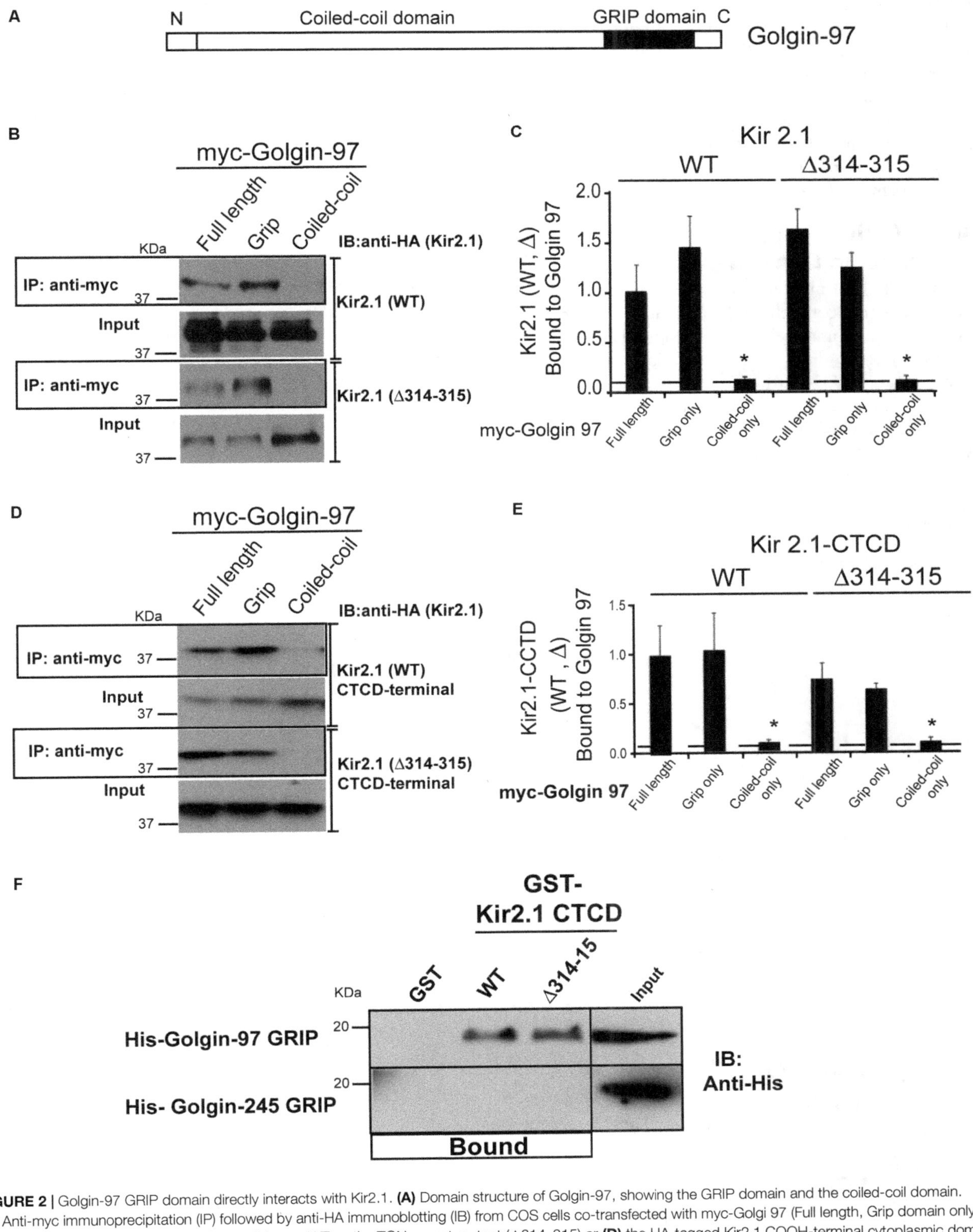

FIGURE 2 | Golgin-97 GRIP domain directly interacts with Kir2.1. **(A)** Domain structure of Golgin-97, showing the GRIP domain and the coiled-coil domain. **(B)** Anti-myc immunoprecipitation (IP) followed by anti-HA immunoblotting (IB) from COS cells co-transfected with myc-Golgi 97 (Full length, Grip domain only, or coiled-coiled domain only) and HA-Kir2.1 wild type, WT, or the TGN-export mutant (Δ314–315) or **(D)** the HA-tagged Kir2.1 COOH-terminal cytoplasmic domain (CTCD). **(C,E)** Quantitative summaries comparing relative amounts of Kir2.1 (WT or Δ314–315) immunoprecipitated with full-length Golgin-97, or GRIP or Coiled-Coil domain, $^{*}P < 0.05$. **(F)** GST pulldowns: GST alone or GST fusion proteins of the Kir2.1 CTCD were used to test for direct interaction with His-tagged GRIP domains of Golgin-97 or Golgin-245 purified from bacteria. Protein bound is shown relative to 5% input.

(**Figure 1B**). By contrast, we were unable co-immunoprecipitate Kir2.1 with antibodies to Golgin-245/p230 (**Figure 1C**), another TGN-localized, GRIP-containing Golgin (Cowan et al., 2002), or GM130 (**Figure 1D**), a member of the Golgin family of coiled-coil proteins that controls membrane tethering between the *cis*-Golgi intermediate compartment and endoplasmic reticulum and that has been implicated in HERG-channel trafficking (Newton-Cheh et al., 2009). Thus, Kir2.1/Golgin-97 interaction appears to be specific, at least amongst the Golgin molecules that were studied.

Golgin-97 GRIP Domain Associates With the Cytoplasmic Domain of Kir2.1

We next sought to determine the protein binding domains that govern the interaction between Kir2.1 and Golgi-97. Golgin-97 contains two major domains, the ~45 residue GRIP domain, which binds to Arl1 to drive Golgi localization (Lu and Hong, 2003; Panic et al., 2003; Derby et al., 2004; Lu et al., 2004; Wu et al., 2004), and a long coiled domain, which provides a tethering function (Wong and Munro, 2014; **Figure 2A**). To test which Golgin-97 domain(s) interact with Kir2.1, COS7 were co-transfected different myc-tagged Golgin-97 constructs and HA-tagged Kir2.1, and anti-myc immunoprecipitations were followed by anti-HA immunoblotting. As shown in **Figure 2** (**Figure 2B** representative gel, **Figure 2C**, summary data, $n = 3$), the isolated GRIP domain of Golgin-97 but not the coiled-coil domain is sufficient for binding to Kir2.1. Both WT Kir2.1 and the TGN-export mutant (Kir2.1 Δ314–315) are able to interact with the GRIP domain.

We considered that the large C-terminal cytoplasmic domain (CTCD) to be the most likely structure in the channel to interact with Golgin-97, and, therefore tested if it was sufficient to interact with Golgin-97. For these studies, the HA-tagged C-terminal domain (WT or the Δ314–315 mutant) was co-expressed in COS7 cells with myc-tagged Golgin-97 (full length or isolated) and myc-antibody immunoprecipitations were performed (**Figure 2D**, summarized in **Figure 2E**). As detected in anti-HA Western blots of the myc-antibody immunoprecipitates, we found the Kir2.1 CTCD is able to interact with full length Golgin-97 through the GRIP domain. The Δ314–315 mutant, which lacks part of the Golgi-export signal (Ma et al., 2011), also supports interaction with the Golgin-97 grip domain. Thus, Kir2.1 cytoplasmic C-terminus has the capacity to orchestrate Golgi-97 binding, independently of TGN-export.

To test if the interaction is direct, His-tagged Golgin GRIP domains of Golgin-97 and Golgin-245 were produced in *E. coli*, purified and tested for binding in GST-affinity

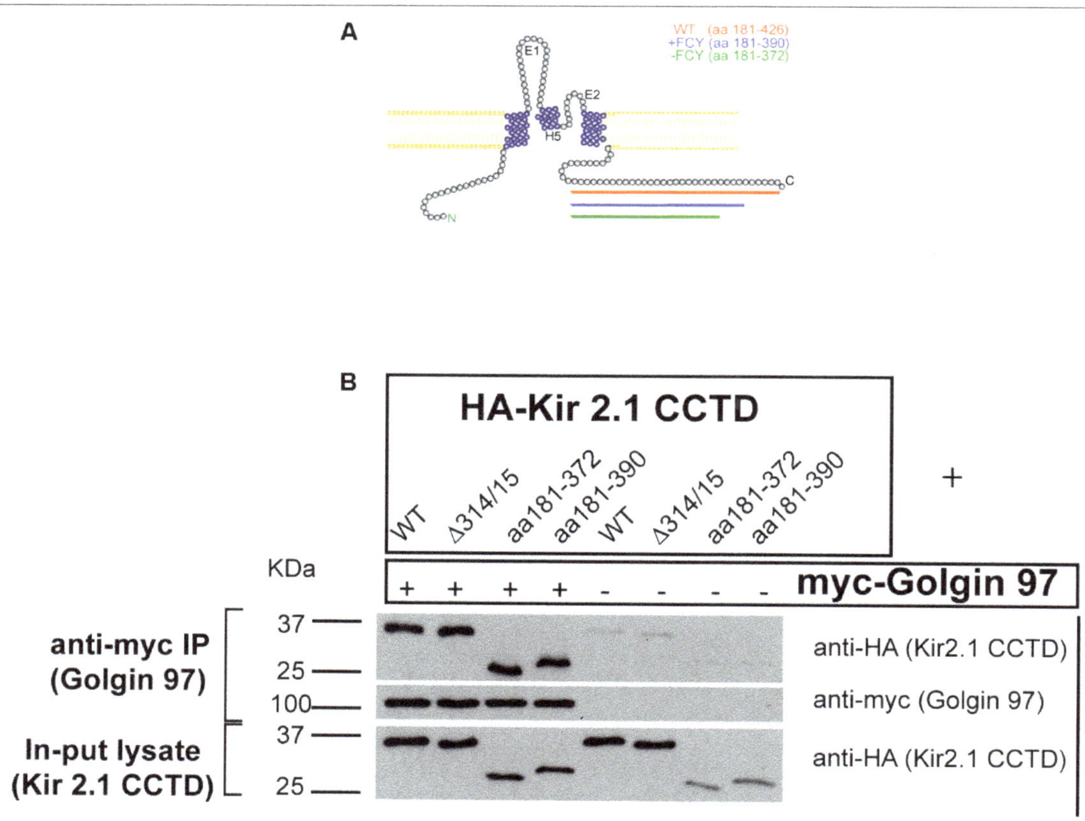

FIGURE 3 | The Kir2.1 C-terminal cytoplasmic domain (CTCD) Interacts with Golgi-97 independently of ER/Golgi export and PDZ-binding signals. **(A)** Topological structure of Kir2.1, depicting C-terminal deletion mutants. **(B)** The HA-tagged Kir2.1 channel CTCD or deletion mutants, including Golgi-export Δ314/15 (aa181–426), ER export -FCY (aa181–372) or -PDZ (181–390), were co-transfected with myc-tagged Golgin-97, and cell lysates were subjected to immunoprecipitation anti-myc and then immunoblotted with anti-HA or anti-myc antibodies.

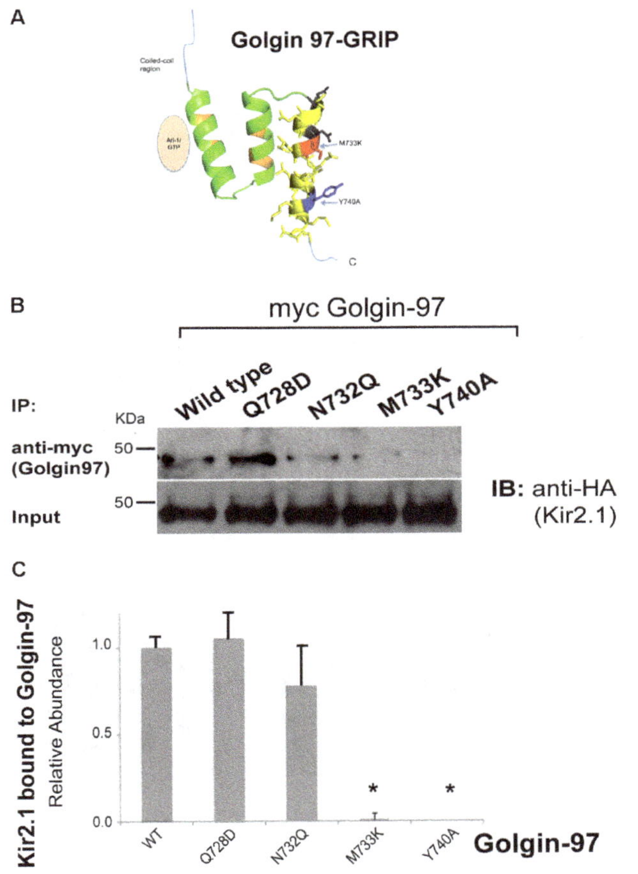

FIGURE 4 | Mapping the residues in GRIP domain involved in Kir2.1 binding. **(A)** Model of the Golgin-97 GRIP domain. First helix directly interacts with Arl1, while the third helix contains residues (M733, Y740) that are necessary for binding to Kir2.1. **(B)** The HA-tagged Kir2.1 channel was co-transfected with myc-tagged Golgin-97 (WT or GRIP domain mutants), and cell lysates were subjected to immunoprecipitation with anti-myc and then immunoblotted with anti-HA to detect Kir2.1 bound. **(C)** Summary Data, Relative to Average WT Kir2.1 immunoprecipitated with wild type (WT) Golgin-97 GRIP. $^{*}P < 0.05$.

chromatography studies with purified GST-fusion proteins of the Kir2.1 C-terminal domain (WT and Δ314–315 mutant). As shown in **Figure 2F**, GST-Kir2.1C (WT and Δ314–315 mutant), but not GST alone, pulled down the Golgin-97 GRIP domain. The interaction appeared to be highly specific because the Golgin-245 grip domain was unable to interact with GST-Kir2.1CTCD; no detectable binding was observed even after prolonged exposure.

We wondered if Golgi-97 might interact with the "FCY" ER-export signal (Ma et al., 2001) or the PDZ binding site (Leonoudakis et al., 2004a) at the extreme C-terminus of Kir2.1. To test this, we transfected COS cells with myc-tagged Golgin-97 and HA-tagged fragments of the Kir2.1 C-terminus (**Figure 3A**), and performed anti-myc immunoprecipitation, anti-HA immunoblots (**Figure 3B**). CTCD fragments, included the full length polypeptide (aa 181–426); a CTCD deletion mutant, lacking the PDZ binding motif (aa 181–390); and another CTCD domain, lacking the FCY ER export signal (181–337). As shown in **Figure 3**, each of the CTCD fragments co-immunoprecipitated with Golgin-97. Because Golgin-97 interacts with Kir2.1, independently of the ER-export signal it unlikely that Golgin-97 controls ER- to-Golgi transport of Kir2.1.

Residues in GRIP Domain Essential for the Interaction With Kir2.1

We hypothesized that Kir2.1 might interact with the Golgin-97 GRIP domain at a site that is distinct from the Arl1-binding domain, and structural homology modeling with Golgin-245 (**Figure 4A**), suggested that the third helix as the most likely channel interaction site. Sequence analysis identified several residues in the third helix of the Golgi-97 GRIP domain that are different from the GRIP domain of Golgin-245. We replaced these residues with the corresponding amino acids found Golgin-245. As evaluated by co-immunoprecipitation, M733K and Y740A point mutations abrogated the binding of the GRIP domain to Kir2.1 (**Figures 4B,C**). Thus, M733 and Y740 are necessary for the interaction, presumably by acting as a direct docking site for Kir2.1.

Interaction of Golgin-97 and Kir2.1 Occurs at the Golgi

We next determined whether the Golgin-97-Kir2.1 interaction is initiated in the Golgi. For these studies, COS7 cells were transfected with two different Kir2.1 trafficking mutants, the ER-export deficient, ΔFCY, (Ma et al., 2001) or the Golgi-export deficient, Δ314–315 (Ma et al., 2011), and the channels were co-localized (**Figure 5A**) or co-immunoprecipitated (**Figure 5B**) with Golgi 97, before and after treatment with brefeldin A (Ward et al., 2001). As shown in **Figure 5**, the ΔFCY mutant channel largely resided in subcellular compartment, typical of the endoplasmic reticulum as shown previously (Ma et al., 2001), and did not appreciably co-localize (**Figure 5A**) or co-immunoprecipitate with Golgin-97 (**Figure 5B**), regardless of BFA treatment. By contrast, a large fraction of the Golgi-export mutant, Kir2.1 Δ314–315, interacted with and co-localized with Golgin-97 in a perinuclear compartment, typical of the Golgi as shown previously (Ma et al., 2011). Treatment with BFA stimulated the absorption of Kir2.1 Δ314–315 and Golgi-97 to the ER, where the two proteins remained co-localized (**Figure 5A**), and co-immunoprecipitated (**Figure 5B**). These observations are consistent with the idea that Golgin-97 channel binds to Golgin-97 in the *cis-* or medial Golgi en route to the TGN, and the proteins remain tightly associated even after BFA treatment.

Knockdown of Golgin-97 Inhibits the Cell Surface Delivery of Kir2.1

To evaluate the functional consequence of the interaction between Kir2.1 and Golgin-97, we assessed the impact of knocking down Golgi-97 on the subcellular localization and expression of Kir2.1 at the plasmalemma. Significant reduction in Golgin-97 protein abundance was achieved upon transfection with Golgin-97 specific siRNA, compared to the scramble

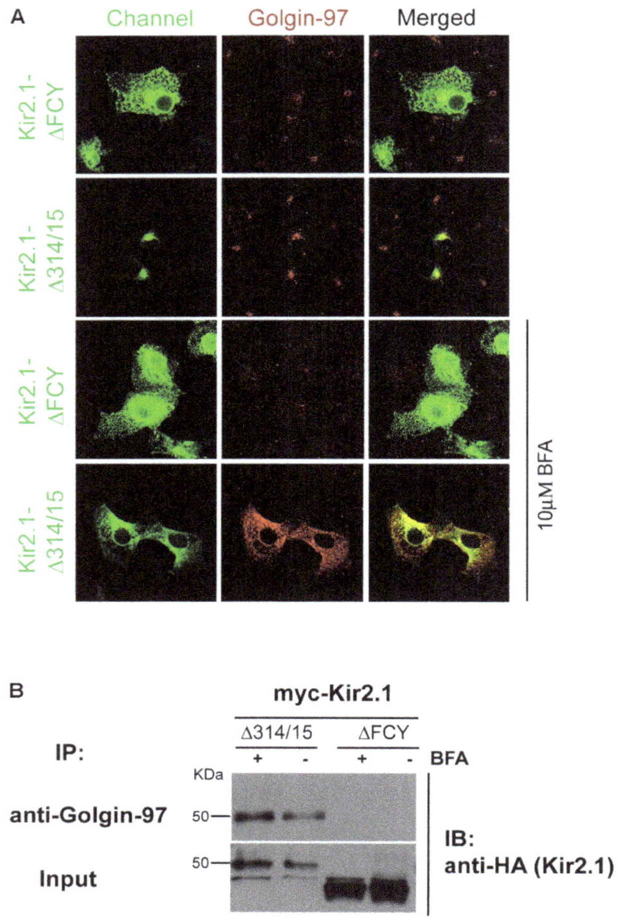

FIGURE 5 | Golgin-97 Interacts with Kir2.1 in the Golgi. **(A)** Confocal images of Kir2.1 (TGN-export mutant (Δ314–315) compared to ER-export mutant ΔFCY) in COS-cells (green) and Golgi-97 (red) before (top) and after 10 min of brefeldin A treatment. **(B)** Anti-Golgin-97 immunoprecipitation (IP) followed by anti-HA immunoblotting (IB) from COS cells transfected with the HA-Kir2.1 mutants and treated with vehicle (–) or Brefeldin (+).

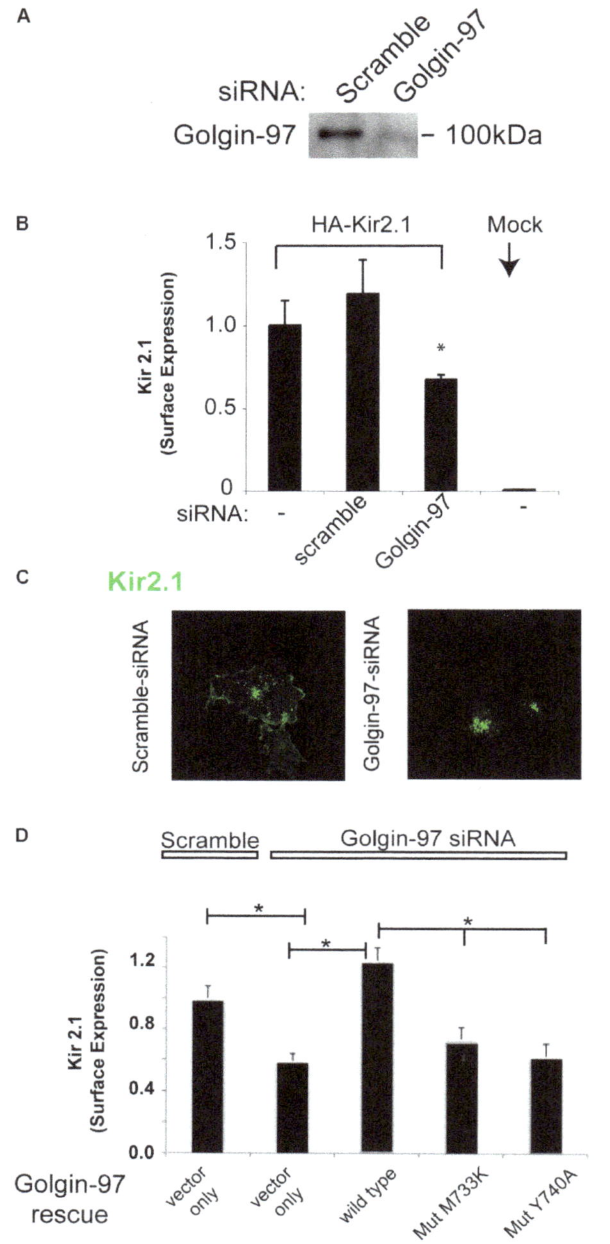

FIGURE 6 | Golgin-97 is required for efficient delivery of Kir2.1 to the cell surface membrane from the Golgi. **(A)** Immunoblot of Golgin-97 from COS cells transfected with scramble or Golgi-97 siRNA. **(B)** Surface Expression of external HA-epitope tagged Kir2.1 in COS cells co-transfected with scramble or Golgi-97 siRNA or nothing. Mock are cells transfected with vector alone. **(C)** Representative confocal microscopy of Kir2.1 in COS cells transfected with scrample, or Golgin-97 siRNA. **(D)** Rescue Studies, Surface Expression of external HA-epitope tagged Kir2.1 in COS cells co-transfected with scramble or Golgi-97 siRNA and Golgin-97 rescue cDNA (WT vs mutant), $^*P < 0.05$.

probe (**Figure 6A**) in COS cells. As measured by surface anti-HA antibody binding and analytical luminometry, Golgin-97 depletion significantly reduced Kir2.1 expression on the surface membrane (**Figure 6B**). Immunocytochemistry and confocal microscopy revealed that Kir2.1 largely accumulated in the Golgi following Golgin-97 knockdown, while the scramble siRNA probe had no effect on the Kir2.1 distribution at the cell surface membrane (**Figure 6C**). We conclude from these studies that Golgin-97 is necessary for Kir2.1 export from the Golgi.

To test whether Golgin-97 drives Kir2.1 channel trafficking in a manner that is dependent on channel interaction, we performed rescue experiments with siRNA-resistant Golgi-97 constructs, and compared the rescue response of WT Golgi-97 to binding deficient (M733K and Y740A) mutants (**Figure 6D**). For these studies, COS-7 cells were co-transfected with the Golgin-97 constructs, Golgin-97 siRNA and the external epitope tagged Kir2.1. As measured by surface anti-HA antibody binding, expression of wild type Golgi-97, but not the binding deficient mutants, rescued the trafficking of Kir2.1 to the surface membrane in Golgin-97 knockdown cells. Thus, trafficking of

Kir2.1 to the cell surface is dependent on Kir2.1 interaction with Golgin-97.

DISCUSSION

This study reveals a previously unappreciated trafficking process that directs potassium channels in the Golgi for delivery to the plasma membrane. It has been generally believed that secretory proteins are sorted in Golgi from resident Golgi proteins and proteins traveling to the ER by virtue of differences in transmembrane spans and lipid partitioning (Patterson et al., 2008). Similar processes have recently have been shown to segregate endolysosomal proteins from plasma membrane-destined proteins in the *cis*-Golgi for transport to distinct exit sites at the TGN (Chen et al., 2017). Our data suggest signal-dependent protein–protein interactions can also drive Golgi sorting processes. Indeed, we identified Golgin-97 as an interacting partner of Kir2.1, and found Gogin-97 is essential for Golgi-trafficking and delivery of Kir2.1 to the cell surface membrane. Because the interaction is initiated in the Golgi, we propose Golgin-97 marks the channel for inclusion in specialized exit sites at the TGN, where the Kir2.1 and related channels are incorporated into clathrin-coated vesicles through AP1 clathrin adaptor interactions (Ma et al., 2011).

The discovery of Golgin-97-dependent Kir2.1 trafficking extends our understanding of the Golgin molecules. Golgin-97 and Golgin p230 belong to a subset of the Golgin family members that interact with TGN membranes (Munro, 2011). Although both Golgins depend on Arl1 for TGN localization (Lu and Hong, 2003; Panic et al., 2003; Derby et al., 2004; Shin et al., 2005), they associate with distinct sets of vesicular carriers (Wong and Munro, 2014) and appear to orchestrate different trafficking processes. For instance, Golgin-p230 is required for TNF secretion (Lieu et al., 2008), whereas Golgi-97 is required for controlling exit of E-cadherin from the TGN (Lock et al., 2005). Golgin specificity is achieved, in part, by differences in vesicle-binding sequences found in the coiled-coil domains (Wong and Munro, 2014; Gillingham and Munro, 2016). In fact, the coiled-coil domain of Golgin-97 contains a specialized binding site for adaptor molecules that associate with donor vesicles (Wong and Munro, 2014). Our observations reveal an additional mechanism. By specifically interacting with Kir2.1 through the GRIP domain, Golgin-97 specifies trafficking at the acceptor membrane. It will be important to learn if other Golgin-97 dependent forward trafficking processes, such as Golgi export of E-cadherin (Lock et al., 2005), are also orchestrated by direct binding interactions at the acceptor membrane.

Although Golgin-97 is required for efficient anterograde trafficking of Kir2.1 and E-cadherin from the TGN (Lock et al., 2005), it also mediates the retrograde transport of endosomes to the TGN (Shin et al., 2017; Wong et al., 2017). We speculate that these seemingly opposite functions are interrelated. Similar to other Golgins, which facilitate endosome-to-Golgi transport to maintain Golgi structure (Derby et al., 2007), Golgin-97 may facilitate retrograde transport of specific endosomes to recycle trafficking machineries and, thereby maintain TGN sub-domains that are competent for the export of Kir2.1 and E-cadherin. Because Kir2.1 (Ma et al., 2011) and E-cadherin (Hase et al., 2013) share a common AP1 clathrin-adaptor dependent Golgi export mechanism, we speculate Golgin-97 mediated endosome-to-TGN transport allows recycling of the appropriate compliment of proteins that are required to nucleate AP1-dependent export carriers, reminiscent of the way that GCC185 recycles AP1 (Derby et al., 2007; Brown et al., 2011).

We found binding site for Golgin-97 is embedded within the large cytoplasmic region of the Kir2.1 C-terminus. Significantly, the binding site is distinct from other known trafficking motifs in the channel, including the Golgi-export signal (Ma et al., 2011), the ER-export signal (Ma et al., 2001), and the PDZ binding motif (Leonoudakis et al., 2004a). The region harbors several residues that are mutated in Andersen-Tawil syndrome (Plaster et al., 2001), and that are known to be required for efficient surface expression (Bendahhou et al., 2003). It will be interesting to learn if these residues form the interaction site for Golgin-97.

There are several limitations of this study that deserve discussion. First, this study focused on membrane trafficking of Kir2.1 in a heterologous expression system. It presently remains to be determined if Golgin-97 controls Kir2.1 in a similar way in tissues where the channel is endogenously expressed, including the heart, skeletal muscle, smooth muscle, and endothelium. Studying endogenous Kir 2.1 trafficking in native tissue is currently not practical, however. Native expression levels are much lower than in experimental expression systems and antibodies are lacking sufficient efficacy to detect the native channel protein with sufficient specificity. Development of new tools will be required to test the Golgi-97 dependent trafficking mechanism in native tissues, such as by engineering an epitope tag on the channel gene, and then studying endogenous tagged-channel in cells isolated from the genetically modified model. Second, these studies were designed to study membrane trafficking of Kir2.1, not necessarily channel activity. It will be interesting for future studies to determine whether Golgi-97 as any direct effects on channel activity.

In summary, Golgin-97 directly interacts with Kir2.1 to control anterograde transport at the Golgi. Signal-dependent interactions with Golgi tethering proteins provide a mechanism to target interacting proteins to specialized TGN sub-domains to facilitate trafficking to appropriate subcellular membrane domains.

AUTHOR CONTRIBUTIONS

TT and DM designed and executed the studies, analyzed the results and prepared the figures. BK executed the studies involving cDNA cloning and mutagenesis. PW designed the studies and prepared the manuscript.

REFERENCES

Ballester, Y., Benson, D. W., Wong, B., Law, I. H., Mathews, K. D., Vanoye, C. G., et al. (2006). Trafficking-competent and trafficking-defective KCNJ2 mutations in Andersen syndrome. *Hum. Mutat.* 27:388.

Bendahhou, S., Donaldson, M. R., Plaster, N. M., Tristani-Firouzi, M., Fu, Y. H., and Ptacek, L. J. (2003). Defective potassium channel Kir2.1 trafficking underlies Andersen-Tawil syndrome. *J. Biol. Chem.* 278, 51779–51785. doi: 10.1074/jbc.M310278200

Brown, C., Schindelhaim, C. H., and Pfeffer, S. R. (2011). GCC185 plays independent roles in Golgi structure maintenance and AP-1-mediated vesicle tethering. *J. Cell Biol.* 194, 779–787. doi: 10.1083/jcb.201104019

Bundis, F., Neagoe, I., Schwappach, B., and Steinmeyer, K. (2006). Involvement of Golgin-160 in cell surface transport of renal ROMK channel: co-expression of Golgin-160 increases ROMK currents. *Cell. Physiol. Biochem.* 17, 1–12. doi: 10.1159/000091454

Chen, Y., Gershlick, D. C., Park, S. Y., and Bonifacino, J. S. (2017). Segregation in the Golgi complex precedes export of endolysosomal proteins in distinct transport carriers. *J. Cell Biol.* 216, 4141–4151. doi: 10.1083/jcb.201707172

Cowan, D. A., Gay, D., Bieler, B. M., Zhao, H., Yoshino, A., Davis, J. G., et al. (2002). Characterization of mouse tGolgin-1 (golgin-245/trans-golgi p230/256 kD golgin) and its upregulation during oligodendrocyte development. *DNA Cell Biol.* 21, 505–517. doi: 10.1089/104454902320219068

Derby, M. C., Lieu, Z. Z., Brown, D., Stow, J. L., Goud, B., and Gleeson, P. A. (2007). The trans-Golgi network golgin, GCC185, is required for endosome-to-Golgi transport and maintenance of Golgi structure. *Traffic* 8, 758–773. doi: 10.1111/j.1600-0854.2007.00563.x

Derby, M. C., van Vliet, C., Brown, D., Luke, M. R., Lu, L., Hong, W., et al. (2004). Mammalian GRIP domain proteins differ in their membrane binding properties and are recruited to distinct domains of the TGN. *J. Cell Sci.* 117(Pt 24), 5865–5874. doi: 10.1242/jcs.01497

Gillingham, A. K., and Munro, S. (2016). Finding the Golgi: Golgin coiled-coil proteins show the way. *Trends Cell Biol.* 26, 399–408. doi: 10.1016/j.tcb.2016.02.005

Han, H., Rosenhouse-Dantsker, A., Gnanasambandam, R., Epshtein, Y., Chen, Z., Sachs, F., et al. (2014). Silencing of Kir2 channels by caveolin-1: cross-talk with cholesterol. *J. Physiol.* 592, 4025–4038. doi: 10.1113/jphysiol.2014.273177

Hase, K., Nakatsu, F., Ohmae, M., Sugihara, K., Shioda, N., Takahashi, D., et al. (2013). AP-1B-mediated protein sorting regulates polarity and proliferation of intestinal epithelial cells in mice. *Gastroenterology* 145, 625–635. doi: 10.1053/j.gastro.2013.05.013

Leonoudakis, D., Conti, L. R., Anderson, S., Radeke, C. M., McGuire, L. M., Adams, M. E., et al. (2004a). Protein trafficking and anchoring complexes revealed by proteomic analysis of inward rectifier potassium channel (Kir2.x)-associated proteins. *J. Biol. Chem.* 279, 22331–22346. doi: 10.1074/jbc.M400285200

Leonoudakis, D., Conti, L. R., Radeke, C. M., McGuire, L. M., and Vandenberg, C. A. (2004b). A multiprotein trafficking complex composed of SAP97, CASK, Veli, and Mint1 is associated with inward rectifier Kir2 potassium channels. *J. Biol. Chem.* 279, 19051–19063. doi: 10.1074/jbc.M400284200

Li, X., Ortega, B., Kim, B., and Welling, P. A. (2016). A common signal patch drives AP-1 dependent Golgi export of inwardly rectifying potassium channels. *J. Biol. Chem.* 291, 14963–14972. doi: 10.1074/jbc.M116.729822

Lieu, Z. Z., Lock, J. G., Hammond, L. A., La Gruta, N. L., Stow, J. L., and Gleeson, P. A. (2008). A trans-Golgi network golgin is required for the regulated secretion of TNF in activated macrophages in vivo. *Proc. Natl. Acad. Sci. U.S.A.* 105, 3351–3356. doi: 10.1073/pnas.0800137105

Lock, J. G., Hammond, L. A., Houghton, F., Gleeson, P. A., and Stow, J. L. (2005). E-cadherin transport from the trans-Golgi network in tubulovesicular carriers is selectively regulated by golgin-97. *Traffic* 6, 1142–1156. doi: 10.1111/j.1600-0854.2005.00349.x

Lu, L., and Hong, W. (2003). Interaction of Arl1-GTP with GRIP domains recruits autoantigens Golgin-97 and Golgin-245/p230 onto the Golgi. *Mol. Biol. Cell* 14, 3767–3781. doi: 10.1091/mbc.e03-01-0864

Lu, L., Tai, G., and Hong, W. (2004). Autoantigen Golgin-97, an effector of Arl1 GTPase, participates in traffic from the endosome to the trans-Golgi network. *Mol. Biol. Cell* 15, 4426–4443. doi: 10.1091/mbc.e03-12-0872

Ma, D., Taneja, T. K., Hagen, B. M., Kim, B. Y., Ortega, B., Lederer, W. J., et al. (2011). Golgi export of the Kir2.1 channel is driven by a trafficking signal located within its tertiary structure. *Cell* 145, 1102–1115. doi: 10.1016/j.cell.2011.06.007

Ma, D., Tang, X. D., Rogers, T. B., and Welling, P. A. (2007). An andersen-Tawil syndrome mutation in Kir2.1 (V302M) alters the G-loop cytoplasmic K+ conduction pathway. *J. Biol. Chem.* 282, 5781–5789. doi: 10.1074/jbc.M608776200

Ma, D., Zerangue, N., Lin, Y. F., Collins, A., Yu, M., Jan, Y. N., et al. (2001). Role of ER export signals in controlling surface potassium channel numbers. *Science* 291, 316–339. doi: 10.1126/science.291.5502.316

Munro, S. (2011). The golgin coiled-coil proteins of the Golgi apparatus. *Cold Spring Harb. Perspect. Biol.* 3:a005256. doi: 10.1101/cshperspect.a005256

Newton-Cheh, C., Johnson, T., Gateva, V., Tobin, M. D., Bochud, M., Coin, L., et al. (2009). Genome-wide association study identifies eight loci associated with blood pressure. *Nat. Genet.* 41, 666–676. doi: 10.1038/ng.361

Panic, B., Perisic, O., Veprintsev, D. B., Williams, R. L., and Munro, S. (2003). Structural basis for Arl1-dependent targeting of homodimeric GRIP domains to the Golgi apparatus. *Mol. Cell* 12, 863–874. doi: 10.1016/S1097-2765(03)00356-3

Patterson, G. H., Hirschberg, K., Polishchuk, R. S., Gerlich, D., Phair, R. D., and Lippincott-Schwartz, J. (2008). Transport through the Golgi apparatus by rapid partitioning within a two-phase membrane system. *Cell* 133, 1055–1067. doi: 10.1016/j.cell.2008.04.044

Plaster, N. M., Tawil, R., Tristani-Firouzi, M., Canun, S., Bendahhou, S., Tsunoda, A., et al. (2001). Mutations in Kir2.1 cause the developmental and episodic electrical phenotypes of Andersen's syndrome. *Cell* 105, 511–519. doi: 10.1016/S0092-8674(01)00342-7

Rubi, L., Koenig, X., Kubista, H., Todt, H., and Hilber, K. (2017). Decreased inward rectifier potassium current IK1 in dystrophin-deficient ventricular cardiomyocytes. *Channels* 11, 101–108. doi: 10.1080/19336950.2016.1228498

Shin, H. W., Kobayashi, H., Kitamura, M., Waguri, S., Suganuma, T., Uchiyama, Y., et al. (2005). Roles of ARFRP1 (ADP-ribosylation factor-related protein 1) in post-Golgi membrane trafficking. *J. Cell Sci.* 118(Pt 17), 4039–4048. doi: 10.1242/jcs.02524

Shin, J. J. H., Gillingham, A. K., Begum, F., Chadwick, J., and Munro, S. (2017). TBC1D23 is a bridging factor for endosomal vesicle capture by golgins at the trans-Golgi. *Nat. Cell Biol.* 19, 1424–1432. doi: 10.1038/ncb3627

Vaidyanathan, R., Van Ert, H., Haq, K. T., Morotti, S., Esch, S., McCune, E. C., et al. (2018). Inward rectifier potassium channels (Kir2.x) and caveolin-3 domain-specific interaction: implications for purkinje cell-dependent ventricular arrhythmias. *Circ. Arrhythm. Electrophysiol.* 11:e005800. doi: 10.1161/CIRCEP.117.005800

Vaidyanathan, R., Vega, A. L., Song, C., Zhou, Q., Tan, B. H., Berger, S., et al. (2013). The interaction of caveolin 3 protein with the potassium inward rectifier channel Kir2.1: physiology and pathology related to long qt syndrome 9 (LQT9). *J. Biol. Chem.* 288, 17472–17480. doi: 10.1074/jbc.M112.43{\break}5370

Ward, T. H., Polishchuk, R. S., Caplan, S., Hirschberg, K., and Lippincott-Schwartz, J. (2001). Maintenance of Golgi structure and function depends on the integrity of ER export. *J. Cell Biol.* 155, 557–570. doi: 10.1083/jcb.200107045

Witkos, T. M., and Lowe, M. (2015). The golgin family of coiled-coil tethering proteins. *Front Cell Dev. Biol.* 3:86. doi: 10.3389/fcell.2015.00086

Wong, M., Gillingham, A. K., and Munro, S. (2017). The golgin coiled-coil proteins capture different types of transport carriers via distinct N-terminal motifs. *BMC Biol.* 15:3. doi: 10.1186/s12915-016-0345-3

Wong, M., and Munro, S. (2014). Membrane trafficking. The specificity of vesicle traffic to the Golgi is encoded in the golgin coiled-coil proteins. *Science* 346:1256898. doi: 10.1126/science.1256898

Wu, M., Lu, L., Hong, W., and Song, H. (2004). Structural basis for recruitment of GRIP domain golgin-245 by small GTPase Arl1. *Nat. Struct. Mol. Biol.* 11, 86–94. doi: 10.1038/nsmb714

4

Arrhythmic Risk in Elderly Patients Candidates to Transcatheter Aortic Valve Replacement: Predictive Role of Repolarization Temporal Dispersion

Gianfranco Piccirillo[1], Federica Moscucci[1], Marcella Fabietti[1], Ilaria Parrotta[1], Fabiola Mastropietri[1], Claudia Di Iorio[1], Teresa Sabatino[1], Davide Crapanzano[1], Giulia Vespignani[1], Marco Valerio Mariani[1], Nicolò Salvi[1] and Damiano Magrì[2]*

[1] Dipartimento di Scienze Cardiovascolari, Respiratorie, Geriatriche, Anestesiologiche e Nefrologiche, Policlinico Umberto I, "La Sapienza" University of Rome, Rome, Italy, [2] Dipartimento di Medicina Clinica e Molecolare, S. Andrea Hospital, "Sapienza" University of Rome, Rome, Italy

***Correspondence:**
Federica Moscucci
federica.moscucci@uniroma1.it

Background/Aim: Degenerative aortic valve stenosis (AS) is associated to ventricular arrhythmias and sudden cardiac death, as well as mental stress in specific patients. In such a context, substrate, autonomic imbalance as well as repolarization dispersion abnormalities play an undoubted role. Aim of the study was to evaluate the increase of premature ventricular contractions (PVC) and complex ventricular arrhythmias during mental stress in elderly patients candidate to the transcatheter aortic valve replacement (TAVR).

Methods: In eighty-one elderly patients with AS we calculated several short-period RR- and QT-derived variables at rest, during controlled breathing and during mild mental stress, the latter being represented by a mini-mental state evaluation (MMSE).

Results: All the myocardial repolarization dispersion markers worsened during mental stress ($p < 0.05$). Furthermore, during MMSE, low frequency component of the RR variability increased significantly both as absolute power (LF_{RR}) and normalized units (LF_{RRNU}) ($p < 0.05$) as well as the low-high frequency ratio (LF_{RR}/HF_{RR}) ($p < 0.05$). Eventually, twenty-four (30%) and twelve (15%) patients increased significantly PVC and, respectively, complex ventricular arrhythmias during the MMSE administration. At multivariate logistic regression analysis, the standard deviation of QTend (QTe_{sd}), obtained at rest, was predictive of increased PVC (odd ratio: 1.54, 95% CI 1.14–2.08; $p = 0.005$) and complex ventricular arrhythmias (odd ratio: 2.31, 95% CI 1.40–3.83; $p = 0.001$) during MMSE. The QTe_{sd} showed the widest sensitive-specificity area under the curve for the increase of PVC (AUC: 0.699, 95% CI: 0.576–0.822, $p < 0.05$) and complex ventricular arrhythmias (AUC: 0.801, 95% CI: 0.648–0.954, $p < 0.05$).

Conclusion: In elderly with AS ventricular arrhythmias worsened during a simple cognitive assessment, this events being a possible further burden on the outcome of TAVR. QTe_{sd} might be useful to identify those patients with the highest risk of ventricular arrhythmias. Whether the TAVR could led to a QTe_{sd} reduction and, hence, to a reduction of the arrhythmic burden in this setting of patients is worthy to be investigated.

Keywords: aortic stenosis, TAVR, QT, QT standard deviation, T peak-T end, QTc, QT variability

INTRODUCTION

Senile degenerative aortic valve stenosis (AS) represents the most relevant valvular heart disease both in terms of prevalence and of prognostic implications in Western countries. Indeed, about 3.4% of over 75 years subjects suffers from this valvulopathy (Osnabrugge et al., 2013) and, after the beginning of symptoms, in absence of surgical or transcatheter replacement, the survival is less than half at 2 years (Lindman et al., 2014; Afilalo et al., 2017). Obviously, the poor prognosis in this setting of patients is strongly influenced by a number of possible comorbidities over the AS. However, a mainly neglected factor possibly impacting the AS patients prognosis is represented by their propensity to the malignant arrhythmias. Myocardial hypertrophy, fibers disarray, fibrosis, necrosis and calcification are all features constituting an optimum structural substrate for arrhythmic sudden cardiac death. Furthermore, sympathetic over-activity, typical in chronic heart failure, could also play an important role as malignant ventricular arrhythmias' trigger. In such a context, there are two previous observations corroborating these claims: it was recently confirmed that the sudden cardiac death during AS remains statistically important (Minamino-Muta et al., 2017) and, some non-invasive electrocardiographic (ECG) markers were found significantly associated to a poor outcome in elderly patients with AS after the transcatheter aortic valve replacement (TAVR) (Piccirillo et al., 2018).

Therefore, the present study evaluated a number of non-invasive markers of myocardial electrical instability in a cohort of elderly patients with AS candidate to the TAVR procedure. Particularly, we analyzed the short period RR- and QT-interval variables (Baumert et al., 2016) at rest, during controlled breathing and during mild mental stress, the latter being represented by a mini-mental state evaluation (MMSE). Thereafter we evaluated a possible MMSE-induced increase in premature ventricular contraction (PVC) or complex ventricular arrhythmias (bigeminy, trigeminy, couplets episodes, R on T phenomena, sustained or non-sustained ventricular tachycardia) (Zanobetti et al., 2017). Eventually, we sought to assess a possible relationship between the abovementioned ECG derived markers obtained during rest and the arrhythmic risk in terms of complex ventricular arrhythmias increase during MMSE.

The major part of these repolarization markers are normalized for RR variability (Baumert Europace 2016; 18, 925–944) (Baumert et al., 2016) and for this reason the patients with frequent premature contractions or atrial fibrillation are frequently excluded from these kind of studies. Notwithstanding, the elderly with AS presented a very high level of supra- or ventricular arrhythmias, consequently we decided to use repolarization indexes only, without RR variability normalization; in this way, we were able to include even patients with atrial fibrillation or with frequent premature atrial or ventricular contractions.

MATERIALS AND METHODS

Participants and Protocol

A total of 92 consecutive symptomatic (NYHA III class) elderly patients who underwent evaluation for TAVR HCM were recruited between September 2017 and July 2018 at Policlinico Umberto I University Hospital in Rome. Patients' characteristics, preoperative echocardiographic issues, a complete functional assessment and ECG-derived data were recorded at time of enrollment.

The functional assessment included the following: Mini-Mental State Examination (MMSE), Activity of Daily Living (ADL), Instrumental Activities of Daily Living (IADL), and Mini-Nutritional Assessment (MNA). Furthermore the Clinical Frailty Scale (Rockwood et al., 2005) and the Essential Frailty Toolset (Afilalo et al., 2017) have been administered.

The ECG study included, for each patients, three distinct and consecutive sessions with a short-period single lead (II) ECG acquired in supine position: the first session during rest (REST); the second session during controlled breathing (15 breaths per minute) (RESP) and the third one during MMSE (MENTAL STRESS). Both the REST and RESP recordings lasted 5 min while the MENTAL STRESS session lasted averagely 10 min (11.5 ± 3.9 min), being the sum of the three recordings equal to 22.1 ± 3.9 min. Contextually, a non-invasive beat-to-beat blood pressure wave recordings (Finometer MIDI, FMS B.V., Amsterdam, Netherlands) has been recorded.

No patient has been excluded from the ECG analysis, being included also those with atrial and ventricular arrhythmias (premature ventricular or atrial contractions, atrial fibrillation, etc.) or pacemaker. Concerning the latter category, the pacing setting during the study was VDD with lower rate well below the patient's lowest intrinsic heart rate so that the physiological atrial tracking under study conditions has been preserved. In patients with bundle branch block, J-T interval was considered in place of QT.

The study was approved by the Ethical Committee of Azienda Universitaria Policlinico Umberto I. Each patients signed an appropriate informed consent. Trial was registered on ClinicalTrial.gov database with number NCT03145376.

Off-Line Data Analysis

To acquire and digitalize the ECG and pressure signals, we used a custom-designed card (National Instruments USB-6008; National Instruments, Austin, TX, United States) with a sampling frequency equal to 500 Hz. The software for data acquisition, storage, and analysis with the LabView program (National Instruments), designed and produced from our research team, follows the technical recommendation of consensus guidance endorsed by European Heart Rhythm Association jointly with the European Society of Cardiology Working Group on cardiac cellular electrophysiology (Baumert et al., 2016). With respect the QT-derived measurements, they were obtained with the template method proposed by Berger et al. (1997).

Each ECG recording undergoes three consecutive processes: rhythm analysis; elimination of ventricular and atrial premature contraction (PVC ad sPVC) from ECG traces; RR and QT interval analysis. During the rhythm analysis, a quantitative evaluation of PVC has been made by dividing the number of PVC every 3 min of each single examined recording thus disclosing the patients with the increase of PVC per minutes during the MENTAL STRESS session. If during the MENTAL STRESS session only, patients showed bigeminy, trigeminy, couplets episodes, R on T phenomenon, sustained or non-sustained ventricular tachycardia, we considered this fact as an increase of arrhythmias (Zanobetti et al., 2017). Secondly, we identified the PVC and sPVC on the traces and we eliminated manually their QRS-T data and also the corresponding following beat (**Figure 1**), as recommended in previous consensus guidance (Baumert et al., 2016). After this preliminary phase, we used three time-series of "cleaned" 256 consecutive QRS-T (REST, RESP, and MENTAL STRESS) to study the repolarization variables. With respect the MENTAL STRESS recording, we focused on the period with the higher sympathetic activity (i.e., the QRS-T data series with lower RR cycle length and then higher heart rate). Short-term myocardial temporal repolarization dispersion measurements were obtained on three different intervals: the interval from Q to end of T wave (QTe); the interval between and the Q and the peak of T wave (QTp); the interval between peak and end of T wave (Te) (**Figure 2**). We then calculated the following QT-derived data: mean and standard deviation of QTe, QTp and Te (QTe_m, QTe_{sd}, QTp_m, QTp_{sd}, Te_m, and Te_{sd}), Te_m and QTe_m ratio (Te_m/QTe_m). We also calculated normalized QTe (QTeVN), QTp (QTpVN) and Te (TeVN) interval variances (Baumert et al., 2016) according to the formulas:

$$QTeVN = {QTe_{sd}}^2/{QeT_m}^2;$$

$$QTpVN = {QTp_{sd}}^2/{QTp_m}^2;$$

$$TeVN = {Te_{sd}}^2/{Te_m}^2.$$

Short term variability of QTe (QTe_{STV}), QTp (QTp_{STV}) and Te (Te_{STV}) (Baumert et al., 2016) was also obtained according to the formulas:

$$QTe_{STV} = \Sigma[QT_{n+1} - QT_n]\ (256 \times \sqrt{}2);$$

$$QTp_{STV} = p\Sigma[QTp_{n+1} - QTp_n]\ (256 \times \sqrt{}2);$$

$$Te_{STV} = [Te_{n+1} - Te_n]\ (256 \times \sqrt{}2).$$

Furthermore, we calculated the spectral coherence between the QTp and Te (Piccirillo et al., 2014b) on the 256 beats in the three different study sessions according to the formula (Baumert et al., 2016):

$$\text{Coherence}^2_{(QTp-Te)}(f);$$

$$\frac{\text{Cross spectral power density}^2_{(QTp-Te)}(f) = |\ \text{Coherence}_{(QTp-Te)}(f)^2}{\text{Spectral density}_{Te}(f)\ \text{Spectral density}_{QTp}(f)}$$

where f was the spectral frequency.

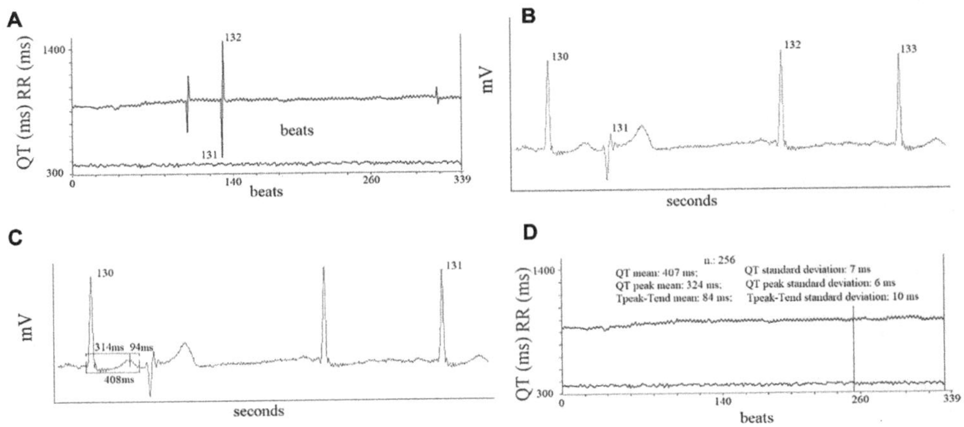

FIGURE 1 | An example of RR and QTe recordings at rest **(A)**, it is possible to observe three PVC in picture, the second PVC is the beat number 131. In the second phase of off-line analysis **(B)**, the computer eliminated the data of PVC (131) and of following beats number 132. Note, the complete flattening of T wave of beat number 132. Therefore, this beats was eliminated from final analysis of data **(C)**. Finally, it was reported the some final analyses in the 256 window data recordings **(D)**.

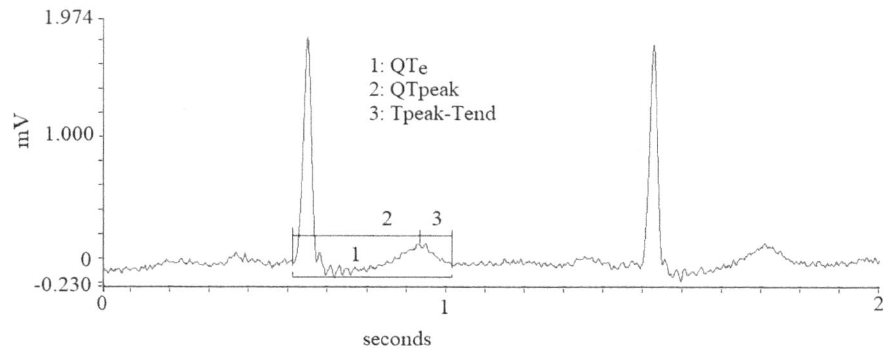

FIGURE 2 | Different repolarization intervals obtained in the study.

The spectral coherence value ranges between 0 and 1 with the high level of coherence being closer to 1 and it indicates the temporal relation between two signals (QTp and Te).

We also measured manually, by means an electronic caliper and applying the tangent method on three consecutive cycles (II lead), the following intervals: QT (from q to end T wave); QRS (from q to end S wave); JT (from J point to end of T wave); Te (from the peak to the end of T wave) and we corrected them on three preceding RR interval with Bazett method (QT_{Bazett}: $QT/RR^{0.5}$; QRS_{Bazett}: $QRS/RR^{0.5}$; JT_{Bazett}: $JT/RR^{0.5}$; $Te_{Bazett}/RR^{0.5}$) (Crow et al., 2003; Rautaharju et al., 2004, 2009).

Eventually, only in those patients with sinus rhythm, excluding those with higher than one PVC per minute, we obtained the spectral and cross-spectral analysis, using the autoregressive method (Task Force of the European Society of Cardiology, and the North American Society of Pacing, and Electrophysiology, 1996; Berger et al., 1997; Baumert et al., 2016) and we reported the following RR and systolic blood pressure (SBP) variables: the total power (TP_{RR}, TP_{SBP}), resulted from the spectral densities included between the 0 and 0.40 Hz; the high-frequency (HF_{RR}, HF_{SBP}) component (from 0.15 to 0.40 Hz); the low-frequency (LF_{RR}, LF_{SBP}) component (from 0.04 to 0.15 Hz Eq); the very-low frequency (VLF_{RR}, VLF_{SBP}) component (below 0.04 Hz Eq) (Task Force of the European Society of Cardiology, and the North American Society of Pacing, and Electrophysiology, 1996; Piccirillo et al., 2009b, 2016). We also calculated the LF (LF_{NU}) and HF (HF_{NU}) normalized units according the following formulas:

$$LF_{NU} = LF_{RR}/(TP_{RR} - VLF_{RR}) \times 100;$$

$$HF_{NU} = HF_{RR}/(TP_{RR} - VLF_{RR}) \times 100.$$

We also measured LF and HF central frequencies and the α index was calculated according to the formulas: (Robbe et al., 1987; Pagani et al., 1988; Piccirillo et al., 2000a,b, 2004b, 2013, 2016).

$$\alpha LF = \sqrt{LF_{RR}}/\sqrt{LF_{SBP}};$$

$$\alpha HF = \sqrt{HF_{RR}}/\sqrt{HF_{SBP}}.$$

Absolute power, LF/HF, α LF and α HF were converted in natural logarithm (ln) (Task Force of the European Society of Cardiology, and the North American Society of Pacing, and Electrophysiology, 1996; Piccirillo et al., 2009b, 2016).

Statistical Analysis

All data with normal distribution were expressed as means ± standard deviation; non-normally distributed variables were expressed as median and inter-quartile range (iqr); categorical variables are presented as frequencies and percentage (%). In normal distributed data one-way repeated-measures ANOVA test has been used to compare the same variable in the three different study session (REST, RESP, and MENTAL STRESS); the variables with non-normal distribution were compared using Friedman test.

Then, we grouped patients in two categories according to the presence or the absence of complex ventricular arrhythmias recorded during the MENTAL STRESS session. The criteria to include a patient in the complex ventricular arrhythmia group were the following rhythm disturbs during the MENTAL STRESS session: bigeminy, trigeminy or couplet episodes, R on T phenomenon, sustained or non-sustained ventricular tachycardia (Zanobetti et al., 2017). Thereafter we also grouped the patients in two other categories according the presence or the absence of an increase PVC per minute during the MENTAL STRESS session. The values of repolarization obtained during REST of these study groups were compared using Student's T and Mann-Whitney U tests, respectively for normal and non-normal distribution data.

Uni- and multivariable forward (A. Wald) stepwise logistic regression analysis were used to determine the association between the increase of the number or the complex ventricular arrhythmias during the MENTAL STRESS session and clinical, hemodynamic, repolarization and spectral data during the REST session. Particularly, we considered covariates the following repolarization data: QTe_m, QTe_{sd}, QTp_m, QTp_{sd}, Te_m, Te_{sd}, Te_m/QTe_m, QTe_{STV}, QTp_{STV}, Te_{STV}, $Coherence_{(QTp-Te)}$,QRS, QT, JT, Te, QRS_{Bazett}, QT_{Bazett}, JT_{Bazett}, Te_{Bazett}, Te/QTe, Te_{Bazett}/QTe_{Bazett}. QTeVN, QTpVN, TeVN were excluded from the present analysis because of their non-normal distribution.

Receiver operating characteristic (ROC) curves were used to determine the sensitivity and specificity of studied parameters predictive of complex ventricular arrhythmias and areas under ROC curves and 95% confidence intervals (CI) were calculated to compare the diagnostic efficiencies. All data were evaluated by use of database SPSS-PC + (SPSS-PC + Inc., Chicago, IL, United States).

RESULTS

From the initial 92 patients' study sample, 11 patients were excluded because the ECG traces' poor quality (No. 4 patients) or because they did not complete the protocols (No. 6 patients). **Table 1** summarized clinical, echocardiographic, cognitive, nutritional and functional data for a total of 81 elderly patients effectively enrolled in the present study.

TABLE 1 | General characteristic of the degenerative aortic valve stenosis.

	N: 81
Age, years	81 ± 7
M/F,	36/45
BMI, kg/m^2	26.7 ± 4.5
Complete right bundle branch block	6(7)
Complete left bundle branch block	10(12)
Aortic peak gradient, mm Hg	73 ± 23
Aortic mean gradient, mm Hg	45 ± 15
Aortic valve area, cm^2/m^2	0.46 ± 0.14
Aortic peak velocity, m/s	4.2 ± 0.8
Ejection fraction,%	51 ± 9
Stroke volume index, ml/m^2	41 ± 17
Left ventricular mass index, g/m^2	143 ± 39
Mini-mental state evaluation	26.3 ± 3.9
Activity of day living	5 ± 1
Instrumental activities of day living	5 ± 2
Clinical frailty scale	4 ± 1
Essential frailty toolset	2 ± 1
Mini-nutritional assessment	23 ± 4
β-blockers, n (%)	43(53)
Verapamil/Diltiazem, n (%)	4(5)
Amiodarone, n (%)	4(5)
Flecainide, n (%)	2(2)
Propafenone, n (%)	1(1)
Ivabradine, n (%)	2(2)
Digoxin, n (%)	4(5)
ACE/sartan, n (%)	47(58)
Dihydropyridine calcium channel blockers, n (%)	26(32)
Furosemide, n (%)	46(57)
Nitrate, n (%)	7(9)
Ranolazine, n (%)	6(7)
Statine, n (%)	37(46)
Antiplatelet therapy, (%)	39(48)
Oral anticoagulants, (%)	26 (32)
Pacemaker, n (%)	5(6)

Data are expressed as mean ± SD or number (n) of patients (%).

The arrhythmic characteristics obtained during the three sessions (REST, RESP, MENTAL STRESS) were reported in the **Table 2**. During the MENTAL STRESS session, an increase of PVC and of arrhythmic ventricular complexity were found in 24 (from 0.3 [2.1] to 0.8 [3.9], $p < 0.001$) and, respectively, in 12 patients (from 0 [0] to 7 ventricular bigeminy or trigemini – 8 ventricular couplets episodes; 3 non-sustained ventricular tachycardia; 3 R on T phenomenon). Remarkably, two patients with an increased complexity of ventricular arrhythmias during MENTAL STRESS did not report any isolated PVC during REST (both of them showed a ventricular couplet episode and, only one of them, an R on T phenomenon, too). Three subjects showed premature ventricular couplets during the RESP session, these type of arrhythmic episodes interesting a total of 11 patients. No significant difference was found between those patients with increased PVC's number or complexity of ventricular arrhythmias and all the other AS patients with respect clinical, cognitive, nutritional, functional and echocardiographic data.

Hemodynamic and Repolarization Data

During MENTAL STRESS, all patients reported a significant increase of heart rate ($p < 0.01$) and, at the same time, they significantly reduced the non-invasively measured stroke volume ($p < 0.001$) and cardiac output ($p < 0.05$) (**Table 3**).

The QTe mean and QTp_m values were steady between REST and MENTAL STRESS session while Te_m significantly increased ($p < 0.05$) (**Table 3**). Moreover the Te_m value increased significantly during the RESP session in comparison to the REST one, too. All markers of myocardial ventricular temporal dispersion, excepted the Te_m/QTe_m, were significantly higher during the MENTAL STRESS in comparison to the REST ($p < 0.05$) and RESP ($p < 0.05$) (**Table 3**). Instead, the $\text{Coherence}_{(QTp-Te)2}$ showed a mirrored trend, this variable decreasing during MENTAL STRESS and RESP in comparison to the REST session ($p < 0.05$) (**Table 3**). Eventually, during the RESP session, in all study patients a significant increase of QTe ($p < 0.001$), Te_m/QTe_m ($p < 0.05$) and QTeVN ($p < 0.05$) in comparison to the REST session have been observed (**Table 3**).

TABLE 2 | Arrhythmic characteristic of study subjects during short term ECG monitoring.

	N: 81
Sinus rhythm	59(73)
Permanent atrial fibrillation	22(27)
Premature supraventricular contraction	17(21)
Premature ventricular contraction	50(62)
>1 Premature ventricular contraction/minute	19(23)
<1 Premature ventricular contraction/minute	31(38)
Complex ventricular arrhythmias	15(19)
Ventricular bigeminy or trigeminy	7(9)
Premature ventricular couplets	11(14)
Non-sustained ventricular tachycardia	3(4)
R on T phenomenon	3(4)
Increasing premature ventricular contractions during mental stress	24(30)
Increasing ventricular arrhythmic complexity during mental stress	12(15)

TABLE 3 | Hemodynamic (Fenometer) and short period repolarization variability data obtained on 256 beats in all study subjects.

	Rest N:81	Controlled breathing N:81	Mental challenge N:81	*P ANOVA*
Variables				
Heart rate, b/m	69 ± 11**	69 ± 11**	72 ± 12	<0.001
Systolic blood pressure, mm Hg	119 ± 23	118 ± 24	116 ± 41	Ns
Diastolic blood pressure, mm Hg	62 ± 11	61 ± 12	62 ± 20	Ns
Stroke volume, ml	39 ± 13**	39 ± 14**	35 ± 18	<0.001
Cardiac output, l/m	2.72 ± 0.94	2.71 ± 0.98*	2.48 ± 1.20	0.032
Peripheral resistance, a.u.	3853 ± 2316	3925 ± 2431	4425 ± 3342	Ns
QTe mean, ms	408 ± 53	412 ± 53	407 ± 50	ns
QTe standard deviation, ms	7 ± 2§§*	8 ± 2*	11 ± 2	<0.001
QTp mean, ms	328 ± 45	326 ± 48	322 ± 45	Ns
QTp standard deviation, ms	7 ± 2*	7 ± 2*	9 ± 5	0.002
Te mean, ms	80 ± 24§*	86 ± 24	85 ± 24	0.026
Te standard deviation, ms	10 ± 2*	10 ± 2*	13 ± 9	<0.001
Te mean/QTe mean	0.22 ± 0.06§*	0.24 ± 0.06	0.24 ± 0.06	0.005
QTeVN	0.28[0.21]§§**	0.33[0.33]**	0.46[0.29]	<0.001
QTpVN	0.56[0.49]**	0.58[0.51]**	0.97[2.00]	<0.001
TeVI	14[21.33]**	14[15]*	21[20]	<0.001
$Coherence_{(QTp-Te)}^2$	0.600 ± 0.139§*	0.555 ± 0.122	0.552 ± 0.115	0.002
QTe_{STV}	14 ± 4§§**	15 ± 4*	19 ± 13	<0.001
QTp_{STV}	14 ± 5*	15 ± 6*	16 ± 6	0.023
Te_{STV}	20 ± 6*	21 ± 8	25 ± 13	0.010

*Values are expressed as mean ± SD or median [interquartile range 75th percentile – 25th percentile]. **p < 0.001 REST or RESP vs. MENTAL STRESS; *p < 0.05 REST or RESP vs. MENTAL STRESS; §§p < 0.001 REST vs. RESP; §p < 0.05 REST vs. RESP.*

During MENTAL STRESS, the repolarization data manually obtained were almost steady (**Table 4**) when corrected for the heart rate (Bazett). Only the Te_{Bazett} value decreased significantly during the MENTAL STRESS with respect the REST and RESP sessions ($p < 0.001$).

RR Spectra Analysis Data

RR and SBP power and cross spectral analysis were obtained in only 59 patients on sinus rhythm. LF, expressed in absolute and normalized power, and LF/HF were significantly higher during MENTAL STRESS (ln LF_{RR}: 4.44 ± 1.35 ms^2; LF NU: 48 ± 17; ln LF/HF; 0.76 ± 1.13) in comparison to REST (ln LF_{RR}: 3.66 ± 1.42, $p < 0.05$; LF_{NU}: 39 ± 20, $p < 0.05$; ln LF/HF; 0.22 ± 1.1.52, $p < 0.05$) and RESP (ln LF_{RR}: 3.63 ± 1.46, $p < 0.001$; LF_{NU}: 34 ± 22, $p < 0.001$; ln LF/HF: -0.14 ± 1.17, $p < 0.001$).

HF_{NU} was significantly lower in REST (HF_{NU}: 35 ± 25, $p < 0.05$) and RESP (HF_{NU}: 39 ± 22, $p < 0.001$) than during MENTAL STRESS (HF_{NU}: 26 ± 18).

TABLE 4 | Manual repolarization data obtained on 3 QRS-T cycles.

	Rest N:81	Controlled breathing N:81	Mental challenge N:81	*P ANOVA*
Variables				
RR, ms	881 ± 150*	873 ± 134*	853 ± 133	0.017
QT, ms	425 ± 54*	424 ± 53*	414 ± 49	0.003
QRS, ms	91 ± 23	91 ± 24	93 ± 40	Ns
JT, ms	334 ± 55*	333 ± 54*	321 ± 64	0.006
Te, ms	92 ± 25*	88 ± 20	86 ± 20	0.034
QT_{Bazett}, ms	455 ± 48	455 ± 51	450 ± 41	Ns
QRS_{Bazett}, ms	98 ± 28	99 ± 29	102 ± 47	Ns
JT_{Bazett}, ms	357 ± 49	356 ± 50	348 ± 61	Ns
Te_{Bazett}, ms	98 ± 28**	95 ± 21*	94 ± 23	<0.001
Te/QTe,	0.21 ± 0.5	0.21 ± 0.5	0.21 ± 0.5	Ns
Te_{Bazett}/QTe_{Bazett}	0.21 ± 0.5	0.21 ± 0.4	0.21 ± 0.4	Ns

*Values are expressed as mean ± SD or median [interquartile range 75th percentile – 25th percentile]. **p < 0.001 REST or RESP vs. MENTAL STRESS; *p < 0.05 REST or RESP vs. MENTAL STRESS.*

Both the α indexes, marker of baroreflex sensitivity, were lower during MENTAL STRESS (α LF: 0.80 ± 0.90; α HF: 0.77 ± 0.91) than REST (α LF: 1.32 ± 0.96, $p < 0.001$; α HF: 1.41 ± 0.96, $p < 0.001$) and RESP (α LF: 1.42 ± 0.79, $p < 0.001$; α HF: 1.44 ± 0.95, $p < 0.001$).

No statistically significant difference have been found between RR variability data obtained at REST and RESP.

Category With PCVs' Increase During the MENTAL STRESS Session

At REST, the 24 patients with an increase of PVC during MENTAL STRESS showed the following repolarization markers significantly higher than other 57 patients: QTe_{SD} (8 ± 2 vs. 7 ± 2 ms^2, $p < 0.05$), QTeVN (0.37[0.22] vs. 0.25 [0.20], $p < 0.05$), QTe_{STV} (15 ± 3 vs. 13 ± 5, $p < 0.05$) (**Figures 3A,C,E**), QRS (102 ± 27 vs. 87 ± 20 ms, $p < 0.05$), QRS_{Bazett} (111 ± 32 vs. 93 ± 25 ms, $p < 0.05$). No other significant differences were observed between these two study groups.

Category With Complex Ventricular Arrhythmias' Increase During the MENTAL STRESS Session

At REST, the 12 patients with an increased complexity of ventricular arrhythmias during MENTAL STRESS showed the following markers significantly higher than other 69 patients: QTe_{sd} (9 ± 2 vs. 7 ± 2 ms^2, $p < 0.001$), Te_m SD (12 ± 3 vs. 10 ± 2 ms^2, $p < 0.05$), QTeVN (0.43[0.49] vs. 0.25 [0.20], $p < 0.001$), QTpVN (0.52[0.56] vs. 0.41 [0.31], $p < 0.05$) and QTe_{STV} (17 ± 5 vs. 13 ± 4, $p < 0.05$) (**Figures 3B,D,F**). Instead $Coherence_{(QTp-Te)2}$ was lower in the arrhythmic patients' group in comparison with the counterpart (0.524 ± 0.119 vs. 0.613, $p < 0.05$). Eventually, excepted the Te/QTe (0.242 ± 0.049 vs. 0.210 ± 0.046 ms, $p < 0.05$) and Te_{Bazett}/QTe_{Bazett} (0.241 ± 0.051 vs. 0.210 ± 0.046, $p < 0.05$), most of the manual repolarization indexes were not significantly different between the study groups.

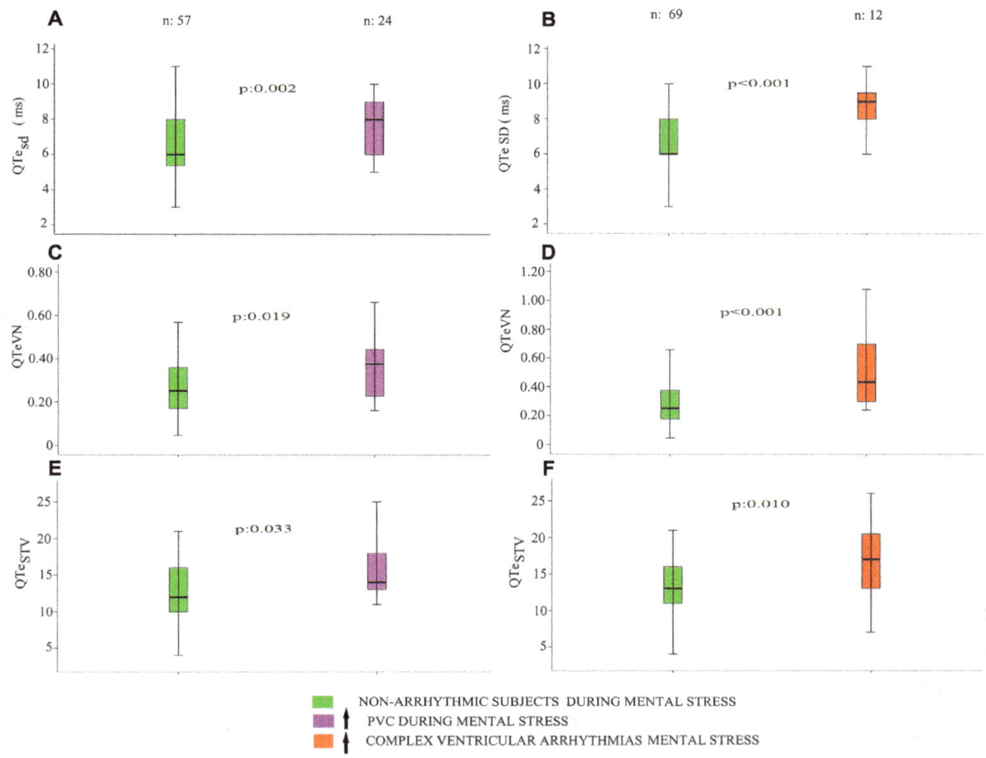

FIGURE 3 | QTe standard deviation QTe_{sd}, QTeVN and QTe_{STV}, obtained at rest, in subjects with an increase of PVC (purple) and complex ventricular arrhythmias (red) during mental stress. At REST, the 24 patients with an increase of PVC during MENTAL STRESS showed the following repolarization markers significantly higher than other 57 patients: QTe_{SD} ($p < 0.05$), QTeVN ($p < 0.05$), QTe_{STV} ($p < 0.05$) (panel **A**, **C**, and **E**). At REST, the 12 patients with an increased complexity of ventricular arrhythmias during MENTAL STRESS showed the following markers significantly higher than other 69 patients: QTe_{sd} ($p < 0.001$), Te_m SD ($p < 0.05$), QTeVN ($p < 0.001$), QTpVN ($p < 0.05$) and QTe_{STV} ($p < 0.05$) (panel **B**, **D**, and **F**).

Relationship Between Ventricular Arrhythmic Risk and Clinical, Hemodynamic and Repolarization Data

Uni- and multivariable logistic regression analysis reported only statistically significant associations between increase of PVC or complex ventricular arrhythmias during MENTAL STRESS and repolarization data at REST (**Table 5**). None of clinical, echocardiographic, non-invasive hemodynamic spectral data showed a significant relationship with the ventricular arrhythmic risk during the MENTAL STRESS session.

The univariable logistic analysis identified the following repolarization variables obtained at REST and the risk factors of PVC increase: QTe_{sd} ($p < 0.05$), QTe_{STV} ($p < 0.05$), QRS ($p < 0.05$), QRS_{Bazett} ($p < 0.05$) (**Table 5**). On the contrary, the same statistical approach detected the following repolarization variables obtained at REST as predictors of complex ventricular arrhythmias during MENTAL STRESS: QTe_{sd} ($p < 0.05$); Te SD ($p < 0.05$); $Coherence_{(QTp-Te)2}$ ($p < 0.05$); QTe_{STV} ($p < 0.05$); Te/QTe; Te_{Bazett}/QTe_{Bazett} (**Table 5**).

Multivariable logistic analysis identified only the QTe_{SD} as risk factor of the increase of PVC (odd ratio: 1.54, 95% CI 1.14–2.08; $p = 0.005$) and complex ventricular arrhythmias (odd ratio: 2.31, 95% CI 1.40–3.83; $p = 0.001$).

Short Period Analysis Versus Manual Measurements: Comparative Study in the Ventricular Arrhythmic Risk Prediction

Although several short period and manual repolarization markers reached a sufficient statistical significance only QTe_{sd} showed the widest sensitivity-specificity area under curve (AUC) for predicting both the increase of PVC (AUC: 0.699, 95% CI: 0.576–0.822, $p < 0.05$) and complex ventricular arrhythmias (AUC: 0.801, 95% CI: 0.648–0.954, $p < 0.05$) during the MENTAL STRESS session (**Figure 4**). Particularly, the other markers with significant area under the curve were: QTeVN (AUC: 0.685, 95% CI 0.565–0.805, $p < 0.05$); QRS (AUC: 0.682, 95% CI 0.556–0.809, $p < 0.05$); QRS_{Bazett} (AUC: 0.673, 95% CI 0.545–0.800, $p < 0.05$); and QTe_{STV} (AUC: 0.664, 95% CI 0.545–0.780, $p < 0.05$) for an increase of PVC during the MENTAL STRESS session (**Figure 4A**). On the contrary, the other variable with statistically significant area under the curve were: QTeVN (AUC: 0.781, 95% CI 0.655–0.908, $p < 0.05$); QTpVN (AUC: 0.694, 95% CI 0.530–0.859, $p < 0.05$),; Te/QTe (AUC: 0.692, 95% CI 0.525–0.859, $p < 0.05$), QTe_{STV} (AUC: 0.688, 95% CI 0.501–0.875, $p < 0.05$), and $Coherence_{(QTp-Te)2}$ (AUC: 0.303, 95% CI 0.154–0.451, $p < 0.05$) (**Figure 4B**).

TABLE 5 | Univariable logistic regression analysis data.

	↑ PVC during mental stress Odds ratio (95% CI) *P*-value	↑ Complex ventricular arrhythmias during mental stress Odds ratio (95% CI) *P*-value
QTe standard deviation, ms	1.540(1.114–2.080) $p = 0.005$	2.153(1.338–3.465) $p = 0.002$
Te standard deviation, ms	p = ns	1.353(1.061–1.726) $p = 0.015$
$\text{Coherence}_{(QTp-Te)}{}^2$	p = ns	0.009(0–0.930) $p = 0.047$
QTe_{STV}	1.131(1.007–1.270) $p = 0.038$	1.207(1.036–1.405) $p = 0.016$
QRS	1.030(1.007–1.053) $p = 0.010$	p = ns
QRS_{Bazett}	1.022(1.004–1.041) $p = 0.016$	p = ns
Te/QTe	p = ns	1.143(1.007–1.297) $p = 0.039$
Te_{Bazett}/QTe_{Bazett}	p = ns	1.136(1.002–1.289) $p = 0.047$

Effects of Possible Confounders (β-Blocker Therapy, Atrial Fibrillation)

A concomitant therapy with β-blocker was present in 43 patients (53%) but this group did not any differences with respect the increase PVC or complex ventricular arrhythmias. The others repolarization markers, as well as clinical and hemodynamic data, did not even change in relation to the β-blocker therapy.

Multivariable logistic analysis confirmed QTe_{sd} as predictive of the complex ventricular arrhythmias' increase also considering sinus rhythm patients alone (odd ratio: 3.17, 95% CI 1.37–7.35; $p = 0.007$), thus excluding from those with atrial fibrillation (odd ratio: 2.92, 95% CI 1.23–6.93; $p = 0.015$). On the contrary, excluding the patients on atrial fibrillation, the same statistical analysis confirmed QTe_{sd} (odd ratio: 1.84, 95% CI 1.59–2.92; $p = 0.01$) predicative only for an increase of PVC during the MENTAL STRESS session.

DISCUSSION

The main finding of the present study was that a non-negligible percentage of elderly patients with degenerative AS group increased the PVC and complex ventricular arrhythmias during a mild mental stress, such as the one represented by a simple MMSE and, notably, it happens regardless a concomitant beta-blockers therapy. The MMSE is usually needed to assess possible cognitive impairment in elderly candidates to a TAVR procedure (Lindman et al., 2014; Otto et al., 2017). It is highly conceivable that this simple standard test might lead, through a mental arithmetical exercise and several other cognitive tests (orientation, registration recall, language, repetition and complex tasks) (Folstein et al., 1975), to an increase of ventricular arrhythmias due to an increase of sympathetic activity and a reduced vagal tone. Supporting the abovementioned hypothesis, we found a significant increase in the explored sympathetic markers at RR power spectral analysis (ln LF_{RR}; LF NU; ln LF/HF) (Task Force of the European Society of Cardiology, and the North American Society of Pacing, and Electrophysiology, 1996; Piccirillo et al., 2009b, 2016) as well a significant reduction in two well-known vagal markers (ln HF_{RR} and ln α HF) (Robbe et al., 1987; Pagani et al., 1988; Piccirillo et al., 2000a,b, 2004b, 2013, 2016).

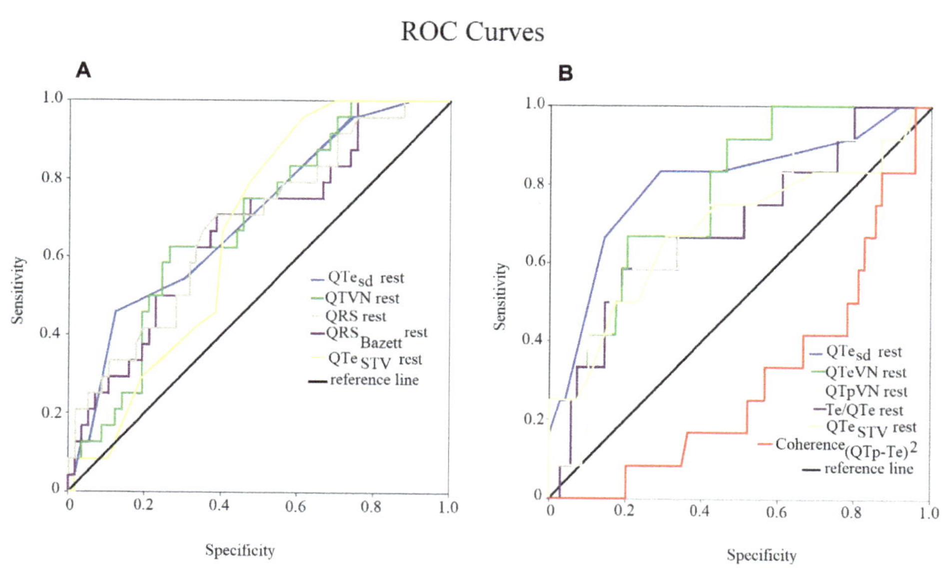

FIGURE 4 | ROC curve of statistical significant examined variables. Sensitivity-specificity of different variables, obtained at rest, to individuate patients with increase of PVC **(A)** and complex ventricular arrhythmias **(B)** during mental stress. QTe standard deviation (QTe_{sd}) had the widest area under the curve in both the diagrams (blue lines).

Another, possibly clinical relevant, finding of the present study was that a simple non-invasive short period myocardial repolarization index, such as the QTe_{sd} obtained at rest, seems to be able to identify those patients with the highest probability to increase ventricular arrhythmias (PVC or complex ventricular arrhythmias) during the MMSE administration. Thus, albeit highly speculative, the QTe_{sd} obtained at rest could be potentially useful in disclosing a general arrhythmias propensity and, accordingly, an increased risk of sudden cardiac death in elderly patients with AS candidate to a TAVR procedure (Massing et al., 2006; Cheriyath et al., 2011; Ataklte et al., 2013; Agarwal et al., 2015; Zanobetti et al., 2017). This clinical feature could frustrate the TAVR's outcomes and, accordingly, should be worthy to be weighted during the screening procedures. Indeed, although the TAVR improves undoubtedly the hemodynamic patient's conditions, the myocardial arrhythmic substrate of AS (hypertrophy, disarray, calcifications, ischemia, fibrosis, necrosis, etc.) remains theoretically and practically still able to induce malignant reentrant ventricular arrhythmias also after the AS resolution. In such a context, we also compared the predicative power of conventional QTe and Te measurements with novel short period repolarization variability markers and we found that the QTe_{sd} demonstrated the best accuracy in disclosing those patients more susceptible to increase ventricular arrhythmias during MMSE. Thus, an easy-to-obtain surface ECG-derived parameter, that is the QTe_{sd} obtained at rest, might be considered in guiding at least a more aggressive treatment in these specific category (i.e., high dosage of β-blockers or amiodarone therapy).

Mental Stress and Sudden Cardiac Death

Emotions are able to trigger malignant ventricular arrhythmias and sudden cardiac death in subjects with known or unknown heart disease and this aspect is particularly relevant in elderly patients. In such a context, retrospective studies highlighted an increase of sudden cardiac death during natural or unnatural thrilling events such as earthquakes (Trichopoulos et al., 1981; Leor et al., 1996; Kario et al., 1997; Kitamura et al., 2013; Kiyohara et al., 2015) bombings (Meisel et al., 1991), terrorist attack (Steinberg et al., 2004) and also football matches (Wilbert-Lampen et al., 2008) or other positive (Phillips et al., 2004) or negative emotional events (Cannon, 2002; Lampert et al., 2002; Williams et al., 2011).

Although no specific data on elderly patients with AS are present in literature, it is easily supposable from a pathophysiologic viewpoint that the simultaneous joint of degenerative valve disease with chronic heart failure and mental stress can exacerbated a tendency for life-threatening arrhythmias. The myocardial hypertrophy and reentrant circuits provide the substratum and electrophysiologic mechanism; the resulting simpato-vagal imbalance, induced by the chronic heart failure, constitutes the "milieu ideal"; and, finally, the sudden sympathetic stimulus, emotion mediated, can easily trigger a fatal arrhythmias. Noteworthy two patients of our study reported ventricular couplets during mental stress without preexistent PVC at rest and one of them reported a R on T phenomenon. Thus it might be hypothesized that the MMSE alone was able to induce a sympathetic overstimulation leading a complex ventricular arrhythmias. Therefore, in these two elderly patients an episode of malignant ventricular arrhythmias could be triggered "like a bolt from the blue" during a high emotional level event. This clinical feature might be clinically relevant in defining the therapeutic strategy: i.e., the elderly patient with AS candidate to a TAVR procedure who shows ventricular complex arrhythmias just during mental stress without any PVC at rest should be aggressively beta-blocked or should receive amiodarone. Clearly, in light of our present data, we strongly recommend the ECG monitoring during MMSE in such patient's category.

Sympatho-Vagal Imbalance, Abnormal Repolarization and Ventricular Malignant Arrhythmias

Myocardial repolarization phase is abnormal in patients with myocardial hypertrophy and it might be non-invasively evaluated by analyzing the QT interval prolongation and its dispersion. The molecular basis of these ECG features are complex (Abriel et al., 2015; Rahm et al., 2018). Briefly, in chronic heart failure the potassium channels (I_{to}, I_{Ks}, I_{Kr} and I_{K1}) are downregulated, sodium channel (I_{Na}) shows a delayed inactivation, finally, calcium handling is deeply altered. Then, chronic heart failure is able to induce a prolonged and inhomogeneous action potential duration both in the time and spatial domain, detectable on ECG as a prolonged and temporal dispersed QT interval. This condition constitutes an optimum "pabulum" for reentry arrhythmias. Several experimental and clinical studies, mostly by our research group reported that the sympathetic stimulation was able to exacerbate the QT temporal dispersion in different clinical setting all characterized by myocardial structural abnormalities (Piccirillo et al., 2009a, 2012, 2013, 2014a; Baumert et al., 2016). However, up to now, specific data in elderly patients with AS were not present. Originally we now supplied data with respect a worsening of all markers of myocardial temporal dispersion of repolarization phases during a mild mental stress. In sush a context, between several conventional manually measurements of myocardial repolarization, only Te and Te_{Bazett} were increased during mental stress. Obviously, the temporal dispersion markers were more sensitive to detect the sympathetic-dependent changes, probably because they were obtained on a longer period (256 cycles) in comparison with the manual measurement (3 cycles). These two ECG parameters followed the trend of all short period markers of QT most likely because the Te interval represents the QT interval subsegment more susceptible to the sympathetic variations (Shimizu and Antzelevitch, 2000; Shimizu et al., 2003; Piccirillo et al., 2012, 2013, 2014a). Indeed, in this last part of repolarization phase, I_{Ks} is capable to modulate the QT duration to RR cycle length and, in chronic heart failure, these channels are downregulated. Thus, a mental stress could be sufficient to trigger this alteration also with conventional QT measurement (Aro et al., 2017; Tse et al., 2017; Piccirillo et al., 2018; Yu et al., 2018).

Autonomic cardiovascular regulation is deeply involved in the pathophysiology of the AS, too. The sympathetic drive's increase and the vagal control alterations are typical of all different stages of this syndrome, together with the baroreflex sensitivity depression. Therefore, RR power spectral analysis shows different spectral pattern according the class impairment and the related therapy. In the first two NYHA classes, the LF spectral component tend to increase (Guzzetti et al., 1995; Yaniv et al., 2014) whereas the most advanced stages are usually associated to a reduction of LF spectral power (Mortara et al., 1994; Guzzetti et al., 1995; Piccirillo et al., 2006, 2009b; Yaniv et al., 2014). The latter changes are also usually observed as quite physiological aging-related changes (Piccirillo et al., 1995, 1998) our sample with symptomatic AS showed a low short period heart rate variability and, consequently LF, in normalize and absolute power, but the patients were still able to increase LF during mental stress; probably this ability could be impaired in comparison with normal age-matched subjects (Piccirillo et al., 1995, 1998). Therefore, the β-blocker treatment can modify all spectral components and LF in particular (Piccirillo et al., 2000a). Nevertheless, chronic heart failure and aging are capable to reduce contextually the HF spectral component (Pagani et al., 1986; Piccirillo et al., 2004a). Eventually, during mental stress, our patients showed a decrease of baroreflex sensitivity indexes (α-index), this behavior mirroring a sympathetic activation and parasympathetic deactivation (Piccirillo et al., 2001a,b; Pinna et al., 2015).

Temporal Repolarization Variability as Markers of Sudden Cardiac Death

Probably the most dreadful AS complication is sudden cardiac death induced by reentrant ventricular arrhythmias.

CONCLUSION

In elderly with AS, ventricular arrhythmias worsened during a simple cognitive assessment, this events could be a further burden on the outcome of TAVR. Although, the TAVR reduces the morbidity and mortality, in some subjects sudden death's risk remains high. Therefore, it could come in handy to stratify the ventricular malignant arrhythmias risk using a non-invasive, not expensive, repeatable and simple test. In such a context, our data enlightened that QTe_{sd}, obtained at rest on 256 consecutive cycles, shows the best accuracy in identifying those patients with AS more prone to develop ventricular arrhythmias. Obviously, in the present study we evaluated the predictive repolarization markers in stratifying the increase of number and complexity of ventricular arrhythmias as a surrogate of major arrhythmic risk (i.e., sudden cardiac death). Then we could reasonably hypothesize that these two markers of electrical ventricular instability could represent the first point of reference waiting more specific data. However, it is reasonable to suggest a more aggressive antiarrhythmic therapy in those patients with AS candidates to TAVR procedures and high QTe_{sd} value at rest.

AUTHOR CONTRIBUTIONS

GP: conceptualization, data curation, formal analysis, and writing. FeM: writing - review and editing. MF, CDI, FaM, TS, DC, MM, NS, and GV: investigation, methodology, and data curation. IP: data curation. DM: supervision, validation, visualization, review, and editing.

REFERENCES

Abriel, H., Rougier, J. S., and Jalife, J. (2015). Ion channel macromolecular complexes in cardiomyocytes: roles in sudden cardiac death. *Circ. Res.* 116, 1971–1988. doi: 10.1161/CIRCRESAHA.116.305017

Afilalo, J., Lauck, S., Kim, D. H., Lefèvre, T., Piazza, N., Lachapelle, K., et al. (2017). Frailty in older adults undergoing aortic valve replacement: the FRAILTY-AVR study. *J. Am. Coll. Cardiol.* 70, 689–700. doi: 10.1016/j.jacc.2017.06.024

Agarwal, S. K., Chao, J., Peace, F., Judd, S. E., Kissela, B., Kleindorfer, D., et al. (2015). Premature ventricular complexes on screening electrocardiogram and risk of ischemic stroke. *Stroke* 46, 1365–1367. doi: 10.1161/strokeaha.114.008447

Aro, A. L., Reinier, K., Rusinaru, C., Uy-Evanado, A., Darouian, N., Phan, D., et al. (2017). Electrical risk score beyond the left ventricular ejection fraction: prediction of sudden cardiac death in the oregon sudden unexpected death study and the atherosclerosis risk in communities study. *Eur. Heart J.* 38, 3017–3025. doi: 10.1093/eurheartj/ehx331

Ataklte, F., Erqou, S., Laukkanen, J., and Kaptoge, S. (2013). Meta-analysis of ventricular premature complexes and their relation to cardiac mortality in general populations. *Am. J. Cardiol.* 112, 1263–1270. doi: 10.1016/j.amjcard.2013.05.065

Baumert, M., Porta, A., Vos, M. A., Malik, M., Couderc, J. P., Laguna, P., et al. (2016). QT interval variability in body surface ECG: measurement, physiological basis, and clinical value: position statement and consensus guidance endorsed by the European Heart Rhythm Association jointly with the ESC working group on cardiac cellular electrophysiology. *Europace* 18, 925–944. doi: 10.1093/europace/euv405

Berger, R. D., Kasper, E. K., Baughman, K. L., Marban, E., Calkins, H., and Tomaselli, G. F. (1997). Beat-to-beat QT interval variability: novel evidence for repolarization lability in ischemic and nonischemic dilated cardiomyopathy. *Circulation* 96, 1557–1565. doi: 10.1161/01.cir.96.5.1557

Cannon, W. B. (2002). "Voodoo" death. American anthropologist, 1942;44(new series):169-181. *Am. J. Public Health* 92, 1593–1596; discussion 1594–1595.

Cheriyath, P., He, F., Peters, I., Li, X., Alagona, P. Jr., Wu, C., et al. (2011). Relation of atrial and/or ventricular premature complexes on a two-minute rhythm strip to the risk of sudden cardiac death (the Atherosclerosis Risk in Communities [ARIC] study). *Am. J. Cardiol.* 107, 151–155. doi: 10.1016/j.amjcard.2010.09.002

Crow, R. S., Hannan, P. J., and Folsom, A. R. (2003). Prognostic significance of corrected QT and corrected JT interval for incident coronary heart disease in a general population sample stratified by presence or absence of wide QRS complex: the ARIC Study with 13 years of follow-up. *Circulation* 108, 1985–1989. doi: 10.1161/01.cir.0000095027.28753.9d

Folstein, M. F., Folstein, S. E., and McHugh, P. R. (1975). "Mini-mental state". A practical method for grading the cognitive state of patients for the clinician. *Psychiatr. Res.* 12, 189–198.

Guzzetti, S., Cogliati, C., Turiel, M., Crema, C., Lombardi, F., and Malliani, A. (1995). Sympathetic predominance followed by functional denervation in the progression of chronic heart failure. *Eur. Heart J.* 16, 1100–1107. doi: 10.1093/oxfordjournals.eurheartj.a061053

Kario, K., Matsuo, T., Kobayashi, H., Yamamoto, K., and Shimada, K. (1997). Earthquake-induced potentiation of acute risk factors in hypertensive elderly patients: possible triggering of cardiovascular events after a major earthquake. *J. Am. Coll. Cardiol.* 29, 926–933. doi: 10.1016/s0735-1097(97)00002-8

Kitamura, T., Kiyohara, K., and Iwami, T. (2013). The great east Japan earthquake and out-of-hospital cardiac arrest. *N. Engl. J. Med.* 369, 2165–2167.

Kiyohara, K., Kitamura, T., Iwami, T., Nishiyama, C., and Kawamura, T. (2015). Impact of the Great East Japan earthquake on out-of-hospital cardiac arrest with cardiac origin in non-disaster areas [corrected]. *J. Epidemiol. Commun. Health* 69, 185–188. doi: 10.1136/jech-2014-204380

Lampert, R., Joska, T., Burg, M. M., Batsford, W. P., McPherson, C. A., and Jain, D. (2002). Emotional and physical precipitants of ventricular arrhythmia. *Circulation* 106, 1800–1805. doi: 10.1161/01.cir.0000031733.51374.c1

Leor, J., Poole, W. K., and Kloner, R. A. (1996). Sudden cardiac death triggered by an earthquake. *N. Engl. J. Med.* 334, 413–419. doi: 10.1056/nejm199602153340701

Lindman, B. R., Alexander, K. P., O'Gara, P. T., and Afilalo, J. (2014). Futility, benefit, and transcatheter aortic valve replacement. *JACC Cardiovasc. Interv.* 7, 707–716. doi: 10.1016/j.jcin.2014.01.167

Massing, M. W., Simpson, R. J. Jr., Rautaharju, P. M., Schreiner, P. J., Crow, R., and Heiss, G. (2006). Usefulness of ventricular premature complexes to predict coronary heart disease events and mortality (from the atherosclerosis risk in communities cohort). *Am. J. Cardiol.* 98, 1609–1612. doi: 10.1016/j.amjcard.2006.06.061

Meisel, S. R., Kutz, I., Dayan, K. I., Pauzner, H., Chetboun, I., Arbel, Y., et al. (1991). Effect of Iraqi missile war on incidence of acute myocardial infarction and sudden death in Israeli civilians. *Lancet* 338, 660–661. doi: 10.1016/0140-6736(91)91234-l

Minamino-Muta, E., Kato, T., Morimoto, T., Taniguchi, T., Shiomi, H., Nakatsuma, K., et al. (2017). Causes of death in patients with severe aortic stenosis: an observational study. *Sci. Rep.* 7:14723. doi: 10.1038/s41598-017-15316-6

Mortara, A., La Rovere, M. T., Signorini, M. G., Pantaleo, P., Pinna, G., Martinelli, L., et al. (1994). Can power spectral analysis of heart rate variability identify a high risk subgroup of congestive heart failure patients with excessive sympathetic activation? A pilot study before and after heart transplantation. *Br. Heart J.* 71, 422–430. doi: 10.1136/hrt.71.5.422

Osnabrugge, R. L., Mylotte, D., Head, S. J., Van Mieghem, N. M., Nkomo, V. T., LeReun, C. M., et al. (2013). Aortic stenosis in the elderly: disease prevalence and number of candidates for transcatheter aortic valve replacement: a meta-analysis and modeling study. *J. Am. Coll. Cardiol.* 62, 1002–1012. doi: 10.1016/j.jacc.2013.05.015

Otto, C. M., Kumbhani, D. J., Alexander, K. P., Calhoon, J. H., Desai, M. Y., Kaul, S., et al. (2017). ACC expert consensus decision pathway for transcatheter aortic valve replacement in the management of adults with aortic stenosis: a report of the american college of cardiology task force on clinical expert consensus documents. *J. Am. Coll. Cardiol.* 69, 1313–1346. doi: 10.1016/j.jacc.2016.12.006

Pagani, M., Lombardi, F., Guzzetti, S., Rimoldi, O., Furlan, R., Pizzinelli, P., et al. (1986). Power spectral analysis of heart rate and arterial pressure variabilities as a marker of sympatho-vagal interaction in man and conscious dog. *Circ. Res.* 59, 178–193. doi: 10.1161/01.res.59.2.178

Pagani, M., Somers, V., Furlan, R., Dell'Orto, S., Conway, J., Baselli, G., et al. (1988). Changes in autonomic regulation induced by physical training in mild hypertension. *Hypertension* 12, 600–610. doi: 10.1161/01.hyp.12.6.600

Phillips, D. P., Jarvinen, J. R., Abramson, I. S., and Phillips, R. R. (2004). Cardiac mortality is higher around Christmas and New Year's than at any other time: the holidays as a risk factor for death. *Circulation* 110, 3781–3788. doi: 10.1161/01.cir.0000151424.02045.f7

Piccirillo, G., Bucca, C., Bauco, C., Cinti, A. M., Michele, D., Fimognari, F. L., et al. (1998). Power spectral analysis of heart rate in subjects over a hundred years old. *Int. J. Cardiol.* 63, 53–61. doi: 10.1016/s0167-5273(97)00282-9

Piccirillo, G., Cacciafesta, M., Viola, E., Santagada, E., Nocco, M., Lionetti, M., et al. (2001a). Influence of aging on cardiac baroreflex sensitivity determined non-invasively by power spectral analysis. *Clin. Sci.* 100, 267–274. doi: 10.1042/cs1000267

Piccirillo, G., Di Giuseppe, V., Nocco, M., Lionetti, M., Moisè, A., Naso, C., et al. (2001b). Influence of aging and other cardiovascular risk factors on baroreflex sensitivity. *J. Am. Geriatr. Soc.* 49, 1059–1065. doi: 10.1046/j.1532-5415.2001.49209.x

Piccirillo, G., Fimognari, F. L., Viola, E., and Marigliano, V. (1995). Age-adjusted normal confidence intervals for heart rate variability in healthy subjects during head-up tilt. *Int. J. Cardiol.* 50, 117–124. doi: 10.1016/0167-5273(95)93680-q

Piccirillo, G., Luparini, R. L., Celli, V., Moisè, A., Lionetti, M., Marigliano, V., et al. (2000a). Effects of carvedilol on heart rate and blood pressure variability in subjects with chronic heart failure. *Am. J. Cardiol.* 86, 1392–1395, A6.

Piccirillo, G., Viola, E., Nocco, M., Durante, M., Tarantini, S., and Marigliano, V. (2000b). Autonomic modulation of heart rate and blood pressure in normotensive offspring of hypertensive subjects. *J. Lab. Clin. Med.* 135, 145–152. doi: 10.1067/mlc.2000.103428

Piccirillo, G., Magrì, D., di Carlo, S., De Laurentis, T., Torrini, A., Matera, S., et al. (2006). Influence of cardiac-resynchronization therapy on heart rate and blood pressure variability: 1-year follow-up. *Eur. J. Heart Fail.* 8, 716–722. doi: 10.1016/j.ejheart.2006.01.008

Piccirillo, G., Magrì, D., Naso, C., di Carlo, S., MoisE, A., De Laurentis, T., et al. (2004a). Factors influencing heart rate variability power spectral analysis during controlled breathing in patients with chronic heart failure or hypertension and in healthy normotensive subjects. *Clin. Sci.* 107, 183–190. doi: 10.1042/cs20030401

Piccirillo, G., Naso, C., Moisè, A., Lionetti, M., Nocco, M., Di Carlo, S., et al. (2004b). Heart rate and blood pressure variability in subjects with vasovagal syncope. *Clin. Sci.* 107, 55–61. doi: 10.1042/cs20030327

Piccirillo, G., Magrì, D., Ogawa, M., Song, J., Chong, V. J., Han, S., et al. (2009a). Autonomic nervous system activity measured directly and QT interval variability in normal and pacing-induced tachycardia heart failure dogs. *J. Am. Coll. Cardiol.* 54, 840–850. doi: 10.1016/j.jacc.2009.06.008

Piccirillo, G., Ogawa, M., Song, J., Chong, V. J., Joung, B., Han, S., et al. (2009b). Power spectral analysis of heart rate variability and autonomic nervous system activity measured directly in healthy dogs and dogs with tachycardia-induced heart failure. *Heart Rhythm.* 6, 546–552. doi: 10.1016/j.hrthm.2009.01.006

Piccirillo, G., Magrì, D., Pappadà, M. A., Maruotti, A., Ogawa, M., Han, S., et al. (2012). Autonomic nerve activity and the short-term variability of the Tpeak-Tend interval in dogs with pacing-induced heart failure. *Heart Rhythm.* 9, 2044–2050. doi: 10.1016/j.hrthm.2012.08.030

Piccirillo, G., Moscucci, F., D'Alessandro, G., Pascucci, M., Rossi, P., Han, S., et al. (2014a). Myocardial repolarization dispersion and autonomic nerve activity in a canine experimental acute myocardial infarction model. *Heart Rhythm.* 11, 110–118. doi: 10.1016/j.hrthm.2013.10.022

Piccirillo, G., Moscucci, F., Persi, A., Di Barba, D., Pappadà, M. A., Rossi, P., et al. (2014b). Intra-QT spectral coherence as a possible noninvasive marker of sustained ventricular tachycardia. *Biomed. Res. Int.* 2014:583035. doi: 10.1155/2014/583035

Piccirillo, G., Moscucci, F., Mastropietri, F., Di Iorio, C., Mariani, M. V., Fabietti, M., et al. (2018). Possible predictive role of electrical risk score on transcatheter aortic valve replacement outcomes in older patients: preliminary data. *Clin. Interv. Aging* 13, 1657–1667. doi: 10.2147/CIA.S170226

Piccirillo, G., Ottaviani, C., Fiorucci, C., Petrocchi, N., Moscucci, F., Di Iorio, C., et al. (2016). Transcranial direct current stimulation improves the QT variability index and autonomic cardiac control in healthy subjects older than 60 years. *Clin. Interv. Aging* 11, 1687–1695. doi: 10.2147/cia.s116194

Piccirillo, G., Rossi, P., Mitra, M., Quaglione, R., Dell'Armi, A., Di Barba, D., et al. (2013). Indexes of temporal myocardial repolarization dispersion and sudden cardiac death in heart failure: any difference? *Ann. Noninvasive Electrocardiol.* 18, 130–139. doi: 10.1111/anec.12005

Pinna, G. D., Maestri, R., and La Rovere, M. T. (2015). Assessment of baroreflex sensitivity from spontaneous oscillations of blood pressure and heart rate: proven clinical value? *Physiol. Meas.* 36, 741–753. doi: 10.1088/0967-3334/36/4/741

Rahm, A. K., Lugenbiel, P., Schweizer, P. A., Katus, H. A., and Thomas, D. (2018). Role of ion channels in heart failure and channelopathies. *Biophys. Rev.* 10, 1097–1106. doi: 10.1007/s12551-018-0442-3

Rautaharju, P. M., Surawicz, B., Gettes, L. S., Bailey, J. J., Childers, R., Deal, B. J., et al. (2009). AHA/ACCF/HRS recommendations for the standardization and interpretation of the electrocardiogram: part IV: the ST segment, T and U waves, and the QT interval: a scientific statement from the American Heart Association Electrocardiography and Arrhythmias Committee, Council on Clinical Cardiology; the American College of Cardiology Foundation; and the Heart Rhythm Society. Endorsed by the International Society for Computerized Electrocardiology. *J. Am. Coll. Cardiol.* 53, 982–991. doi: 10.1016/j.jacc.2008.12.014

Rautaharju, P. M., Zhang, Z. M., Prineas, R., and Heiss, G. (2004). Assessment of prolonged QT and JT intervals in ventricular conduction defects. *Am. J. Cardiol.* 93, 1017–1021. doi: 10.1016/j.amjcard.2003.12.055

Robbe, H. W., Mulder, L. J., Rüddel, H., Langewitz, W. A., Veldman, J. B., and Mulder, G. (1987). Assessment of baroreceptor reflex sensitivity by means of spectral analysis. *Hypertension* 10, 538–543. doi: 10.1161/01.hyp.10.5.538

Rockwood, K., Song, X., MacKnight, C., Bergman, H., Hogan, D. B., McDowell, I., et al. (2005). A global clinical measure of fitness and frailty in elderly people. *CMAJ* 173, 489–495. doi: 10.1503/cmaj.050051

Shimizu, W., and Antzelevitch, C. (2000). Differential effects of beta-adrenergic agonists and antagonists in LQT1, LQT2 and LQT3 models of the long QT syndrome. *J. Am. Coll. Cardiol.* 35, 778–786. doi: 10.1016/s0735-1097(99)00582-3

Shimizu, W., Noda, T., Takaki, H., Kurita, T., Nagaya, N., Satomi, K., et al. (2003). Epinephrine unmasks latent mutation carriers with LQT1 form of congenital long-QT syndrome. *J. Am. Coll. Cardiol.* 41, 633–642. doi: 10.1016/s0735-1097(02)02850-4

Steinberg, J. S., Arshad, A., Kowalski, M., Kukar, A., Suma, V., Vloka, M., et al. (2004). Increased incidence of life-threatening ventricular arrhythmias in implantable defibrillator patients after the World Trade Center attack. *J. Am. Coll. Cardiol.* 44, 1261–1264. doi: 10.1016/j.jacc.2004.06.032

Task Force of the European Society of Cardiology, and the North American Society of Pacing, and Electrophysiology (1996). Heart rate variability Standards of measurement, physiological interpretation, and clinical use. *Eur. Heart J.* 17, 354–381. doi: 10.1093/oxfordjournals.eurheartj.a014868

Trichopoulos, D., Katsouyanni, K., Zavitsanos, X., Tzonou, A., and Dalla-Vorgia, P. (1981). Psychological stress and fatal heart attack: the Athens earthquake natural experiment. *Lancet* 1, 441–444. doi: 10.1016/s0140-6736(83)91439-3

Tse, G., Gong, M., Wong, W. T., Georgopoulos, S., Letsas, K. P., Vassiliou, V. S., et al. (2017). The Tpeak - Tend interval as an electrocardiographic risk marker of arrhythmic and mortality outcomes: a systematic review and meta-analysis. *Heart Rhythm.* 14, 1131–1137. doi: 10.1016/j.hrthm.2017.05.031

Wilbert-Lampen, U., Leistner, D., Greven, S., Pohl, T., Sper, S., Völker, C., et al. (2008). Cardiovascular events during World Cup soccer. *N. Engl. J. Med.* 358, 475–483. doi: 10.1056/NEJMoa0707427

Williams, B. R., Zhang, Y., Sawyer, P., Mujib, M., Jones, L. G., Feller, M. A., et al. (2011). Intrinsic association of widowhood with mortality in community-dwelling older women and men: findings from a prospective propensity-matched population study. *J. Gerontol. A Biol. Sci. Med. Sci.* 66, 1360–1368. doi: 10.1093/gerona/glr144

Yaniv, Y., Lyashkov, A. E., and Lakatta, E. G. (2014). Impaired signaling intrinsic to sinoatrial node pacemaker cells affects heart rate variability during cardiac disease. *J. Clin. Trials* 4:152.

Yu, Z., Chen, Z., Wu, Y., Chen, R., Li, M., Chen, X., et al. (2018). Electrocardiographic parameters effectively predict ventricular tachycardia/fibrillation in acute phase and abnormal cardiac function in chronic phase of ST-segment elevation myocardial infarction. *J. Cardiovasc. Electrophysiol.* 29, 756–766. doi: 10.1111/jce.13453

Zanobetti, A., Coull, B. A., Kloog, I., Sparrow, D., Vokonas, P. S., Gold, D. R., et al. (2017). Fine-scale spatial and temporal variation in temperature and arrhythmia episodes in the VA Normative aging study. *J. Air Waste Manag. Assoc.* 67, 96–104. doi: 10.1080/10962247.2016.1252808

5

Visualizing Mutation-Specific Differences in the Trafficking-Deficient Phenotype of Kv11.1 Proteins Linked to Long QT Syndrome Type 2

*Allison R. Hall[1], Corey L. Anderson[2], Jennifer L. Smith[1], Tooraj Mirshahi[3], Claude S. Elayi[4], Craig T. January[2] and Brian P. Delisle[1]**

[1] *Department of Physiology, University of Kentucky, Lexington, KY, United States,* [2] *Cellular and Molecular Arrhythmia Research Program, University of Wisconsin–Madison, Madison, WI, United States,* [3] *Department of Molecular and Functional Genomics, Genomic Medicine Institute, Geisinger Clinic, Danville, PA, United States,* [4] *Department of Cardiology, Gill Heart Institute, University of Kentucky, Lexington, KY, United States*

***Correspondence:**
Brian P. Delisle
brian.delisle@uky.edu

KCNH2 encodes the Kv11.1 α-subunit that underlies the rapidly activating delayed-rectifier K^+ current in the heart. Loss-of-function *KCNH2* mutations cause long QT syndrome type 2 (LQT2), and most LQT2-linked missense mutations inhibit the trafficking of Kv11.1 channel protein to the cell surface membrane. Several trafficking-deficient LQT2 mutations (e.g., G601S) generate Kv11.1 proteins that are sequestered in a microtubule-dependent quality control (QC) compartment in the transitional endoplasmic reticulum (ER). We tested the hypothesis that the QC mechanisms that regulate LQT2-linked Kv11.1 protein trafficking are mutation-specific. Confocal imaging analyses of HEK293 cells stably expressing the trafficking-deficient LQT2 mutation F805C showed that, unlike G601S-Kv11.1 protein, F805C-Kv11.1 protein was concentrated in several transitional ER subcompartments. The microtubule depolymerizing drug nocodazole differentially affected G601S- and F805C-Kv11.1 protein immunostaining. Nocodazole caused G601S-Kv11.1 protein to distribute into peripheral reticular structures, and it increased the diffuse immunostaining of F805C-Kv11.1 protein around the transitional ER subcompartments. Proteasome inhibition also affected the immunostaining of G601S- and F805C-Kv11.1 protein differently. Incubating cells in MG132 minimally impacted G601S-Kv11.1 immunostaining, but it dramatically increased the diffuse immunostaining of F805C-Kv11.1 protein in the transitional ER. Similar results were seen after incubating cells in the proteasome inhibitor lactacystin. Differences in the cellular distribution of G601S-Kv11.1 and F805C-Kv11.1 protein persisted in transfected human inducible pluripotent stem cell derived cardiomyocytes. These are the first data to visually demonstrate mutation-specific differences in the trafficking-deficient LQT2 phenotype, and this study has identified a novel way to categorize trafficking-deficient LQT2 mutations based on differences in intracellular retention.

Keywords: K^+ channel, trafficking, long QT syndrome, arrhythmia, Kv11.1, hERG

INTRODUCTION

Long QT syndrome (LQTS) is a disorder characterized by delayed ventricular repolarization, prolongation of the QT interval on an electrocardiogram (ECG), and an increased risk for the ventricular arrhythmia Torsades de Pointes (Crotti et al., 2008). LQT2 is a major form of LQTS, which is caused by loss-of-function (LOF) mutations in the *KCNH2* gene (a.k.a the *human ether-a-go-go related gene* or *hERG*) (Curran et al., 1995; Sanguinetti et al., 1996; Smith et al., 2016). *KCNH2* encodes the pore-forming Kv11.1 α-subunits that conduct the rapidly activating delayed-rectifier K^+ current (I_{Kr}) in the heart (Trudeau et al., 1995).

The majority of LQT2-linked mutations are missense, and heterologous expression studies demonstrate that ~90% of LQT2 missense mutations decrease the intracellular transport (trafficking) of Kv11.1 channels to the cell surface membrane (Zhou et al., 1998a; Ficker et al., 2000a; Anderson et al., 2006, 2014). Trafficking-deficient LQT2 mutations are postulated to disrupt Kv11.1 α-subunit protein folding/assembly and cellular quality control (QC) mechanisms in endoplasmic reticulum (ER) prevent their trafficking early in the secretory pathway (Zhou et al., 1998a, 1999; Ficker et al., 2003; Delisle et al., 2005; Gong et al., 2005; Walker et al., 2007, 2010; Foo et al., 2016). A key finding is several drugs that bind to Kv11.1 channels and block I_{Kr} (e.g., E-4031) can act as "pharmacological chaperones" to improve the trafficking and functional expression for many LQT2 channels (pharmacological correction) (Zhou et al., 1999; Ficker et al., 2002; Anderson et al., 2006, 2014). This is an important finding because it indicates that some trafficking-deficient LQT2 channels are promising targets for therapeutic intervention to improve delivery of channels to the surface membrane. Data suggest that pharmacological chaperones bind to the high affinity drug-binding site in the Kv11.1 pore to stabilize Kv11.1 channel conformations suitable for ER export into the secretory pathway (Zhou et al., 1999; Ficker et al., 2002; Ellgaard and Helenius, 2003; Delisle et al., 2005; Gong et al., 2006).

We previously studied the cellular QC mechanisms that prevent the trafficking of the LQT2-linked missense mutations Gly601Ser (G601S) early in the secretory pathway. In control conditions, most of the G601S-Kv11.1 protein is excluded from ER exit sites (ERES) and sequestered in a microtubule-sensitive ER compartment that contains the transitional ER protein BAP31 (Furutani et al., 1999; Ficker et al., 2002; Wakana et al., 2008; Smith et al., 2011, 2013). This transitional ER compartment did not contain other ER or ER Golgi Intermediate proteins, including calnexin, proteins with the ER retention KDEL sequence, the ER-associated degradation (ERAD) protein derlin-1, the ERES protein Sec31, or the ER-Golgi intermediate compartment 53 kDa protein (ERGIC-53). Importantly, we found that incubating cells in the pharmacological chaperone E-4031 directly increased the trafficking of the sequestered G601S-Kv11.1 channels to the cell surface membrane (Smith et al., 2013). In this study we investigate the cellular QC control mechanisms that prevent the trafficking of the LQT2-linked missense mutation F805C (Ficker et al., 2002). Unlike G601S (which is located on the extracellular side of the Kv11.1 α-subunit in the pore domain), F805C is located on the intracellular portion of the Kv11.1 α-subunit in the cyclic nucleotide-binding domain (CNBD) and does not undergo pharmacological correction with E-4031 because it likely impairs Kv11.1 tetramer assembly (Ficker et al., 2002; Delisle et al., 2003). We tested the hypothesis that the ER QC control mechanisms that prevent the trafficking of G601S- and F805C-Kv11.1 proteins are different.

MATERIALS AND METHODS

Cell Lines and Drug Exposure

The Human Embryonic Kidney 293 (HEK293) cells used in this study stably express Kv11.1 channel proteins (wild type or WT, G601S, R752W, or F805C) and they have been previously described (Zhou et al., 1998b; Delisle et al., 2003; Anderson et al., 2006). Cells are cultured at 37°C (5% CO_2) in MEM supplemented with 10% Fetal Bovine Serum (FBS, Invitrogen, Carlsbad, CA, United States) and geneticin. The data shown in **Figures 1–4, 5B** are obtained from stably expressing cell lines. For some experiments we transiently transfected G601S- or F805C-Kv11.1 plasmid cDNA in HEK293 cells. Transfections were performed similar to that previously described (Anson et al., 2004), 3 μg of Kv11.1 plasmid cDNA was transfected with the Superfect Transfection Reagent (Qiagen, Germantown, MD, United States). The data for **Figure 5A** are from transiently expressing HEK293 cells. We also used transiently transfected iCell Cardiomyocytes (Cellular Dynamics International, Madison, WI, United States). iCell Cardiomyocytes were transiently transfected with green fluorescent protein (GFP) tagged Kv11.1 cDNA plasmids (3 μg) using the Viafect (Promega, Madison, WI, United States) transfection reagent and the protocol for iCell Cardiomyocytes. The GFP cDNA is located in-frame and upstream of the Kv11.1 protein start site. For pharmacological studies, we incubated cells in nocodazole (20 μM) (Millipore, Sigma, St. Louis, MO, United States), bortezomib, lactacystin, and MG132 (Millipore, Sigma, St. Louis, MO, United States), or E-4031 (10 μM) (Alomone Laboratories, Jerusalem, Israel). Nocodazole, bortezomib, lactacystin or MG132 were dissolved in DMSO and added to the MEM (final DMSO concentration was <0.1%). E-4031 was dissolved in water. Control studies were done in parallel with equivalent amounts of vehicle (DMSO or water) only.

Immunocytochemistry and Confocal Imaging

Immunocytochemistry and confocal imaging experiments were done similar to those previously described (Smith et al., 2011, 2013). HEK293 cells or iCell Cardiomyocytes were plated in 35 mm tissue culture plates containing collagen-coated coverslips. Cells were fixed with 4% buffered paraformaldehyde for 10 min, permeabilized with triton X-100 (0.1%) for 10 min, and rinsed in 0.75% glycine buffer for 10 min to quench background fluorescence. The cells were incubated with 2 mL blocking solution (10% goat serum in PBS) for 1 h to block non-specific binding sites, and

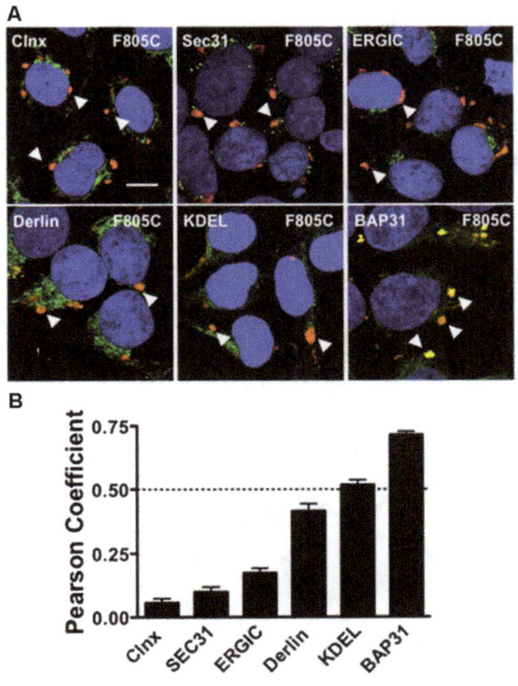

FIGURE 1 | F805C selectively co-localizes with BAP31. **(A)** Representative confocal images of HEK293 cells expressing F805C-Kv11.1 protein showing the overlap between anti-Kv11.1 and anti-ER/ERGIC protein immunostaining. Anti-Kv11.1 immunostaining is shown in red; anti-calnexin (n = 12 images), anti-Sec31 (n = 19 images), anti-ERGIC-53 (n = 19 images), anti-derlin-1 (n = 18 images), anti-KDEL (n = 15 images), or anti-BAP31 (n = 17 images) is shown as green; overlapping immunostaining of red and green signals of similar intensities is shown as yellow; and the cell nuclei are labeled blue. The arrowheads highlight the distinct immunostaining pattern of F805C-Kv11.1 protein, and the scale bar represents 10 μm. **(B)** The mean Costes' Pearson Coefficient (PC) for the image data sets are shown. PC values at or below the dashed line are (PC = 0.5) indicative of weak or no co-localization. Two independent cultures were tested for each condition.

the cells were subsequently incubated with the appropriate primary antibodies: anti-Kv11.1 (1:1000, Alomone Laboratories, Jerusalem, Israel), anti-calnexin (1:1000, Abcam, Cambridge, MA, United States), anti-KDEL (1:1000, Abcam, Cambridge, MA, United States), anti-Sec31a (1:100, BD Labs, Franklin Lakes, NJ, United States), anti-Bap31 (1:500, Abcam, Cambridge, MA, United States), and anti-ERGIC-53 (1:1000, Alexis Biochemicals, Plymouth Meeting, PA, United States) mixed with blocking solution at room temperature. Excess antibody was washed off with three 10 min long rinses of blocking solution. The cells were then incubated for 1 h with the appropriate Highly Cross-absorbed Alexa Fluor antibodies (1:500, Invitrogen Inc., Carlsbad, CA, United States). The cells were washed four times for 10 min with blocking solution alone. After the final wash, the coverslips were mounted onto a slide using ProLong Gold with DAPI mounting medium (Invitrogen, Carlsbad, CA, United States). For iCell Cardiomyocytes experiments, we prepared the cells as described above but utilized the fluorescence signal from GFP for imaging analyses. Imaging was performed at the University of Kentucky Imaging Facility using a Leica TSP SP5 confocal microscope (Leica, Wetzler, Germany). HEK293 cells or iCell Cardiomyocytes did not show any labeling with any of the secondary antibodies when used alone (data not shown). Data are shown as representative single z-scan images for each fluorescence signal (fluorescent images). Overlapping signals of similar intensities colored as red and green are shown as yellow and green and purple are shown as white.

Co-localization analyses were performed using ImageJ[1]. We calculated the Pearson Coefficient (PC) and the Manders Colocalization Coefficients (MCC) for some experiments. The PC is the goodness of fit for the linear regression describing the relation between overlapping signal intensities. We calculated the coefficients using the intensity thresholds defined by the Costes' approach to minimize the contribution of noise. Using the Costes PC approach, the values range between 0 (no co-localization) to 1 (100% co-localization). Weak co-localization is defined as having PC values < 0.5 (Bolte and Cordelieres, 2006). The MCC calculates the fraction of overlap between the signals even if the intensities of the signals are very different from one another. The MCC also vary from 0 (no overlap) to 1 (complete overlap) and are calculated for both signals (M1 and M2). We use the MCC to describe the fraction of Kv11.1 signal in compartments containing the BAP31 signal (M1), or to describe the fraction of BAP31 signal in compartments containing Kv11.1 signal (M2).

Statistics

A one-way ANOVA was performed on data sets. In order to identify which experimental groups differed from control, *post hoc* Bonferroni's tests on selected data sets were performed (Prism, La Jolla, CA, United States). Significance was reported at $p < 0.05$.

RESULTS

F805C-Kv11.1 Protein Selectivity Co-localizes With BAP31

We initially tested whether the trafficking-deficient F805C-Kv11.1 protein co-localized with different ER/ERGIC proteins (**Figure 1A**) in HEK293 cells by calculating the Costes PC. Confocal data showed that F805C-Kv11.1 protein immunostaining localized into several discrete compartments throughout the cell. Based on the PC analysis, the F805C-Kv11.1 protein did not (or only weakly) co-localize with the ER lectin chaperone calnexin (Hammond et al., 1994), the ER Golgi Intermediate Complex (ERGIC) protein ERGIC-53 (Schweizer et al., 1993), the ERES protein Sec31 (Salama et al., 1997), the ERAD protein derlin-1 (Lilley and Ploegh, 2004), or ER proteins that contain the KDEL ER retention signal sequence (Munro and Pelham, 1987) (**Figure 1B**). However, F805C-Kv11.1 protein co-localized with the transitional ER protein BAP31. These data suggest that F805C-Kv11.1 protein is concentrated in the transitional ER.

[1] https://imagej.nih.gov

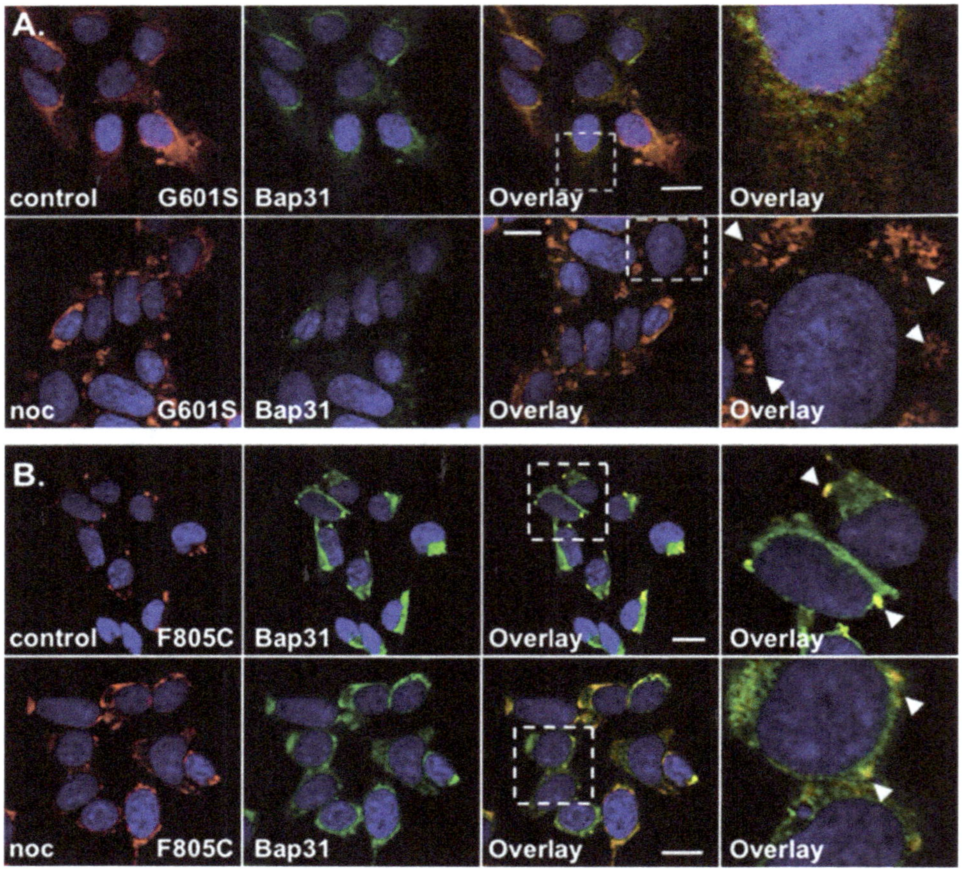

FIGURE 2 | G601S- and F805C-Kv11.1 proteins show distinct immunostaining patterns. Shown are representative confocal images of HEK293 cells expressing **(A)** G601S- or **(B)** F805C-Kv11.1 protein immunostained with anti-Kv11.1 (red, first column), anti-Bap31 (green, second column) in control conditions (top row; $n = 13$ images for G601S and $n = 17$ images for F805C) or after incubation in nocodazole (bottom row; $n = 15$ images for G601S and $n = 16$ images for F805C). The overlay images are also shown (overlapping immunostaining is yellow, third column), and the white dashed box portion of the overlay image is shown in larger detail (fourth column). The nuclei are labeled blue. The arrowheads in **(A)** highlight the reticular immunostaining pattern of G601S-Kv11.1 protein after nocodazole treatment, the arrowheads in **(B)** highlight the unique immunostaining pattern of F805C-Kv11.1 protein, and the scale bar represents 10 μm. Two independent cultures were tested for each condition.

G601S- and F805C-Kv11.1 Proteins Show Differences in Protein Immunostaining

We previously showed that G601S-Kv11.1 protein is sequestered in microtubule-dependent ER QC compartment with BAP31 (Smith et al., 2011, 2013). We directly compared the anti-Kv11.1 protein immunostaining pattern of HEK293 cells expressing G601S-Kv11.1 or F805C-Kv11.1 protein in control conditions or after treatment in the microtubule depolymerizing agent nocodazole (20 μM) for 2 h. Similar to what was previously reported, cells expressing G601S-Kv11.1 protein showed a peri-nuclear immunostaining pattern that diffused into the cell periphery and co-localized with BAP31 in control conditions (**Figure 2A**; PC = 0.62 ± 0.02 in control $n = 13$ images) (Smith et al., 2011, 2013). Incubating cells in nocodazole caused G601S-Kv11.1 and BAP31 protein to redistribute together into several peripheral reticulated membrane compartments (PC = 0.72 ± 0.02 after nocodazole, $n = 15$ images). In control conditions, the F805C-Kv11.1 protein immunostaining pattern was qualitatively different than the G601S-Kv11.1 protein immunostaining pattern (**Figure 2B**). Similar to **Figure 1A**, the F805C-Kv11.1 protein immunostaining was concentrated in several compartments that co-localized with BAP31 protein (PC = 0.71 ± 0.01 in control $n = 17$ images). Nocodazole treatment did not cause F805C-Kv11.1 protein to redistribute to reticulated membrane compartments, but it modestly increased the amount of diffuse F805C-Kv11.1 protein immunostaining, still co-localizing with BAP31 (PC = 0.77 ± 0.02 after nocodazole, $n = 16$ images). We conclude that unlike G601S-Kv11.1 protein, F805C-Kv11.1 protein likely concentrates to distinct sub-compartments in the transitional ER.

F805C-Kv11.1 Protein Immunostaining Is Disrupted by Proteasome Inhibition

The WT Kv11.1 α-subunit is synthesized in the ER as a ~135 kDa N-linked glycoprotein, and once the WT-Kv11.1 α-subunit

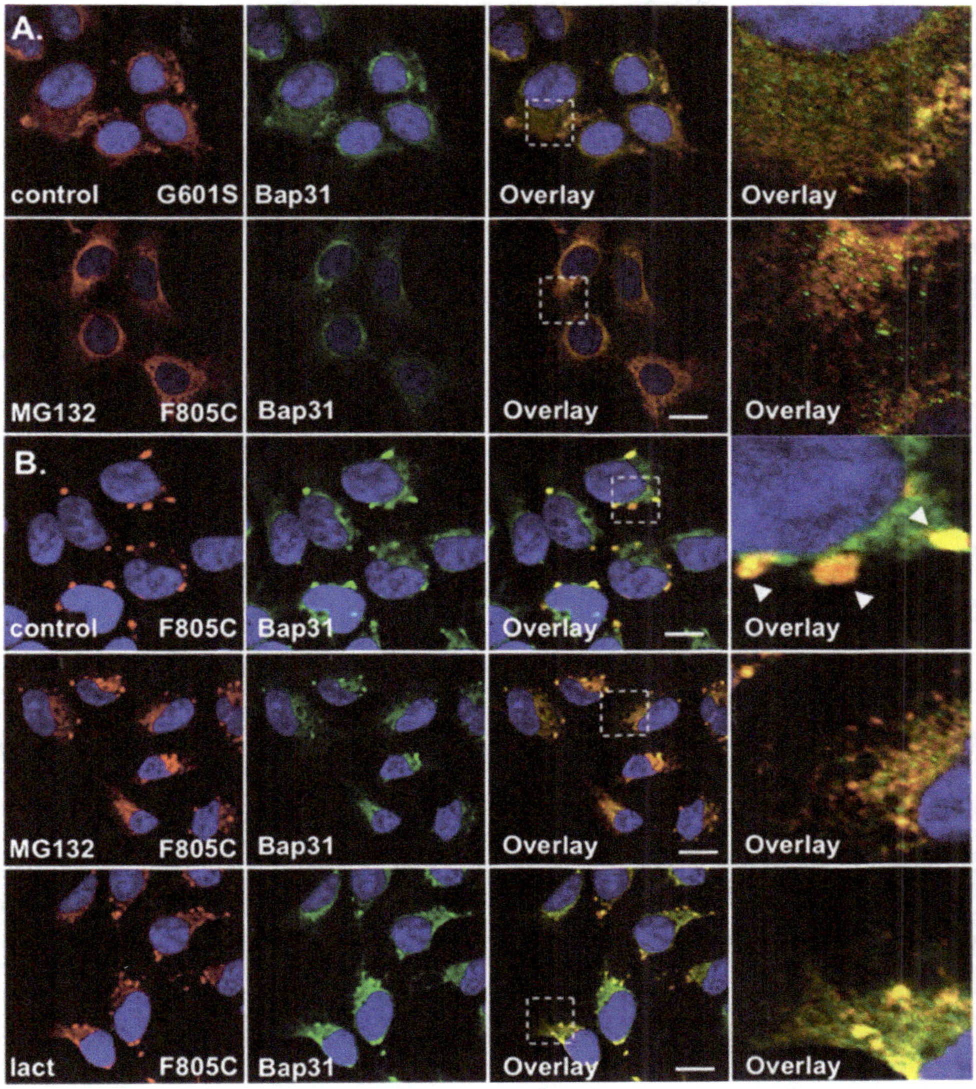

FIGURE 3 | F805C-Kv11.1 protein immunostaining is sensitive to proteasome inhibition. Shown are representative images of HEK293 cells expressing **(A)** G601S- or **(B)** F805C-Kv11.1 protein immunostained with anti-Kv11.1 (red, first column), anti-Bap31 (green, second column), the overlay (co-localization is shown as yellow, third column), and the white dashed box portion of the overlay in more detail (fourth column). The nuclei are shown in blue and the scale bars represent 10 μm. The top row of images in **(A,B)** show control conditions (n = 13 images for G601S and n = 17 images for F805C) and the second row of images in **(A,B)** show cells after incubation in 5 μM MG132 for 5 h (n = 15 images for G601S and n = 17 images for F805C). The arrowheads in **(B)** highlight the immunostaining pattern of F805C-Kv11.1 protein in control conditions. The bottom row of images show F805C-Kv11.1 protein immunostaining after incubation in 5 μM lactacystin (n = 17 images) for 5 h. Two independent cultures were tested for each condition.

traffics to the Golgi apparatus, it is terminally glycosylated to a ~155 kDa glycoprotein (Zhou et al., 1998b; Petrecca et al., 1999). Studies show that only 60% of the 135 kDa WT-Kv11.1 protein is processed to the terminally glycosylated 155 kDa form. The fraction of WT-Kv11.1 protein that fails to mature is degraded via the ERAD (ubiquitin-proteasome) pathway (Gong et al., 2005). In the presence of proteasome inhibitors, there is an increase in the immature form of WT-Kv11.1 protein, and a decrease in the efficiency in the ER dislocation of WT-Kv11.1 protein in ERAD pathway (Gong et al., 2005). Therefore, we tested whether the proteasome inhibitor MG132 impacted G601S- or F805C-Kv11.1 protein immunostaining. We incubated HEK293 cells expressing G601S- or F805C-Kv11.1 protein in the proteasome inhibitor MG132 (5 μM) for 5 h (**Figures 3A,B**). This incubation time is based on previous reports that investigated the impact that proteasome inhibitors had on the ER retention of proteins in other studies (Kamhi-Nesher et al., 2001; Spiliotis et al., 2002; Wakana et al., 2008). Compared to control cells, incubating cells in MG132 did not appear to alter G601S-Kv11.1 protein immunostaining or its co-localization with BAP31 (PC = 0.57 ± 0.02 after MG132, n = 15 images). In contrast,

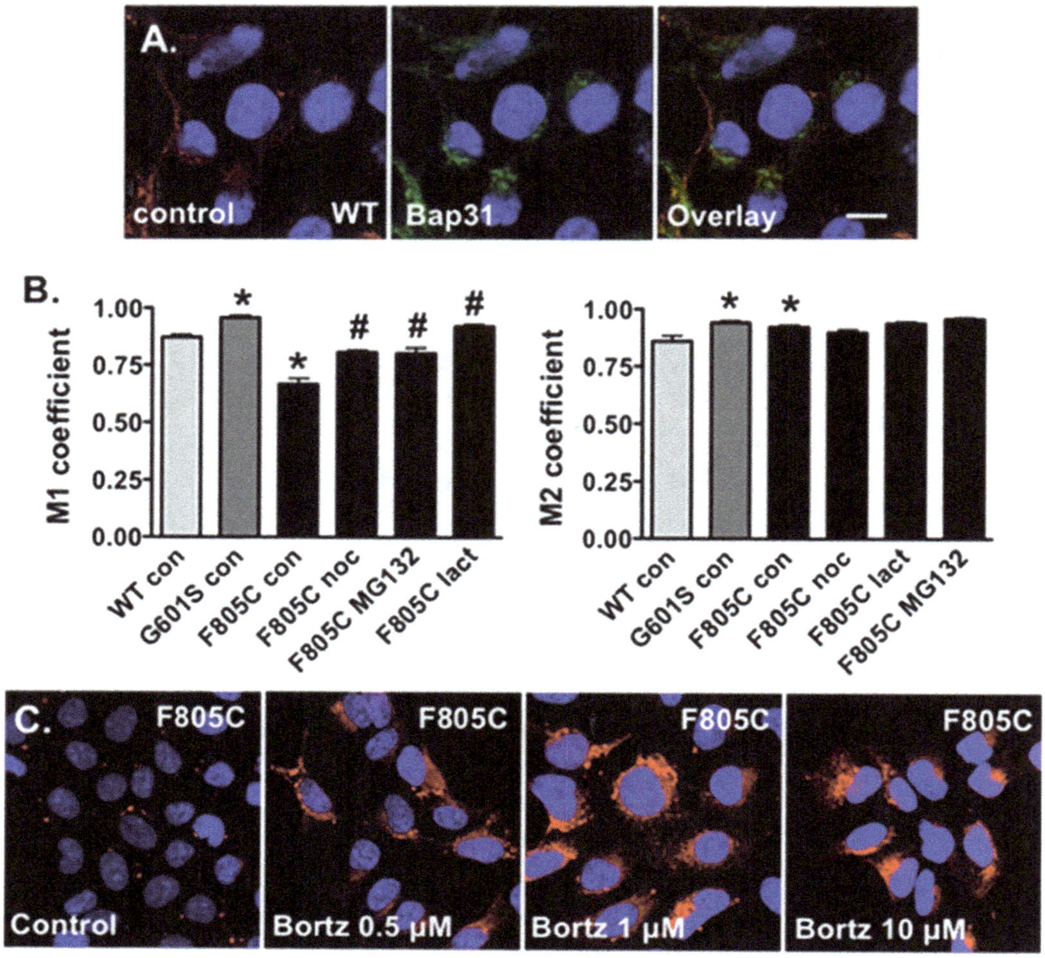

FIGURE 4 | Proteasome inhibition increases the fraction of Kv11.1 signal overlapping with BAP31 signal. **(A)** Shown are representative confocal images of HEK293 cells expressing WT-Kv11.1 protein immunostained with anti-Kv11.1 (red, first column), anti-Bap31 (green, second column) in control conditions. The nuclei are labeled blue, and the scale bar represents 10 μm. **(B)** Shown is the graph for the MCC that describes the fraction of Kv11.1 signal in compartments containing the BAP31 signal (M1, left graph), as well as the fraction of BAP31 signal in compartments containing Kv11.1 signal (M2, right graph). We compared M1 and M2 for cells stably expressing WT-, G601S-, or F805C-Kv11.1 protein in control conditions (n = 19, 13, and 17 images, respectively, $^{*}p < 0.05$ compared to cells expressing WT-Kv11.1 in control conditions). We also compared the M1 or M2 in cells expressing F805C-Kv11.1 in control conditions to cells incubated in nocodazole (F805C noc, n = 16 images), MG132 (F805C MG132, n = 17 images), or lactacystin (F805C lact, n = 17 images). At least two independent cultures were tested for each condition ($^{\#}p < 0.05$) compared to cells expressing F805C-Kv11.1 protein in control conditions. **(C)** Shown are representative images of cells expressing F805C-Kv11.1 protein immunostained with anti-Kv11.1 (red) in control conditions or in different concentrations of bortezomib for 5 h. The nuclei are labeled blue. The effect of bortezomib on F805C-Kv11.1 immunostaining was confirmed in two independent test cultures (n = 5–11 images per condition).

treating cells expressing F805C-Kv11.1 protein dramatically transformed the protein immunostaining pattern from several compartments to a peri-nuclear pattern that diffused into the cell periphery (**Figure 3B**). Although incubating cells in MG132 dramatically altered the distribution of F805C-Kv11.1 protein, the F805C-Kv11.1 protein still co-localized with BAP31 (PC = 0.78 ± 0.02 after MG132, n = 17 images). We next determined if another proteasome inhibitor similarly affected the immunostaining pattern of cells expressing F805C-Kv11.1 protein. Incubating cells expressing F805C-Kv11.1 protein in the proteasome inhibitor lactacystin for 5 h also altered the F805C-Kv11.1 protein immunostaining pattern similar to cells incubated with MG132 (**Figure 3B**). Moreover, incubating cells in lactacystin did not alter F805C-Kv11.1 protein co-localization with BAP31 (PC = 0.72 ± 0.03 after lactacystin, n = 17 images). These data indicate that F805C-Kv11.1 protein concentrates in sub-compartments of the transitional ER that are sensitive to proteasome inhibition.

Nocodazole, Lactacystin, and MG132 Increase the Fractional Overlap of F805C-Kv11.1 Protein With BAP31 and Immunostaining

The Costes' PC quantifies the co-localization between Kv11.1 and BAP31 protein immunostaining by measuring the goodness of

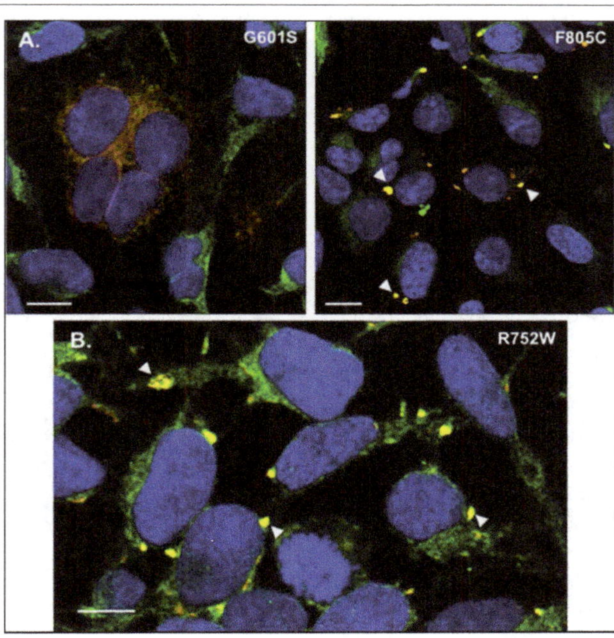

FIGURE 5 | Transient transfection of G601S- or F805C-Kv11.1 does not alter mutation-specific differences in immunostaining pattern, and cells stably expressing R752W-Kv11.1 protein show similar immunostaining patterns as cells expressing F805C-Kv11.1 protein. **(A)** Representative confocal images of HEK293 cells transiently expressing G601S-Kv11.1 (left) or F805C-Kv11.1 (right) protein showing the overlapped anti-Kv11.1 (red) and anti-BAP31 immunostaining (green) (n = 12 images for each, from 2 independent cultures). Overlapping immunostaining of red and green signal of similar intensities is shown as yellow and the cell nuclei are labeled blue. The transfection efficiency is <100%, so not all cells were expressing Kv11.1 protein. **(B)** Representative confocal images of HEK293 cells stably expressing R752W-Kv11.1 protein showing the overlap between anti-Kv11.1 (red) and anti-BAP31 immunostaining (green). Overlapping immunostaining of red and green signal of similar intensities is shown as yellow and the cell nuclei are labeled blue. The arrowheads highlight the immunostaining pattern of R752W-Kv11.1 protein, and the scale bar represents 10 μm. The mean Costes' Pearson Coefficient (PC) for the image data is 0.65 ± 0.01 (n = 11 images from 2 independent cultures).

fit for the relation between overlapping signal intensities. An additional approach for confocal image analysis is to calculate the MCC, which provides a measure of how much one signal overlaps with a second signal. Qualitatively, the major effect of incubating cells expressing F805C-Kv11.1 protein in nocodazole (**Figure 2B**), MG132, or lactacystin (**Figure 3B**) was to increase the overlap of Kv11.1 protein with BAP31 immunostaining, therefore we quantified the MCC between Kv11.1 protein and BAP31.

Manders Colocalization Coefficients analyses have not been done for cells expressing Kv11.1 proteins. Therefore we imaged cells stably expressing WT-Kv11.1 protein (**Figure 4A**) and compared the M1 and M2 with cells expressing G601S- or F805C-Kv11.1 protein. The data show the M1 for cells expressing WT-Kv11.1 protein is smaller than that of cells expressing G601S-Kv11.1 protein (**Figure 4B**). In other words, cells expressing WT-Kv11.1 protein show less overlap of Kv11.1 protein with BAP31 compared to cells expressing G601S-Kv11.1 protein. These data are consistent with more G601S-Kv11.1 protein retained in the transitional ER compartment. In contrast, the M1 for cells expressing WT-Kv11.1 protein is greater than F805C-Kv11.1 protein. This is because F805C-Kv11.1 protein concentrates in several small transitional ER subcompartments. We conclude that mutation-specific differences in the trafficking-deficient LQT2 phenotype can be quantified by differences in the fraction of Kv11.1 protein overlapping with BAP31.

In contrast the M2 for cells expressing WT-Kv11.1 protein is smaller than cells expressing G601S- or F805C-Kv11.1 protein (**Figure 4B**). This means that more BAP31 overlapped with Kv11.1 protein in cells expressing G601S- or F805C-Kv11.1 protein. This is because cells expressing WT-Kv11.1 protein appear to have more Kv11.1 protein in the cell surface membrane (**Figure 4A**).

We next determined how incubating cells expressing F805C-Kv11.1 protein in nocodazole or the proteasome inhibitors affected the M1 and M2 (**Figure 4B**). Compared to control cells expressing F805C-Kv11.1, incubating cells expressing F805C-Kv11.1 protein in the proteasome inhibitors increased M1. These data demonstrate that nocodazole and the proteasome inhibition increased the amount of F805C-Kv11.1 protein in the larger transitional ER compartment. We did not see any significant changes in M2, indicating that incubating cells in nocodazole or proteasome inhibitors did affect the high amount of BAP31 overlap with F805C-Kv11.1 protein.

The effect of proteasome inhibitors on the immunostaining patterns of F805C-Kv11.1 protein was striking. Inhibiting the proteasome pathway is an approach in the treatment of certain cancers, including myeloma and mantle cell lymphoma (Chen et al., 2011). Bortezomib is the first FDA approved proteasome inhibitor to be implemented in cancer treatment. Therefore, we also determined the impact that different concentrations of bortezomib had on the immunostaining pattern of F805C-Kv11.1 protein (**Figure 4C**). We found that, similar to MG132 and lactacystin, incubating cells in different concentrations of bortezomib for 5 h transformed the F805C-Kv11.1 protein immunostaining pattern to a diffuse peri-nuclear pattern.

G601S- and F805C-Kv11.1 Proteins Show Differences in Protein Immunostaining in Transiently Transfected Cells

One possible reason for the immunostaining difference between the cell lines expressing G601S- and F805C-Kv11.1 could be due to differences in protein expression. The unique immunostaining pattern of F805C-Kv11.1 protein might be because the mutant protein levels are too high for a normal functioning of the cellular QC system. Therefore we immunostained HEK293 cells transiently transfected with equal amounts of G601S- or F805C-Kv11.1 plasmid DNA. Importantly, the mutation-specific immunostaining pattern of G601S- and F805C-Kv11.1 proteins were similar to what was seen in stably expressing cells (**Figure 5A**). These data suggest that the mutation-specific difference in immunostaining was not due to differences in mutant Kv11.1 cDNA levels.

We previously showed that cells stably expressing different LQT2-linked mutations in the Kv11.1 pore region (A614V- or N629D-Kv11.1) exhibit a diffuse immunostaining pattern that co-localizes with BAP31 similar to G601S-Kv11.1 protein (Smith et al., 2013). We determined whether R752W-Kv11.1 (another LQT2-linked mutation that is located intracellular CNBD, impairs Kv11.1 tetramer assembly, and does not undergo pharmacological correction with E-4031) exhibited a similar immunostaining pattern as cells expressing F805C-Kv11.1 protein. Imaging cells stably expressing R752W-Kv11.1 protein showed that it also concentrated in transitional ER subcompartments (**Figure 5B**). Together, the data demonstrate that the immunostaining pattern seen in cells expressing of F805C-Kv11.1 protein is also seen in cells expressing other LQT2-linked mutant proteins in the CNBD.

G601S and F805C Show Distinct Immunostaining Patterns in iPSC-CMs

We next determined whether the mutation-specific immunostaining patterns of G601S- or F805C-Kv11.1 proteins persisted in human inducible pluripotent stem cell derived cardiomyocytes (iPSC-CMs). This will help to determine if mutation-specific differences occurs in a more native-like cell that expresses endogenous WT-Kv11.1 protein (including the shorter Kv11.1b subunit) (Jones et al., 2004, 2014). iPSC-CMs were transfected with WT-, G601S- or F805C-Kv11.1 proteins tagged with GFP on the Kv11.1 amino-terminus to distinguish between heterologously expressed and endogenous WT-Kv11.1 or WT-Kv11.1b protein. We immunostained the cells for BAP31. Similar to what we previously showed in HEK293 cells, WT-Kv11.1-GFP protein expressed in iPSC-CMs did not co-localize with BAP31 (**Figures 6A,D**) (Smith et al., 2013). G601S-Kv11.1-GFP expressed in iPSC-CMs co-localized with BAP31, and importantly, this co-localization was decreased in iPSC-CMs treated with the pharmacological chaperone E-4031 for 24–48 h (**Figures 6B,D**). In most iPSC-CMs, F805C-Kv11.1-GFP protein concentrated in discrete compartments (although the co-localization with BAP31 was not as strong as it was in HEK293 cells) (**Figures 6C,D**). These data confirm that the differences in subcellular localization of WT-, G601S-, and F805C-Kv11.1 proteins persisted in a cell model of human cardiomyocytes.

DISCUSSION

In this study we demonstrate that the trafficking-deficient LQT2 missense mutation F805C generated Kv11.1 protein that accumulates in discrete ER subcompartments. In HEK293 cells F805C-Kv11.1 protein did not co-localize with several ER/ERGIC marker proteins, but it did co-localize with the transitional ER protein BAP31. The immunostaining pattern of F805C-Kv11.1 protein was sensitive to the microtubule depolymerizing drug nocodazole, as well as the proteasome inhibitors MG132 or lactacystin. Interestingly, these drugs did not alter F805C-Kv11.1 protein co-localization with BAP31, but they all caused the F805C-Kv11.1 protein to become more diffuse and increased the overlapping immunostaining between F805C-Kv11.1 and BAP31. In contrast, G601S-Kv11.1 protein did not accumulate in distinct subcompartments and its immunostaining pattern was insensitive to proteasome inhibition. Importantly, the mutation-specific differences in the subcellular patterns of G601S- and Kv11.1-Kv11.1 protein were also present in human iPSC-CMs. We conclude that distinct QC mechanisms in the ER regulate the retention of G601S- and F805C-Kv11.1 protein.

Mutation-specific differences in trafficking-deficient phenotype for LQT2 mutations have long been recognized (Ficker et al., 2000b; Anderson et al., 2006, 2014; Smith et al., 2016). For example, there are mutation-specific differences in pharmacological correction, intragenic suppression, and dominant negative effects on the trafficking of WT-Kv11.1 protein, suggesting that different mutations likely disrupt different steps in the native Kv11.1 protein folding pathway (e.g., co-assembly of α-subunits, formation of the voltage-sensor/pore domains, increasing the proximity of the NH_2 and COOH termini, etc.) (Ficker et al., 2000a; Delisle et al., 2005; Anderson et al., 2006; Smith et al., 2016). However, this is the first study to investigate mutation specific differences in cellular mechanisms associated with ER retention. Although we focus only on two different mutations, we found that other trafficking-deficient LQT2-linked proteins have immunostaining/co-localization patterns similar to cells expressing G601S-Kv11.1 (A614V and N629D) (Smith et al., 2013) or F805C-Kv11.1 protein (R752W, **Figure 5B**). Therefore, this study has identified a novel way to categorize subgroups of trafficking-deficient LQT2 mutations. We expect these findings will help identify new drugs that improve LQT2 protein trafficking by targeting mutation-specific ER QC mechanisms.

The exact mechanism by which proteasome inhibitors alter F805C-Kv11.1 protein immunostaining remains unclear. Previous studies show that retrotranslocation of misfolded proteins into the cytosol likely occurs concurrently with their degradation by the proteasome, and that upon inhibition of proteasomal activity, misfolded proteins remain intact in the secretory pathway (Hirsch and Ploegh, 2000). Consistent with this concept, studies show that inhibition of the proteasome decreases the efficiency of WT-Kv11.1 protein dislocation from the ER (Gong et al., 2005). However, F805C-Kv11.1 protein did not co-localize with the ERAD protein derlin-1, and surprisingly, we found that longer-term proteasome inhibition did not improve Kv11.1 protein trafficking but actually appeared to inhibit it (data not shown).

An intriguing implication to the findings in this study is that, because different immunostaining patterns of different LQT2-linked mutant proteins can be easily visualized with microtubule depolymerizing agents or proteasome inhibitors, cell lines expressing these trafficking-deficient Kv11.1

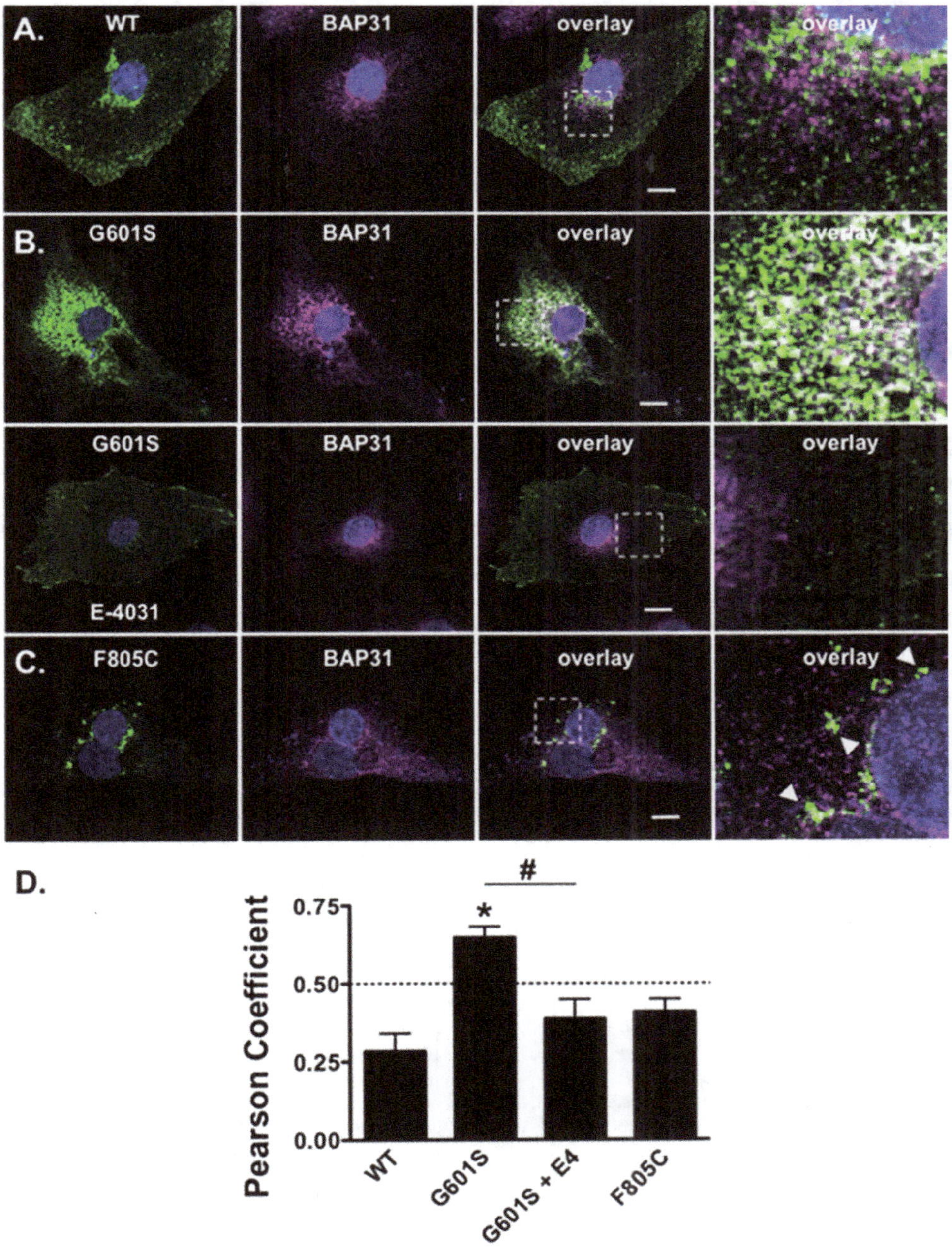

FIGURE 6 | G601S- and F805C-Kv11.1 proteins show distinct immunostaining patterns in iPSC-CMs. Shown are representative images of iPSC-CMs expressing **(A)** WT-Kv11.1-GFP, **(B)** G601S-Kv11.1-GFP, or **(C)** F805C-Kv11.1-GFP (green, first column), immunostained with anti-BAP31 (purple, second column). Also shown are the overlays (co-localization is shown as white, third column) and the white dashed box portion of the overlay in more detail (fourth column). The nuclei are stained in blue and the scale bar represents 10 μm. The row in **(A)**, top row in **(B)**, and row in **(C)** show iPSC-CMs in control conditions. The arrowheads in **(C)** highlight the unique fluorescence pattern of cells expressing F805C-Kv11.1-GFP. The bottom row in **(B)** shows images from iPSC-CMs expressing G601S-Kv11.1-GFP after incubation in 10 μM E-4031 (E4) for ~24 h. **(D)** The mean Costes' Pearson Coefficient (PC) for the iPSC-CMs expressing WT-GFP (n = 16 images), G601S-GFP (n = 20 images), G601S-GFP after incubation in 10 μM E-4031 (n = 19 images), or F805C-GFP (n = 14 images) ($^*p < 0.05$ compared to WT, $^{\#}p < 0.05$ compared to G601S con). Two independent cultures were tested for each condition.

proteins might be used as a novel drug-screening platform to identify new anti-neoplastic agents that have microtubule depolymerization properties or inhibit the proteasome activity.

There are several limitations to this study. We primarily used HEK293 cells for most of the experiments in the study, however, we confirmed similar mutation-specific differences in the subcellular localization of G601S- and F805C-Kv11.1 proteins in iPSC-CMs. Interestingly the co-localization of F805C-Kv11.1 and BAP31 protein was decreased in iPSC-CM. We suspect that this difference might be due to cell type specific differences. For example, the subcellular localization of mutant F805C-Kv11.1 protein may be altered by endogenous WT-Kv11.1 proteins (including the Kv11.1b protein). However, F805C-Kv11.1 is not expected to co-assemble with other Kv11.1 subunits (Ficker et al., 2002). Another possibility is that the larger size of iPSC-CMs might help to better resolve the spatial differences between F805C-Kv11.1 protein and BAP31. Regardless, the data clearly show that both G601S- and F805C-Kv11.1 proteins have unique localization patterns in both cell types, suggesting they are regulated by different QC pathway interactions.

AUTHOR CONTRIBUTIONS

AH, JS, and BD performed the experiments and data analysis. CA, CE, TM, CJ, and BD contributed to the writing, interpretation, editing, and presentation of the manuscript.

REFERENCES

Anderson, C. L., Delisle, B. P., Anson, B. D., Kilby, J. A., Will, M. L., Tester, D. J., et al. (2006). Most LQT2 mutations reduce Kv11.1 (hERG) current by a class 2 (trafficking-deficient) mechanism. *Circulation* 113, 365–373. doi: 10.1161/CIRCULATIONAHA.105.570200

Anderson, C. L., Kuzmicki, C. E., Childs, R. R., Hintz, C. J., Delisle, B. P., and January, C. T. (2014). Large-scale mutational analysis of Kv11.1 reveals molecular insights into type 2 long QT syndrome. *Nat. Commun.* 5:5535. doi: 10.1038/ncomms6535

Anson, B. D., Ackerman, M. J., Tester, D. J., Will, M. L., Delisle, B. P., Anderson, C. L., et al. (2004). Molecular and functional characterization of common polymorphisms in HERG (KCNH2) potassium channels. *Am. J. Physiol. Heart Circ. Physiol.* 286, H2434–H2441. doi: 10.1152/ajpheart.00891.2003

Bolte, S., and Cordelieres, F. P. (2006). A guided tour into subcellular colocalization analysis in light microscopy. *J. Microsc.* 224, 213–232. doi: 10.1111/j.1365-2818.2006.01706.x

Chen, D., Frezza, M., Schmitt, S., Kanwar, J., and Dou, Q. P. (2011). Bortezomib as the first proteasome inhibitor anticancer drug: current status and future perspectives. *Curr. Cancer Drug Targets* 11, 239–253. doi: 10.2174/156800911794519752

Crotti, L., Celano, G., Dagradi, F., and Schwartz, P. J. (2008). Congenital long QT syndrome. *Orphanet J. Rare Dis.* 3:18. doi: 10.1186/1750-1172-3-18

Curran, M. E., Splawski, I., Timothy, K. W., Vincent, G. M., Green, E. D., and Keating, M. T. (1995). A molecular basis for cardiac arrhythmia: HERG mutations cause long QT syndrome. *Cell* 80, 795–803. doi: 10.1016/0092-8674(95)90358-5

Delisle, B. P., Anderson, C. L., Balijepalli, R. C., Anson, B. D., Kamp, T. J., and January, C. T. (2003). Thapsigargin selectively rescues the trafficking defective LQT2 channels G601S and F805C. *J. Biol. Chem.* 278, 35749–35754. doi: 10.1074/jbc.M305787200

Delisle, B. P., Slind, J. K., Kilby, J. A., Anderson, C. L., Anson, B. D., Balijepalli, R. C., et al. (2005). Intragenic suppression of trafficking-defective KCNH2 channels associated with long QT syndrome. *Mol. Pharmacol.* 68, 233–240. doi: 10.1124/mol.105.012914

Ellgaard, L., and Helenius, A. (2003). Quality control in the endoplasmic reticulum. *Nat. Rev. Mol. Cell Biol.* 4, 181–191. doi: 10.1038/nrm1052

Ficker, E., Dennis, A. T., Obejero-Paz, C. A., Castaldo, P., Taglialatela, M., and Brown, A. M. (2000a). Retention in the endoplasmic reticulum as a mechanism of dominant-negative current suppression in human long QT syndrome. *J. Mol. Cell Cardiol.* 32, 2327–2337. doi: 10.1006/jmcc.2000.1263

Ficker, E., Dennis, A. T., Wang, L., and Brown, A. M. (2003). Role of the cytosolic chaperones Hsp70 and Hsp90 in maturation of the cardiac potassium channel HERG. *Circ. Res.* 92, e87–e100. doi: 10.1161/01.RES.0000079028.31393.15

Ficker, E., Obejero-Paz, C. A., Zhao, S., and Brown, A. M. (2002). The binding site for channel blockers that rescue misprocessed human long QT syndrome type 2 ether-a-gogo-related gene (HERG) mutations. *J. Biol. Chem.* 277, 4989–4998. doi: 10.1074/jbc.M107345200

Ficker, E., Thomas, D., Viswanathan, P. C., Dennis, A. T., Priori, S. G., Napolitano, C., et al. (2000b). Novel characteristics of a misprocessed mutant HERG channel linked to hereditary long QT syndrome. *Am. J. Physiol. Heart Circ. Physiol.* 279, H1748–H1756.

Foo, B., Williamson, B., Young, J. C., Lukacs, G., and Shrier, A. (2016). hERG quality control and the long QT syndrome. *J. Physiol.* 594, 2469–2481. doi: 10.1113/JP270531

Furutani, M., Trudeau, M. C., Hagiwara, N., Seki, A., Gong, Q., Zhou, Z., et al. (1999). Novel mechanism associated with an inherited cardiac arrhythmia: defective protein trafficking by the mutant HERG (G601S) potassium channel. *Circulation* 99, 2290–2294. doi: 10.1161/01.CIR.99.17.2290

Gong, Q., Jones, M. A., and Zhou, Z. (2006). Mechanisms of pharmacological rescue of trafficking-defective hERG mutant channels in human long QT syndrome. *J. Biol. Chem.* 281, 4069–4074. doi: 10.1074/jbc.M511765200

Gong, Q., Keeney, D. R., Molinari, M., and Zhou, Z. (2005). Degradation of trafficking-defective long QT syndrome type II mutant channels by the ubiquitin-proteasome pathway. *J. Biol. Chem.* 280, 19419–19425. doi: 10.1074/jbc.M502327200

Hammond, C., Braakman, I., and Helenius, A. (1994). Role of N-linked oligosaccharide recognition, glucose trimming, and calnexin in glycoprotein folding and quality control. *Proc. Natl. Acad. Sci. U.S.A.* 91, 913–917. doi: 10.1073/pnas.91.3.913

Hirsch, C., and Ploegh, H. L. (2000). Intracellular targeting of the proteasome. *Trends Cell Biol.* 10, 268–272. doi: 10.1016/S0962-8924(00)01768-2

Jones, D. K., Liu, F., Vaidyanathan, R., Eckhardt, L. L., Trudeau, M. C., and Robertson, G. A. (2014). hERG 1b is critical for human cardiac repolarization. *Proc. Natl. Acad. Sci. U.S.A.* 111, 18073–18077. doi: 10.1073/pnas.1414945111

Jones, E. M., Roti Roti, E. C., Wang, J., Delfosse, S. A., and Robertson, G. A. (2004). Cardiac IKr channels minimally comprise hERG 1a and 1b subunits. *J. Biol. Chem.* 279, 44690–44694. doi: 10.1074/jbc.M408344200

Kamhi-Nesher, S., Shenkman, M., Tolchinsky, S., Fromm, S. V., Ehrlich, R., and Lederkremer, G. Z. (2001). A novel quality control compartment derived from the endoplasmic reticulum. *Mol. Biol. Cell* 12, 1711–1723. doi: 10.1091/mbc.12.6.1711

Lilley, B. N., and Ploegh, H. L. (2004). A membrane protein required for dislocation of misfolded proteins from the ER. *Nature* 429, 834–840. doi: 10.1038/nature02592

Munro, S., and Pelham, H. R. (1987). A C-terminal signal prevents secretion of luminal ER proteins. *Cell* 48, 899–907. doi: 10.1016/0092-8674(87)90086-9

Petrecca, K., Atanasiu, R., Akhavan, A., and Shrier, A. (1999). N-linked glycosylation sites determine HERG channel surface membrane expression. *J. Physiol.* 515(Pt 1), 41–48. doi: 10.1111/j.1469-7793.1999.041ad.x

Salama, N. R., Chuang, J. S., and Schekman, R. W. (1997). Sec31 encodes an essential component of the COPII coat required for transport vesicle budding from the endoplasmic reticulum. *Mol. Biol. Cell* 8, 205–217. doi: 10.1091/mbc.8.2.205

Sanguinetti, M. C., Curran, M. E., Spector, P. S., and Keating, M. T. (1996). Spectrum of HERG K+-channel dysfunction in an inherited cardiac arrhythmia. *Proc. Natl. Acad. Sci. U.S.A.* 93, 2208–2212. doi: 10.1073/pnas.93.5.2208

Schweizer, A., Ericsson, M., Bachi, T., Griffiths, G., and Hauri, H. P. (1993). Characterization of a novel 63 kDa membrane protein. Implications for the organization of the ER-to-Golgi pathway. *J. Cell Sci.* 104(Pt 3), 671–683.

Smith, J. L., Anderson, C. L., Burgess, D. E., Elayi, C. S., January, C. T., and Delisle, B. P. (2016). Molecular pathogenesis of long QT syndrome type 2. *J. Arrhythm.* 32, 373–380. doi: 10.1016/j.joa.2015.11.009

Smith, J. L., Mcbride, C. M., Nataraj, P. S., Bartos, D. C., January, C. T., and Delisle, B. P. (2011). Trafficking-deficient hERG K channels linked to long QT syndrome are regulated by a microtubule-dependent quality control compartment in the ER. *Am. J. Physiol. Cell Physiol.* 301, C75–C85. doi: 10.1152/ajpcell.00494.2010

Smith, J. L., Reloj, A. R., Nataraj, P. S., Bartos, D. C., Schroder, E. A., Moss, A. J., et al. (2013). Pharmacological correction of long QT-linked mutations in KCNH2 (hERG) increases the trafficking of Kv11.1 channels stored in the transitional endoplasmic reticulum. *Am. J. Physiol. Cell Physiol.* 305, C919–C930. doi: 10.1152/ajpcell.00406.2012

Spiliotis, E. T., Pentcheva, T., and Edidin, M. (2002). Probing for membrane domains in the endoplasmic reticulum: retention and degradation of unassembled MHC class I molecules. *Mol. Biol. Cell* 13, 1566–1581. doi: 10.1091/mbc.01-07-0322

Trudeau, M. C., Warmke, J. W., Ganetzky, B., and Robertson, G. A. (1995). HERG, a human inward rectifier in the voltage-gated potassium channel family. *Science* 269, 92–95. doi: 10.1126/science.7604285

Wakana, Y., Takai, S., Nakajima, K., Tani, K., Yamamoto, A., Watson, P., et al. (2008). Bap31 is an itinerant protein that moves between the peripheral endoplasmic reticulum (ER) and a juxtanuclear compartment related to ER-associated Degradation. *Mol. Biol. Cell* 19, 1825–1836. doi: 10.1091/mbc.E07-08-0781

Walker, V. E., Atanasiu, R., Lam, H., and Shrier, A. (2007). Co-chaperone FKBP38 promotes HERG trafficking. *J. Biol. Chem.* 282, 23509–23516. doi: 10.1074/jbc.M701006200

Walker, V. E., Wong, M. J., Atanasiu, R., Hantouche, C., Young, J. C., and Shrier, A. (2010). Hsp40 chaperones promote degradation of the HERG potassium channel. *J. Biol. Chem.* 285, 3319–3329. doi: 10.1074/jbc.M109.024000

Zhou, Z., Gong, Q., Epstein, M. L., and January, C. T. (1998a). HERG channel dysfunction in human long QT syndrome. Intracellular transport and functional defects. *J. Biol. Chem.* 273, 21061–21066.

Zhou, Z., Gong, Q., and January, C. T. (1999). Correction of defective protein trafficking of a mutant HERG potassium channel in human long QT syndrome. Pharmacological and temperature effects. *J. Biol. Chem.* 274, 31123–31126. doi: 10.1074/jbc.274.44.31123

Zhou, Z., Gong, Q., Ye, B., Fan, Z., Makielski, J. C., Robertson, G. A., et al. (1998b). Properties of HERG channels stably expressed in HEK 293 cells studied at physiological temperature. *Biophys. J.* 74, 230–241.

6

Beat-to-Beat Patterning of Sinus Rhythm Reveals Non-Linear Rhythm in the Dog Compared to the Human

N. Sydney Moïse[1], Wyatt H. Flanders[2] and Romain Pariaut[1]*

[1] College of Veterinary Medicine, Department of Clinical Sciences, Cornell University, Ithaca, NY, United States, [2] Department of Physics, University of Washington, Seattle, WA, United States

***Correspondence:**
N. Sydney Moïse
nsm2@cornell.edu*

The human and dog have sinus arrhythmia; however, the beat-to-beat interval changes were hypothesized to be different. Geometric analyses (R–R interval tachograms, dynamic Poincaré plots) to examine rate changes on a beat-to-beat basis were analyzed along with time and frequency domain heart rate variability from 40 human and 130 canine 24-h electrocardiographic recordings. Humans had bell-shaped beat-interval distributions, narrow interval bands across time with continuous interval change and linear changes in rate. In contrast, dogs had skewed non-singular beat distributions, wide interval bands {despite faster average heart rate of dogs [mean (range); 81 (64–119)] bpm compared to humans [74.5 (59–103) $p = 0.005$]} with regions displaying a paucity of intervals (*zone of avoidance)* and linear plus non-linear rate changes. In the dog, dynamic Poincaré plots showed linear rate changes as intervals prolonged until a point of divergence from the line of identity at a mean interval of 598.5 (95% CI: 583.5–613.5) ms (*bifurcation interval*). The dog had bimodal beat distribution during sleep with slower rates and greater variability than during active hours that showed singular interval distributions, higher rates and less variability. During sleep, Poincaré plots of the dog had clustered or branched patterns of intervals. A slower rate supported greater parasympathetic modulation with a branched compared to the clustered distribution. Treatment with atropine eliminated the non-linear patterns, while hydromorphone shifted the bifurcated branching and beat clustering to longer intervals. These results demonstrate the unique non-linear nature of beat-to-beat variability in the dog compared to humans with increases in interval duration (decrease heart rate). These results provoke the possibility that changes are linear with a dominant sympathetic modulation and non-linear with a dominant parasympathetic modulation. The abrupt bifurcation, zone of avoidance and beat-to-beat patterning are concordant with other studies demonstrating the development of exit block from the sinus node with parasympathetic modulation influencing not only the oscillation of the pacing cells, but conduction to the atria. Studies are required to associate the *in vivo* sinus node beat patterns identified in this study to the mapping of sinus impulse origin and exit from the sinus node.

Keywords: sinus arrhythmia, heart rate variability, Poincaré plots, Holter monitoring, parasympathetic, sinus node, non-linear, autonomic nervous system

INTRODUCTION

Arising from the normal sinus node the relationship of each beat to that of the next is dependent on the intrinsic characteristics of the pacing cells (Gao et al., 2010; Nicolini et al., 2012; Monfredi et al., 2013; Yaniv et al., 2014a,b; Valente et al., 2018) and the external forces of the autonomic nervous system (Billman, 2011). Recent studies reveal that the stochastic (unpredictable) (Yaniv et al., 2014b) and chaotic (deterministic) (Nicolini et al., 2012; Yaniv et al., 2014b; Zhang et al., 2015) mechanisms that regulate the beating heart are caused by the complexity of structure (Fedorov et al., 2009; Ambrosi et al., 2012) and function of the sinus node in both the dog and human (Fedorov et al., 2009, 2010, 2012; Glukhov et al., 2013; Csepe et al., 2016; Kalyanasundaram et al., 2019). The sinus node is not simply a cluster of the most rapidly depolarizing cells of the heart. Instead, it is a central core surrounded by a transitional region of specialized cells, fibrous tissue, and atrial myocytes. After spontaneous depolarization a sinus impulse traverses specialized conduction pathways to depolarize the atria (Kalyanasundaram et al., 2019). The rhythm so recognized in the dog of sinus arrhythmia results from dynamic inputs of sympathetic and parasympathetic systems triggered by a combination of central medullary influences, cardiovascular reflexes, and mechanics of respiration (Boineau et al., 1980; Goldberger et al., 1994; Roossien et al., 1997; Brodde et al., 1998; Yasuma and Hayano, 2004; Billman, 2011, 2013; Krohova et al., 2018).

Long-term electrocardiographic (Holter) recordings have permitted the appraisal of rhythm during variation of autonomic input throughout the day. Time, (Malik et al., 1996; Shaffer and Ginsberg, 2017) frequency, (Csepe et al., 2016) and geometric (tachograms, histograms, Poincaré plots) (Esperer et al., 2008; Khandoker et al., 2013; Borracci et al., 2018) domain indices are often used in the assessment of heart rate (sinus) variability (Malik et al., 1996; Billman, 2011; Billman et al., 2015b; Shaffer and Ginsberg, 2017). Furthermore, to understand better the complexity of biophysical oscillators like the sinus node, advanced methods have been developed to analyze heart rate variability such as measures of fractal-like behavior (long-term analysis), detrended fluctuation (Stein et al., 2005) (short-term analysis), disorder (approximate and sample entropy), non-linear dynamical systems (multiscale Poincaré plots) (Henriques et al., 2015; Shaffer and Ginsberg, 2017) and chaotic behavior (Nicolini et al., 2012; Sassi et al., 2015; Zhang et al., 2015; Behar et al., 2018b; Valente et al., 2018).

The dog and human exhibit sinus arrhythmia; however, the variation between beat intervals is greater in the dog (Behar et al., 2018a,b; Kalyanasundaram et al., 2019). The complexity and mechanism for the dramatic variation in the beat intervals so unique to the dog is explained inadequately. The explanation of high parasympathetic tone does not elucidate the underlying mechanism for the variation, nor does it explain the different patterns of sinus arrhythmia commonly identified on the canine electrocardiogram. The integration of G-protein coupled receptors that with activation reduce the heart rate and regulators of G-protein signaling that attenuate the parasympathetic signaling acting through M2 muscarinic and adenosine receptors that control ion channels responsible for the autorhythmic depolarization of the sinus node cells (Mighiu and Heximer, 2012) is key in the dog with normal or abnormal sinus node function.

We, and others, have observed the unique beat patterning of changes in heart rate in the dog using geometric heart rate variability (Moïse et al., 2010; Gladuli et al., 2011; Blake et al., 2018). However, as the heart rhythm is non-stationary and two-dimensional methods do not permit thorough examination, expanded techniques are required to understand the dynamics of heart rate variability. In the observational portion of the study herein, we used new methodologies (three-dimensional tachograms, dynamic Poincaré plots, three-dimensional histographic Poincaré plots) to glean new insights into our understanding of sinus arrhythmia in the dog as it compares to the human. Our observations led to the following hypotheses. We hypothesized that our new methods to examine beat-to-beat dynamics during sinus arrhythmia would reveal a unique non-linear beat patterning in the dog that differed from humans. We hypothesized that particular beat patterning of sinus arrhythmia is associated with different levels of parasympathetic input as indirectly reflected by indices of heart rate variability and through studies in the dog whereby parasympatholytic and parasympathomimetic drugs altered the beat-to-beat patterns. We further hypothesized that the rate at which the beat-to-beat interval in the dog deviates from a linear slowing (bifurcation interval) approximates the intrinsic rate of oscillation of the canine sinus node. Finally, from our data on 130 dogs and 40 humans with clinically normal sinus node function, we propose hypotheses for future studies concerning the mechanistic difference in the patterning of sinus arrhythmia between these two species.

MATERIALS AND METHODS

Human Holter Recording Database

The 24-h ambulatory ECG recordings (Holter recordings) from 200 healthy adult humans were accessed from the Telemetric and Holter ECG Warehouse (THEW) maintained by the University of Rochester Medical Center, Rochester, NY, United States. Permission to use these data was approved by the review board after submission of proposal for use via http://www.thew-project.org/. Reasons for performing the Holter recordings were not given for this database. The enrollment criteria for selection from this data set included the following: no overt cardiovascular disease, no history of cardiovascular disease, no systemic hypertension or chronic illnesses, adults > 18-years of age, normal physical examination, no medications that would interfere with sinus rate, normal echocardiographic examination, no pregnancy, no diagnosis of sinus node dysfunction, no sinus

Abbreviations: RMSSD, square root of the mean squared successive interval differences; R–R intervals or beat-to-beat intervals, duration between two QRS complexes (R–R intervals or beat-to-beat intervals) and verified surrogate for P–P intervals for this study; SACP, sinoatrial conduction pathways; SDANN, standard deviation of all 5-min beat interval means; SDNN, Standard deviation of all beat intervals; SDNNIn, mean of all 5-min beat interval standard deviations (index).

pauses > 2500 ms, < 3.0% or < 4000 ventricular ectopic complexes, < 0.25% atrial ectopic complexes and no abnormal symptoms during Holter recording. It is noted that the only difference in the criteria between the human and dog concerns the duration of sinus pauses. None of the humans had pause durations > 2500 ms. However, this is a common finding in the dog. The goal of these criteria was not to select recordings devoid of any abnormalities, but to select those for which sinus node function was deemed normal and the presence of arrhythmias not of clinical importance.

Canine Holter Recording Database

Holter recordings of dogs were retrieved from the database of the Section of Cardiology Holter Laboratory at the College of Veterinary Medicine, Cornell University, Ithaca, NY, United States (analyzing canine recordings since 1988). A database of > 5000 Holter recordings between 2009 and 2014 was examined to identify only those performed using Forest Medical Holter recorders (Trillium 5000/5900) (Syracuse, NY, United States). Each recording was required to have a minimum of 22 h with 99% artifact free data. All recordings were from clinical patients. Recordings in these dogs were performed to screen for arrhythmias, to determine if suspected arrhythmias identified by either auscultation or during electrocardiographic monitoring were of clinical importance, or to investigate cause of syncope or seizure. Recordings were selected only if sinus node function was determined to be normal. The enrollment criteria for this data set included the following: no overt cardiovascular disease (including myocardial failure or congestive heart failure), no systemic diseases, adult dog > 1-year of age, no physical abnormalities that would affect sinus rate, no medications that would influence sinus rate, no pregnancy, no diagnosis of sinus node dysfunction, no sinus pauses > 5500 ms, no more than 3 pauses > 4000 ms, < 3.0% or < 4000 ventricular ectopic complexes, < 0.25% atrial ectopic complexes and no abnormal clinical signs during Holter recording. Additionally, any Holters that had evidence of vasovagal reflex or Bezold-Jarisch reflex in association with a history of syncope were excluded. Therefore, the goal of these criteria was not to select recordings devoid of any abnormalities (so that aged dogs could be included), but to select those for which sinus node function was deemed normal and the presence of arrhythmias not of clinical importance. Clinical sinus node dysfunction in the dog is characterized by an average heart rate < 60 bpm, minimum heart rate < 30 bpm, time with heart rate < 50 bpm > 350 min, number of pauses > 2 s > 1500, longest sinus pause > 5500 ms and > 3 pauses > 4 s. All 24-h electrocardiographic recordings were performed with the dogs in the home environment.

Owners were given a detailed diary form to complete so that sleep-wake cycles could be documented. The Forest Medical Holter recorders (Trillium® 5000/5900) provide 256 Hz sampling frequency signals (4 ms time resolution) with 8-bit amplitude resolution (5 μV amplitude resolution). Leads were positioned for a 3-lead modified orthogonal X, Y, Z configuration. After downloading the raw data, a technician trained in cardiac rhythm and Holter analysis edited the recordings. All recordings were then over-read by a veterinary cardiologist (NSM) to ensure > 99% accuracy for the identification and classification of P and QRS waves given the importance for heart rate variability analysis (Peltola, 2012). It is emphasized that a veterinary cardiologist with extensive experience in the analysis of canine electrocardiographic recordings reviewed all electrocardiograms to ensure that identified complexes were sinus in origin and not atrial premature complexes. Others unfamiliar with the rhythms of the dog mistakenly identify normal sinus beats as atrial premature complexes because of the prominent sinus arrhythmia. To implement these analyses, software from Forest Medical (Trillium®), was used for the QRS detection, beat annotations, time domain and frequency domain heart rate variability. Additionally, Forest Medical permitted access to the raw data (R–R intervals and annotations) for the development of additional software (WHF).

Sinus Rate Determination

For both the human and canine recordings, the files were examined to ensure that the R–R intervals represented the P–P intervals. Throughout this manuscript the term R–R interval will be used as a surrogate for P–P interval. When referring to the relationship between an R–R interval and the next, the term beat-to-beat interval will be used. Any recordings with atrioventricular conduction block, QRS complexes not preceded by a P wave (e.g., junctional origin) or any other arrhythmias that would be annotated as a normal complex, were not included in the analyses for the assessment of sinus node rate and rhythm. Descriptive data for sinus rate were determined including the average, minimum and maximum rate, time with rate < 50 bpm, time with rate > 120 bpm, number of pauses > 2 s and the longest pause. The density of specific R–R intervals was shown as histograms for each hour and summed for the full 24-h. Additionally, heart rate over time was graphically displayed across time with heart rate tachograms and two- and three-dimensional R–R interval tachograms. On the heart rate tachogram the rolling eight-beat average rate was shown between the minimum and maximum rate for each segment. The two-dimensional tachogram plotted the R–R interval for each hour and over 24-h. Importantly, because each recording contained approximately 100,000 data points, an overlay of points did not permit an appreciation of interval density (number of intervals with same or similar values inadequately identified) and this prompted the development of customized software (WHF).

Heart Rate Variability Analyses

Based on the guidelines for heart rate variability analysis time, (Malik et al., 1996; Shaffer and Ginsberg, 2017) frequency, and geometric domain analyses were performed (Trillium®). Time domain methods included (1) estimate of overall heart rate variability using standard deviation of all beats (SDNN), (2) estimate of long-term components of heart rate variability using standard deviation of all 5-min beat interval means (SDANN) and (3) cycles shorter than 5 min were assessed by the mean of all 5-min beat interval standard deviations (SDNNIn), (4) estimate of short-term components of heart rate variability using the square root of the mean squared successive interval differences

TABLE 1 | Heart rate and heart rate variability comparisons.

(A) Comparisons of populations and 24-h heart rate characteristics boxer versus non-boxer (31 other dog breeds represented). Data shown as median (range) and *p*-value from Wilcoxon Test with Bonferroni correction.

Parameter	Boxer (n = 69)	Non-boxer (n = 61)	p-value
Age	5 (1–12)	9 (1.5–16)	<0.0001
Weight (kg)	27 (16–38)	15 (4–61)	<0.0001
Heart rate (bpm)	81 (66–112)	82 (64–119)	1.0
Minimum heart rate (bpm)	40 (29–59)	41 (32–69)	1.0
Maximum heart rate (bpm)	240 (182–333)	236 (163–301)	1.0
Heart rate < 50 (min)	27 (0–312)	3 (0–432)	1.0
Heart rate > 120 (min)	102 (16–444)	90 (0–726)	1.0
Longest pause (s)	3.2 (2–5.5)	2.6 (0–5.5)	<0.001
Number of pauses > 2 s	157 (2–2737)	40 (0–2082)	<0.001

(B) Comparisons of 24-h heart rate dog versus human heart rate. Data shown as median (range) and *p*-value from Wilcoxon Test with Bonferroni correction.

	Dog (n = 130)	Human (n = 40)	p-value
Heart rate (bpm)	81 (64–119)	74.5 (59–103)	0.005
Minimum heart rate (bpm)	41 (29–69)	51 (34–67)	<0.001
Maximum heart rate (bpm)	236 (163–333)	132 (98–187)	<0.001

(C) Comparisons of 24-h time domain heart rate variability between boxers, non-boxers, and humans. Heart rate variability parameters corrected for heart rate (see text). Data shown are mean and standard deviation. Groups with letter (a–c) in common are not different from each other at $p > 0.05$.

	Boxer (n = 69)	Non-boxer (n = 61)	Human (n = 40)
SDNN (ms)	0.457 (0.056)[a]	0.396 (0.008)[b]	0.176 (0.010)[c]
SDANNIn (ms)	0.376 (0.054)[a]	0.314 (0.079)[b]	0.077 (0.022)[c]
SDANN (ms)	0.249 (0.046)[a]	0.215 (0.068)[b]	0.157 (0.048)[c]
RMSSD (ms)	0.475 (0.075)[a]	0.412 (0.132)[b]	0.045 (0.021)[c]

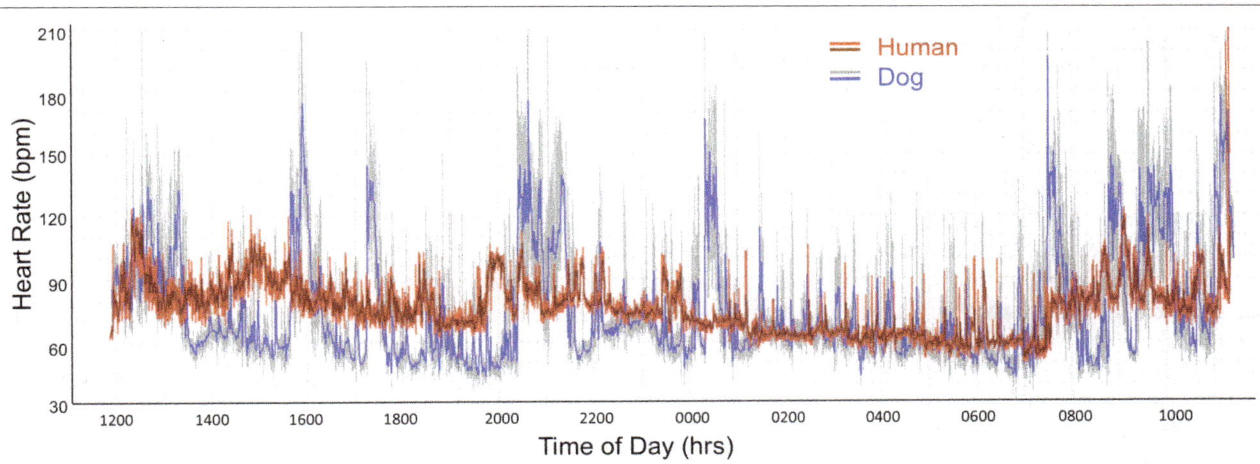

FIGURE 1 | Heart rate tachogram from a human (red/magenta) and dog (gray/blue). The representative patterns exhibited in these two subjects were similar to all. The tachogram shows the heart rate over the course of a 24-h day. The inner magenta (human) and blue (dog) colors indicate the average heart rate as determined by a rolling average of 8 beats. The red (human) and gray (dog) colors indicate the maximum and minimum heart rate during that time. Between the hours of 0100 and 0730 a nocturnal dip (slowing of heart rate) is seen in both the human and dog. In the dog other periods have a similar heart rate slowing associated with sleep as indicated by the diary kept by the owners. The dog has a wider range of heart rates. From the two-dimensional heart rate tachogram the beat-to-beat distribution cannot be determined.

(RMSSD). The frequency domain parameters analyzed were total power and high frequency. For the frequency domain analyses a window of 512 beats with a Hamming filter applied was used. Total power density was determined with frequencies < 0.4 Hz and high frequency was in the range of 0.15–0.4 Hz. During the hour-windows of the frequency analysis, the 512 beat window

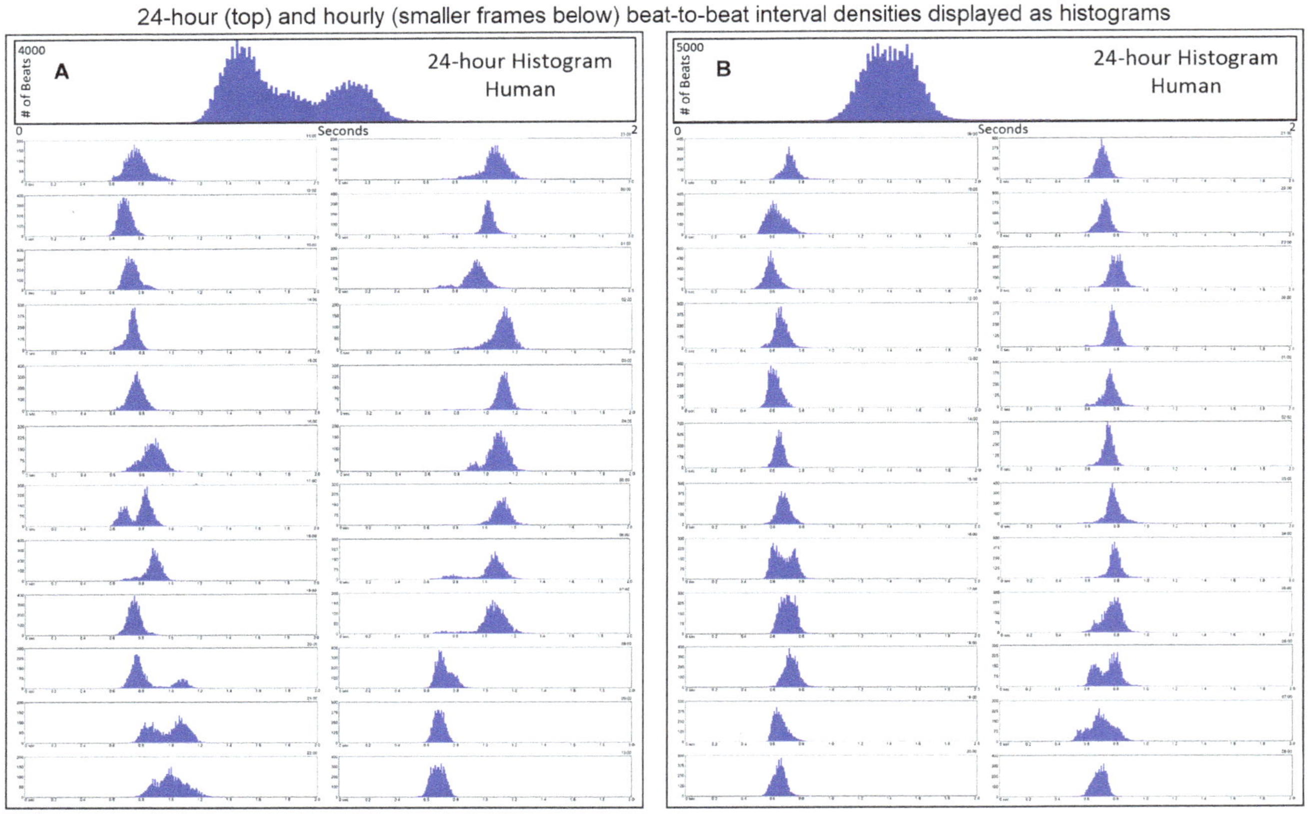

FIGURE 2 | R–R interval histograms from 24-h ECG recordings from two different humans. All of the human R–R interval histograms were either similar to these two individuals or a mixture of these two types of distributions. The top expanded frame is the summation of all R–R intervals over the 24 h. Note the different density distribution of R–R intervals (thus, heart rates) in these two individuals. The individual in frame **(A)** has more time at longer R–R intervals compared to the individual in frame **(B)**. Below the 24-h summary frames the corresponding 1-h histograms for each individual are shown. The summation of these 24 single 1-h histograms form the composite shown at the top for each individual. In general, depending on physiologic needs, the heart rate over a 1-h period primarily has a Gaussian-shaped distribution. Some hours have more than one Gaussian-shaped distribution. This type of distribution exists likely because the heart rate decreases and increases linearly.

was initially selected at the midpoint in the hour so long as the average heart rate approximated that of the average for that hour ± 5 bpm. The window was moved from the midpoint before or after until this heart rate was found. During sleep hours with stable rate and rhythm, time and frequency domain parameters were corrected for heart rate. To correct for the mathematical influence of rate on variability, time domain indices were divided by the average interval of the examined period and frequency domain indices were divided by the square of the average interval in seconds (Sacha and Pluta, 2008; Billman, 2013; Sacha et al., 2013; Billman et al., 2015b).

Beat-to-Beat and Three-Dimensional Analyses

All Holter recordings were examined using geometric domain heart rate variability to identify beat-to-beat patterns. Two-dimensional Poincaré plots were constructed for each hour and 24-h by plotting an R–R interval on the x-axis and the next interval (R–R + 1 interval) on the y-axis. In order to examine the beat-to-beat patterning it was necessary to create the ability to select periods for analysis such as hours of activity or stable sleep hour, while also having the ability to visualize the formation of the Poincaré plots in two and three-dimensions. Therefore, advanced geometric domain analyses including dynamic Poincaré plots, three-dimensional histographic Poincaré and three-dimensional R–R interval tachograms were developed by one of us (WHF) using JavaScript HTML and GLSL[1,2], after integration with the time series R–R intervals. Three-dimensional histographic Poincaré plots were generated by sorting the interval data and logarithmically adding onto a GPU based on different regions. A user interface was developed for a web-based amalgamation to permit interval and time selection. The dynamic Poincaré plots were used to specifically follow the patterns during acceleration and slowing of the heart rate. Examination of these plots, in addition to the R–R interval tachograms, prompted the development

[1] http://wyattflanders.com/poincare/

[2] http://wyattflanders.com/poincareplot/

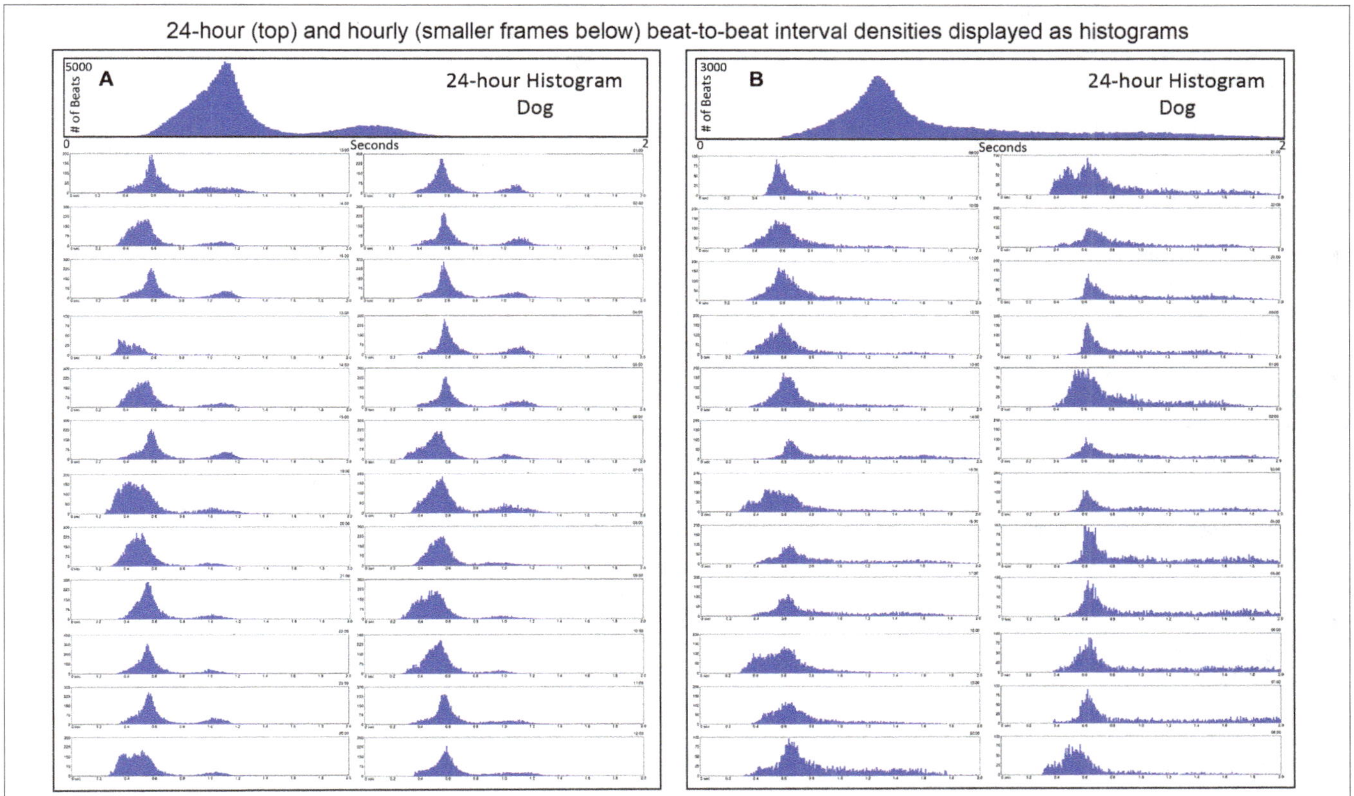

FIGURE 3 | R–R interval histograms from 24-h electrocardiographic recordings from two different dogs. These two dogs represented the basic patterns seen in all dogs. The top expanded frame is the summation of all R–R intervals over the 24-h. Note the different density distribution of R–R intervals (thus, heart rates) in these two examples. Below the 24-h summary frames, the corresponding single 1-h histograms for each dog are shown. The summation of these 24 single 1-h histograms form the composite shown at the top for each dog. Note the more complicated beat distribution of the dog when compared to the human. Dog **(A)** tends to have different distributions within a given hour. Shorter R–R intervals (more leftward distribution) tend to merge with the dominant distribution centered at approximately 550 ms (109 bpm) with a paucity of beats centered at approximately 800 ms (75 bpm). A small number of beats (but not time spent at these intervals) with the distribution centered at approximately 1050 ms (57 bpm) is seen. Dog **(B)** has a dominant distribution of R–R intervals centered at 600 ms (100 bpm) with a tail of more diffusely distributed long R–R intervals. Dog **(A)** was a boxer and dog **(B)** a Doberman pincher.

of pattern classification that then led to further analyses and comparisons.

(1) Regions with a paucity (also coined as a 'zone of avoidance') (Moïse et al., 2010) of R–R intervals seen on the tachograms and beat-to-beat intervals seen on the Poincaré plots.
(2) Regions with clustered beat-to-beat intervals (defined as discontinuous and isolated intervals on the Poincaré plots coupled with dense banding separated by a paucity of R–R intervals on the tachogram and bimodal distribution on histograms) (13 boxers/12 non-boxers).
(3) Regions with branched beat-to-beat intervals (defined as continuous intervals on the Poincaré plots coupled with broad spreading of R–R intervals on the tachogram and rightward-skewed distribution on histograms) (13 boxers/12 non-boxers).
(4) R–R interval bifurcation (this interval determined as the average of the three shortest intervals during a stable sleep hour in 25 boxers and 25 non-boxers).

Parasympatholytic and Parasympathomimetic Drug Effects

The findings of beat patterning during spontaneous sinus rhythm in the dog strongly suggested the influence of the parasympathetic nervous system. After approval from the Institutional Animal Care and Use Committee, 8 beagles had 24-h electrocardiographic recordings to assess the geometric beat-to-beat patterning as influenced by parasympatholytic and parasympathomimetic agents. Atropine (0.04 mg/kg intravenously) and hydromorphone (0.2 mg/kg intravenously) were administered on separate days after a baseline recording was obtained. Regions of the recordings associated with these treatments were analyzed for beat-to-beat patterns. The corresponding time of the baseline recording served as the control period.

Statistical Analysis

The following comparisons were made (1) 24-h data for boxer dog breed, non-boxer breeds and human (2) hour for all dogs with bimodal versus singular interval density, and (3) stable

TABLE 2 | Comparisons of bimodal versus singular histogram distributions within dog and clustered versus branched beat-to-beat interval patterns between dogs.

(A) Within dog (n = 128) (paired data) comparison of an hour with a large paucity of beats resulting in a bimodal distribution and an hour with a small paucity of beats characterized as a single distribution. Heart rate variability parameters corrected for heart rate (see text). Data shown as median (range) and p-value from Wilcoxon Signed Rank Test with Bonferroni correction.

Parameter	Bimodal	Singular	p-value
Average heart rate (bpm)	68 (50–130)	110 (75–163)	<0.001
Beat-to-beat interval (ms)	882 (462–1200)	546 (368–800)	<0.001
Minimum heart rate (bpm)	48 (32–139)	69 (34–108)	<0.001
Maximum heart rate (bpm)	147 (80–236)	199 (123–313)	<0.001
SDNN (ms)	0.38 (0.22–0.58)	0.27 (0.07–1.35)	<0.001
SDANNIn (ms)	0.34 (0.15–0.49)	0.20 (0.05–0.55)	<0.001
SDANN (ms)	0.11 (0.03–0.50)	0.16 (0.03–0.59)	0.032
RMSSD (ms)	0.47 (0.18–0.69)	0.24 (0.04–0.57)	<0.001
Frequency domain total power (ms^2)	24486 (1379–66913)	4493 (335–31063)	<0.001
Frequency domain HRV-HF (ms^2)	19311 (33–59924)	312 (14–10770)	<0.001

(B) Comparison of beat patterning (clustered versus branched) during a single sleep hour in 50 dogs (13/12 boxers/non-boxers each group). Heart rate variability parameters corrected for rate/interval (see text). Data shown as median (range) and p-value from Wilcoxon Test with Bonferroni correction.

	Clustered (n = 25)	Branched (n = 25)	p-value
Average heart rate (bpm)	71 (57–93)	54 (46–92)	<0.001
Beat-to-beat interval (ms)	845 (645–1053)	1111 (652–1304)	<0.001
Minimum heart rate (bpm)	55 (42–68)	41 (34–71)	<0.001
Maximum heart rate (bpm)	144 (103–196)	137 (112–174)	0.99
Number of pauses	1 (0–16)	24 (0–374)	0.006
SDNN (ms)	0.349 (0.156–0.468)	0.409 (0.273–0.467)	0.008
SDANNIn (ms)	0.312 (0.128–0.424)	0.369 (0.245–0.426)	0.02
SDANN (ms)	0.099 (0.049–0.205)	0.118 (0.038–0.226)	0.36
RMSSD (ms)	0.477 (0.167–0.619)	0.481 (0.373–0.686)	0.99
Frequency domain total power (ms^2)	19036 (6352–59061)	33541 (11492–86423)	<0.001
Frequency domain HRV-HF (ms^2)	15856 (4107–55894)	19741 (5205–44501)	0.2

sleep hour with clustered versus branched interval distribution in the dogs. Additionally, the bifurcation interval in the dog was examined relative to age, average heart rate and time domain indices of heart rate variability SDNN (the latter after correction for heart rate). Distribution of all continuous variables was assessed for normality. Difference between groups for variables with normal distribution were analyzed using a t-test and data is presented as mean and standard deviation. Differences between those variables showing a non-normal distribution were analyzed with non-parametric methods (Wilcoxon Rank Sum test, also called Mann–Whitney-Test) and data is presented as median and range. Adjustments for p-values controlling for multiple comparisons was done using Bonferroni correction. The relationship between variables of heart rate and heart rate variability with age for each group (boxers, non-boxers, and humans) was examined by a regression analysis with slopes and standard error reported. Differences in the time domain parameters between these groups was tested with a one-way ANOVA followed with a *post hoc* multiple comparisons with Tukey correction. Differences between groups for categorical variables were tested using Fisher's exact test. Differences for paired data (singular/bimodal distribution) within a category (boxer, non-boxer) were achieved with paired data non-parametric Wilcoxon Signed Rank test. Correlation between continuous variables was explored by using Pearson correlation for parametric data and Spearman for non-parametric. To determine relationship bivariate analysis was performed for specific variables. All analyses were performed in JMP (v.12.0.1 and v. 14.0.0, SAS Institute, Cary, NC, United States).

RESULTS

Human and Canine Holter Recordings

After review of recordings in THEW, Holter recordings from 40 humans were studied that met the criteria. It is noted that none of the reviewed recordings in the bank had pauses > 2.5 s. Equal numbers of males and females were included with a median age of 41.7 years (range 18–80 years). Holter recordings from 130 dogs were studied. Canine recordings included 69 boxers (41 females/28 males) and 61 (32 females/29 males) non-boxers (no difference in sex distribution; p-value = 0.32). Of the 61 non-boxers, 31 different breeds were represented. Those with more than one dog per breed included eight mixed breed, six Shi Tzu, four Labrador retrievers, four miniature schnauzers, three great Danes, three Doberman pinschers, and two dachshunds. Boxers were overrepresented

Still frame dynamic 2-dimensional Poincaré plots of 5 humans and 5 dogs as rate slows

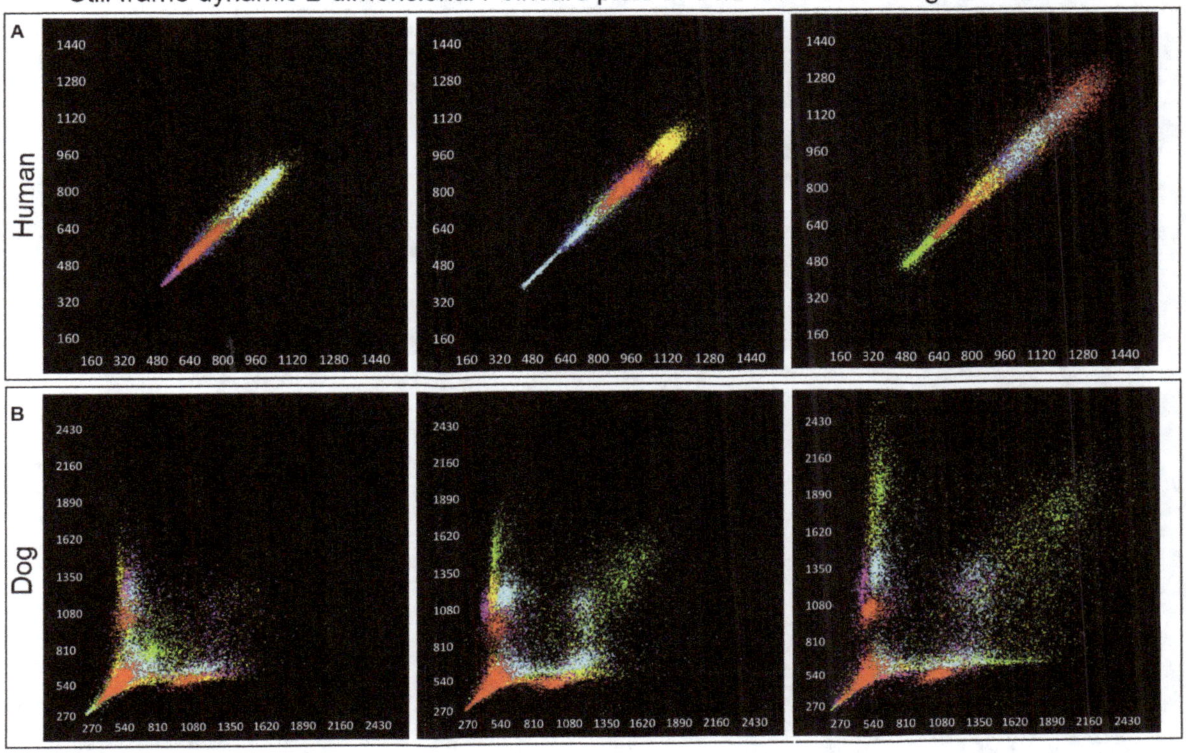

FIGURE 6 | (**Supplementary Videos 1, 2**) Examination that is limited to still frames of two-dimensional geometric heart rate variability restricts understanding of the beat-to-beat dynamics. Here, frames captured from dynamic/animated two-dimensional Poincaré plots of five humans **(A)** and five dogs **(B)** provide the ability to examine heart rate dynamics in the human and dog.http://wyattflanders.com/poincare/ Each individual dog or human is represented by a different color. The R–R interval (X axis) and R–R + 1 interval (Y-axis) (intervals are in 'ms') are plotted with the ability to change the number of intervals represented (for clarity, labeling for these axes is omitted). The associated videos (**Supplementary Videos 1, 2**) for these frames illustrate the difference between the dog and human concerning the beat-to-beat increasing and decreasing of heart rate and associated beat-to-beat changes. In the human, these changes occur primarily along the line of identity (diagonal line from lower left corner to upper right corner). In the dog as the beat-to-beat intervals increase they do so along the line of identity until approximately 600 ms when a bifurcation develops resulting in two 'branches' or 'clusters' along the X and Y axes. In the dog, a paucity of beats is noted for certain beat-to-beat intervals (zone of avoidance). The latter will not be evident if an excessive number of beats are shown. Additionally, some dogs develop a 'cloud' of long–long R–R intervals with an upper border along the line of identity. These videos can also have lines added and the speed adjusted so that the exact beat-to-beat interval relationships are seen (see **Figure 8** and **Supplementary Videos 3–6**). **Supplementary Videos 1, 2** correspond with this figure.

R–R Interval Tachograms Human Versus Dog

R–R interval tachograms showed consistent differences between humans and dogs (**Figures 4, 5**). The patterns shown in these figures represent those that were seen for all subjects. Each dot represents an R–R interval. Tachograms in humans had the appearance of a narrow band that would move up and down as the intervals lengthened and shortened (**Figure 4**). In contrast, the patterns in dogs were more complex. Three general features characterized the tachograms of the dogs (**Figure 5**):

(1) Broader spread of longer intervals. This region of longer intervals varied in its spread between dogs or within dog depending on the wake-sleep cycle. The greatest spread occurred during documented sleep.
(2) Regions of lower beat density (infrequent R–R intervals) that looked like a 'white-band' separating shorter and longer R–R intervals. Often this low beat density band was consistent over the day (this region identified as the zone of avoidance). Two general characteristics were noted: (1) low beat density separated by two distinct wide bands of R–R intervals and (2) region of lower beat density with more diffuse band at longer R–R intervals. During times of heart rate change, these banding characteristics were less distinct.
(3) A denser region of shorter R–R intervals that appeared as a 'dark-band' that also was consistent over the day. This band tended to have the appearance of a 'line' demarcating the shortest intervals. Shorter intervals did interrupt this 'line' and correlated with abrupt increases in heart rate (shorter intervals), and often associated with artifact indicating body movement (exercise/excitement).

Beat-to-Beat Analyses: Poincaré Plots

Two-Dimensional Poincaré Plots

To gain a better understanding of the unique patterns identified in the dog when compared to the human, beat-to-beat analyses were performed. As shown in **Figures 4, 5**, the two-dimensional

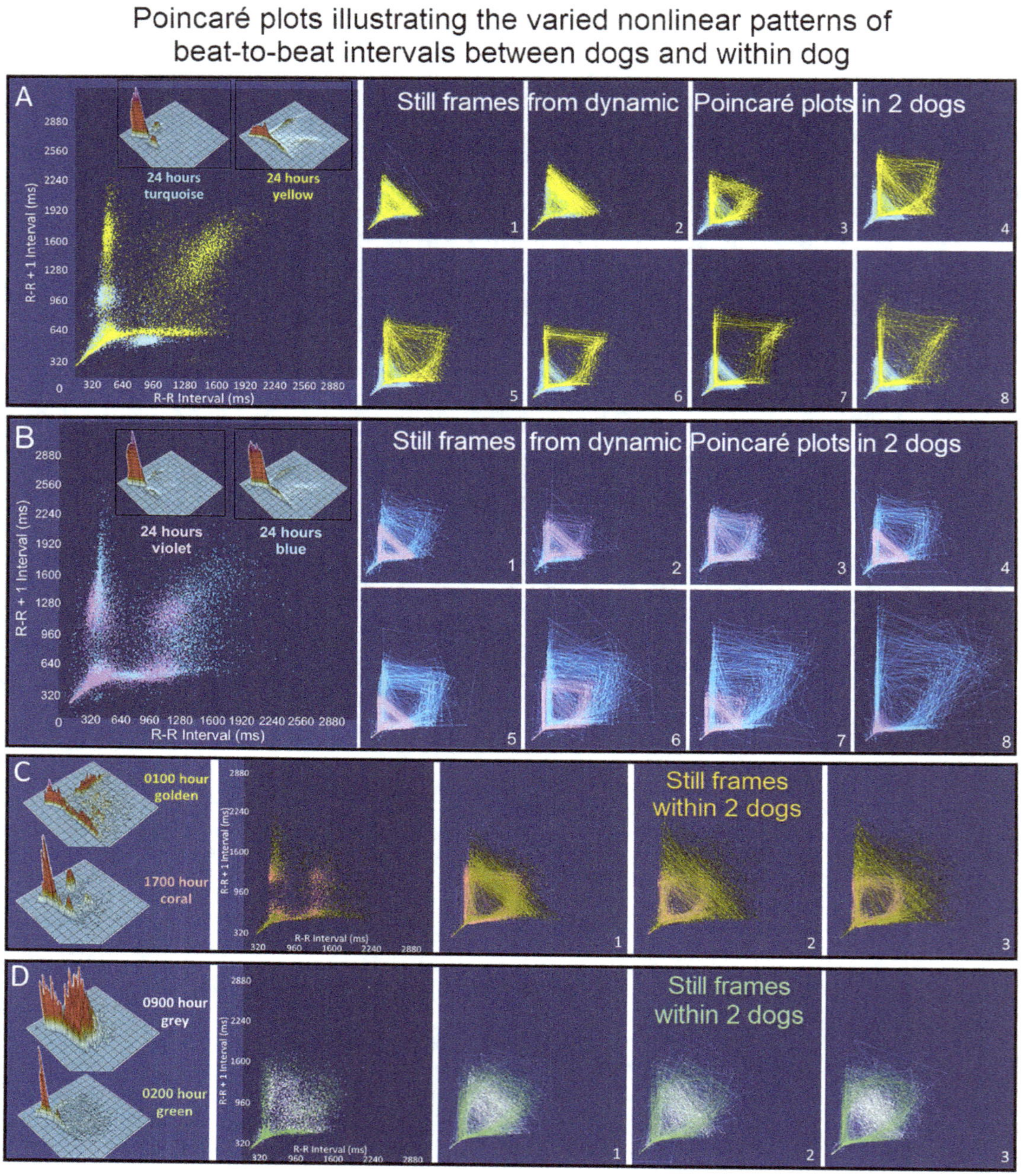

FIGURE 7 | (**Supplementary Videos 3–6**) Still frames from dynamic Poincaré plots (http://wyattflanders.com/poincareplot/) of six different dogs demonstrate the varied R–R interval patterns between dogs (frames **A,B**) and within dogs (frames **C,D**). In frames **(A,B)** large Poincaré plots without connecting lines contain 10,000 beat intervals and above this plot, the corresponding three-dimensional histographic Poincaré plots of the entire 24-h are shown. Below the three-dimensional histographic plots, a color code is stated for that dog that corresponds with the animated Poincaré plot in this figure and in the accompanying **Supplementary Videos**. To the right of this panel, from the dynamic two-dimensional Poincaré plots still frames of 1000 intervals with lines, the beat-to-beat relationships are presented. The still frames were captured at different time points during 24-h electrocardiographic recordings (Frames **1–8**). In frame **(A)**, the dog in aqua (boxer) has a clustered pattern with no long–long intervals while the dog in yellow (small mixed-breed) has a long-branched pattern with a long–long R–R interval cloud. Compare the beat density of the dog in yellow (Frame **A**) to the dog in blue (Frame **B**). In frame **(B)** a boxer with a clustered pattern (color violet) also has the central cloud of long–long intervals. The Doberman pinscher in blue shows a large variation in long–long intervals. Frames **(C,D)** illustrate the varied patterns within dog. The hour of the day and color representing that hour for the dynamic Poincaré plots are indicated to the right of the three-dimensional histographic Poincaré plot for each dog. The pattern of sinus arrhythmia can change over time with varying autonomic input. This also shows that if the entire 24 h is considered at one time the true dynamics of the interval relationships can be masked. The dog in frame **(C)** (boxer) during the sleep hour 0100 (golden) has a 'branched' pattern with slower rates; however, a more clustered pattern with faster rate is identified during an hour of wakefulness (coral). The dog in frame **(C)** (Wheaton Terrier) during the 0900 h (gray) was noted to have wide swings in heart rate associated with different activities as documented in the diary. This resulted in many transitions of rate with a more dense pattern; however, during the sleep hour (green) a different pattern was identified with the zone of avoidance evident. **Supplementary Videos 3–6** provided with this figure.

Comparison in dogs of singular, clustered and branched beat-to-beat interval distributions as identified by histograms, tachograms and Poincaré plots

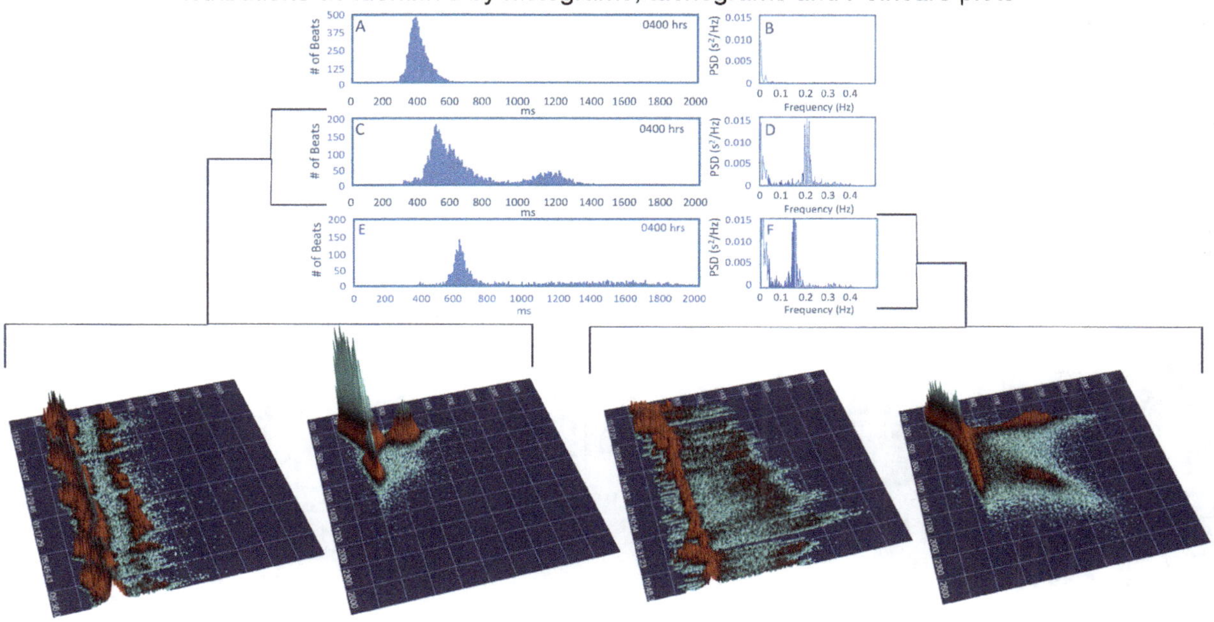

FIGURE 8 | To assist in understanding some of the geometric patterns identified in the dog analyses were performed after visual inspection to categorize major beat-to-beat patterns. Initially, the hourly R–R interval histograms were inspected to identify those with a single Gaussian-shaped distributions and those with two or more distributions apparent that also had a region with a paucity of beats (Frames **A,C,E**). Statistics regarding time domain and frequency domain characteristics are provided in **Table 2**. In this figure, examples of the two-dimensional histogram and corresponding power spectrum/frequency domain profile of heart rate variability (Frames **B,D,F**) are shown. The three-dimensional R–R interval tachograms and histographic Poincaré plots for the two different dogs shown in frames **(C,D)** and frames **(E,F)** are bracketed below. Each of these dogs was a boxer.

Poincaré plots of the human and dog are distinctly different. In the human, as the heart rate changes with shorter to longer intervals the beat-to-beat changes occur along the line of identity of the Poincaré plot. In **Figure 4D** a three-dimensional histographic Poincaré plot more clearly illustrates the beat-to-beat distribution along the line of identity and the three-dimensional tachogram shows the change in beat intervals throughout the day. Importantly, is the notation that these graphs show number intervals; however, this does not give a representation of the amount of time and at shorter versus longer intervals. That is, the lower density of the longer intervals should not be interpreted as minimal or infrequent because the 'time spent' may be greater. In contrast, two-dimensional Poincaré plots in the dog (**Figure 5**) illustrate that beat intervals occur along the line of identity until a point at which a bifurcation occurs resulting in a wide spread corresponding to long–short and short–long intervals. In the dog, two-dimensional Poincaré plots could be described as branched or clustered (see section "Materials and Methods") with a paucity of interval beats of varying degree. Because these plots were a summation of the entire 24-h, it was necessary to examine shorter times to understand the formation of these patterns.

Dynamic Poincaré Plots

Dynamic (animated) Poincaré plots were developed to examine both human and canine data sets (**Figure 6** and **Supplementary Videos 1, 2**). This new methodology illustrated the difference in the increasing and decreasing of heart rate on a beat-to-beat basis between the human and dog. Humans consistently changed rate in a linear fashion, but dogs had a visual bifurcation at a relatively stable point on the graph. However, the spread of beat intervals after the bifurcation point differed amongst the dogs (**Figures 7, 8**). Examination of individual hours with lines connecting each successive beat interval provided the ability to see the sequence of heartbeat intervals (**Figure 9**). From these data it was apparent that dogs had different patterns after the bifurcation from the consistent shorter intervals (**Figures 7A,B** and **Supplementary Videos 3, 4**). Moreover, an individual dog could have different patterns throughout the day (**Figure 7C** and **Supplementary Videos 5, 6**). The dynamic Poincaré plots with lines illustrating sequence clearly showed the paucity of beats/zone of avoidance for both clustered and branched R–R interval distributions.

Three-Dimensional Tachograms and Histographic Poincaré Plots

Three-dimensional plots revealed a truer representation of beat distributions (**Figures 4, 8**) permitting selection of 25 clustered and 25 branched R–R interval patterns (**Figure 8**). Time domain and frequency domain analyses of heart rate variability revealed slower heart rates and mixed evidence of greater parasympathetic modulation with beat distribution characterized as branched

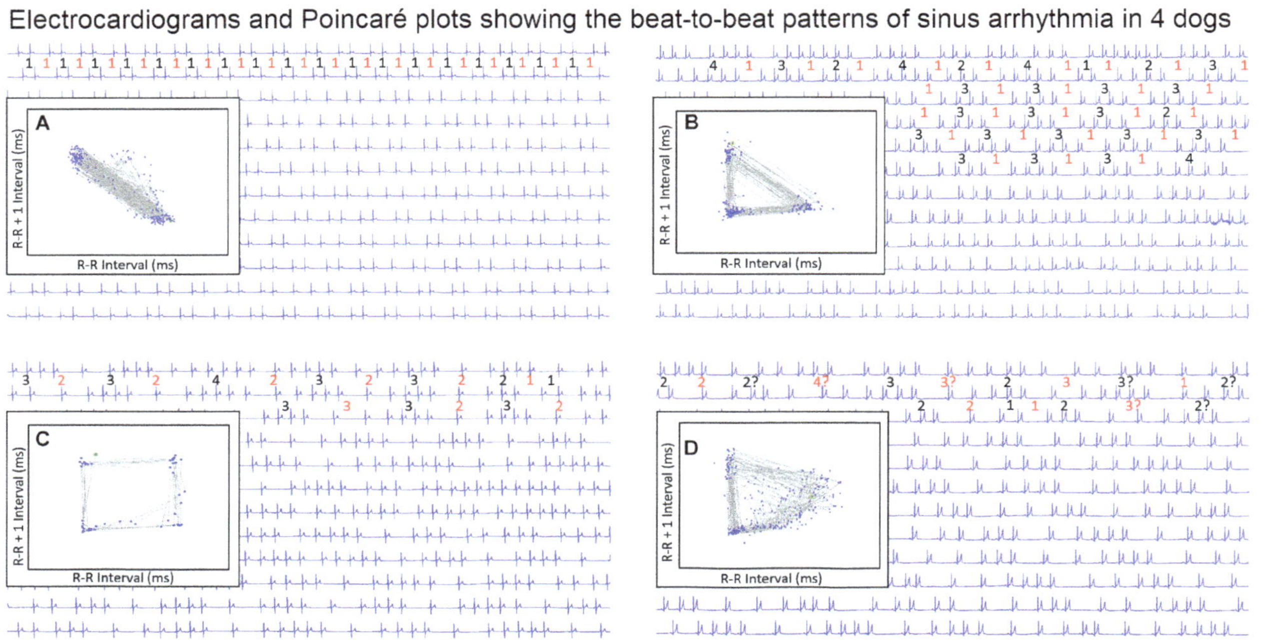

FIGURE 9 | During stable sleep hours, focused intervals were identified on the electrocardiogram and compared to the Poincaré plots. This figure illustrates four common patterns. Each line is 30 s. The inset is the Poincaré plot of the ECG frame shown (for clarity the specific R–R interval in milliseconds is omitted). Frame **(A)** shows the Poincaré plot when the sinus arrhythmia has primarily a ratio of one-short R–R interval to one-long R–R interval. Because there are no consecutive short-short R–R intervals, no clusters of intervals are seen in the lower left region of the Poincaré plot. Frame **(B)** shows the Poincaré plot when the primary ratio is one-long R–R interval to two to four-short R–R intervals. The short-short intervals are in the lower left region and the single long interval between the clusters of short intervals results in a triangular shape (long–short interval followed by short intervals followed by short–long interval). Frame **(C)** shows the pattern when the sinus arrhythmia has primarily two-long R–R intervals with clusters of short intervals. The long–long intervals result in a cloud in the upper right region beginning at the line of identity. The resulting shape is that of a polygon. Frame **(D)** illustrates the shape of the Poincaré plot with more variability in the R–R intervals creating a long–long cloud of intervals. From frame **(D)** the R–R intervals before the speeding of the rate are more variable than the long R–R interval that follows the short sequence. That is, with sinus arrhythmia the long interval after the faster rate is more consistent then the long interval before the faster rate. It is important to note that these examples were taken during a time when each of the dogs was displaying a sinus arrhythmia with presumed high parasympathetic tone and not interrupted by marked increases in sympathetic tone. Without a sympathetic surge note that none of the short-short intervals goes below a specific point. Although for clarity the scale is omitted, this was approximately 600 ms. This corresponds to the limit of the R–R interval seen on the R–R interval tachogram (see **Figure 7** and **Table 3**). For each frame, the numbers in red are long R–R intervals and numbers in black are short R–R intervals. If a '?' follows the number, this indicates that some uncertainty exists concerning the exact number of intervals defined as long or short (e.g., R–R interval duration is medium).

versus clustered (**Figure 8** and **Table 2B**). Beats clustered more with a sequence of short–long intervals. That is, the last beat sequence of short–long intervals was more consistent than that of a long–short interval. When examining these plots it is important to keep in mind that the interval density mathematically will show a greater density for the short intervals rather than the longer intervals, but this does not reflect the 'time' the heart spent at shorter or longer rates.

Electrocardiographic Relationship to Beat-to-Beat Patterns

Beat-to-Beat Pattern With Slowing Heart Rate

To understand the beat patterns identified in the dog the dynamic Poincaré plots were examined in conjunction with visualization of the electrocardiogram. **Figure 9** illustrates this examination of four dogs during a stable sleep hour revealing the differing patterns of sinus arrhythmia and corresponding Poincaré plots. Note that during these stable sleep times with likely low sympathetic input, no short-short R–R intervals along the line of identity are present (compare with **Figures 7**, **8**). However, the bifurcation point is consistent and is identified in the dog when the heart rate slows after a sympathetic stimulation associated with excitement (**Figure 10** and **Supplementary Video 7**). The human heart rate slows linearly throughout the full range of beat intervals; however, although the dog heart slows initially along the line of identity when the heart rate slows to a particular interval, a bifurcation develops. This interval was coined the 'bifurcation interval.' An additional finding from the comparison of the Poincaré plots with the electrocardiogram is the 'cloud' of longer intervals. The cloud associated with long–long (**Figure 5D**) intervals in many dogs formed a mass effect of intervals widely spread around the line of identity.

Bifurcation Interval/Zone

It was noted that amongst dogs the bifurcation interval was visually within a narrow range of beat-to-beat intervals. Moreover, this bifurcation interval or zone corresponded

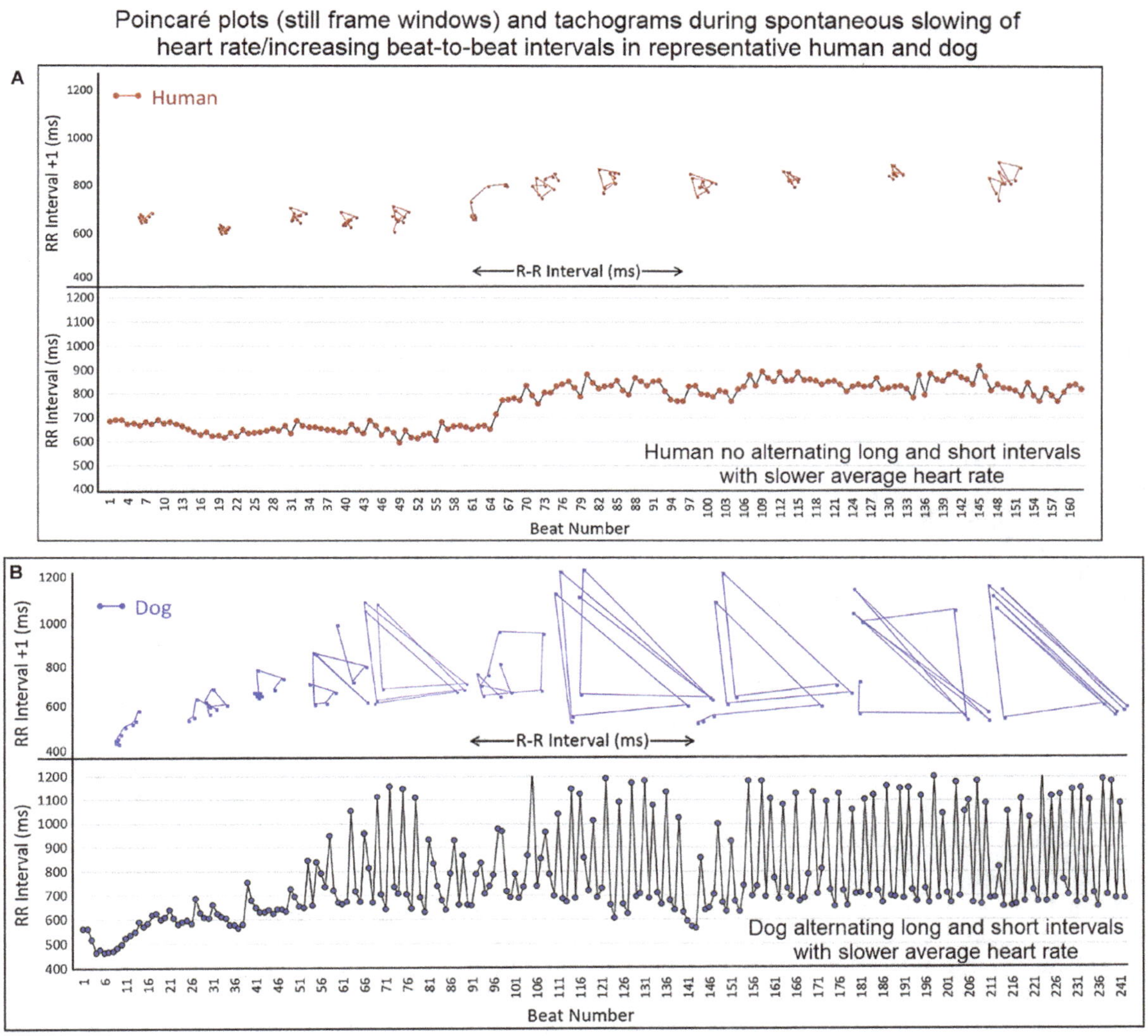

FIGURE 10 | (Supplementary Video 7) This figure illustrates the slowing of the sinus rhythm in the human and dog. As the human sinus node slows the beat-to-beat variation is confined along the line of identity (Frame **A**). As the dog sinus node slows (Frame **B**), the rate slows along the line of identity, just as in the human, until approximately 600 ms when a bifurcation occurs with long–short R–R intervals. This is shown in the Poincaré plots as well as the tachogram in this focused illustration. For clarity, the scale for Poincaré plots on the x-axis is not shown. **Supplementary Video 7** complements this figure.

to the same visual point identified on the tachogram as a 'line' of 'usually' shortest-intervals during stable sleep (see **Figure 5**). Therefore, measurement from the canine data set during a stable sleep hour in 25 boxers and 25 non-boxers was performed to determine the range for the bifurcation interval, its relationship to overall heart rate and its relationship to a measure of parasympathetic modulation using the overall time domain variable, SDNN corrected for heart rate. Data were normally distributed with results in **Table 3**. The average heart rate during the sleep hour was correlated modestly with the bifurcation interval and rate corrected SDNN; that is, the longer the bifurcation interval, the slower the heart rate and the higher the SDNN. The bifurcation interval had a 95% confidence interval (**Table 3**) that was equivalent to a heart rate range of 97.8–102.8 bpm. The bifurcation interval was not correlated with SDNN.

Parasympatholytic and Parasympathomimetic Drug Effects

The beat-to-beat patterns after both atropine and hydromorphone were compared to baseline during and following the peak of drug effects (**Figures 11–14** and **Supplementary Videos 8, 9**). After treatment with the parasympatholytic drug atropine, the heart rate increased (decrease in beat-to-beat interval) as expected. Additionally, the beat-to-beat interval did change below the identified bifurcation interval in a linear fashion. Over time, dynamic Poincaré plots and tachograms revealed that as the parasympatholytic effects waned

TABLE 3 | Pairwise correlation of bifurcation interval measured during stable sleep hour in 50 dogs* with heart rate, R–R-interval, rate corrected SDNN, and age.

Parameter	Mean	*SD*	95% CI
Bifurcation interval (ms)	598.5	54.3	583.5–613.5
Age (years)	6.5	3.32	5.6–7.4
Average heart rate (bpm)	63.6	11.1	60.4–66.7
Average R–R-interval (ms)	971	164	924–1018
SDNN (ms)	0.364	0.07	0.343–0.386

Variable	By variable	Correlation *r*	95% CI of *r*	*p*-value
Bifurcation interval (ms)	Age (years)	−0.102	−0.367 to 0.182	0.48
Bifurcation interval (ms)	Average heart rate (bpm)	−0.572	−0.733 to −0.349	<0.001
Bifurcation interval	SDNN (ms)	−0.235	−0.482 to 0.05	0.10
Average heart rate (bpm)	SDNN (ms)	−0.342	−0.566 to −0.070	0.02

*CI, confidence interval. *Boxers and non-boxers were combined because data for each of these variables were not different for these data.*

a bifurcation and non-linear slowing of the heart rate (increase in beat-to-beat interval) developed (**Figures 11, 12, 14** and **Supplementary Video 8**). Treatment with hydromorphone with its parasympathomimetic effects (Deo et al., 2008) not only showed a slowing of rate with an increase in the beat-to-beat interval, but also a loss of linear heart rate changes. The zone of avoidance or paucity of beats as seen on the Poincaré plots was expanded (**Figures 11, 13, 14** and **Supplementary Video 9**). Each of the features described above was noted in all eight dogs.

DISCUSSION

The present study investigated the unique beat-to-beat patterning of sinus rhythms in the dog compared to the human. To accomplish the study objectives, additional tools of geometric beat-to-beat analyses were developed. The major findings in this study include: (1) During sinus arrhythmia the dog has a unique non-Gaussian and non-linear patterning when compared to humans as revealed by interval distributions (histograms and tachograms) and beat-to-beat maps (two- and three-dimensional and dynamic Poincaré plots). (2) Dogs have distinctive beat-to-beat distributions with regions of low beat density (zone of avoidance) and patterns (clustered and branched) associated with potentially different parasympathetic and sympathetic influence as reflected by qualitative assessment of time and frequency domain indices of heart rate variability. Furthermore, administration of parasympatholytic and parasympathomimetic drugs supported the role of the parasympathetic system in dictating the patterns identified. (3) The patterns of beat-to-beat variability in the dog evidenced by the dynamic Poincaré plots revealed a consistent region or zone (bifurcation interval) at which the long- and short- intervals of sinus arrhythmia became non-linear. Moreover, the results of this study in a clinical population of dogs under the influence of spontaneous changes in autonomic input, is congruent with the hypotheses of experimental canine studies (Fedorov et al., 2009, 2010; Glukhov et al., 2013; Lou et al., 2013, 2014; Kalyanasundaram et al., 2019) of the sinus node that demonstrate the likelihood of parasympathetic influence on the sinoatrial conduction pathways (SACPs). Finally, these studies serve as a background to the potential understanding of not only normal sinus node function in the dog, but of potential mechanisms of sinus node dysfunction.

Different Ways to Speed and Slow

Each of the geometric heart rate indices used in the assessment of beat-to-beat changes in rate showed clear differences between the human and dog. The unique pattern identified in the dog may be related to key structural components of the sinus node complex and the electrophysiologic consequences of parasympathetic modulation and how these target the key receptors of spontaneous depolarization of pacing cells and the exit to the surrounding atrial tissue. Numerous investigations of structure and function of the sinus node conclude a similarity between the human and dog (Fedorov et al., 2009, 2010, 2012; Nikolaidou et al., 2012; Csepe et al., 2015, 2016; Kalyanasundaram et al., 2019) however, the influence of vagal modulation may be more profound in the dog. In contrast to smaller species (e.g., mouse, rabbit) with a thinner atrium and a sinus node that functions more similarly to a two-dimensional structure, the canine and human have a three-dimensional structure (Fedorov et al., 2009, 2010, 2012; Nikolaidou et al., 2012; Li et al., 2017). In the larger hearts, specific SACP connect the sinus node to the atrium (Fedorov et al., 2009, 2010, 2012; Nikolaidou et al., 2012; Glukhov et al., 2013; Lou et al., 2014; Csepe et al., 2015; Li et al., 2017; Kalyanasundaram et al., 2019). These discrete exit pathways (2–5 in the dog) have been identified by thorough investigations of structure and function using high-resolution optical mapping, action potential morphologies, immunostaining and histologic confirmation (Opthof, 2000). Because these narrow SACP slow the impulse velocity from the pacing cells, charge accumulates to overcome the source-sink mismatch between the sinus node and atria. These studies and others have demonstrated that the stimulation of the heart beat is the result of not only the pacing cells within the complex compartmentalized sinus node, but also dependent on the conduction of these impulses reaching the atrial myocardium through the SACP. Just as the spontaneous depolarization rate shifts in the location of the

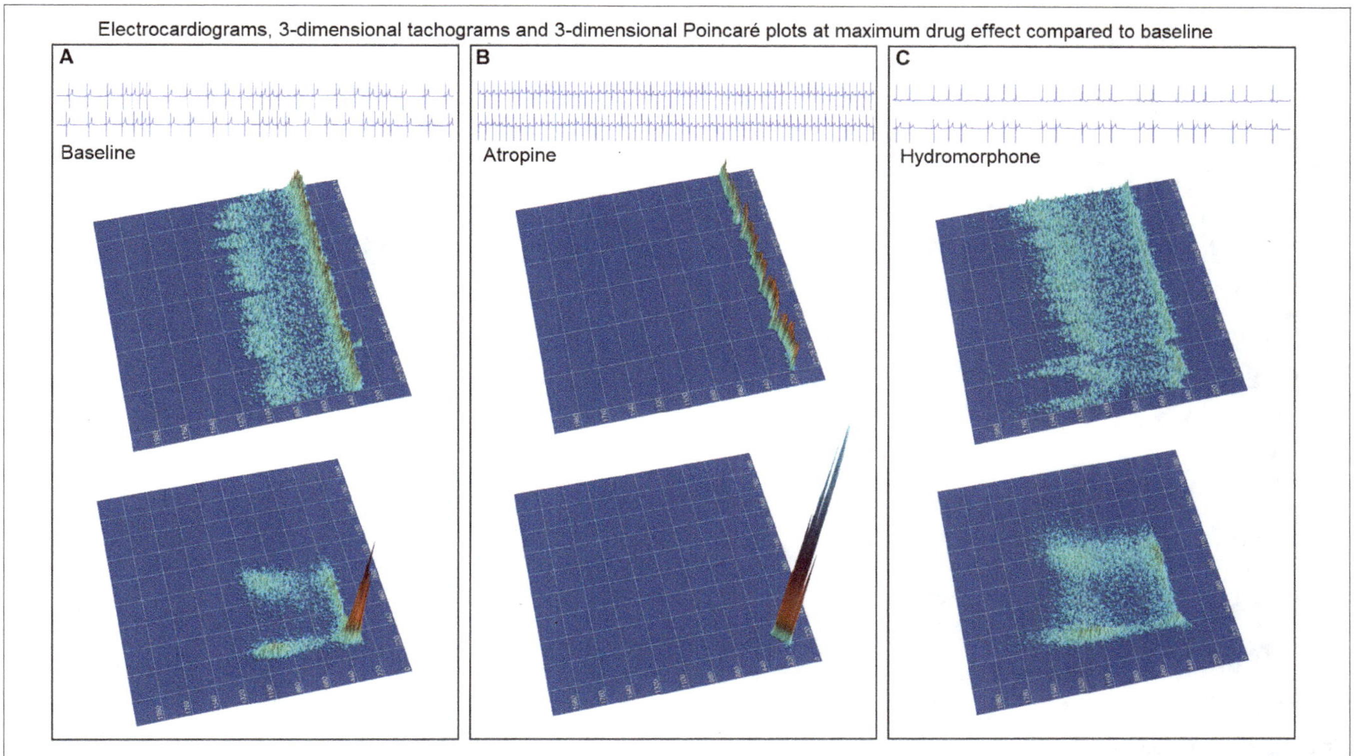

FIGURE 11 | The peak effects of atropine (0.04 mg/kg given intravenously) (Frame **A**) and hydromorphone (0.2 mg/kg given intravenously) (Frame **B**) compared to baseline (Frame **C**) are shown in the electrocardiograms, three-dimensional tachograms and Poincaré plots of beagle 5. During the baseline recording the sinus arrhythmia has a pattern with a paucity of beat intervals that can be identified on both the tachogram and Poincaré plots. At the longest intervals a cloud appears near the line of identity. After the administration of atropine (Frame **B**) that results in a decrease in parasympathetic modulation, the heart rate not only increases with a loss of sinus arrhythmia but the pattern of beat-to-beat intervals becomes linear. After the administration of hydromorphone (Frame **C**) that results in an increase in parasympathetic modulation, the heart rate slows and the bifurcation interval increases with a paucity of beat intervals (zone of avoidance). Scaling of all images is the same to show proportionality.

leading sinus pacing cells, SACP are substantially influenced by mediators of autonomic tone. For example, depending on the dose of adenosine or acetylcholine, not only are the membrane (I_f current) and voltage (Ca^{2+}) clocks suppressed to slow depolarization (Gao et al., 2010; Lou et al., 2013; Li et al., 2017), but conduction through the SACP is slowed (Opthof, 2000; Fedorov et al., 2009, 2010, 2012; Nikolaidou et al., 2012; Glukhov et al., 2013; Lou et al., 2013, 2014; Kalyanasundaram et al., 2019). Exit block through the SACP can develop in the dog with high levels of acetylcholine corresponding to high vagal tone potentially obtained during sleep (Glukhov et al., 2013; Kalyanasundaram et al., 2019). Although the intrinsic sinus rate of the dog (Evans et al., 1990; Du et al., 2017) and human (Opthof, 2000; Li et al., 2017) are similar, the higher parasympathetic tone in the dog is associated with a more pronounced sinus arrhythmia that we hypothesize based on the identified patterning of intervals in this study is, in part, the consequence of a more profound effect on the SACP resulting in exit block. Moreover, although variations in the non-linear patterns of sinus rhythm were seen in the dog, those with greater clustering of beats with 'shorter' short-long intervals had less variability than those with greater branching suggesting a possible difference in the balance between the rhythmicity of the parasympathetic and sympathetic tone. Of course, further studies are require to confirm these hypotheses.

SACP and Bifurcation Interval

Detailed and expansive studies of the canine sinus node support the existence of SACP that are subject to exit block during certain perturbations that mimic parasympathetic modulation. Moreover, the potential for decremental conduction would support modulation of exit block and this would then explain the inexact multiples and clustering of intervals. Experimental studies show that acetylcholine or adenosine can influence pacing cell depolarization and conduction through the SACP (Fedorov et al., 2009, 2010, 2012; Glukhov et al., 2013; Lou et al., 2013, 2014). Therefore, it is reasonable to hypothesize that our results, which demonstrate clustered and branched patterns related to the ratio of short- and long- intervals in the dog, could follow the same modulation of rate and rhythm via exit block through the SACP and slowed phase four-depolarization of pacing cells. In dogs with the longer beat-to-beat intervals a 'cloud' widely surrounding the line of identity may indicate a more profound effect of impulse initiation rather than conduction out the SACP. This type of pattern

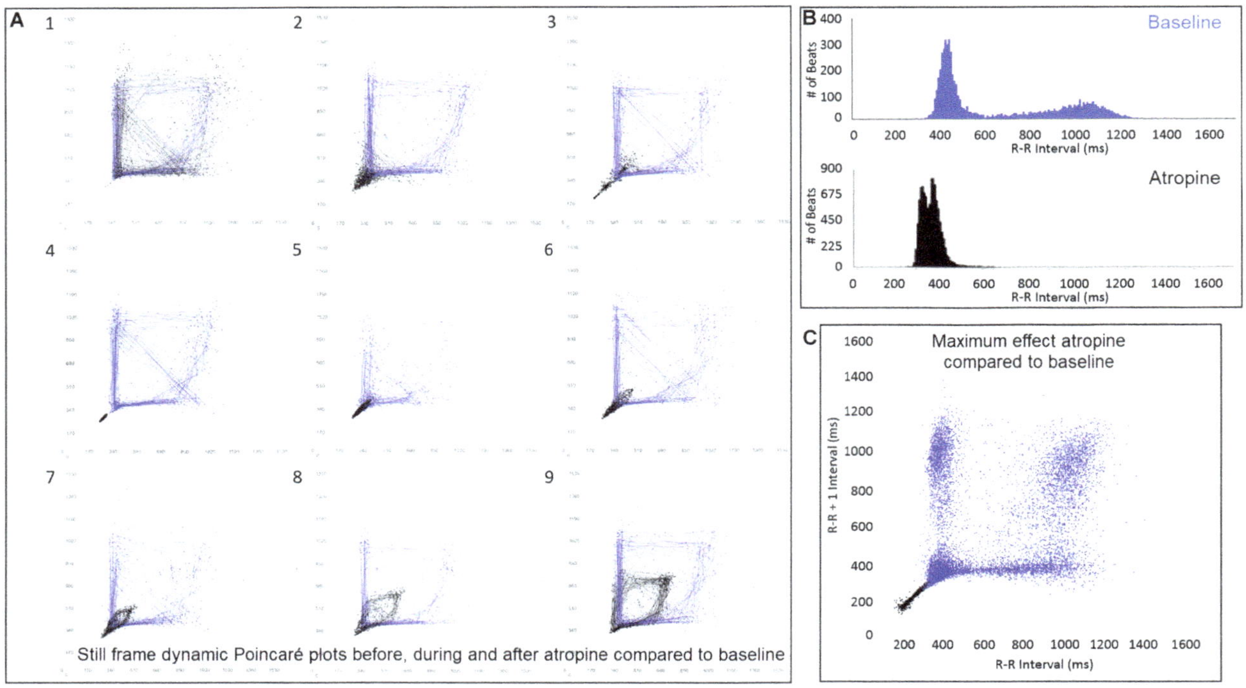

FIGURE 12 | (**Supplementary Video 8**) Still frames from dynamic Poincaré plots (Frame **A1–9**) from the electrocardiographic recordings from two different days during a stable rest period (blue) and just before, during and after administration of atropine (black) (0.04 mg/kg given intravenously) in beagle 8. Dots represent the beat-to-beat interval (R–R interval surrogate for P–P interval with all these verified to be sinus in origin) with lines connecting the next beat-to-beat interval. Each frame shows 500 beat-to-beat intervals. After atropine, the parasympatholytic effects result in the beat-to-beat intervals becoming shorter (Frames **1–4**) and as parasympathetic modulation returns, the beat-to-beat intervals become longer (Frames **5–9**). Note that after treatment with atropine the beat-to-beat patterning characterized by a bifurcation collapses to short intervals that hug the line of identity. When the heart rate slows (longer beat-to-beat intervals) with the decreasing drug effect, the bifurcation is identified again. In frame **(B)**, the number of beats at a particular beat interval are shown for the stable rest time (blue) and during treatment with atropine (black). The double peak during the atropine treatment represents the faster rate during the intravenous injection followed by the true drug effect and its short beat-to-beat intervals. In frame **(C)**, the Poincaré plot illustrates a comparison without the connecting lines of the entire baseline period and the time of maximum effect of atropine. **Supplementary Video 8** complements this figure.

was identified in all dogs administered hydromorphone which is known to have a parasympathomimetic effect on the sinus node. This observation maybe concordant with saturation of the parasympathetic effect on the sinus node decreasing the respiratory modulation of heart rate variability. The latter is identified in trained athletes (Goldberger et al., 1994). We corrected for the mathematical biased inherent in time and frequency analyses by dividing by the standard deviation or standard deviation squared, respectively (Sacha and Pluta, 2008; Billman, 2011, 2013; Billman et al., 2015b; Sacha et al., 2013). Finally, it is intriguing that the bifurcation interval at which point slowing of the heart rate in the dog becomes non-linear, a very narrow 95% confidence range of 97.8–102.8 beats per minute (583.5–613.5 ms) approximates the intrinsic sinus node rate of the adult and older dog. The intrinsic rate of the sinus node is that which is inherent to spontaneous depolarization of the sinus node cells without autonomic input (Billman et al., 2015a). How autonomic input is subtracted (e.g., pharmacological blockade, surgical denervation, explanted heart) influences this value (Evans et al., 1990). Also, age is an important determinant of the intrinsic rate with young dogs (168 ± 11 bpm) having faster rates compared to adults (120 ± 9 beats per minute) and elderly (88 ± 9 bpm) dogs (Du et al., 2017).

Heart Rate Variability

Heart rate variability is influenced by multiple inputs of central and peripheral parasympathetic and sympathetic modulation (Evans et al., 1990; Goldberger et al., 1994; Cerutti et al., 1995; Roossien et al., 1997; Stein et al., 2005; Billman, 2011, 2013; Billman et al., 2015b; Shaffer and Ginsberg, 2017; Behar et al., 2018a,b). The variability results from complex interactions and cannot be simplified to say that high variability universally indicates high parasympathetic modulation (Goldberger et al., 1994; Costa et al., 2017; Shaffer and Ginsberg, 2017; Hayano and Yuda, 2019). Both groups of dogs in this study had greater variability using traditional time domain indices than in humans. Traditional methods to evaluate the variability of the sinus node driven rate in humans have meaningful limitations particularly when evaluating disease states and this has prompted advanced methods (Hayano and Yuda, 2019). Some indices used in the evaluation of the rhythm in humans are not applicable to the dog. For example, the percentage of successive R–R intervals that differ by more than 50 ms

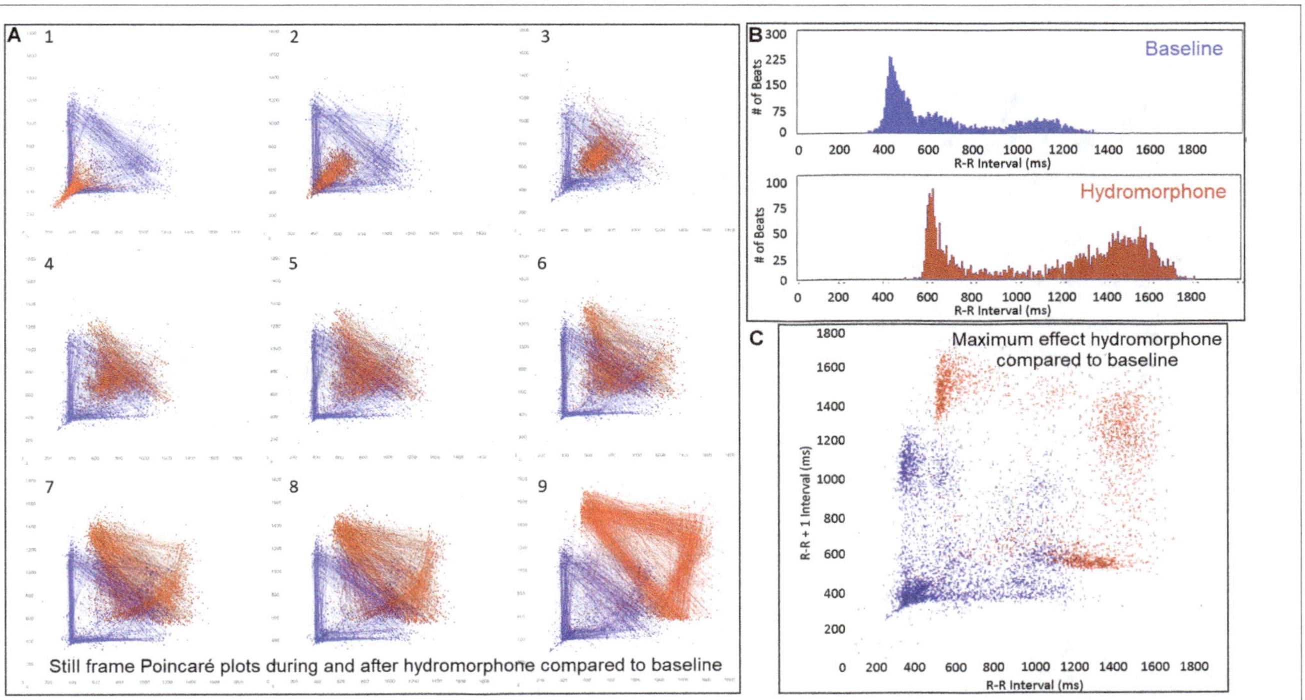

FIGURE 13 | (**Supplementary Video 9**) Still frames from dynamic Poincaré plots (Frame **A1–9**) derived from intervals of 24-h electrocardiographic recordings from two different days during a stable rest period (blue) and just before and after administration of hydromorphone (red) (0.2 mg/kg given intravenously) given to beagle 1. Dots represent the beat-to-beat interval (R–R interval surrogate for P–P interval with all these verified to be sinus in origin) with lines connecting the next beat-to-beat interval. Each frame shows 1500 beat-to-beat intervals. After hydromorphone the beat-to-beat intervals become longer. In frames (**1–5**) the heart rate is faster because the dog is excited during the intravenous administration and then calms as the drug takes effect. The heart rate and beat-to-beat interval pattern changes with increasing drug effect. The characteristic pattern with a paucity of beat intervals (zone of avoidance) and beat intervals that do not hover around the line of identity are seen in the dog with high parasympathetic modulation induced by the hydromorphone. In frame **(B)** the number of beats at a particular beat interval are shown for the stable rest period (blue) and during treatment with hydromorphone (red). In frame **(C)**, the Poincaré plot illustrates a comparison without the connecting lines of the entire baseline period and the time of maximum effect of hydromorphone. **Supplementary Video 9** complements this figure.

(pNN50) because this difference is too small for the dog. The triangular index is not applicable because the dog does not have a singular Gaussian distribution (Shaffer and Ginsberg, 2017). Furthermore, some of the linear measurements used in the evaluation of Poincaré plots in humans are also not valid in the dog because they are derived from the studies of linear changes along the line of identity (Shaffer and Ginsberg, 2017). These include the area of the ellipse (width/length), which represents total heart rate variability, the standard deviation perpendicular to the line of identity and the standard deviation along the line of identity. Newly developed methods to better understand the variability in the sinus rhythm have been developed and deserve further evaluation in different species (Costa et al., 2017).

Beyond Visual Geometric Analyses

Although this study used dynamic Poincaré plots and three-dimensional imaging to demonstrate a difference in beat-to-beat intervals between the dog and human these visual indices are inadequate (Esperer et al., 2008). Moreover, linear quantification are inappropriate, thus non-linear analyses demand exploration. These may include approximate or sample entropy, detrended fluctuation analyses and fractal measures, as well as the development of new methodologies through computer modeling of the beat-to-beat variation (Esperer et al., 2008; Nicolini et al., 2012; Khandoker et al., 2013; Burykin et al., 2014; Yaniv et al., 2014b; Henriques et al., 2015; Shaffer and Ginsberg, 2017; Borracci et al., 2018; Valente et al., 2018). In humans, slowing of the heart rate is a continuum with some having slower rates (e.g., athletes), but in the normal dog slowing of the heart is not a continuous process. We hypothesize that the dog has greater potential for alterations of conduction in the SACP that is linked to the parasympathetic modulation. This hypothesis is supported by the (1) abrupt change of beat-to-beat intervals, (2) paucity and grouping of beats rather than a continuum of beat intervals, and (3) relatively consistent bifurcation interval during basal conditions.

Clinical Relevance

Both humans and dogs can be afflicted with sinus node dysfunction. Such dysfunction may be intrinsic, extrinsic or both. Alterations in the parasympathetic nervous system or molecular targets likely play an important role, thus understanding the relationship of the sinus node complex with the inclusion of the SACP is likely vital to differentiating disease that results in exit block versus those with disease from impulse formation.

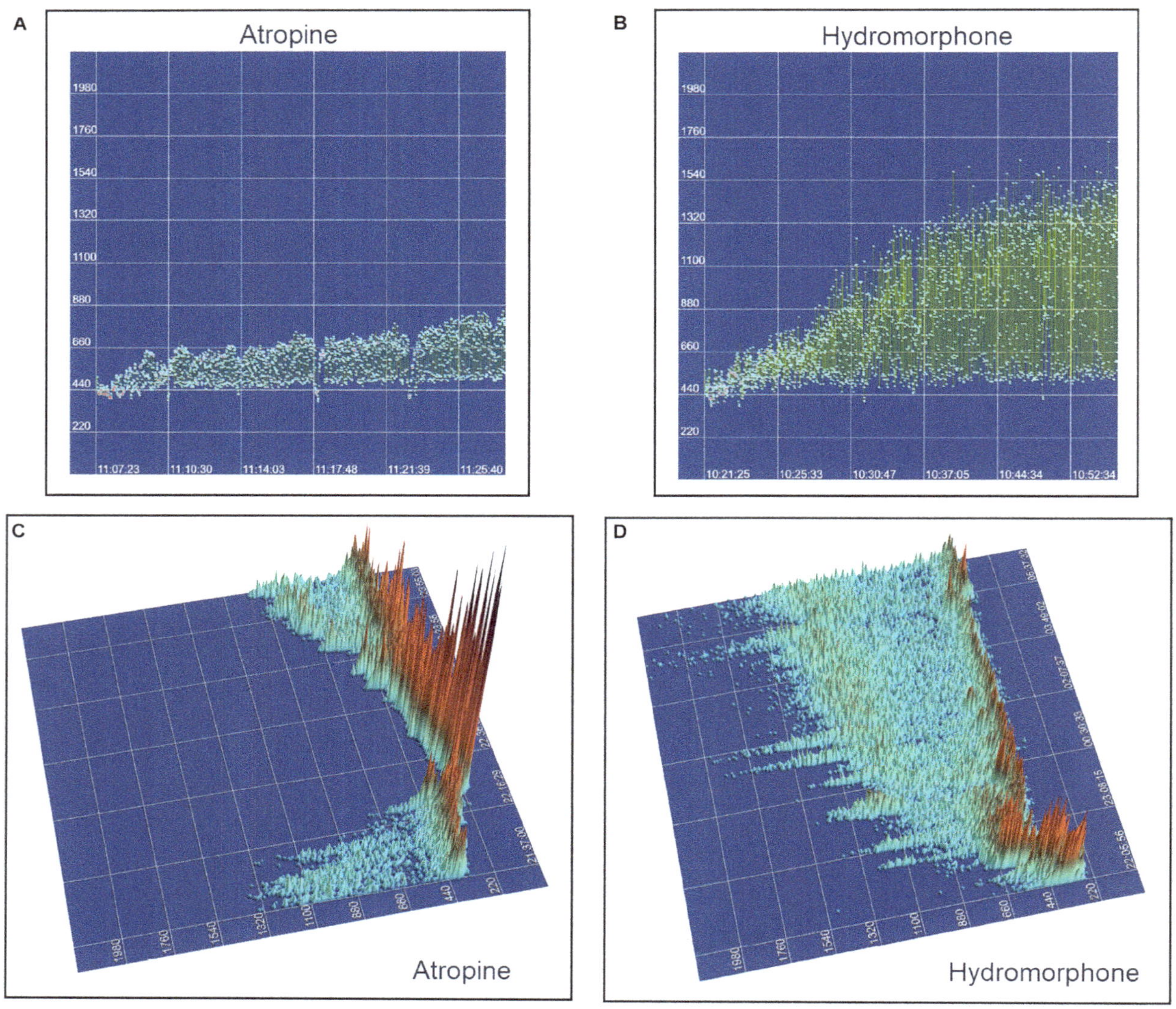

FIGURE 14 | This figure uses two-dimensional **(A,B)** and three-dimensional **(C,D)** tachograms to show the pattern and density of sinus intervals before, during, and after treatment to decrease and increase parasympathetic modulation. Recordings were from two different days for each treatment. Frame **(A)** (beagle 1) illustrates the interval changes (turquoise dots represent interval duration and yellow lines connect sequential intervals) as the drug effects of atropine (0.04 mg/kg given intravenously) dissipate. The decreasing and increasing interval duration associated with the increasing and decreasing drug effects of atropine are seen in frame **(C)** (beagle 1). As the effects of atropine subside the bifurcation interval increases with an increased paucity of beats as sinus arrhythmia returns. Frame **(B,D)** (beagle 8) show increasing interval duration associated with the increasing drug effects of hydromorphone (0.2 mg/kg given intravenously). The effects of hydromorphone result in an increased paucity of beats, an increase in the bifurcation interval and a greater spread of long intervals. Scaling for frames **(C,D)** are equal to show proportionality of the interval density.

The use of the techniques illustrated herein may be valuable in this differentiation.

Limitations

Our study is limited to the surface electrocardiogram without direct assessment of the multiplicity of inputs that control the sinus rhythm. However, the patterning observed supports experimental studies of the sinus node in the dog. The study population of dogs and humans included a wide range of ages; however, the range in age between boxers and non-boxers was different and likely responsible for the difference in the relationship of age to time domain indices of heart rate variability. Equating dog age to human age is known to be difficult, non-linear and highly variable depending on the breed of dog (Cotman and Head, 2008). Consequently, attempts to compare the influence of age between the dog and human from our study is not possible. It is known that sinus node function varies with age, and, thus, this must be taken into consideration. Additionally, because 32 different breeds were studied of varied sizes with 108 dogs neutered, comparison to humans by weight or sex was not undertaken. Although the only entry criteria that differed between the dogs and humans was the duration that defined a sinus pause, this did not impact the difference in beat-to-beat patterning because the non-linear change occurred at intervals that were more than 1000 ms shorter than the defined pause. It is stressed that autonomic activity was not directly measured, and heart rate variability provides only an indirect qualitative assessment of cardiac parasympathetic activity. More advanced analyses need to be undertaken to further investigate the potential mechanisms for the unique patterning of sinus arrhythmia in the dog.

CONCLUSION

Our study demonstrated distinctive differences in beat-to-beat sinus rhythms in the dog compared to humans. Specific patterns within and between dog were associated with differences in heart rate, time and frequency domain variability. Treatment with atropine as a parasympatholytic agent resulted in small variation in beat intervals that were along the line of identity while treatment with hydromorphone as a parasympathomimetic agent resulted in an expansion and exaggeration of the patterns identified without linear variation in the beat-to-beat intervals. The non-linear rhythms of sinus arrhythmia in the dog require assessment using analyses appropriate to the dynamics. The multiplicity of input that results in the beat-to-beat dynamics identified in the normal canine are concordant with the possibility of not only alterations in the initiation of sinus impulses, but also variable exit block within the SACP. Furthermore, these results may offer insight to the possible mechanisms for sinus node dysfunction seen in the dog that has a disease footprint similar to humans.

AUTHOR CONTRIBUTIONS

NM designed the study, analyzed the data, created all the images, interpreted the data, and wrote the manuscript. WF created the software for the analysis and contributed to the interpretation of the data. RP contributed to the interpretation of the data and reviewed the manuscript.

ACKNOWLEDGMENTS

We wish to sincerely thank Drs. Sabine Mann and Françoise Vermeylen for assistance with statistical analyses; Shari Hemsley for assistance with editing of 24-h Holter recordings; and Kelsey Kearns, Andrea Gladuli, Ellen Gunzel, Emily Herrold, and Caitlin Hokanson for assistance with data management. We are also grateful to Don Greenfield and Forest Medical, Syracuse, NY, United States for permitting us access to the raw Holter data for our investigation. We are appreciative of the investigators who established and maintain the Telemetric and Holter ECG Warehouse (THEW) at the University of Rochester Medical Center, Rochester, NY, United States. Special appreciation is given to Dr. George Billman for critical input.

REFERENCES

Ambrosi, C. M., Fedorov, V. V., Schuessler, R. B., Rollins, A. M., and Efimov, I. R. (2012). Quantification of fiber orientation in the canine atrial pacemaker complex using optical coherence tomography. *J. Biomed. Opt.* 17:071309. doi: 10.1117/1.JBO.17.7.071309

Behar, J. A., Rosenberg, A. A., Shemla, O., Murphy, K. R., Koren, G., Billman, G. E., et al. (2018a). A universal scaling relation for defining power spectral bands in mammalian heart rate variability analysis. *Front. Physiol.* 9:1001. doi: 10.3389/fphys.2018.01001

Behar, J. A., Rosenberg, A. A., Weiser-Bitoun, I., Shemla, O., Alexandrovich, A., Konyukhov, E., et al. (2018b). PhysioZoo: a novel open access platform for heart rate variability analysis of mammalian electrocardiographic data. *Front. Physiol.* 9:1390. doi: 10.3389/fphys.2018.01390

Billman, G. E. (2011). Heart rate variability? A historical perspective. *Front. Physiol.* 2:86. doi: 10.3389/fphys.2011.00086

Billman, G. E. (2013). The effect of heart rate on the heart rate variability response to autonomic interventions. *Front. Physiol.* 4:222. doi: 10.3389/fphys.2013.00222

Billman, G. E., Cagnoli, K. L., Csepe, T., Li, N., Wright, P., Mohler, P. J., et al. (2015a). Exercise training-induced bradycardia: evidence for enhanced parasympathetic regulation without changes in intrinsic sinoatrial node function. *J. Appl. Physiol.* 118, 1344–1355. doi: 10.1152/japplphysiol.01111.2014

Billman, G. E., Huikuri, H. V., Sacha, J., and Trimmel, K. (2015b). An introduction to heart rate variability: methodological considerations and clinical applications. *Front. Physiol.* 6:55. doi: 10.3389/fphys.2015.00055

Blake, R. R., Shaw, D. J., Culshaw, G. J., and Martinez-Pereira, Y. (2018). Poincaré plots as a measure of heart rate variability in healthy dogs. *J. Vet. Cardiol.* 20, 20–32. doi: 10.1016/j.jvc.2017.10.006

Boineau, J. P., Schuessler, R. B., Hackel, D. B., Miller, C. B., Brockus, C. W., and Wylds, A. C. (1980). Widespread distribution and rate differentiation of the atrial pacemaker complex. *Am. J. Physiol. Circ. Physiol.* 239, H406–H415. doi: 10.1152/ajpheart.1980.239.3.H406

Borracci, R. A., Montoya Pulvet, J. D., Ingino, C. A., Fitz Maurice, M., Hirschon Prado, A., and Dominé, E. (2018). Geometric patterns of time-delay plots from different cardiac rhythms and arrhythmias using short-term EKG signals. *Clin. Physiol. Funct. Imaging* 38, 856–863. doi: 10.1111/cpf.12494

Brodde, O. E., Konschak, U., Becker, K., Rüter, F., Poller, U., Jakubetz, J., et al. (1998). Cardiac muscarinic receptors decrease with age. In vitro and in vivo studies. *J. Clin. Invest.* 101, 471–478. doi: 10.1172/JCI1113

Burykin, A., Costa, M. D., Citi, L., and Goldberger, A. L. (2014). Dynamical density delay maps: simple, new method for visualising the behaviour of complex systems. *BMC Med. Inform. Decis. Mak.* 14:6. doi: 10.1186/1472-6947-14-6

Cerutti, S., Bianchi, A. M., and Mainardi, L. T. (1995). "Spectral analysis of the heart rate variability signal," in *Heart Rate Variability*, eds M. Malik, and A. J. Camm, (Wiley, NJ: Wiley).

Costa, M. D., Davis, R., and Goldberger, A. L. (2017). Heart rate fragmentation: a new approach to the analysis of cardiac interbeat interval dynamics. *Front. Physiol.* 8:255. doi: 10.3389/fphys.2017.00255

Cotman, C. W., and Head, E. (2008). The canine (dog) model of human aging and disease: dietary, environmental and immunotherapy approaches. *J. Alzheimers Dis.* 15, 685–707. doi: 10.3233/JAD-2008-15413

Csepe, T. A., Kalyanasundaram, A., Hansen, B. J., Zhao, J., and Fedorov, V. V. (2015). Fibrosis: a structural modulator of sinoatrial node physiology and dysfunction. *Front. Physiol.* 6:37. doi: 10.3389/fphys.2015.00037

Csepe, T. A., Zhao, J., Hansen, B. J., Li, N., Sul, L. V., Lim, P., et al. (2016). Human sinoatrial node structure: 3D microanatomy of sinoatrial conduction pathways. *Prog. Biophys. Mol. Biol.* 120, 164–178. doi: 10.1016/j.pbiomolbio.2015.12.011

Deo, S., Barlow, M., Gonzalez, L., Yoshishige, D., and Caffrey, J. (2008). Cholinergic location of δ-opioid receptors in canine atria and SA node. *Am. J. Physiol. Hear. Circ. Physiol.* 294, H829–H838.

Du, J., Deng, S., Pu, D., Liu, Y., Xiao, J., and She, Q. (2017). Age-dependent down-regulation of hyperpolarization-activated cyclic nucleotide-gated channel 4 causes deterioration of canine sinoatrial node function. *Acta Biochim. Biophys. Sin.* 49, 400–408. doi: 10.1093/abbs/gmx026

Esperer, H. D., Esperer, C., and Cohen, R. J. (2008). Cardiac arrhythmias imprint specific signatures on Lorenz plots. *Ann. Noninvasive Electrocardiol.* 13, 44–60. doi: 10.1111/j.1542-474X.2007.00200.x

Evans, J. M., Randall, D. C., Funk, J. N., and Knapp, C. F. (1990). Influence of cardiac innervation on intrinsic heart rate in dogs. *Am. J. Physiol. Circ. Physiol.* 258, H1132–H1137. doi: 10.1152/ajpheart.1990.258.4.H1132

Fedorov, V. V., Chang, R., Glukhov, A. V., Kostecki, G., Janks, D., Schuessler, R. B., et al. (2010). Complex interactions between the sinoatrial node and atrium during reentrant arrhythmias in the canine heart. *Circulation* 122, 782–789. doi: 10.1161/CIRCULATIONAHA.109.935288

Fedorov, V. V., Glukhov, A. V., and Chang, R. (2012). Conduction barriers and pathways of the sinoatrial pacemaker complex: their role in normal rhythm and atrial arrhythmias. *Am. J. Physiol. Circ. Physiol.* 302, H1773–H1783. doi: 10.1152/ajpheart.00892.2011

Fedorov, V. V., Schuessler, R. B., Hemphill, M., Ambrosi, C. M., Chang, R., Voloshina, A. S., et al. (2009). Structural and functional evidence for discrete exit pathways that connect the canine sinoatrial node and atria. *Circ. Res.* 104, 915–923. doi: 10.1161/CIRCRESAHA.108.193193

Gao, Z., Chen, B., Joiner, M. A., Wu, Y., Guan, X., Koval, O. M., et al. (2010). I(f) and SR Ca(2+) release both contribute to pacemaker activity in canine sinoatrial node cells. *J. Mol. Cell. Cardiol.* 49, 33–40. doi: 10.1016/j.yjmcc.2010.03.019

Gladuli, A., Moïse, N. S., Hemsley, S. A., and Otani, N. F. (2011). Poincaré plots and tachograms reveal beat patterning in sick sinus syndrome with supraventricular tachycardia and varying AV nodal block. *J. Vet. Cardiol.* 13, 63–70. doi: 10.1016/j.jvc.2010.12.001

Glukhov, A. V., Hage, L. T., Hansen, B. J., Pedraza-Toscano, A., Vargas-Pinto, P., Hamlin, R. L., et al. (2013). Sinoatrial node reentry in a canine chronic left ventricular infarct model. *Circ. Arrhythmia Electrophysiol.* 6, 984–994. doi: 10.1161/CIRCEP.113.000404

Goldberger, J. J., Ahmed, M. W., Parker, M. A., and Kadish, A. H. (1994). Dissociation of heart rate variability from parasympathetic tone. *Am. J. Physiol. Circ. Physiol.* 266, H2152–H2157. doi: 10.1152/ajpheart.1994.266.5.H2152

Hayano, J., and Yuda, E. (2019). Pitfalls of assessment of autonomic function by heart rate variability. *J. Physiol. Anthropol.* 38:3. doi: 10.1186/s40101-019-0193-2

Henriques, T. S., Mariani, S., Burykin, A., Rodrigues, F., Silva, T. F., and Goldberger, A. L. (2015). Multiscale Poincaré plots for visualizing the structure of heartbeat time series. *BMC Med. Inform. Decis. Mak.* 16:17. doi: 10.1186/s12911-016-0252-0

Kalyanasundaram, A., Li, N., Hansen, B. J., Zhao, J., and Fedorov, V. V. (2019). Canine and human sinoatrial node: differences and similarities in the structure, function, molecular profiles, and arrhythmia. *J. Vet. Cardiol.* 22, 2–19. doi: 10.1016/j.jvc.2018.10.004

Khandoker, A. H., Karmakar, C., Brennan, M., Voss, A., and Palaniswami, M. (2013). *Poincaré Plot Methods for Heart Rate Variability Analysis.* New York, NY: Springer Science+Business Media.

Krohova, J., Czippelova, B., Turianikova, Z., Lazarova, Z., Wiszt, R., Javorka, M., et al. (2018). Information domain analysis of respiratory sinus arrhythmia mechanisms. *Physiol. Res.* 67, S611–S618.

Li, N., Hansen, B. J., Csepe, T. A., Zhao, J., Ignozzi, A. J., Sul, L. V., et al. (2017). Redundant and diverse intranodal pacemakers and conduction pathways protect the human sinoatrial node from failure. *Sci. Transl. Med.* 9:eaam5607. doi: 10.1126/scitranslmed.aam5607

Lou, Q., Glukhov, A. V., Hansen, B., Hage, L., Vargas-Pinto, P., Billman, G. E., et al. (2013). Tachy-brady arrhythmias: the critical role of adenosine-induced sinoatrial conduction block in post-tachycardia pauses. *Hear. Rhythm* 10, 110–118. doi: 10.1016/j.hrthm.2012.09.012

Lou, Q., Hansen, B. J., Fedorenko, O., Csepe, T. A., Kalyanasundaram, A., Li, N., et al. (2014). Upregulation of adenosine A1 receptors facilitates sinoatrial node dysfunction in chronic canine heart failure by exacerbating nodal conduction abnormalities revealed by novel dual-sided intramural optical mapping. *Circulation* 130, 315–324. doi: 10.1161/CIRCULATIONAHA.113.007086

Malik, M., Bigger, J. T., Camm, A. J., Kleiger, R. E., Malliani, A., Moss, A. J., et al. (1996). Heart rate variability: standards of measurement, physiological interpretation, and clinical use. *Eur. Heart J.* 17, 354–381.

Mighiu, A., and Heximer, S. (2012). Controlling parasympathetic regulation of heart rate: a gatekeeper role for RGS proteins in the sinoatrial node. *Front. Physiol.* 3:204. doi: 10.3389/fphys.2012.00204

Moïse, N. S., Gladuli, A., Hemsley, S. A., and Otani, N. F. (2010). "Zone of avoidance": RR interval distribution in tachograms, histograms, and Poincaré plots of a Boxer dog. *J. Vet. Cardiol.* 12, 191–196. doi: 10.1016/j.jvc.2010.07.001

Monfredi, O., Maltseva, L. A., Spurgeon, H. A., Boyett, M. R., Lakatta, E. G., and Maltsev, V. A. (2013). Beat-to-beat variation in periodicity of local calcium releases contributes to intrinsic variations of spontaneous cycle length in isolated single sinoatrial node cells. *PLoS One* 8:e67247. doi: 10.1371/journal.pone.0067247

Nicolini, P., Ciulla, M. M., de Asmundis, C., Magrini, F., and Brugada, P. (2012). The prognostic value of heart rate variability in the elderly, changing the perspective: from sympathovagal balance to chaos theory. *Pacing Clin. Electrophysiol.* 35, 621–637. doi: 10.1111/j.1540-8159.2012.03335.x

Nikolaidou, T., Aslanidi, O. V., Zhang, H., and Efimov, I. R. (2012). Structure-function relationship in the sinus and atrioventricular nodes. *Pediatr. Cardiol.* 33, 890–899. doi: 10.1007/s00246-012-0249-0

Opthof, T. (2000). The normal range and determinants of the intrinsic heart rate in man. *Cardiovasc. Res.* 45, 177–184.

Peltola, M. A. (2012). Role of editing of R–R intervals in the analysis of heart rate variability. *Front. Physiol.* 3:148. doi: 10.3389/fphys.2012.00148

Roossien, A., Brunsting, J. R., Nijmeijer, A., Zaagsma, J., and Zijlstra, W. G. (1997). Effects of vasoactive intestinal polypeptide on heart rate in relation to vagal cardioacceleration in conscious dogs. *Cardiovasc. Res.* 33, 392–399.

Sacha, J., Barabach, S., Statkiewicz-Barabach, G., Sacha, K., Müller, A., Piskorski, J., et al. (2013). How to strengthen or weaken the HRV dependence on heart rate–Description of the method and its perspectives. *Int. J. Cardiol.* 168, 1660–1663. doi: 10.1016/j.ijcard.2013.03.038

Sacha, J., and Pluta, W. (2008). Alterations of an average heart rate change heart rate variability due to mathematical reasons. *Int. J. Cardiol.* 128, 444–447. doi: 10.1016/j.ijcard.2007.06.047

Sassi, R., Cerutti, S., Lombardi, F., Malik, M., Huikuri, H. V., Peng, C.-K., et al. (2015). Advances in heart rate variability signal analysis: joint position statement by the e-Cardiology ESC working group and the european heart rhythm association co-endorsed by the Asia Pacific Heart Rhythm Society. *Europace* 17, 1341–1353. doi: 10.1093/europace/euv015

Shaffer, F., and Ginsberg, J. P. (2017). An overview of heart rate variability metrics and norms. *Front. Public Heal.* 5:258. doi: 10.3389/fpubh.2017.00258

Stein, P. K., Domitrovich, P. P., Hui, N., Rautaharju, P., and Gottdiener, J. (2005). Sometimes higher heart rate variability is not better heart rate variability: results of graphical and nonlinear analyses. *J. Cardiovasc. Electrophysiol.* 16, 954–959. doi: 10.1111/j.1540-8167.2005.40788.x

Valente, M., Javorka, M., Porta, A., Bari, V., Krohova, J., Czippelova, B., et al. (2018). Univariate and multivariate conditional entropy measures for the characterization of short-term cardiovascular complexity under physiological stress. *Physiol. Meas.* 39:014002. doi: 10.1088/1361-6579/aa9a91

Yaniv, Y., Ahmet, I., Liu, J., Lyashkov, A. E., Guiriba, T.-R., Okamoto, Y., et al. (2014a). Synchronization of sinoatrial node pacemaker cell clocks and its autonomic modulation impart complexity to heart beating intervals. *Hear. Rhythm* 11, 1210–1219. doi: 10.1016/j.hrthm.2014.03.049

Yaniv, Y., Lyashkov, A. E., Sirenko, S., Okamoto, Y., Guiriba, T.-R., Ziman, B. D., et al. (2014b). Stochasticity intrinsic to coupled-clock mechanisms underlies beat-to-beat variability of spontaneous action potential firing in sinoatrial node pacemaker cells. *J. Mol. Cell. Cardiol.* 77, 1–10. doi: 10.1016/j.yjmcc.2014.09.008

Yasuma, F., and Hayano, J.-I. (2004). Respiratory sinus arrhythmia: why does the heartbeat synchronize with respiratory rhythm? *Chest* 125, 683–690. doi: 10.1378/chest.125.2.683

Zhang, L., Guo, T., Xi, B., Fan, Y., Wang, K., Bi, J., et al. (2015). Automatic recognition of cardiac arrhythmias based on the geometric patterns of Poincaré plots. *Physiol. Meas.* 36, 283–301. doi: 10.1088/0967-3334/36/2/283

7

Cardiac Arrhythmias and Antiarrhythmic Drugs: An Autophagic Perspective

*Joanne J. A. van Bavel, Marc A. Vos and Marcel A. G. van der Heyden**

Department of Medical Physiology, Division of Heart and Lungs, University Medical Center Utrecht, Utrecht, Netherlands

***Correspondence:**
Marcel A. G. van der Heyden
m.a.g.vanderheyden@umcutrecht.nl

Degradation of cellular material by lysosomes is known as autophagy, and its main function is to maintain cellular homeostasis for growth, proliferation and survival of the cell. In recent years, research has focused on the characterization of autophagy pathways. Targeting of autophagy mediators has been described predominantly in cancer treatment, but also in neurological and cardiovascular diseases. Although the number of studies is still limited, there are indications that activity of autophagy pathways increases under arrhythmic conditions. Moreover, an increasing number of antiarrhythmic and non-cardiac drugs are found to affect autophagy pathways. We, therefore, suggest that future work should recognize the largely unaddressed effects of antiarrhythmic agents and other classes of drugs on autophagy pathway activation and inhibition.

Keywords: autophagy, AMPK, antiarrhythmic drugs, arrhythmias, mTOR, heart

INTRODUCTION

Degradation of cellular material occurs mainly via two pathways: the ubiquitin-proteasome system (UPS) and the autophagy-lysosome pathway. The UPS targets mainly short-lived or misfolded proteins, whereas autophagy includes the degradation, digestion and recycling of autophagy substrates, by lysosomes (Li et al., 2012). In healthy conditions, autophagy acts principally as a protective and control mechanism by maintaining cellular growth, proliferation, survival, and clearance of dying cells (Cremonese Filipi-Chiela et al., 2016). Over the last decade, an increasing amount of research has focused on autophagy and attention has been paid to the association between autophagy and cardiac diseases, including ischemia and hypertrophy. Thus far, a potential link between arrhythmic conditions and changes in autophagy activity has gained little attention, although the evidence for such interaction currently expands. There remains a need for increased research focus on the association between pro- and antiarrhythmic drugs and autophagy pathways in the heart. We review the link between cardiac autophagy and arrhythmic conditions, and the limitations regarding the effect of antiarrhythmic drugs on autophagy. Only a few years from now we can determine whether the current niche of arrhythmias and autophagy research will emerge in a mature field of investigation.

AUTOPHAGY TYPES AND TARGETS

Autophagy substrates (referred to as cellular material) include proteins, proteasomes, lysosomes, endoplasmic reticulum (ER), mitochondria, lipid droplets, polyribosomes, peroxisomes, bacteria, viruses and ruptured phagosomes. These substrates are targeted for degradation as long as they are freely accessible in the cytosol (Galluzzi et al., 2017). Three types of autophagic targeting are recognized (**Figure 1A**). Microautophagy is the least studied type of autophagy, which involves the direct uptake of soluble cellular substrates from the cytoplasm by invaginations in lysosomal membranes (Li et al., 2012). Macroautophagy, the best characterized variant of autophagy, is used synonymous with the term autophagy. It refers to both selective and non-selective capture of cellular components in double-membraned vesicles in the cytosol, and subsequent transport of the content to lysosomes (Feng et al., 2014). Chaperone-mediated autophagy (CMA) is a selective autophagic mechanism, which is mediated by the recognition of a peptide sequence in substrate proteins by chaperones, e.g. hsc70 (Cuervo and Wong, 2014). The substrate binds to lysosome-associated membrane protein 2A (LAMP-2A) and translocates into the lysosome for degradation. The main and most important function of the strictly organized process of autophagy is to maintain cellular homeostasis (Singh and Cuervo, 2011). Autophagy can act selectively, which includes the degradation of specific cargo selected by receptor proteins, and non-selectively by maintenance of intracellular nutrient supply with starvation as its main trigger (Svenning and Johansen, 2013). Besides small cellular components, selective autophagy can target specific cell components, e.g. mitochondria (mitophagy), ER (reticulophagy), ribosomes (ribophagy), lipids (lipophagy), and ion channels (channelophagy, as suggested by Klionsky et al., 2007; Kondratskyi et al., 2017). Autophagic processes are either continuously active (constitutive) or triggered (inducible). The primary stimulus of autophagy in yeast is nutrient withdrawal, whereas in mammals several stimuli can trigger autophagy, of which the most important are nutritional changes (e.g. starvation), organelle damage, hormonal regulation, infectious agents, hypoxia (such as in cardiac ischemia), and intracellular accumulation of toxic products (e.g. some antiarrhythmic drugs; Kudenchuk et al., 1984; Singh and Cuervo, 2011; Reggiori and Klionsky, 2013). The first reports on autophagic processes appeared in 1955. Christian de Duve coined the term "autophagy" in 1963, which was based on the discovery of self-eating lysosomes in rat hepatic cells (De Duve et al., 1955). The following decades, research focused on studying molecular autophagy mechanisms in yeast, which differ from autophagy processes in mammals (Matsuura et al., 1997; Reggiori and Klionsky, 2013). Furthermore, genetic screens revealed the existence of AuTophaGy-related (ATG) genes, of which the role in autophagy is associated to various processes in health and disease (Feng et al., 2014; Schneider and Cuervo, 2014). Recently, the field of autophagy was honored by a Nobel Prize awarded to Yoshinori Ohsumi in 2016 (Levine and Klionsky, 2017).

AUTOPHAGY-RELATED PROTEINS AND THEIR USE AS THERAPEUTICAL TARGETS

ATG proteins are mainly described in macroautophagy because of its best-known machinery, and are illustrated in **Figure 1B**. Two important regulators of autophagy initiation are AMP-activated protein kinase (AMPK) and mechanistic target of rapamycin complex 1 (mTORC1). Active AMPK stimulates autophagy initiation, whereas mTORC1 inhibits autophagy (Kim et al., 2011). In autophagy stimulation, the ULK1/2-Atg13-FIP200 complex becomes active, ATG proteins are recruited and a phagophore is formed (Xie et al., 2015). The class III phosphatidylinositol 3-kinase (PI3KCIII) complex (beclin-1, VPS34, VPS15, and Atg14L) mediates nucleation of the phagophore (Baskaran et al., 2014). Different ubiquitin-like conjugation systems (Atg12-Atg5 and Atg8/LC3) are central in the next autophagic step; elongation of the phagophore, and proteins and lipids involved in autophagosome formation and maturation are recruited by the PI3KCIII complex (Feng et al., 2014; Xie et al., 2015). Beclin-1 is part of the PI3KCIII complex, and plays a key role in autophagosome formation and maturation (Xie et al., 2015). Mature autophagosomes move along microtubules and fuse with lysosomes in a process that involves gamma-aminobutyric acid receptor-associated proteins (GABARAP) and soluble NSF attachment protein receptor (SNARE) family proteins (Nair et al., 2011; Itakura et al., 2012). Autophagy's final step is degradation of the autophagolysosome cargo by different types of proteases (Kaminskyy and Zhivotovsky, 2012). Detailed overviews of the macroautophagy machinery are given by Feng et al. (2014) and Xie et al. (2015).

Inability to maintain cellular homeostasis due to defective autophagy associates with a variety of systemic diseases, such as cancer, neurodegeneration, liver disease and (cardio-) myopathies (Schneider and Cuervo, 2014). Distinct ATG proteins are considered as interesting targets for autophagy modulation (**Figure 1B**, **Table 1**), in which the field of cancer therapy progressed furthest (Mulcahy Levy et al., 2017). Rapamycin and its analogs (rapalogs) inhibit mTORC1 resulting in autophagy activation, and are used in certain cancer treatments (Li J. et al., 2014). Other recognized mTORC1 inhibitors are perhexiline (antianginal agent), niclosamide (used in treating worm infections), and rottlerin (natural product, known to open potassium channels) (Balgi et al., 2009). Activation of autophagy can also result from AMPK activators, such as commonly used antidiabetic agents metformin and phenformin, and AMP analog 5-aminoimidazole-4-carboxamide-1-β-D-ribofuranoside (AICAR) (Zhou et al., 2001; Yang et al., 2013; Ducommon et al., 2014). Common inhibitors of AMPK include adenine 9-beta-D-arabinofuranoside (Ara-A, or vidarabine) and compound C (Zhou et al., 2001; Pelletier et al., 2005). Antitumor drug wogonin can affect the next step in the autophagy pathway (phagophore nucleation) by targeting the beclin-1/PI3K complex, and thereby

Abbreviations: AF, atrial fibrillation; AMPK, AMP-activated protein kinase; AICAR, 5-aminoimidazole-4-carboxamide-1-β-D-ribofuranoside; Ara-A, adenine 9-beta-D-arabinofuranoside; ATG, AuTophaGy related; CMA, chaperone-mediated autophagy; Cx43, connexin43; EPG5, ectopic P-granules autophagy protein 5; ER, endoplasmic reticulum; GABARAP, gamma-aminobutyric acid receptor-associated proteins; GSK3β, glycogen synthase kinase 3β; HAT, histone acetyltransferase; HDAC, histone deacetylase; hERG, human ether-a-go-go-related gene; hsc70, heat shock-cognate protein of 70 kDa; IP_3, inositol 1,4,5-triphosphate; I/R, ischemia/reperfusion; LAMP-2A, lysosome-associated membrane protein 2A; LC3-II, microtubule-associated protein 1A/1B chain 3 phosphatidylethanolamine conjugate; LTCC, L-type calcium channel; mTOR, mechanistic target of rapamycin; mTORC1, mTOR complex 1; NAD^+, nicotinamide adenine dinucleotide; P-AMPK, phosphorylated AMPK; PI3KCIII, class III phosphatidylinositol 3-kinase; PKA, protein kinase A; RAP, rapid atrial pacing; SNARE, soluble NSF attachment protein receptor; TAC, transverse aortic constriction; TdP, torsade de pointes; TP53, transcription factor 53; ULK1/2, unc-51-like kinase 1 and 2; UPS, ubiquitin proteasome system.

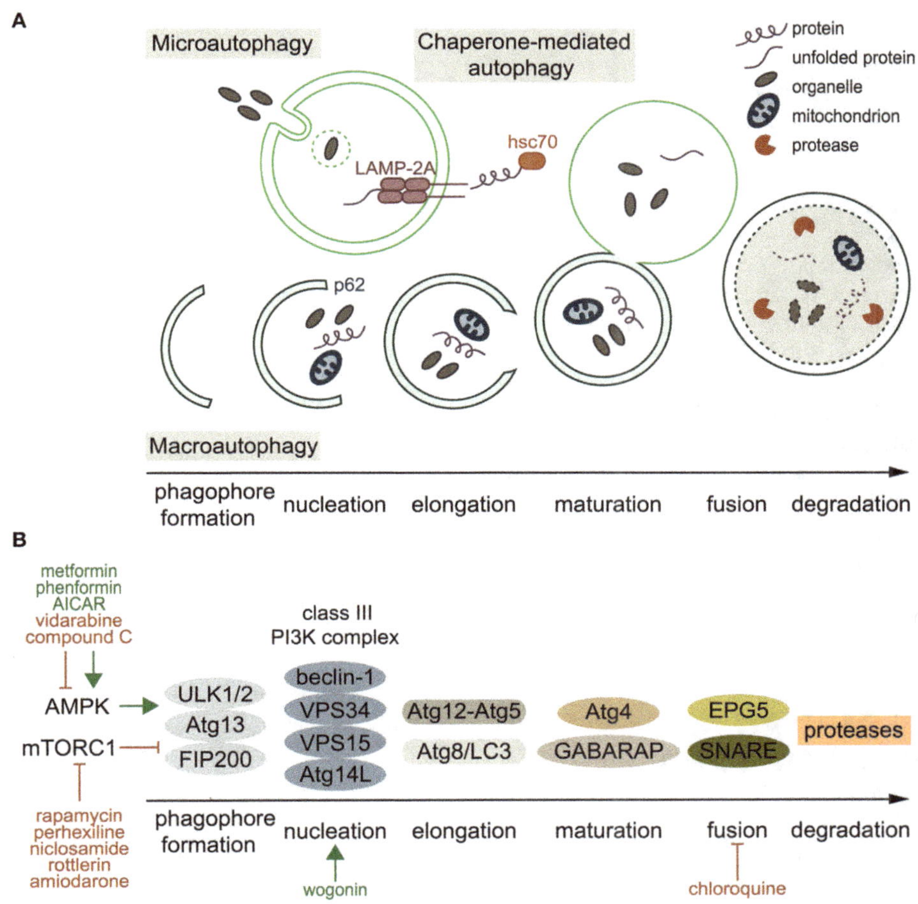

FIGURE 1 | Autophagy types, processes, molecular players and pharmacological regulators. **(A)** Schematic presentation of the three autophagy types. Microautophagy refers to the direct uptake of soluble cellular substrates from the cytoplasm by invaginations in lysosomal membranes. Chaperone-mediated autophagy includes targeting of a specific motif in a substrate protein, translocation of the substrate to the lysosome by heat shock-cognate protein of 70 kDa (hsc70), and translocation into the lysosome by lysosome-associated membrane protein 2A (LAMP-2A) on the lysosomal membrane. Macroautophagy starts with formation of a double-membraned phagophore, at which proteins and lipids are recruited by, among others, p62 (nucleation). Then, the phagophore elongates, matures, and the autophagosome fuses with a lysosome. **(B)** Overview of the mediators involved in macroautophagy and some of their stimulators/inhibitors (green and red respectively). Autophagy initiation occurs by activated AMPK, which phosphorylates the ULK1/2-Atg13-FIP200 complex. mTORC1 inhibits this complex. Once the autophagy pathway is activated, a phagophore is formed and the class III PI3K complex is responsible for nucleation. Two different conjugation systems are important for elongation of the phagophore (Atg12-Atg5 and Atg8/LC3). GABARAP and Atg4 are involved in autophagosome maturation, and fusion of the autophagosome with a lysosome is mediated by EPG5 and SNARE proteins. Finally, the cargo is degraded by proteases.

inducing autophagy in human pancreatic cancer cells (Li et al., 2016). The antimalarial and anti-inflammatory agent chloroquine targets the last step in the autophagy pathway by inhibiting fusion of autophagosomes and lysosomes (Yoon et al., 2010). Although certain compounds seem to target autophagy pathways effectively, former mentioned compounds can act directly with a positive effect (e.g., tumor regression), as well as indirectly causing side effects.

AUTOPHAGY IN THE HEART: SOME LESSONS FROM GENE DEFECTS

Autophagy is important for maintenance of the highly organized cardiac structure, function and homeostasis. Nutrient insufficient conditions lead to the inactivation of mTORC1: rapamycin interacts with and inhibits mTORC1 activating unc-51-like kinase 1 and 2 (ULK1 and ULK2), leading to autophagy induction (Lavandero et al., 2013). Activation of sensitive nutrient sensor AMPK occurs when ATP/AMP levels decrease due to exercise, ischemia or lack of glucose, resulting in autophagy initiation (Hardie et al., 2012). Other important autophagy mediators in the cardiovascular system include inositol 1,4,5-triphosphate (IP_3), transcription factor 53 (TP53), cyclic AMP-dependent protein kinase A (PKA), histone acetyltransferases (HATs) and histone deacetylases (HDACs), glycogen synthase kinase 3β (GSK3β), nicotinamide adenine dinucleotide (NAD^+) and microRNAs, which can initiate and inhibit autophagy, as reviewed by Lavandero et al. (2013). Impaired autophagy pathway signaling, due to ATG protein deficiency, may cause cardiac pathologies.

Mice with Atg5 and Atg7 deficiency, ATG proteins involved in phagophore elongation, displayed dilated cardiomyopathy and contractile dysfunction, and accumulation of defective proteins and organelles, respectively (Komatsu et al., 2005; Nakai et al., 2007). Ectopic P-granules autophagy protein 5 (EPG5), important in translocation of autophagosomes to lysosomes, deficient individuals suffer from the Vici syndrome; a multisystem disorder with autophagy malfunction (Cullup et al., 2013). Cardiac symptoms, predominantly hypertrophy and left ventricular dilatation, are present in 90% of the Vici syndrome patients (Byrne et al., 2016). Deficiency of LAMP-2, required for the fusion of autophagosomes with endosomes and lysosomes (Endo et al., 2015), leads to Danon disease causing intellectual disability, skeletal myopathy and severe cardiomyopathy (D'souza et al., 2014). LAMP-2 deficient mice have a high mortality rate, show autophagosome accumulation in the pancreas, liver, kidney, skeletal muscle and heart, and possess cardiomyocytes filled with large vacuoles. The latter might be the cause of a reduced heart muscle contractility observed in these mice (Tanaka et al., 2000). Apart from the reductive, but instructive, ATG deficient models, most studies however focus on ischemia/reperfusion (I/R) and hypertrophy models to examine the role of cardiac autophagy (Lavandero et al., 2013).

AUTOPHAGY IN CARDIAC ISCHEMIA/REPERFUSION AND HYPERTROPHY MODELS

Both protective (clearance and removal of misfolded proteins and roles in energy homeostasis) and detrimental (massive digestion of cellular components and cross-talk to other forms of cell death) functions of autophagy have been presented in ischemic and hypertrophy models (Sciarretta et al., 2011). In the ischemic heart, upregulation of autophagy associates with a reduction in infarct size and apoptosis, and vice versa, suggested to work cardioprotective by maintaining energy levels (Sciarretta et al., 2014). In this situation, the drop in ATP levels during ischemia activates AMPK leading to an upregulation of autophagy activation (Takagi et al., 2007). In mice hearts however that underwent I/R, when oxygen and nutrient supply is impaired and subsequently restored, AMPK is inactivated, mTOR is upregulated, and beclin-1 is highly upregulated, suggesting an inhibition of autophagy (Matsui et al., 2007). Remarkably, these mice showed an increase in autophagosome levels and a decrease in apoptosis.

Cardiac hypertrophy is associated with an upregulation of autophagy. Weng et al. (2014) presented an increase in autophagic gene (Atg5 and Atg16) expression, and increased beclin-1 and microtubule-associated protein 1A/1B chain 3 phosphatidylethanolamine conjugate (LC3-II) levels in transverse aortic constriction (TAC), to induce pressure overload, operated mice. Furthermore, AMPK induces autophagy in TAC operated hearts by regulating the mTORC1 pathway, leading to inhibition of cardiac hypertrophy and improved cardiac function (Li Y. et al., 2014). Cardiac-specific knockout of mTOR showed an impaired hypertrophic response and enhanced heart failure progression after TAC mediated pressure-overload in mice, suggesting detrimental effects when mTOR is lacking (Zhang et al., 2010). However, pharmacologic inhibition of mTOR indicates a cardiac protective effect: rapamycin treatment in TAC operated mice showed an inhibitory effect on cardiac hypertrophy development (McMullen et al., 2004). Moreover, treatment of rapamycin in cardiac transplant recipients resulted in reduced left ventricular mass and improved diastolic function (Raichlin et al., 2008). Altogether, current evidence states that regulation of autophagy levels is crucial in protecting cardiomyocytes under ischemic and hypertrophic conditions.

INCREASED AUTOPHAGY ACTIVATION IN ARRHYTHMIC CONDITIONS

Connexin43 (Cx43) proteins form gap junctions, which are responsible for the propagation of cardiac action potentials between cardiomyocytes. In the recent years, literature has been growing regarding the role of autophagy in degradation of Cx43 (Falk et al., 2014). A lowered expression of Cx43 was also linked to arrhythmias: among others, (Shu et al., 2017) showed a lowered Cx43 protein expression in a canine model with atrial fibrillation (AF) induced by rapid atrial pacing (RAP). It remains to be identified if a lowered Cx43 expression in arrhythmic conditions was mediated by autophagic degradation. As an indication of autophagy activation, levels of autophagy mediators have been examined in several arrhythmic conditions. A RAP canine model, vulnerable to AF, showed an increase in LC3B-II (LC3 family member) and phosphorylated AMPK (p-AMPK) protein levels (Yuan et al., 2014). Moreover, in the same study, it was presented that these autophagy mediators were increased in human patients suffering from AF. Furthermore, beclin-1 and LC3B-II expression levels were increased in I/R-injured fibrillated mouse hearts (Meyer et al., 2013). The increased levels of these autophagy mediators suggest increased autophagy activation in response to arrhythmias. Although the number of autophagic vacuoles was elevated in patients who underwent coronary artery bypass grafting with postoperative AF, decreased levels of LC3B-II levels were found in these patients (Garcia et al., 2012). A decrease in vesicle degradation and an impaired autophagic flow can clarify the elevated vesicle levels and the decreased LC3B-II levels, respectively (Garcia et al., 2012). These exciting findings, albeit just a few, appear to outpoint that autophagy pathways are becoming activated in arrhythmic conditions, and are therefore of interest as potential therapeutic targets. Nonetheless, the exact mechanistic relationship between autophagy and cardiac arrhythmias clearly remains to be elucidated.

ANTIARRHYTHMIC DRUGS AFFECT AUTOPHAGY PATHWAYS

Along with limited research into autophagy occurrence and regulation in arrhythmic conditions, only a few studies have thus far focused on the effect of antiarrhythmic drugs on autophagy activation and the results are interesting. **Table 1** demonstrates the effect on autophagic regulation, the effective concentrations

TABLE 1 | The effect of the discussed compounds on autophagy activation, their effective concentration on autophagy regulation, their therapeutic plasma concentrations, and their potential link to arrhythmic conditions.

Compound	Autophagic activation	Concentrations		Associated with arrhythmias[a]	References
AICAR	↑	AMPK activation Plasma levels	500 μM not reported	+ hERG inhibition	Zhou et al., 2001; Almilaji et al., 2013
Amiodarone	↑	mTORC1 inhibition Plasma levels	>10 μM 0.8–3.9 μM	+ QT prolongation	Balgi et al., 2009; Tarapués et al., 2014; Hrudikova Vyskocilova et al., 2017.
Chloroquine	↓	Autolysosome fusion ↓ Mean peak plasma level	120 μM 0.4 μM	+ at high dose	Walker et al., 1983; White, 2007; Yoon et al., 2010
Compound C	↓	AMPK inhibition Plasma levels	20 μM not reported	↓(potentially) by hERG activation	Zhou et al., 2001; Almilaji et al., 2013
Dronedarone	↑	Autophagy activation Steady-state plasma levels	2 μM 0.15–0.3 μM	+ QT prolongation	Wadhani et al., 2006; Patel et al., 2009; Piccoli et al., 2011
Metformin	↑	AMPK activation Steady-state plasma levels	>2 μM 10–40 μM	↓AF in DM patients	Zhou et al., 2001; Chang et al., 2014
Niclosamide	↑	mTORC1 inhibition Serum concentration range	1 μM 0.76–18.32 μM	Not reported	Andrews et al., 1982; Balgi et al., 2009
Nifedipine	↑	Autophagy activation Mean peak plasma level	10 μM 0.35 μM	↓ LTCC blocker	Van Bortel et al., 1989; Redfern et al., 2003; Pushparaj et al., 2015
Paliperidone	↑	Downstream effector mTOR Mean plasma level	not reported 84.4 nM	+ hERG inhibition	Nazirizadeh et al., 2010; Vigneault et al., 2011; Mas et al., 2015
Pentamidine	↑	Kir2.1 degradation Plasma levels	5–10 μM 0.5–2.4 μM	+ Risk for TdP	Waalkes et al., 1970; Antoniou and Gough, 2005; Nalos et al., 2011
Perhexiline	↑	mTORC1 inhibition Serum concentration range	1–10 μM 0.8–3.8 μM	+ hERG inhibition	Plicher et al., 1985; Walker et al., 1999; Balgi et al., 2009
Phenformin	↑	AMPK activation Plasma level	>0.3 mM 0.27 μM	+ hERG inhibition	Marchetti et al., 1987; Almilaji et al., 2013; Vincent et al., 2015
PI3K inhibitors[b]	↑	AMPK activation[c] Mean peak plasma level[c]	5 μM 3.6 μM	+ APD prolongation	Fava et al., 2008; Yu et al., 2013; Cohen et al., 2017
Propranolol	↓	Late block in autophagy Plasma levels	10 μM 20–428 μM	↓shorter QT in LQT1	Castleden et al., 1975; Farah et al., 2014; Ahn et al., 2017
Ranolazine	↑	Autophagy activation Mean steady-state level	1 μM 6 μM	↓ AF episodes	CV Therapeutics Inc., 2007; Huang et al., 2010; Guerra et al., 2017
Rapamycin	↑	mTORC1 inhibition Target concentration range	0.5–100 nM 4–22 nM	+ >28 nM	Stenton et al., 2005; Foster and Toschi, 2009; Karakas et al., 2016
Rottlerin	↑	mTORC1 inhibition Plasma levels	1–3 μM not reported	+ APD shortening	Lu et al., 2008; Balgi et al., 2009
Verapamil	↑	Autophagy activation Mean peak plasma level	1 μM 0.8 μM	+ LTCC and hERG inhibition	Frishman et al., 1982; Redfern et al., 2003; Williams et al., 2008
Vidarabine	↓	AMPK inhibition Mean peak plasma level	>0.5 mM 3.7 μM	–	Whitley et al., 1980; Pelletier et al., 2005; Wada et al., 2016
Wogonin	↑	Beclin-1/PI3K activation Plasma levels	40 μM not reported	↓ in ischemic model	Lee et al., 2011; Li et al., 2016

AF, atrial fibrillation; APD, action potential duration; DM, diabetes mellitus; LQT1, long QT syndrome 1; LTCC, L-type calcium channel; TdP, Torsade de Pointes; Compound association with arrhythmias (+), no association (–), preventive effect (↓) or "not reported."

[a] Arrhythmic associations tested in human, animal, or in vitro models.

[b] PI3K inhibitor examples are, as mentioned in the text, nilotinib, dasatinib, and sunitinib.

[c] Nilotinib concentration.

affecting autophagy, the clinical effective concentrations, and a possible association with arrhythmias of the compounds discussed in this perspective. The effective concentrations of the compounds on autophagy regulation, although tested *in vitro* with limited concentration ranges, can be compared to drug plasma levels in patients. Overlapping concentrations indicate that a number of clinically used compounds are likely to influence authophagy regulation. Antiarrhythmic drugs are classified by the effect on the targets whose actions form the cardiac action potential. Class I drugs block Na^+ channels, class II drugs are adrenergic receptor antagonists, class III drugs are K^+ channel blockers, and the AV-node conduction is slowed down by class IV drugs usually by blockage of L-type calcium channels (LTCCs). The antiarrhythmic effects of Na^+ channel blocker ranolazine, initially developed as antianginal agent, are convincing (Gupta et al., 2015). Huang et al. (2010) showed induced autophagy activation after ranolazine treatment in HL-1 cells and isolated rat cardiomyocytes. Commonly used beta-blocker propranolol is reported as autophagy inhibitor: increased LC3-II levels, autophagosome formation, and p62 (which degrades during autophagy stimulation) levels were measured in HepG2 cells, suggesting an inhibition of hepatic autophagy by propranolol at a later stage due to reduced degradation (Farah et al., 2014). Class III antiarrhythmic drug amiodarone inhibits mTORC1 leading to stimulation of the autophagy pathway, which was explored *in vitro* (Balgi et al., 2009). In another *in vitro* study, we indicated lysosomal impairment by amiodarone and its synthetic analog dronedarone, which resulted in increased inward rectifier potassium channel $K_{ir}2.1$ expression and intracellular accumulation (Ji et al., 2017a). The well-known drawback of amiodarone is its high incidence of side effects, including thyroid toxicity, pulmonary toxicity, hepatic toxicity, neurological toxicity, which seem to be related to the lifetime cumulative dose of the drug (Santangeli et al., 2012). However, pharmacological activation of autophagy by amiodarone has been shown to improve liver regeneration after partial hepatectomy in mice (Lin et al., 2015). LTCC blocker nifedipine, used as arterial vasodilator, increases autophagic flow, as shown by increased presence of autophagosomes and LC3-II levels, and lower p62 levels in isolated rat cardiomyocytes (Pushparaj et al., 2015). LTCC blocker verapamil, used in treating angina and arrhythmias, increases autophagic flux, which was shown by elevated LC3-II levels in PC12 cells and in a series of human cell lines, in which the latter also included increased development of autophagic vacuoles (Williams et al., 2008; Kania et al., 2017). These studies, although limited in number, clearly represent the existing link between antiarrhythmic drugs and autophagy, and the direct outcomes can be both activation and inhibition of autophagy.

NON-CARDIAC DRUGS CAN ACT PROARRHYTHMIC AND AFFECT AUTOPHAGY

As well as antiarrhythmic compounds, non-cardiac drugs can have the tendency to act proarrhythmic, e.g. by prolonging the QT interval with an increased risk for Torsade de Pointes (TdP) arrhythmias (Bossu et al., 2016), and they can affect the autophagic pathway. Many compounds with increased proarrhythmic risk are clinically used, or only reached phase I of clinical trials, to treat various disease areas. The former discussed drug chloroquine, which increases the lysosomal pH and thereby prevents the degradation of certain autophagy substrates, is reported as proarrhythmic. Accumulated levels of $K_{ir}2.1$ were found intracellularly and I_{K1} densities increased due to chloroquine treatment (Jansen et al., 2008). From an autophagic perspective these results can be linked to the chloroquine-induced QT prolongation, conduction disturbances and cardiomyopathy at high doses, as reviewed by White (2007). The proarrhythmic effect of antiprotozoal drug pentamidine has been firstly reported in 1987 by the description of two case reports with occurrence of TdP arrhythmias after administration of pentamidine, which results have been confirmed later on (Wharton et al., 1987; Antoniou and Gough, 2005). We suggested a link between pentamidine and autophagy, in which pentamidine may induce lysosomal degradation of potassium channel $K_{ir}2.1$ (Nalos et al., 2011). Pentamidine analogs have been, and still are, tested to finally develop efficient and specific $K_{ir}2.x$ ion-channel-carried inward rectifier current (I_{k1}) inhibitors for treating atrial fibrillation and short QT syndrome type 3 (Takanari et al., 2013; Ji et al., 2017b). Antipsychotic drug paliperidone, which inhibits human ether-a-go-go-related gene (hERG) K^+ channel, has also been characterized to increase the QT interval and increase the risk for TdP arrhythmia (Vigneault et al., 2011; Hagiwara et al., 2016). It may be assumed that it also affects autophagy, since mTOR was identified as a downstream effector of paliperidone-induced extrapyramidal symptoms (side effect of antipsychotics), as observed in a network analysis of gene expression (Mas et al., 2015). The role of autophagy in cancer has been characterized as paradoxical because of its pro-survival and pro-death outcomes (Helgason et al., 2013). A frequently altered pathway in cancer includes PI3K and its inhibitors seem to treat solid tumors and hematologic malignancies (Mayer and Arteaga, 2016). Nilotinib, dasatinib and sunitinib are examples of PI3K inhibitors, which are approved by the FDA to treat certain cancer types, and are shown to induce autophagy pathways in cancer cell models (Le et al., 2010; Yu et al., 2013; Wang et al., 2017). However, a recent study by Cohen et al. (2017), presented a prolongation of the action potential by former named PI3K inhibitors, and thereby clearly suggests that drug safety testing should be improved. The compounds discussed in this paragraph, either approved by the FDA or currently in clinical trials, seem to affect the autophagy pathway and cardiac action potential, while their original purpose is not to affect those. Causality however, needs to be demonstrated.

CONCLUSION AND FUTURE PERSPECTIVES

Autophagy regulation is crucial in basal and diseased conditions, and has been shown to act both protective and detrimental in cardiac disease models. Up to now, evidence has brought forward that autophagy activation changes in arrhythmic conditions of the heart. In addition, some antiarrhythmic drugs have been shown to affect autophagy pathways and this may associate with adverse effects. The direct effects and deciphering of the complex underlying mechanisms of antiarrhythmic drugs on autophagy mediation in the heart remain to be determined. Ion channels are crucial in maintaining a regular cardiac rhythm and some are also involved in autophagy regulation, as reviewed by Kondratskyi et al. (2017), indicating a possible direction of future research. Another research aim should be to understand the dependent role of remodeling on autophagy in cardiac arrhythmic conditions. Gene defect models and arrhythmia-induced models are promising in understanding the mechanistic relationship between autophagy and arrhythmias. We also suggest that future work should include the examination of autophagy effects in exploring the effectiveness of antiarrhythmic drugs. This may improve drug development to provide safer antiarrhythmic drugs by removal of autophagy pathway disturbances. Antiarrhythmic drugs may then not further worsen autophagy dysregulation in arrhythmic conditions. Beyond doubt, from an autophagic perspective; focus should increase on its regulation under arrhythmic conditions, and on the effects of its unknown targeting by antiarrhythmic compounds and other drugs.

AUTHOR CONTRIBUTIONS

All authors listed, have made substantial, direct and intellectual contribution to the work, and approved it for publication.

REFERENCES

Ahn, J., Kim, H. J., Choi, J. I., Lee, K. N., Shim, J., Ahn, H. S., et al. (2017). Effectiveness of beta-blockers depending on the genotype of congenital long-QT syndrome: a meta-analysis. *PLoS ONE* 12:e0185680. doi: 10.1371/journal.pone.0185680

Almilaji, A., Munoz, C., Elvira, B., Fajol, A., Pakladok, T., Honisch, S., et al. (2013). AMP-activated protein kinase regulates hERG potassium channel. *Eur. J. Physiol.* 465, 1573–1582. doi: 10.1007/s00424-013-1299-8

Andrews, P., Thyssen, J., and Lorke, D. (1982). The biology and toxicology of molluscicides, bayluscide. *Pharmacol. Ther.* 19, 245–295. doi: 10.1016/0163-7258(82)90064-X

Antoniou, T., and Gough, K. A. (2005). Early-onset pentamidine-associated second-degree heart block and sinus bradycardia: case report and review of the literature. *Pharmacotherapy* 25, 899–903. doi: 10.1592/phco.2005.25.6.899

Balgi, A. D., Fonseca, B. D., Donohue, E., Tsang, T. C. F., Lajoie, P., Proud, C. G., et al. (2009). Screen for chemical modulators of autophagy reveals novel therapeutic inhibitors of mTORC1 signaling. *PLoS ONE* 4:e7124. doi: 10.1371/journal.pone.0007124

Baskaran, S., Carlson, L., Stjepanovic, G., Young, L. N., Kim, D. J., Grob, P., et al. (2014). Architecture and dynamics of the autophagic phosphatidylinositol 3-kinase complex. *Elife* 3:e05115. doi: 10.7554/eLife.05115

Bossu, A., Van der Heyden, M. A. G., De Boer, T. P., and Vos, M. A. (2016). A 2015 focus on preventing drug-induced arrhythmias. *Expert Rev. Cardiovasc. Ther.* 14, 245–253. doi: 10.1586/14779072.2016.1116940

Byrne, S., Dionisi-Vici, C., Smith, L., Gautel, M., and Jungbluth, H. (2016). Vici syndrome: a review. *Orphanet J. Rare Dis.* 11:21. doi: 10.1186/s13023-016-0399-x

Castleden, C. M., Kaye, C. M., and Parsons, R. L. (1975). The effect of age on plasma levels of propranolol and practolol in man. *Br. J. Clin. Pharmacol.* 2, 303–306.

Chang, S., Wu, L., Chiou, M., Liu, J., Yu, K., Kuo, C., et al. (2014). Association of metformin with lower atrial fibrillation risk among patients with type 2 diabetes mellitus: a population-based dynamic cohort and *in vitro* studies. *Cardiovasc. Diabetol.* 13:123. doi: 10.1186/014-0123-x

Cohen, I. S., Lin, R. Z., and Ballou, L. M. (2017). Acquired long QT syndrome and phosphoinositide 3-kinase. *Trends Cardiovasc. Med.* 27, 451–459. doi: 10.1016/j.tcm.2017.05.005

Cremonese Filipi-Chiela, E., Viegas, M. S., Paulo Thome, M., Buffon, A., Wink, M. R., and Lenz, G. (2016). Modulation of autophagy by calcium signalosome in human disease. *Mol. Pharmacol.* 90, 371–384. doi: 10.1124/mol.116.105171

Cuervo, A. M., and Wong, E. (2014). Chaperone-mediated autophagy: roles in disease and aging. *Cell Res.* 24, 92–104. doi: 10.1038/cr.2013.153

Cullup, T., Kho, A. L., Dionisi-Vici, C., Brandmeier, B., Smith, F., Urry, Z., et al. (2013). Recessive mutations in EPG5 cause Vici syndrome, a multisystem disorder with defective autophagy. *Nat. Genet.* 45, 83–87. doi: 10.1038/ng.2497

CV Therapeutics Inc. (2007). *Data from: Ranexa (Ranolazine) Tablet, Film Coated, Extended Release.* Available online at: https://dailymed.nlm.nih.gov/dailymed/archives/fdaDrugInfo.cfm?archiveid=5376

De Duve, C., Pressman, B. C., Gianetto, R., Wattiaux, R., and Appelmans, F. (1955). Tissue fractionation studies. 6. Intracellular distribution patterns of enzymes in rat-liver tissue. *Biochem. J.* 60, 604–717.

D'souza, R. S., Levandowski, C., Slavov, D., Graw, S. L., Allen, L. A., Adler, E., et al. (2014). Danon disease: clinical features, evaluation, and management. *Circ. Heart Fail.* 7, 843–849. doi:10.1161/CIRCHEARTFAILURE.114.001105

Ducommon, S., Ford, R. J., Bultot, L., Deak, M., Bertrand, L., Kemp, B. E., et al. (2014). Enhanced activation of cellular AMPK by dual-small molecule treatment: AICAR and A769662. *Am. J. Physiol. Endocrinol. Metab.* 306, 688–696. doi: 10.1152/ajpendo.00672.2013

Endo, Y., Furuta, A., and Nishino, I. (2015). Danon disease: a phenotypic expression of LAMP-2 deficiency. *Acta Neurophatol.* 129, 391–398. doi: 10.1007/s00401-015-1385-4

Falk, N. M., Kells, R. M., and Berthoud, V. M. (2014). Degradation of connexins and gap junctions. *FEBS Lett.* 588, 1221–1229. doi: 10.1016/j.febslet.2014.01.031

Farah, B. L., Sinha, R. A., Wu, Y., Singh, B. K., Zhou, J., Bay, B. H., et al. (2014). B-adrenergic agonist and antagonist regulation of autopahgy in HepG2 cells, primary mouse hepatocytes and mouse liver. *PLoS ONE* 9:e98155. doi: 10.1371/journal.pone.0098155

Fava, C., Kantarjian, H., Cortes, J., and Jabbour, E. (2008). Development and targeted use of nilotinib in chronic myeloid leukemia. *Drug Des. Devel. Ther.* 2, 233–243.

Feng, Y., He, D., Yao, Z., and Klionsky, D. J. (2014). The machinery of macroautophagy. *Cell Res.* 24, 24–41. doi: 10.1038/cr.2013.168

Foster, D. A., and Toschi, A. (2009). Targeting mTOR with rapamycin: one dose does not fit all. *Cell Cycle* 8, 1026–1029. doi: 10.4161/cc.8.7.8044

Frishman, W., Kirsten, E., Klein, M., Pine, M., Johnson, S. M., Hillis, L. D., et al. (1982). Clinical relevance of verapamil plasma levels in stable angina pectoris. *Am. J. Cardiol.* 50, 1180–1184. doi: 10.1016/0002-9149(82)90440-4

Galluzzi, L., Baehrecke, E. H., Ballabio, A., Boya, P., Bravo-San Pedro, J. M., Cecconi, F., et al. (2017). Molecular definitions of autophagy and related processes. *EMBO J.* 36, 1811–1836. doi: 10.15252/embj.201796697

Garcia, L., Verdejo, H. E., Kuzmicic, J., Zalaquett, R., Gonzalez, S., Lavandero, S., et al. (2012). Impaired cardiac autophagy in patients developing postoperative atrial fibrillation. *J. Thorac. Cardiovasc. Surg.* 143, 451–459. doi: 10.1016/j.jtcvs.2011.07.056

Guerra, F., Romandini, A., Barbarossa, A., Belardinelli, L., and Capucci, A. (2017). Ranolazine for rhythm control in atrial fibrillation: a systemic review and meta-analysis. *Int. J. Cardiol.* 15, 284–291. doi: 10.1016/j.ijcard.2016.11.103.

Gupta, T., Khera, S., Kolte, D., Aronow, W. S., and Iwai, S. (2015). Antiarrhythmic properties of ranolazine: a review of the current evidence. *Int. J. Cardiol.* 187, 66–74. doi: 10.1016/j.ijcard.2015.03.324

Hagiwara, M., Kambayashi, R., Aimoto, M., Nagasawam, Y., and Takahara, A. (2016). *In vivo* analysis of torsadogenic potential of an antipsychotic drug paliperidone using the acute atrioventricular block rabbit as a proarrhythmia model. *J. Pharmacol. Sci.* 132, 48–54. doi: 10.1016/j.jphs.2016.05.001

Hardie, D. G., Ross, F. A., and Hawly, S. A. (2012). AMPK: a nutrient and energy sensor that maintains energy homeostasis. *Nat. Rev. Mol. Cell Biol.* 13, 251–262. doi: 10.1038/nrm3311

Helgason, G. V., Holyoake, T. L., and Ryan, K. M. (2013). Role of autophagy in cancer prevention, development and therapy. *Essays Biochem.* 55, 133–151. doi: 10.1042/bse0550133

Hrudikova Vyskocilova, E., Grundmann, M., Duricova, J., and Kacirova, I. (2017). Therapeutic monitoring of amiodarone: pharmacokinetics and evaluation of the relationship between effect and dose/concentration. *Biomed. Pap. Med. Fac. Univ. Palacky. Olomouc. Czech. Repub.* 161, 134–143. doi: 10.5507/pb.2017.016

Huang, C., Yitzhaki, S., Perry, C. N., Liu, W., Giricz, Z., Mentzer, R. M., et al. (2010). Autophagy induced by ischemic preconditioning is essential for cardioprotection. *J. Cardiacvasc. Transl. Res.* 3, 365–373. doi: 10.1007/s12265-010-9189-3

Itakura, E., Kishi-Itakura, C., and Mizushima, N. (2012). The hairpin-type tail-anchored SNARE syntaxin 17 targets to autophagosomes for fusion with endosomes/lysosomes. *Cell* 151, 1256–1269. doi: 10.1016/j.cell.2012.11.001

Jansen, J. A., De Boer, T. P., Wolswinkel, R., van Veen, T. A. B., Vos, M. A., van Rijen, H. V. M., et al. (2008). Lysosome mediated Kir2.1 breakdown directly influences inward rectifier current density. *Biochem. Biophys. Res. Commun.* 367, 686–692. doi: 10.1016/j.bbrc.2007.12.168

Ji, Y., Takanari, H., Qile, M., Nalos, L., Houtman, M. J. C., Romunde, F. L., et al. (2017a). Class III antiarhythmic drugs amiodarone and dronedarone impair Kir2.1 backward trafficking. *J. Cell. Mol. Med.* 21, 2514–2523. doi: 10.1111/jcmm.13172

Ji, Y., Veldhuis, M. G., Zandvoort, J., Romunde, F. L., Houtman, M. J. C., Duran, K., et al. (2017b). PA-6 inhibits inward rectifier currents carried by V93I and D172N gain-of-function Kir2.1 channels, but increases channel protein expression. *J. Biomed. Sci.* 24:44. doi: 10.1186/s12929-017-0352-x

Kaminskyy, V., and Zhivotovsky, B. (2012). Proteases in autophagy. *Biochim. Biophys. Acta* 1824, 44–50. doi: 10.1016/j.bbapap.2011.05.013

Kania, E., Pajak, B., O'Prey, J., Sierra Gonzalez, P., Litwiniuk, A., Urbanska, K., et al. (2017). Verapamil treatment induces cytoprotective autophagy by modulating cellular metabolism. *FEBS J.* 284, 1370–1387. doi: 10.1111/febs.14064

Karakas, N. M., Erdogan, I., Ozdemir, B., and Sezgin, A. (2016). Pain syndrome and ventricular arrhythmia induced by sirolimus and resolved by dosage adjustment in a child after heart transplant: a case report. *Exp. Clin. Transplant.* doi: 10.6002/ect.2015.0320. [Epub ahead of print].

Kim, J., Kundu, M., Viollet, B., and Guan, K. (2011). AMPK and mTOR regulate autophagy through direct phorphorylation of Ulk1. *Nat. Cell Biol.* 13, 132–141. doi: 10.1038/ncb2152

Klionsky, D. J., Cuervo, A. M., Dunn, W. A. Jr., Levine, B., Van der Klei, I. J., and Seglen, P. O. (2007). How shall I eat thee? *Autophagy* 3, 413–416. doi: 10.4161/auto.4377

Komatsu, M., Waguri, S., Ueno, T., Iwata, J., Murata, S., Tanida, I., et al. (2005). Impairment of starvation-induced and consitutive autophagy in Atg7-deficient mice. *J. Cell Biol.* 169, 425–434. doi: 10.1083/jcb.200412022

Kondratskyi, A., Kondratska, K., Skryma, R., Klionsky, D. J., and Prevarskaya, N. (2017). Ion channels in the regulation of autophagy. *Autophagy* 5,1–19. doi: 10.1080/15548627.2017.1384887

Kudenchuk, P. J., Pierson, D. J., Greene, H. L., Graham, E. L., Sears, G. K., and Trobaugh, G. B. (1984). Prospective evaluation of amiodarone pulmonary toxicity. *Chest* 86, 541–548. doi: 10.1378/chest.86.4.541

Lavandero, S., Tronscoso, R., Rothermel, B. A., Martinet, W., Sadoshima, J., and Hill, J. A. (2013). Cardiovascular autophagy: concepts, controversies, and perspectives. *Autophagy* 9, 1455–1466. doi: 10.4161/auto.25969

Le, X., Mao, W., Lu, Z., Carter, B., and Bast, R. C. (2010). Dasatinib induces autophagic cell death in human ovarian cancer. *Cancer* 116, 4980–4990. doi: 10.1002/cncr.25426

Lee, Y. M., Cheng, P. Y., Chen, S. Y., Chung, M. T., and Sheu, J. R. (2011). Wogonin suppresses arrhythmias, inflammatory responses, and apoptosis induced by myocardial ischemia/reperfusion in rats. *J. Cardiovasc. Pharmacol.* 58, 133–142. doi: 10.1097/FJC.0b013e31821a5078

Levine, B., and Klionsky, D. J. (2017). Autophagy wins the 2016 nobel prize in physiology or medicine: breakthroughs in baker's yeast fuel advances in biomedical research. *Proc. Natl. Acad. Sci. U.S.A.* 114, 201–205. doi: 10.1073/pnas.1619876114

Li, J., Kim, S. G., and Blenis, J. (2014). Rapamycin: one drug, many effects. *Cell Metab.* 19, 373–379. doi: 10.1016/j.cmet.2014.01.001

Li, S., Sun, S., Gao, J., and Sun, F. (2016). Wogonin induces Beclin-1/PI3K and reactive oxygen species-mediated autophagy in human pancreatic cancer cells. *Oncol. Lett.* 12, 5059–5067. doi: 10.3892/ol.2016.5367

Li, W., Li, J., and Bao, J. (2012). Microautophagy: lesser-known self-eating. *Cell. Mol. Life Sci.* 69, 1125–1136. doi: 10.1007/s00018-011-0865-5

Li, Y., Chen, C., Yao, F., Su, Q., Liu, D., Xue, R., et al. (2014). AMPK inhibits cardiac hypertrophy by promoting autophagy via mTORC1. *Arch. Biochem. Biophys.* 558, 79–86. doi: 10.1016/j.abb.2014.06.023

Lin, C., Chen, Y., Lin, C., Chen, Y., Lo, G., Lee, P., et al. (2015). Amiodarone as an autophagy promotor reduces liver injury and enhances liver regeneration and survival in mice after partial hepatectomy. *Sci. Rep.* 5:15807. doi: 10.1038/srep15807

Lu, H. R., Vlaminckx, E., Hermans, A. N., Rohrbacher, J., Van Ammel, K., Towart, R., et al. (2008). Predicting drug-induced changes in QT interval and arrhythmias: QT-shortening drugs point to gaps in the ICHS7B guidelines. *Br. J. Pharmacol.* 154, 1427–1438. doi: 10.1038/bjp.2008.191

Marchetti, P., Benci, L., Cecchetti, P., Giannarelli, R., Boni, C., Ciociaro, D., et al. (1987). Plasma biguanide levels are correlated with metabolic effects in diabetic patients. *Clin. Pharmacol. Ther.* 41, 450–454. doi: 10.1038/clpt.1987.55

Mas, S., Gasso, P., Parellada, E., Bernardo, M., and Lafuente, A. (2015). Network analysis of gene expression in peripheral blood identifies mTOR and NF-kB pathways involved in antipsychotic-induced extrapyramidal symptoms. *Pharmacogenomics J.* 15, 452–460. doi: 10.1038/tpj.2014.84

Matsui, Y., Takagi, H., Qu, X., Abdellatif, M., Sakoda, H., Asano, T., et al. (2007). Distinct roles of autophagy in the heart during ischemia and reperfusion: roles of AMP-activated protein kinase and Beclin 1 in mediating autophagy. *Circ. Res.* 100, 914–922. doi: 10.1161/01.RES.0000261924.76669.36

Matsuura, A., Tsukada, M., Wada, Y., and Ohsumi, Y. (1997). Apg1p, a novel protein kinase required for the autophagic process in *Saccharomyces cerevisiae*. *Gene* 192, 245–250. doi: 10.1016/S0378-1119(97)00084-X

Mayer, I. A., and Arteaga, C. L. (2016). The PI3K/AKT pathway as a target for cancer treatment. *Annu. Rev. Med.* 67, 11–28. doi: 10.1146/annurev-med-062913-051343

McMullen, J. R., Sherwood, M. C., Tarnavski, O., Zhang, L., Dorfman, A. L., Shioi, T., et al. (2004). Inhibition of mTOR signaling with rapamycin regresses established cardiac hypertrophy induced pressure overload. *Circulation* 109, 3050–3055. doi: 10.1161/01

Meyer, G., Czompa, A., Reboul, C., Csepanyi, E., Czegledi, A., Bak, I., et al. (2013). The cellular autophagy markers beclin-1 and LC3B-II are increased during reperfusion in fibrillated mouse hearts. *Curr. Pharm. Des.* 19, 6912–6918. doi: 10.2174/138161281939131127122510

Mulcahy Levy, J. M., Towers, C. G., and Thorburn, A. (2017). Targeting autophagy in cancer. *Nat. Rev. Cancer* 17, 528–542. doi: 10.1038/nrc.2017.53

Nair, U., Jotwani, A., Geng, J., Gammoh, N., Richerson, D., Yen, W., et al. (2011). SNARE proteins are required for macroautophagy. *Cell* 146, 290–302. doi: 10.1016/j.cell.2011.06.022

Nakai, A., Yamaguchi, O., Takeda, T., Higuchi, Y., Hikoso, S., Taniike, M., et al. (2007). The role of autophagy in the basal state and in response to hemodynamic stress. *Nat. Med.* 13, 619–624. doi: 10.1038/nm1574

Nalos, L., De Boer, T. P., Houtman, M. J. C., Rook, M. B., Vos, M. A., and Van der Heyden, M. A. G. (2011). Inhibition of lysosomal degradation rescues pentamidine-mediated decreases of K(ir)2.1 ion channel expression but not of K(v)11.1. *Eur. J. Pharmacol.* 652, 96–103. doi: 10.1016/j.ejphar.2010.10.093

Nazirizadeh, Y., Vogel, F., Bader, W., Haen, E., Pfuhlmann, B., Gründer, G., et al. (2010). Serum concentrations of paliperidone versus risperidone and clinical effects. *Eur. J. Pharmacol.* 66, 797–803. doi: 10.1007/s00228-010-0812-7

Patel, C., Yan, G. X., and Kowey, P. R. (2009). Dronedarone. *Circulation* 120, 636–644. doi: 10.1161/CIRCULATIONNAHA.109.858027

Pelletier, A., Joly, E., Prentki, M., and Coderre, L. (2005). Adenosine 5'-monophosphate-activated protein kinase and p38 mitogen-activated protein kinase participate in the stimulation of glucose uptake by dinitrophenol in adult cardiomyocytes. *Endocrinology* 146, 2285–2294. doi: 10.1210/en.2004-1565

Piccoli, E., Nadai, M., Caretta, C. M., Bergonzini, V., Del Vecchio, C., Ha, H. R., et al. (2011). Amiodarone impairs trafficking through late endosomes inducing a Niemann-Pick C-like phenotype. *Biochem. Pharmacol.* 82, 1234–1249. doi: 10.1016/j.bcp.2011.07.090

Plicher, J., Cooper, J. D., Turnell, D. C., Matenga, J., Paul, R., and Lockhart, J. D. (1985). Investigations of long-term treatment with perhexiline maleate using therapeutic monitoring and electromyography. *Ther. Drug. Monit.* 7, 54–60.doi: 10.1097/00007691-198503000-00009

Pushparaj, C., Das, A., Purroy, R., Nager, M., Herreros, J., Pamplona, R., et al. (2015). Voltage-gated calcium channel blockers deregulate macroautophagy in cardiomyocytes. *Int. J. Biochem. Cell Biol.* 68, 166–175. doi: 10.1016/j.biocel.2015.09.010

Raichlin, E., Chandrasekaran, K., Kremers, W. K., Frantz, R. O., Clavelli, A. L., Pereira, N. L., et al. (2008). Sirolimus as primary immunosuppressant reduces left ventricular mass and improves diastolic function of the cardiac allograft. *Transplantation* 86, 1395–1400. doi: 10.1097/TP.0b013e318189049a

Redfern, W. S., Carlsson, L., Davis, A. S., Lynch, W. G., Machkenzie, I., Palethorpe, S., et al. (2003). Relationships between preclinical cardiac electrophysiology, clinical QT interval prolongation and torsade de pointes for a broad range of drugs: evidence for a provisional safety margin in drug development. *Cardiovasc. Res.* 58, 32–45. doi: 10.1016/S0008-6363(02)00846-5

Reggiori, F., and Klionsky, D. J. (2013). Autophagic processes in yeast: mechanism, machinery and regulation. *Genetics* 194, 341–361. doi: 10.1534/genetics.112.149013

Santangeli, P., Di Biase, L., Burkhardt, J. D., Bai, R., Mohanty, P., Pump, A., et al. (2012). Examining the safety of amiodarone. *Expert Opin. Drug Saf.* 11, 191–214. doi: 10.1517/14740338.2012.660915

Schneider, J. L., and Cuervo, A. M. (2014). Autophagy and human disease: emerging themes. *Curr. Opin. Genet. Dev.* 26, 16–23. doi: 10.1016/j.gde.2014.04.003

Sciarretta, S., Hariharan, N., Monden, Y., Zablocki, D., and Sadoshima, J. (2011). Is autophagy in response to ischemia and reperfusion protective or detrimental for the heart? *Pediatr. Cardiol.* 32, 275–281. doi: 10.1007/s00246-010-9855-x

Sciarretta, S., Yee, D., Shenoy, V., Nagarajan, N., and Sadoshima, J. (2014). The importance of autophagy in cardioprotection. *High Blood Press. Cardiovasc. Prev.* 21, 21–28. doi: 10.1007/s40292-013-0029-9

Shu, C., Huang, W., Zeng, Z., He, Y., Luo, B., Liu, H., et al. (2017). Connexin 43 is involved in the sympathetic atrial fibrillation in canine and canine atrial myocytes. *Anatol. J. Cardiol.* 18, 3–9. doi: 10.14744/AnatolJCardiol.2017.7602

Singh, R., and Cuervo, A. M. (2011). Autophagy in the cellular energetic balance. *Cell Metab.* 13, 495–504. doi: 10.1016/j.cmet.2011.04.004

Stenton, S. B., Partovi, N., and Ensom, M. H. H. (2005). Sirolimus. *Clin. Pharmacokinet.* 44, 769–786. doi: 10.2165/00003088-200544080-00001

Svenning, S., and Johansen, T. (2013). Selective autophagy. *Essays Biochem.* 55, 79–92. doi: 10.1042/bse0550079

Takagi, H., Matsui, Y., Hirotani, S., Sakoda, H., Asano, T., and Sadoshima, J. (2007). AMPK mediates autophagy during myocardial ischemia *in vivo*. *Autophagy* 3, 405–407. doi: 10.4161/auto.4281

Takanari, H., Nalos, L., Stary-Weinzinger, A., De Git, K. C. G., Varkevisser, R., Linder, T., et al. (2013). Efficient and specific cardiac Ik1 inhibition by a new pentamidine analogue. *Cardiovasc. Res.* 99, 203–214. doi: 10.1093/cvr/cvt103

Tanaka, Y., Guhde, G., Suter, A., Eskelinen, E., Hartmann, D., Lullmann-Rauch, R., et al. (2000). Accumulation of autophagic vacuoles and cardiomyopathy in LAMP-2-deficient mice. *Nature* 406, 902–906. doi: 10.1038/35022595

Tarapués, M., Cereza, G., Arellano, A. L., Montané, E., and Figueras, A. (2014). Serious QT interval prolongation with ranolazine and amiodarone. *Int. J. Cardiol.* 172, e60–e61. doi: 10.1016/j.ijcard.2013.12.061

Van Bortel, L., Böhm, R., Mooij, J., Schiffers, P., and Rahn, K. H. (1989). Total and free steady-state plasma levels and pharmacokinetics of nifedipine in patients with terminal renal failure. *Eur. J. Clin. Pharmacol.* 37, 185–189.

Vigneault, P., Kaddar, N., Bourgault, S., Caillier, B., Pilote, S., Patoine, D., et al. (2011). Prolongation of cardiac ventricular repolarization under paliperidone: how and how much? *J. Cardiovasc. Pharmacol.* 57, 690–695. doi: 10.1097/FJC.0b013e318217d941

Vincent, E. E., Coelho, P. P., Blagih, J., Griss, T., Viollet, B., and Jones, R. G. (2015). Differential effects of AMPK agonists on cell growth and metabolism. *Oncogene* 34, 3627–3639. doi: 10.1038/onc.2014.301

Waalkes, T. P., Denham, C., and DeVita, V. T. (1970). Pentamidine: clinical pharmacologic correlations in man and mice. *Clin. Pharmacol. Ther.* 11, 505–512. doi: 10.1002/cpt1970114505

Wada, T., Nakamura, Y., Cao, X., Ohara, H., Izumi-Nakaseko, H., Nakazato, Y., et al. (2016). Antiviral drug vidarabine possessing cardiac type 5 adenylyl cyclase inhibitory property did not affect cardiohemodynamic or electrophysiological variables in the halothane-anesthetized dogs. *J. Toxicol. Sci.* 41, 115–122. doi: 10.2131/jts.41.115

Wadhani, N., Sarma, J. S. M., Singh, B. N., Radzik, D., and Gaud, C. (2006). Dose-dependent effects of oral dronedarone on the circadian variation of RR and QT intervals in healthy subjects: implications for antiarrhythmic actions. *J. Cardiovasc. Pharmacol. Ther.* 11, 184–190. doi: 10.1177/1074248406290678

Walker, B. D., Valenzuela, S. M., Singleton, C. B., Tie, H., Bursill, J. A., Wyse, K. R., et al. (1999). Inhibition of HERG channels stably expressed in a mammalian cell line by the antianginal agent perhexiline maleate. *Br. J. Pharmacol.* 127, 243–251. doi: 10.1038/sj.bjp.0702502

Walker, O., Dawodu, A. H., Adeyokunnu, A. A., Salako, L. A., and Alvan, G. (1983). Plasma chloroquine and desethylchloroquine concentrations in children during and after chloroquine treatment for malaria. *Br. J. Clin. Pharmac.* 16, 701–705.

Wang, B., Lu, D., Xuan, M., and Hu, W. (2017). Antitumor effect of sunitinib in human prostate cancer cells functions via autophagy. *Exp. Ther. Med.* 13, 1285–1294. doi: 10.3892/etm.2017.4134

Weng, L., Zhang, W., Ye, Y., Yin, P., Yuan, J., Wang, X., et al. (2014). Aliskerin ameliorates pressure overload-induced heart hypertrophy and fibrosis in mice. *Acta Pharmacol. Sin.* 35, 1005–1014. doi: 10.1038/aps.2014.45

Wharton, J. M., Demopulos, P. A., and Goldschlager, N. (1987). Torsade de pointes during administration of pentamidine isethionate. *Am. J. Med.* 83, 571–576. doi: 10.1016/0002-9343(87)90774-1

White, N. J. (2007). Cardiotoxicity of antimalarial drugs. *Lancet Infect. Dis.* 7, 549–558. doi: 10.1016/S1473-3099(07)70187-1

Whitley, R. J., Tucker, B. C., Kinkel, A. W., Barton, N. H., Pass, R. F., Whelchel, J. D., et al. (1980). Pharmacology, tolerance, and antiviral activity of vidarabine monophosphate in humans. *Antimicrob. Agents Chemother.* 18, 709–715.

Williams, A., Sarkar, S., Cuddon, P., Ttofi, E. K., Saiki, S., Siddiqi, F. H., et al. (2008). Novel targets for Huntington's disease in an mTOR-independent autophagy pathway. *Nat. Chem. Biol.* 4, 295–305. doi: 10.1038/nchembio.79

Xie, Y., Kang, R., Sun, X., Zhong, M., Huang, J., Klionsky, D. J., et al. (2015). Posttranslational modification of autophagy-related proteins in macroautophagy. *Autophagy* 11, 28–45. doi: 10.4161/15548627.2014.984267

Yang, L., Sha, H., Davisson, R. L., and Qi, L. (2013). Phenformin activates the unfolded protein response in an AMP-activated protein kinase (AMPK)-dependent manner. *J. Biol. Chem.* 288, 13631–13638. doi: 10.1074/jbc.M113.462762

Yoon, Y. H., Cho, K. S., Hwang, J. J., Lee, S., Choi, J. A., and Koh, J. (2010). Induction of lysosomal degradation, arrested autophagy, and cell death by chloroquine in cultured ARPE-19 cells. *Invest. Ophthalmol. Vis. Sci.* 51, 6030–6037. doi: 10.1167/iovs.10-5278

Yu, H., Lin, C., Tai, W., Liu, C., Shiau, C., and Chen, K. (2013). Nilotinib induces autophagy in hepatocellular carcinoma through AMPK activation. *J. Biol. Chem.* 288, 18249–18259. doi: 10.1074/jbc.M112.446385

Yuan, Y., Zhao, J., Yan, S., Wang, D., Zhang, S., Yun, F., et al. (2014). Autophagy: a potential novel mechanistic contributor to atrial fibrillation. *Int. J. Cardiol.* 172, 492–494. doi: 10.1016/j.ijcard.2014.01.027

Zhang, D., Contu, R., Latronico, M. V. G., Zhang, J. L., Rizzi, R., Catalucci, D., et al. (2010). MTORC1 regulates cardiac function and myocyte survival through 4E-BP1 inhibition in mice. *J. Clin. Invest.* 120, 2805–2816. doi: 10.1172/JCI43008

Zhou, G., Myers, R., Li, Y., Chen, Y., Shen, X., Fenyk-Melody, J., et al. (2001). Role of AMP-activated protein kinase in mechanism of metformin action. *J. Clin. Invest.* 108, 1167–1174. doi: 10.1172/JCI 13505

8

Autonomic Control of the Heart and its Clinical Impact: A Personal Perspective

*Maria Teresa La Rovere[1], Alberto Porta[2,3] and Peter J. Schwartz[4]**

[1]Department of Cardiology, IRCCS Istituti Clinici Scientifici Maugeri, Montescano (Pavia), Italy, [2]Department of Biomedical Sciences for Health, University of Milan, Milan, Italy, [3]Department of Cardiothoracic, Vascular Anesthesia and Intensive Care, IRCCS Policlinico San Donato, Milan, Italy, [4]Center for Cardiac Arrhythmias of Genetic Origin and Laboratory of Cardiovascular Genetics, Istituto Auxologico Italiano, IRCCS, Milan, Italy

***Correspondence:**
Peter J. Schwartz
p.schwartz@auxologico.it

This essay covers several aspects of the autonomic control of the heart, all relevant to cardiovascular pathophysiology with a direct impact on clinical outcomes. Ischemic heart disease, heart failure, channelopathies, and life-threatening arrhythmias are in the picture. Beginning with an overview on some of the events that marked the oscillations in the medical interest for the autonomic nervous system, our text explores specific areas, including experimental and clinical work focused on understanding the different roles of tonic and reflex sympathetic and vagal activity. The role of the baroreceptors, not just for the direct control of circulation but also because of the clinical value of interpreting alterations (spontaneous or induced) in their function, is discussed. The importance of the autonomic nervous system for gaining insights on risk stratification and for providing specific antiarrhythmic protection is also considered. Examples are the interventions to decrease sympathetic activity and/or to increase vagal activity. The non-invasive analysis of the RR and QT intervals provides additional information. The three of us have collaborated in several studies and each of us contributes with very specific and independent areas of expertise. Here, we have focused on those areas to which we have directly contributed and hence speak with personal experience. This is not an attempt to provide a neutral and general overview on the autonomic nervous system; rather, it represents our effort to share and provide the readers with our own personal views matured after many years of research in this field.

Keywords: heart rate variability, QT interval, baroreflex sensitivity, autonomic nervous system, sympathetic nervous system, vagal activity, long QT syndrome, sudden death

INTRODUCTION

One of the characteristics of the autonomic nervous system is the waxing and waning of its activity, both afferent and efferent. Similarly, the last 50 years have witnessed the waxing and waning of its interest for clinical cardiologists dealing with cardiac arrhythmias, sudden death, and heart failure.

Especially in the 1970s, but also later, much effort was devoted to the study of neural activity through the recording of single fibers in the sympathetic and vagal nerves (Malliani et al., 1969, 1973; Kunze, 1972; Cerati and Schwartz, 1991), which allowed the description of important autonomic reflexes (Schwartz et al., 1973). In the 1970s, 1980s, and 1990s, interest for the autonomic nervous system peaked. Some investigators focused on the stimulation of nerves directed to the heart trying to derive information for potential clinical translation (Schwartz, 1985), others focused on various aspects of the analysis of heart rate, either at rest (Kleiger et al., 1987) or in response to stimuli (Billman, 2009); these analyses of tonic or reflex autonomic activity had post-myocardial infarction (post-MI) and heart failure risk stratification as one significant objective (Schwartz et al., 1992a; Mortara et al., 1997; La Rovere et al., 1998, 2003). During the last 20 years, there was a surge of interest for the possibility of modulating autonomic activity, especially the vagal one, also in chronic conditions such as heart failure (Schwartz et al., 2008a, 2015; De Ferrari et al., 2011); however, the combination of unsatisfactory results and superficial analyses (Hauptman et al., 2012; Gold et al., 2016) has somewhat cooled down these hopes. One area where clinical success has fueled interest is the one related to the prevention of life-threatening events by cardiac sympathetic denervation (Schwartz, 2014).

Here, the three of us, who have collaborated in a number of studies, present our unabashed views on some of these topics.

INITIAL OVERVIEW

The neural control of the heart is accomplished throughout a multilevel neural network within the central nervous system and peripheral extracardiac and cardiac ganglia that exert their influence *via* the sympathetic and parasympathetic nervous systems (Levy and Schwartz, 1994; Shivkumar et al., 2016). Cardiac diseases may profoundly affect central and peripheral mechanisms of neural control of cardiac function, thus resulting in maladaptive responses that may be critically involved in the progression of the disease or in the development of arrhythmias. Neural sensory information from the heart (Paintal, 1963; Schwartz et al., 1973), blood vessels, and other organs is processed at different levels within the neuraxis with a first level of integration represented by the intrinsic cardiac nervous system located in the cardiac ganglia within the heart. The intrinsic cardiac nervous system processes sensory information and provides efferent input to the myocardium under the tonic modulation of the extrinsic sympathetic and parasympathetic input. Arterial baroreceptors play a paramount role in the neural control of the cardiovascular system (Eckberg and Sleight, 1992). Arterial baroreceptors are stretch receptors embedded in the adventitia of the carotid sinus and aortic wall. Increases in arterial blood pressure will result in an increased rate of impulse firing to the nucleus tractus solitarius, which modulates sympathetic and parasympathetic output to the cardiovascular system. The baroreflex control of circulatory homeostasis occurs on a negative feedback basis. Thus, the attending reflex decrease in sympathetic activity and increase in vagal activity will reduce heart rate, cardiac contractility, and peripheral resistance. Opposite changes are associated with an arterial pressure decrease.

By complex interactions between the main neurotransmitters [namely, noradrenaline, acetylcholine, and neuropeptide Y; (Dusi et al., 2020)] and their effects on specific receptors of cardiac cells in the sinoatrial node, atrioventricular node, and left ventricle, the autonomic nervous system affects several aspects of cardiac electrophysiology. At the sinus node level, efferent vagal activity decreases while sympathetic activity increases the spontaneous depolarization rate of sinus node cells.

Furthermore, it has been known for many years that sympathetic nervous system stimulation may be pro-arrhythmic, particularly in conditions of acute myocardial ischemia (Harris et al., 1971; Schwartz and Vanoli, 1981; Janse et al., 1985; Schwartz et al., 1985), while vagal nerve stimulation may reduce the potential for lethal arrhythmias (Kent et al., 1973; Vanoli et al., 1991). Thus, by controlling the autonomic traffic to the heart, the baroreceptors are involved in the susceptibility to ventricular and supraventricular arrhythmias. Moreover, by controlling the hemodynamic adjustments to blood pressure changes, they also play a role in the clinical response to sustained rhythm disorders (De Ferrari et al., 1995; Landolina et al., 1997).

Damage to cardiac sensory nerve endings caused by acute myocardial infarction and left ventricular remodeling directly affects the baroreceptor system. The attending reflex autonomic dysfunction, characterized by reduced parasympathetic and increased sympathetic activity coupled with neural remodeling and nerve sprouting (Cao et al., 2000), promotes arrhythmogenesis.

The prominent neurohumoral mechanism at play in heart failure is the sympathetic nervous system whose increased activity coupled with vagal withdrawal is initiated by the arterial baroreflex (Hartupee and Mann, 2017). Although other mediators, including sympatho-excitatory reflexes, humoral factors, and central mechanisms (Floras and Ponikowski, 2015) contribute to the development of sympathetic-parasympathetic imbalance in heart failure, an impairment of baroreflex control of heart rate is a prominent characteristic of the heart failure syndrome and a reliable marker of the severity of the disease (Mortara et al., 1997).

Relevant insights into the pathophysiological implications of heart disease-related baroreflex impairment date back to the early 1970s when it was recognized that baroreceptor reflexes can be modulated by cardiac afferent sympathetic activity activated by mechanical and chemical stimuli (Malliani et al., 1973; Schwartz et al., 1973). An animal model provided the first evidence that reduction in cardiac parasympathetic control is associated with an increased risk for sudden death. In this canine model (Billman et al., 1982; Schwartz et al., 1984), baroreflex sensitivity (BRS) was impaired by myocardial infarction, with the greatest impairment noted in animals particularly susceptible to sudden death (Schwartz et al., 1988). Similarly in humans, a tight relationship between reduced baroreceptor activity and heart disease state was first reported by Eckberg et al. (1971) and was subsequently found to be associated with an increased risk of cardiac mortality and sudden cardiac death in post-MI and heart failure patients (Mortara et al., 1997; La Rovere et al., 1998, 2001).

The initial results with BRS led some investigators to consider the possibility that powerful baroreceptive reflex would imply that the attendant increase in vagal activity to the sinus node would extend to the ventricles as well. The high specificity of the cardiac innervation (Pagani et al., 1974; Randall, 1984), the central organization of cardiovascular reflexes (Wurster, 1984), and the important report by Inoue and Zipes (1987) indicate clearly that such an extrapolation would be both naïve and unwarranted. Indeed, a heart-rate response indicative of increased vagal activity does not exclude the possibility of a dominant sympathetic activity at ventricular level (e.g., the diving reflex, hypoxia, and inferior myocardial ischemia). Nonetheless, the most frequent reflex response is synergistic, i.e., one limb of the autonomic nervous system is excited with simultaneous inhibition of the other (Wurster, 1984), and the reduction in heart rate produced by the baroreflex is accompanied by a reflex withdrawal of sympathetic activity that is generalized and extends to the ventricles. In the sudden death animal model that played such an important role in the development of the clinical interest for BRS (Schwartz et al., 1984), the dogs with higher BRS were also those with larger heart rate reductions during acute myocardial ischemia despite continuation of exercise (Schwartz et al., 1984). One logical implication is that the animals responding with strong vagal reflexes to blood pressure increases are likely to respond similarly to acute myocardial ischemia. The animals with the greatest sinus node response to the baroreflex test are less prone to sudden death during myocardial ischemia, and conversely, those with the most reduced BRS are more vulnerable to ventricular fibrillation. This does not mean that the baroreflex test predicts the autonomic changes at the ventricular level during myocardial ischemia but indicates that it can often predict the outcome during an ischemic episode, which is what really matters. Although, as correctly stated (Inoue and Zipes, 1987), the use of spontaneous or reflex changes in heart rate as an indicator of what might happen at the ventricular level would certainly be naive, their use to identify individuals at varying risk of life-threatening events is a rational exploitation of the current understanding of cardiovascular pathophysiology.

ASSESSMENT OF CARDIAC AUTONOMIC FUNCTION

As the baroreflex affects the balance between parasympathetic inhibition and sympathetic excitation of the sinoatrial node of the heart, sinus node activity (either spontaneous or in response to a provocation) can provide information on the underlying regulatory system.

Assessment of Arterial Baroreflex Control

Several methods have been developed so far to evaluate arterial baroreflex control in humans (La Rovere et al., 2008; Pinna et al., 2017). The reference method in clinical and research applications entails the assessment of the heart rate response to a physiological provocation (Smyth et al., 1969; La Rovere et al., 2008). In the original method, intravenous injections of small boluses of phenylephrine are used to raise blood pressure transiently, and the resultant reflex bradycardia (expressed as the following heart periods) is used as an index of BRS. A wealth of non-invasive indicators of the arterial-cardiac baroreceptor reflex sensitivity can be obtained by the joint analysis of beat-to-beat spontaneous fluctuations of systolic blood pressure and RR interval series (La Rovere et al., 2008). These methods include: model-free techniques (Robbe et al., 1987; Pinna et al., 2002), interactions among heart period and systolic arterial pressure (Porta et al., 2000; Nollo et al., 2005; Milan-Mattos et al., 2018), models searching for specific patterns of baroreflex origin (Bertinieri et al., 1985) or heart rate responses to systolic pressure changes (Bauer et al., 2010), and others merely requiring a certain degree of association between spontaneous heart period and systolic arterial pressure variations (Westerhof et al., 2004). Some methods lead to an indirect estimate of BRS *via* analysis of the bi-phasic response of the sinus node to a premature ventricular contraction (named heart rate turbulence) that is largely dependent on the baroreflex (Schmidt et al., 1999; La Rovere et al., 2011). Despite indices of baroreflex control derived from spontaneous variability cannot be considered fully equivalent to the interventional ones (Diaz and Taylor, 2006), their value in clinical setting has been proved (La Rovere et al., 2008; Pinna et al., 2017). The reliability of these non-invasive indices has been recently reviewed (Pinna et al., 2015) with special attention to their predictive value (Pinna et al., 2017).

Assessment of Heart Rate Variability

Since the seminal study by Akselrod et al. (1981), autonomic function has been non-invasively inferred from the variability of sinus RR interval obtained from surface electrocardiogram (ECG). The disappearance of RR variability after vagal blockade by high dose atropine not only proved the predominance of vagal over sympathetic cardiac modulation in humans at rest (Pomeranz et al., 1985; Montano et al., 1998) but also confirmed that RR interval variability was related to autonomic control. Indeed, in humans at rest, the primacy of the vagal versus the sympathetic drive leads to a heart rate lower than the intrinsic heart rate of the isolated heart (Jose and Collison, 1970).

The RR mean provides an indication of the tonic balance between sympathetic and vagal mean neural activities (Malik et al., 2019b), while the magnitude of the RR variations about its mean is linked to the balance of the spontaneous variations of vagal and sympathetic neural activities about their correspondent means, usually referred to as vagal and sympathetic modulations (Task Force of the European Society of Cardiology and the North American Society of Pacing and Electrophysiology, 1996; Pagani et al., 1997; Bauer et al., 2017; Malik et al., 2019a). A number of techniques have been developed to quantify the RR interval variability in order to evaluate cardiac autonomic regulation. The measurement of RR interval variability was initially based on simple statistics, such as the standard deviation of RR interval variation and its derivative, and on power spectral analysis that separates and quantifies the various oscillations that exist in the RR interval signal. At variance with the conventional measures of RR interval variability, complexity markers and fractal measures of HRV account for the inherent irregularity, long range correlation, and scale invariance of the spontaneous fluctuations of RR interval (Goldberger, 1996; Porta et al., 2009).

It has been recently stressed that RR variability markers might be biased proxies of autonomic modulation as a result of the nonlinear relation between mean RR and magnitude of RR changes (Opthof et al., 1984; Boyett et al., 2019; Malik et al., 2019a). The rate-dependency of RR variability markers is the consequence of the direct effect of acetylcholine concentration on the diastolic depolarization rate of the sinus node pacemaker cells producing larger variations of the cycle length if the cycle length is longer (Zaza and Lombardi, 2001). This relation might limit the value of RR variability markers expressed in absolute units because an augmented modulation of the autonomic activity increases RR variability indices but a greater fluctuations of RR might be simply a consequence of bradycardia, regardless of whether it is of autonomic origin or due to modifications of the properties of sinus node pacemaker cells [e.g., I_f modifications; Zaza and Lombardi, (2001); Da Silva et al. (2015); Boyett et al. (2019)]. Since this effect is the mere consequence of the sinus node transduction process, it could affect any marker based on RR changes including BRS. Therefore, the possibility of interpreting RR variability markers as proxies of autonomic modulation is fully preserved as long as the compared populations and/or experimental conditions exhibit the same RR mean. Alternatively, it was suggested to use RR variability indices that feature an intrinsic normalization (Zaza and Lombardi, 2001; Da Silva et al., 2015). Among those indices, normalized high frequency (HF) powers and the low frequency (LF)/HF ratio can be exploited (Pagani et al., 1997). Especially whether the RR mean varies among groups and experimental conditions and, thus, the genuine role of an altered neural modulation is not warranted, it is recommended to check for the potential variations of the LF/HF ratio before concluding that RR variability indices expressed in absolute units indicate modifications of the autonomic control.

Concurrent Assessment of RR and QT Variability

The difficulty in the assessment of the sympathetic modulation from RR variability is a direct consequence of the vagal nature of the spontaneous fluctuations of RR (Eckberg, 1997), especially when the magnitude of the RR changes is assessed in absolute units (Montano et al., 1994). This observation, in association with the clinical importance of the non-invasive inference of cardiac sympathetic modulation, has led to search for possible alternatives, still obtained from the ECG, to the sole analysis of RR variability.

An important one, in our opinion, is the study of the QT interval variability (Malik, 2008; Berger, 2009; Baumert et al., 2016). Its interest lies in the fact that the amplitude of the QT changes has been related to the magnitude of sympathetic control. Indeed, the higher the sympathetic drive and its variations about its mean value such as during an orthostatic challenge, mental stress, or advanced age, the greater the magnitude of the QT variations in healthy individuals (Negoescu et al., 1997; Porta et al., 1998a, 2010, 2011; Yeragani et al., 2000a; Piccirillo et al., 2001, 2006; Boettger et al., 2010; Baumert et al., 2016; El-Hamad et al., 2019). This link holds even in pathological conditions characterized by a high sympathetic drive (Berger et al., 1997; Yeragani et al., 2000b; Bär et al., 2007; Baumert et al., 2008, 2011) and provides new clues for stratifying the risk of arrhythmic events (Atiga et al., 1998; Piccirillo et al., 2007; Segerson et al., 2008; Chen et al., 2011; Dobson et al., 2011; Oosterhoff et al., 2011; Tereshchenko et al., 2012; Porta et al., 2015).

These observations suggested a possible strategy to separately quantify vagal and sympathetic modulations in humans *via* the concomitant analysis of RR and QT variabilities (Porta et al., 2015). Vagal modulation is inferred from the respiratory sinus arrhythmia, namely the portion of the RR variability in the HF (from 0.15 to 0.5 Hz) band (Hirsch and Bishop, 1981; Pomeranz et al., 1985). Sympathetic modulation is inferred from the power of the QT variability in the LF (from 0.04 to 0.15 Hz) band (Porta et al., 2011; Baumert et al., 2016). This choice is more robust than the mere exploitation of the QT variance because it prevents the bias produced by non-autonomic influences such as cardiac axis movements leading to periodical artifacts which would affect the QT measurement at the respiratory rate (Lombardi et al., 1996; Porta et al., 1998b). The interpretation of QT variability markers is made more complex by the QT-RR relation (Bazett, 1920), which mirrors on the surface ECG the adaptation of action potential duration to the cycle length observed at the cellular level (Conrath and Opthof, 2006), and by the influences of the autonomic nervous system on the QT-RR relation (Zaza et al., 1991; Porta et al., 1998a; Magnano et al., 2002). Modeling approaches can describe the dynamic dependence of QT on previous RR variations (Zaza et al., 1991; Porta et al., 1998a, 2010) and even account for confounding factors such as respiration (Porta et al., 2017). Alternative approaches excluding the influences of cardiac neural control directed to the sinus node on the regulation of the QT dynamics and preventing the need of hypothesizing any *a priori* defined, and arbitrary, QT-RR relation (Pueyo et al., 2004) are based on gating the QT variability analysis at similar RR mean (Browne et al., 1983) or on the normalization of QT variability markers to the magnitude of RR changes (Berger et al., 1997; Baumert et al., 2016).

Complexity of the Cardiac Autonomic Control

Complexity analysis is an additional approach for the assessment of cardiac control with an inherent normalization given that it is fully independent of the amplitude of spontaneous RR and QT changes (Pincus and Goldberger, 1994; Porta et al., 2009). Under normal conditions, the simultaneous action of multiple regulatory mechanisms operating with slightly different frequencies within the LF and HF bands produces irregular changes of RR and QT intervals. Disease and aging impair the sinus node responsiveness and decrease the level of irregularity of the RR and QT beat-to-beat dynamics (Goldberger, 1996). Complexity analyses of RR and QT variabilities provide non-redundant information. Indeed, the larger irregularity of the QT variability compared to that of the RR variability points to the greater complexity of the neural control directed to the ventricles than that to the sinus node (Inoue and Zipes, 1987; Lewis and Short, 2007; Baumert et al., 2012; Bari et al., 2014a). The decreased complexity of the RR variability during vagal withdrawal and sympathetic activation induced by orthostatic challenge (Porta et al., 2007; Turianikova et al., 2011; Baumert et al., 2014) is interpreted as a consequence of the reduction of the respiratory sinus arrhythmia and of the increase of a dominant LF component limiting the spectral content of the RR variability series (Porta et al., 2012). Therefore, complexity indices derived from RR variability are mainly under vagal control (Porta et al., 2012). Indeed, low-pass filtering approach canceling respiratory sinus arrhythmia from the RR variability prevented the increase of RR variability complexity during nighttime and under β-blockers (Bari et al., 2014a). At difference with the complexity of RR variability, the complexity of the QT variability in healthy individuals during orthostatic challenge and in pathological populations featuring a dominant sympathetic drive remains high (Baumert et al., 2014; Li et al., 2019) or even increases (Sosnowski et al., 2001; Nahshoni et al., 2004; Porta et al., 2010; Li et al., 2015) compared to basal condition or control subjects. Senescence in a healthy population is accompanied by an increase of QT variability complexity (Boettger et al., 2010). The dynamics of QT variability become more irregular during sympathetic activation due to the prevailing action of inputs driving QT independently of RR changes (Porta et al., 2010). The decrease of the T-wave amplitude with sympathetic activation is likely to play a role in increasing the beat-to-beat irregularity of QT by making the process of delineation of the T-wave offset more difficult (Baumert et al., 2016). Therefore, the complexity of the QT variability could largely represent the sympathetic control directed to the ventricles, largely unrelated to the cardiac autonomic regulation impinging on the sinus node. We suggested that a limited complexity of the QT variability might be protective against arrhythmic risk (Bari et al., 2014a,b).

RISK STRATIFICATION

Effective risk stratification for patients who might develop life-threatening ventricular arrhythmia and sudden cardiac death is one of the main unsolved areas in clinical cardiology. Arrhythmic risk represents the sum of several different risk-augmenting processes and factors. Understanding the relation between changes in autonomic activity and cardiac electrophysiological properties has led to the view that the autonomic nervous system modulates interactions between triggering factors and the underlying electrophysiologic substrate. This points to a significant potential prognostic value of markers of autonomic activity.

Since the 1990s, the analysis of BRS has been considered as a tool that might help identifying "high-risk" patients. A multicenter study on more than 1,200 post-infarction patients demonstrated the incremental prognostic value provided by an impaired BRS when combined to left ventricular ejection function and to the potential trigger of non-sustained ventricular tachycardia (La Rovere et al., 1998, 2001). Specifically, a depressed BRS, a reduced left ventricular ejection fraction, and the presence of non-sustained ventricular tachycardia were all independent predictors of mortality, but depressed BRS almost doubled the risk of death provided by the other two markers. Moreover, among patients with either reduced or preserved left ventricular function but without signs of electrical instability, mortality differed significantly according to the presence or absence of preserved autonomic function (La Rovere et al., 2001; De Ferrari et al., 2007).

The role of baroreflex-mediated responses in the control of hemodynamic stability is particularly relevant during the course of a sustained ventricular rhythm. Inadequate baroreflex-mediated sympatho-excitation during a sustained ventricular tachycardia in post-infarction patients was the leading cause of an unfavorable hemodynamic profile leading to circulatory collapse (Landolina et al., 1997).

Randomized trials, demonstrating that among post-infarction patients mortality can be effectively reduced by prophylactic implantation of a cardioverter defibrillator, established a paradigm shift in risk stratification through the assessment of left ventricular ejection fraction as the gold standard risk predictor. However, this does not deprive autonomic markers of their clinical value (Wellens et al., 2014). It is now clear that left ventricular ejection fraction measurement has both limited sensitivity and specificity as a tool for arrhythmic risk stratification and that the field of risk stratification should move from the "high-risk ejection fraction" to the broader concept of the "high-risk patients" (Chugh, 2017). This transition implies a novel opportunity for autonomic markers to be re-evaluated in their involvement in the pathogenesis of arrhythmic risk and incorporated in novel prediction models. Moreover, novel ECG-based risk markers that quantify sympathetic activity-associated repolarization instabilities are promising in their ability to guide decisions about the prophylactic implantation of a cardioverter defibrillator (Bauer et al., 2019). The markers tested by Bauer et al. (2019) are framed in an emerging area of biomedical signal processing aiming at monitoring relevant electrocardiographic fiducial points and time intervals under the hypothesis such that their evolution over time might provide information about cardiac control.

In a founder population of long QT syndrome type 1 (LQT1), which avoids the confounding factors due to different mutations and segregates the malignant *KCNQ1*-A341V mutation (Brink et al., 2005; Crotti et al., 2007; Brink and Schwartz, 2009), the characterization of cardiac autonomic control and baroreflex function was found to be useful to improve the risk stratification of arrhythmic events (Schwartz et al., 2008b; Crotti et al., 2012; Bari et al., 2014a,b, 2015; Porta et al., 2015). In this population which is at the highest risk of fatal events in situations of high sympathetic drive (Schwartz et al., 2001), it was found that subjects who did not experience arrhythmic events, namely the asymptomatic mutation-carriers, have a completely different autonomic profile compared to those experiencing syncope or cardiac arrest requiring resuscitation. Indeed, asymptomatic individuals exhibited longer RR (Schwartz et al., 2008b), lower BRS (Schwartz et al., 2008b), higher QT variability in the LF band during daytime (Porta et al., 2015), lower respiratory sinus arrhythmia during nighttime and under β-blockers (Porta et al., 2015), slower heart rate recovery after exercise test (Crotti et al., 2012), and lower QT variability complexity (Bari et al., 2014a,b, 2015). These findings suggested that, besides RR lengthening, the combination of a more reactive sympathetic drive to the ventricles (i.e., adapting more rapidly QT to RR changes and limiting irregularity of QT changes during a sympathetic stressor) and of a sluggish vagal responsiveness after exercise represents a protective mechanism. Remarkably, non-mutation carriers belonging to the same family line (Brink et al., 2005; Brink and Schwartz, 2009) have an autonomic profile more similar to symptomatic patients than asymptomatic ones, thus suggesting that there are peculiar traits of the autonomic control that might be key for survival because they reduce the severity of the disease (Schwartz et al., 2008b; Porta et al., 2015).

NEUROMODULATION

Vagal Neuromodulation

One relevant aspect of several abnormalities related to the baroreceptors and autonomic nervous system pathophysiology is that they are often correctable by treatment. While β-blockers are the mainstay in the management of autonomic imbalance, device technology and advances in neuromodulatory techniques paved the way to directly target the autonomic nervous system. Baroreflex activation therapy (BAT), providing chronic baroreflex activation through electrical stimulation of the carotid sinus, has been initially developed for the treatment of resistant hypertension. Clinical studies have underlined the potential of BAT to improve blood pressure control and reduce the need of anti-hypertensive therapy at cost of few side effects despite the invasiveness of the procedure (Bolignano and Coppolino, 2018). BAT is currently being evaluated in heart failure with reduced ejection fraction. Initial studies support the hypothesis that baroreflex activation can add significant therapeutic benefit on top of guideline-directed medical therapy in patients with advanced heart failure. A randomized controlled trial (the BeAT-HF trial) is actively recruiting an estimated sample size of 480 patients with New York Heart Association functional class II heart failure but excluding patients actively receiving cardiac resynchronization therapy; its completion is expected by April 2021 (Mann and Abraham, 2019).

Experimental studies in an established conscious canine model of post-MI sudden cardiac death (Schwartz et al., 1984) demonstrated that vagus nerve stimulation (VNS) was effective in preventing ventricular fibrillation induced by acute myocardial ischemia (Vanoli et al., 1991). The initially promising translation of animal studies to the clinical setting of patients with HF and reduced ejection fraction (Schwartz et al., 2008a; De Ferrari et al., 2011) did not show consistent results in randomized trials (Zannad et al., 2015; Gold et al., 2016). In the debate following these studies, several critical issues (patient selection, proper titration of VNS therapy, effective markers for therapy, and pattern of vagal fibers stimulation) have been identified that would require further assessment.

Transcutaneous electrical stimulation of the auricular branch of the vagus nerve located at the tragus, which is effective in stimulating afferent vagal nerve fibers, has been suggested to represent an alternative access path to the same neuronal network without invasiveness and common side effects including hoarseness, sore throat, shortness of breath, and coughing, even though it is likely to lead to a smaller release of ACh compared to direct vagal efferent stimulation. In a study based on spontaneous variability, in young healthy subjects, transcutaneous VNS acutely reduced resting heart rate and the response to orthostatic stress (Tobaldini et al., 2019). Transcutaneous VNS is being studied for a number of pathological conditions including ventricular arrhythmias, heart failure, and myocardial infarction. Experimental and clinical data recently suggested that chronic intermittent VNS lasting 2 h/day for 2 months reduced inducibility of ventricular arrhythmias (Zhu et al., 2019).

Sympathetic Neuromodulation

The fact that acute myocardial ischemia is often associated with life-threatening arrhythmias was recognized from the early days (Harris et al., 1971). When it was shown that acute myocardial ischemia also elicits a powerful excitatory sympathetic reflex within seconds (Malliani et al., 1969), thus increasing the release of norepinephrine at the ventricular level, the link was established. One obvious consequence was the rationale for the use of β-adrenergic blocking agents to prevent cardiac arrhythmias in ischemic heart disease. Another consequence was the concept that if arrhythmias are triggered by an abrupt release of norepinephrine, the section of the nerves mediating this release might have had a protective effect (Schwartz, 2014).

Given the quantitative dominance of the left sided cardiac sympathetic nerves at the ventricular level, the interest went immediately to the potential effects of left cardiac sympathetic denervation (LCSD). Thus, a series of experiments, mostly performed in the 1970s, provided the necessary information. It was shown that LCSD prevents arrhythmias associated with acute myocardial ischemia in normal hearts (Schwartz et al., 1976b) and in hearts with a healed myocardial infarction (Schwartz and Stone, 1980), that it does not impair cardiovascular performance during exercise (Schwartz and Stone, 1979), that it does increase the capability of the coronary bed to dilate (Schwartz and Stone, 1977), and that it does not cause denervation supersensitivity (Schwartz and Stone, 1982). However, the most important effect in terms of clinical relevance is the increase produced by LCSD on the threshold for ventricular fibrillation (Schwartz et al., 1976a). This makes it less likely that a heart will fibrillate and, together with the overall reduction in the norepinephrine release, constitutes the primary rationale for the use of LCSD in several conditions in which the risk for ventricular fibrillation is high.

The evidence for a powerful antifibrillatory effect of LCSD is now firmly established (Schwartz, 2014) and has been observed at clinical level in three different sets of patients: post-MI patients at high risk for sudden death (Schwartz et al., 1992b), long QT syndrome patients (Schwartz et al., 2004), and patients with catecholamine polymorphic ventricular tachycardia (CPVT) syndrome (De Ferrari et al., 2015). Whenever there is a recurrence after LCSD, which is not common for LQTS and CPVT patients, it is reasonable to perform right cardiac sympathetic denervation as well, as we started to do in the 1990s (Schwartz et al., 1991, 2004). There are growing data suggesting that bilateral cardiac sympathetic denervation can be useful in patients with recurrent ventricular tachycardia related to either ischemic heart disease or dilated cardiomyopathy (Vaseghi et al., 2014). Different views exist on the timing for ablating the right cardiac sympathetic nerves; namely, whether together with the left or just in case of failure of unilateral left cardiac sympathetic denervation. Our view is to follow the time-honored precepts of medicine which suggest to begin by the lowest effective dose and to increase it whenever this fails. An implication is that for a number of patients, unilateral left cardiac sympathetic denervation will be sufficient (Schwartz, 2014).

Overall, it is now clear that cardiac sympathetic denervation can save lives while preserving adequate quality of life (Antiel et al., 2016; Schwartz, 2016) and that there is not always the need to rush toward an implantable cardioverter defibrillator.

Renal Denervation

Renal sympathetic nerve activity plays a crucial role in the control of cardiovascular homeostasis and is involved not only in the pathogenesis of hypertension but also in other cardiovascular processes such as heart failure, and perhaps cardiac arrhythmias. Renal afferent and efferent nerves function in a reflex loop where afferent input from the kidney to the central nervous system is integrated with inputs from other neural reflexes to determine the level of sympathetic outflow to individual organs. Renal denervation (RDN) as a method of modulating sympathetic activity by interrupting afferent and efferent sympathetic nerve signaling appears to be an attractive therapeutic target in patients with cardiovascular disease triggered by sympathetic overactivity such as hypertension, heart failure, and – according to some – even atrial or ventricular arrhythmias. RDN has been initially introduced to reduce blood pressure in subjects with resistant hypertension (Mahfoud et al., 2013). While initial clinical trial results failed to reach a consensus on the efficacy of RDN in this context (Bhatt et al., 2014), three subsequent sham-controlled studies that were carefully designed and rigorously conducted have shown that RDN significantly reduces blood pressure regardless of the use of antihypertensive drugs (Townsend et al., 2017; Azizi et al., 2018; Kandzari et al., 2018). Notably, the use of multi-electrode catheter and more ablations per artery have definitely improved the RDN procedure in the more recent studies that also took into account the distribution of the sympathetic nerves among the renal arteries.

Clinical implications of RDN are well beyond blood pressure control. Interestingly, a recent meta-analysis including 17 studies revealed that RDN improved a number of cardiovascular markers of organ damage including left ventricular mass index, central augmentation index, and carotid-femoral pulse wave velocity independent of blood pressure (Kordalis et al., 2018). Moreover, several clinical RDN studies report beneficial effects on ventricular and supraventricular arrhythmias (Ukena et al., 2012; Pokushalov et al., 2014). In the recently reported ERADICATE-AF trial that randomized 302 patients with paroxysmal atrial fibrillation and hypertension, RDN added to catheter ablation, compared with catheter ablation alone, significantly increased the likelihood of freedom from atrial fibrillation at 12 months (Steinberg et al., 2020). While we report these studies and their claims, we cannot help expressing a certain degree of skepticism on the rationale by which RD should provide protection against life-threatening cardiac arrhythmias. The underlying concept seems to be that reduction or elimination of renal afferent would decrease the efferent sympathetic activity directed to the heart, which is mediated by the stellate ganglia. We find it difficult to conceive how this "reduction" could be greater than that produced by the direct section of these nerves, as it is produced by the cardiac sympathetic denervation performed by removing the lower half of the stellate ganglion/ganglia with the first four thoracic ganglia.

RDN has been reported to exert beneficial effects on cardiac function and remodeling in animal models of heart failure (Sharp et al., 2018), but the results in patients are largely inconsistent due in part to limited power with small sample sizes. In a meta-analysis including two controlled (80 patients) and two uncontrolled studies (21 patients) (Fukuta et al., 2017), 6 months after RDN, there was a greater increase in left ventricular ejection fraction and a greater decrease in left ventricular end-diastolic diameter in the RDN group than in the control group. No serious adverse events such as acute renal artery stenosis and dissection occurred.

CONCLUSIONS

A paper like this one does not really need a traditional conclusion, which would merely be a pale summary of what has been a serious effort to share with the interested reader our experience and our views. Our hope is that more and more young investigators will be attracted by this fascinating field of research, which is endowed with so many areas of clinical relevance.

AUTHOR CONTRIBUTIONS

PS, AP, and MR contributed to the conception and design of research, drafted the manuscript, edited and revised critically the manuscript, and approved the final version of the manuscript.

ACKNOWLEDGMENTS

The authors are grateful to Pinuccia De Tomasi for expert editorial support.

REFERENCES

Akselrod, S., Gordon, D., Ubel, F. A., Shannon, D. C., Berger, A. C., and Cohen, R. J. (1981). Power spectrum analysis of heart rate fluctuation: a quantitative probe of beat-to-beat cardiovascular control. *Science* 213, 220–222. doi: 10.1126/science.6166045

Antiel, R. M., Bos, J. M., Joyce, D. D., Owen, H. J., Roskos, P. L., Moir, C., et al. (2016). Quality of life after videoscopic left cardiac sympathetic denervation in patients with potentially life-threatening cardiac channelopathies/cardiomyopathies. *Heart Rhythm.* 13, 62–69. doi: 10.1016/j.hrthm.2015.09.001

Atiga, W. L., Calkins, H., Lawrence, J. H., Tomaselli, G. F., Smith, J. M., and Berger, R. D. (1998). Beat-to-beat repolarization lability identifies patients at risk for sudden cardiac death. *J. Cardiovasc. Electrophysiol.* 9, 899–908. doi: 10.1111/j.1540-8167.1998.tb00130.x

Azizi, M., Schmieder, R. E., Mahfoud, F., Weber, M. A., Daemen, J., Davies, J., et al. (2018). Endovascular ultrasound renal denervation to treat hypertension (RADIANCE-HTN SOLO): a multicentre, international, single-blind, randomised, sham-controlled trial. *Lancet* 391, 2335–2345. doi: 10.1016/S0140-6736(18)31082-1

Bär, K.-J., Koschke, M., Boettger, M. K., Berger, S., Kabisch, A., Sauer, H., et al. (2007). Acute psychosis leads to increased QT variability in patients suffering from schizophrenia. *Schizophr. Res.* 95, 115–123. doi: 10.1016/j.schres.2007.05.034

Bari, V., Girardengo, G., Marchi, A., De Maria, B., Brink, P. A., Crotti, L., et al. (2015). A refined multiscale self-entropy approach for the assessment of cardiac control complexity: application to long QT syndrome type 1 patients. *Entropy* 17, 7768–7785. doi: 10.3390/e17117768

Bari, V., Marchi, A., De Maria, B., Girardengo, G., George, A. L., Brink, P. A., et al. (2014a). Low-pass filtering approach via empirical mode decomposition improves short-scale entropy-based complexity estimation of QT interval variability in long QT syndrome type 1 patients. *Entropy* 16, 4839–4854. doi: 10.3390/e16094839

Bari, V., Valencia, J. F., Vallverdú, M., Girardengo, G., Marchi, A., Bassani, T., et al. (2014b). Multiscale complexity analysis of the cardiac control identifies asymptomatic and symptomatic patients in long QT syndrome type 1. *PLoS One* 9:e93808. doi: 10.1371/journal.pone.0093808

Bauer, A., Camm, A. J., Cerutti, S., Guzik, P., Huikuri, H., Lombardi, F., et al. (2017). Reference values of heart rate variability. *Heart Rhythm.* 14, 302–303. doi: 10.1016/j.hrthm.2016.12.015

Bauer, A., Klemm, M., Rizas, K. D., Hamm, W., von Stülpnagel, L., Dommasch, M., et al. (2019). Prediction of mortality benefit based on periodic repolarisation dynamics in patients undergoing prophylactic implantation of a defibrillator: a prospective, controlled, multicentre cohort study. *Lancet* 394, 1344–1351. doi: 10.1016/S0140-6736(19)31996-8

Bauer, A., Morley-Davies, A., Barthel, P., Muller, A., Ulm, K., Malik, M., et al. (2010). Bivariate phase-rectified signal averaging for assessment of spontaneous baroreflex sensitivity: pilot study of the technology. *J. Electrocardiol.* 43, 649–653. doi: 10.1016/j.jelectrocard.2010.05.012

Baumert, M., Czippelova, B., Ganesan, A., Schmidt, M., Zaunseder, S., and Javorka, M. (2014). Entropy analysis of RR and QT interval variability during orthostatic and mental stress in healthy subjects. *Entropy* 16, 6384–6393. doi: 10.3390/e16126384

Baumert, M., Javorka, M., Seeck, A., Faber, R., Sanders, P., and Voss, A. (2012). Multiscale entropy and detrended fluctuation analysis of QT interval and heart rate variability during normal pregnancy. *Comput. Biol. Med.* 42, 347–352. doi: 10.1016/j.compbiomed.2011.03.019

Baumert, M., Lambert, G. W., Dawood, T., Lambert, E. A., Esler, M. D., McGrane, M., et al. (2008). QT interval variability and cardiac norepinephrine spillover in patients with depression and panic disorder. *Am. J. Phys.* 295, H962–H968. doi: 10.1152/ajpheart.00301.2008

Baumert, M., Porta, A., Vos, M. A., Malik, M., Couderc, J.-P., Laguna, P., et al. (2016). QT interval variability in body surface ECG: measurement, physiological basis, and clinical value: position statement and consensus guidance endorsed by the European Heart Rhythm Association jointly with the ESC Working Group on cardiac cellular electrophsiology. *Europace* 18, 925–944. doi: 10.1093/europace/euv405

Baumert, M., Schlaich, M. P., Nalivaiko, E., Lambert, E., Sari, C. I., Kaye, D. M., et al. (2011). Relation between QT interval variability and cardiac sympathetic activity in hypertension. *Am. J. Phys.* 300, H1412–H1427. doi: 10.1152/ajpheart.01184.2010

Bazett, H. C. (1920). An analysis of the time-relations of electrocardiograms. *Heart* 7, 353–370.

Berger, R. D. (2009). QT interval variability is it a measure of autonomic activity? *J. Am. Coll. Cardiol.* 54, 851–852. doi: 10.1016/j.jacc.2009.06.007

Berger, R. D., Kasper, E. K., Baughman, K. L., Marban, E., Calkins, H., and Tomaselli, G. F. (1997). Beat-to-beat QT interval variability: novel evidence for repolarization lability in ischemic and nonischemic dilated cardiomyopathy. *Circulation* 96, 1557–1565. doi: 10.1161/01.CIR.96.5.1557

Bertinieri, G., di Rienzo, M., Cavallazzi, A., Ferrari, A. U., Pedotti, A., and Mancia, G. (1985). A new approach to analysis of the arterial baroreflex. *J. Hypertens.* 3, S79–S81.

Bhatt, D. L., Kandzari, D. E., O'Neill, W. W., D'Agostino, R., Flack, J. M., Katzen, B. T., et al. (2014). A controlled trial of renal denervation for resistant hypertension. *N. Engl. J. Med.* 370, 1393–1401. doi: 10.1056/NEJMoa1402670

Billman, G. E. (2009). Cardiac autonomic neural remodeling and susceptibility to sudden cardiac death: effect of endurance exercise training. *Am. J. Phys.* 297, H1171–H1193. doi: 10.1152/ajpheart.00534.2009

Billman, G. E., Schwartz, P. J., and Stone, H. L. (1982). Baroreceptor reflex control of heart rate: a predictor of sudden cardiac death. *Circulation* 66, 874–880. doi: 10.1161/01.CIR.66.4.874

Boettger, M. K., Schulz, S., Berger, S., Tancer, M., Yeragani, V. K., Voss, A., et al. (2010). Influence of age on linear and nonlinear measures of autonomic cardiovascular modulation. *Ann. Noninvasive Electrocardiol.* 15, 165–174. doi: 10.1111/j.1542-474X.2010.00358.x

Bolignano, D., and Coppolino, G. (2018). Baroreflex stimulation for treating resistant hypertension: ready for the prime-time? *Rev. Cardiovasc. Med.* 19, 89–95. doi: 10.31083/j.rcm.2018.03.3185

Boyett, M., Wang, Y., and D'Souza, A. (2019). CrossTalk opposing view: heart rate variability as a measure of cardiac autonomic responsiveness is fundamentally flawed. *J. Physiol.* 597, 2599–2601. doi: 10.1113/JP277501

Brink, P. A., Crotti, L., Corfield, V., Goosen, A., Durrheim, G., Hedley, P., et al. (2005). Phenotypic variability and unusual clinical severity of congenital long-QT syndrome in a founder population. *Circulation* 112, 2602–2610. doi: 10.1161/CIRCULATIONAHA.105.572453

Brink, P. A., and Schwartz, P. J. (2009). Of founder populations, long QT syndrome, and destiny. *Heart Rhythm.* 6, S25–S33. doi: 10.1016/j.hrthm.2009.08.036

Browne, K. F., Prystowsky, E., Heger, J. J., Chilson, D. A., and Zipes, D. P. (1983). Prolongation of the Q-T interval in man during sleep. *Am. J. Cardiol.* 52, 55–59. doi: 10.1016/0002-9149(83)90068-1

Cao, J. M., Chen, L. S., KenKnight, B. H., Ohara, T., Lee, M. H., Tsai, J., et al. (2000). Nerve sprouting and sudden cardiac death. *Circ. Res.* 86, 816–821. doi: 10.1161/01.RES.86.7.816

Cerati, D., and Schwartz, P. J. (1991). Single cardiac vagal fiber activity, acute myocardial ischemia, and risk for sudden death. *Circ. Res.* 69, 1389–1401. doi: 10.1161/01.RES.69.5.1389

Chen, X., Hu, Y., Fetics, B. J., Berger, R. D., and Trayanova, N. A. (2011). Unstable QT interval dynamics precedes ventricular tachycardia onset in patients with acute myocardial infarction: a novel approach to detect instability in QT interval dynamics from clinical ECG. *Circ. Arrhythm. Electrophysiol.* 4, 858–866. doi: 10.1161/CIRCEP.110.961763

Chugh, S. S. (2017). Sudden cardiac death in 2017: spotlight on prediction and prevention. *Int. J. Cardiol.* 237, 2–5. doi: 10.1016/j.ijcard.2017.03.086

Conrath, C. E., and Opthof, T. (2006). Ventricular repolarization: an overview of (patho)physiology, sympathetic effects and genetic aspects. *Prog. Biophys. Mol. Biol.* 92, 269–307. doi: 10.1016/j.pbiomolbio.2005.05.009

Crotti, L., Spazzolini, C., Porretta, A. P., Dagradi, F., Taravelli, E., Petracci, B., et al. (2012). Vagal reflexes following an exercise stress test: a simple clinical tool for gene-specific risk stratification in the long QT syndrome. *J. Am. Coll. Cardiol.* 60, 2515–2524. doi: 10.1016/j.jacc.2012.08.1009

Crotti, L., Spazzolini, C., Schwartz, P. J., Shimizu, W., Denjoy, I., Schulze-Bahr, E., et al. (2007). The common long-QT syndrome mutation KCNQ1/A341V causes unusually severe clinical manifestations in patients with different ethnic backgrounds: toward a mutation-specific risk stratification. *Circulation* 116, 2366–2375. doi: 10.1161/CIRCULATIONAHA.107.726950

Da Silva, V. J. D., Tobaldini, E., Rocchetti, M., Wu, M. A., Malfatto, G., Montano, N., et al. (2015). Modulation of sympathetic activity and heart rate variability by Ivabradine. *Cardiovasc. Res.* 108, 31–38. doi: 10.1093/cvr/cvv180

De Ferrari, G. M., Crijns, H. J. G. M., Borggrefe, M., Milasinovic, G., Smid, J., Zabel, M., et al. (2011). Chronic vagus nerve stimulation: a new and promising therapeutic approach for chronic heart failure. *Eur. Heart J.* 32, 847–855. doi: 10.1093/eurheartj/ehq391

De Ferrari, G. M., Dusi, V., Spazzolini, C., Bos, J. M., Abrams, D. J., Berul, C. I., et al. (2015). Clinical management of catecholaminergic polymorphic ventricular tachycardia: the role of left cardiac sympathetic denervation. *Circulation* 131, 2185–2193. doi: 10.1161/CIRCULATIONAHA.115.015731

De Ferrari, G. M., Landolina, M., Mantica, M., Manfredini, R., Schwartz, P. J., and Lotto, A. (1995). Baroreflex sensitivity, but not heart rate variability, is reduced in patients with life-threatening ventricular arrhythmias long after myocardial infarction. *Am. Heart J.* 130, 473–480. doi: 10.1016/0002-8703(95)90354-2

De Ferrari, G. M., Sanzo, A., Bertoletti, A., Specchia, G., Vanoli, E., and Schwartz, P. J. (2007). Baroreflex sensitivity predicts long-term cardiovascular mortality after myocardial infarction even in patients with preserved left ventricular function. *J. Am. Coll. Cardiol.* 50, 2285–2290. doi: 10.1016/j.jacc.2007.08.043

Diaz, T., and Taylor, J. A. (2006). Probing the arterial baroreflex: is there a 'spontaneous' baroreflex? *Clin. Auton. Res.* 16, 256–261. doi: 10.1007/s10286-006-0352-5

Dobson, C. P., La Rovere, M. T., Pinna, G. D., Goldstein, R., Olsen, C., Bernardinangeli, M., et al. (2011). QT variability index on 24-hour Holter independently predicts mortality in patients with heart failure: analysis of Gruppo Italiano per Lo tudio Della Sopravvivenza Nell'Insufficienza Cardiaca (GISSI-HF) trial. *Heart Rhythm.* 8, 1237–1242. doi: 10.1016/j.hrthm.2011.03.055

Dusi, V., De Ferrari, G. M., and Schwartz, P. J. (2020). There are 100 ways by which the sympathetic nervous system can trigger life-threatening arrhythmias. *Eur. Heart J*, ehz950. doi: 10.1093/eurheartj/ehz950 (in press).

Eckberg, D. L. (1997). Sympathovagal balance: a critical appraisal. *Circulation* 96, 3224–3232. doi: 10.1161/01.CIR.96.9.3224

Eckberg, D. L., Drabinsky, M., and Braunwald, E. (1971). Defective cardiac parasympathetic control in patients with heart disease. *N. Engl. J. Med.* 285, 877–883. doi: 10.1056/NEJM197110142851602

Eckberg, D. L., and Sleight, P. (1992). *Human baroreflexes in health and disease.* Oxford: Clarendon Press.

El-Hamad, F., Javorka, M., Czippelova, B., Krohova, J., Turianikova, Z., Porta, A., et al. (2019). Repolarization variability independent of heart rate during sympathetic activation elicited by head-up tilt. *Med. Biol. Eng. Comput.* 57, 1753–1762. doi: 10.1007/s11517-019-01998-9

Floras, J. S., and Ponikowski, P. (2015). The sympathetic/parasympathetic imbalance in heart failure with reduced ejection fraction. *Eur. Heart J.* 36, 1974–1982. doi: 10.1093/eurheartj/ehv087

Fukuta, H., Goto, T., Wakami, K., and Ohte, N. (2017). Effects of catheter-based renal denervation on heart failure with reduced ejection fraction: a systematic review and meta-analysis. *Heart Fail. Rev.* 22, 657–664. doi: 10.1007/s10741-017-9629-0

Gold, M. R., Van Veldhuisen, D. J., Hauptman, P. J., Borggrefe, M., Kubo, S. H., Lieberman, R. A., et al. (2016). Vagus nerve stimulation for the treatment of heart failure: the INOVATE-HF trial. *J. Am. Coll. Cardiol.* 68, 149–158. doi: 10.1016/j.jacc.2016.03.525

Goldberger, A. L. (1996). Non-linear dynamics for clinicians: chaos theory, fractals, and complexity at the bedside. *Lancet* 347, 1312–1314. doi: 10.1016/S0140-6736(96)90948-4

Harris, A. S., Otero, H., and Bocage, A. J. (1971). The induction of arrhythmias by sympathetic activity before and after occlusion of a coronary artery in the canine heart. *J. Electrocardiol.* 4, 34–43. doi: 10.1016/S0022-0736(71)80048-1

Hartupee, J., and Mann, D. L. (2017). Neurohormonal activation in heart failure with reduced ejection fraction. *Nat. Rev. Cardiol.* 14, 30–38. doi: 10.1038/nrcardio.2016.163

Hauptman, P. J., Schwartz, P. J., Gold, M. R., Borggrefe, M., Van Veldhuisen, D. J., Starling, R. C., et al. (2012). Rationale and study design of the increase of vagal tone in heart failure study: INOVATE-HF. *Am. Heart J.* 163, 954–962. doi: 10.1016/j.ahj.2012.03.021

Hirsch, J. A., and Bishop, B. (1981). Respiratory sinus arrhythmia in humans: how breathing pattern modulates heart rate. *Am. J. Phys.* 241, H620–H629. doi: 10.1152/ajpheart.1981.241.4.H620

Inoue, H., and Zipes, D. P. (1987). Changes in atrial and ventricular refractoriness and in atrioventricular nodal conduction produced by combinations of vagal and sympathetic stimulation that result in a constant spontaneous sinus cycle length. *Circ. Res.* 60, 942–951. doi: 10.1161/01.RES.60.6.942

Janse, M. J., Schwartz, P. J., Wilms-Schopman, F., Peters, R. J., and Durrer, D. (1985). Effects of unilateral stellate ganglion stimulation and ablation on electrophysiologic changes induced by acute myocardial ischemia in dogs. *Circulation* 72, 585–595.

Jose, A. D., and Collison, D. (1970). The normal range and determinants of the intrinsic heart rate in man. *Cardiovasc. Res.* 4, 160–167. doi: 10.1093/cvr/4.2.160

Kandzari, D. E., Böhm, M., Mahfoud, F., Townsend, R. R., Weber, M. A., Pocock, S., et al. (2018). Effect of renal denervation on blood pressure in the presence of antihypertensive drugs: 6-month efficacy and safety results from the SPYRAL HTN-ON MED proof-of-concept randomised trial. *Lancet* 391, 2346–2355. doi: 10.1016/S0140-6736(18)30951-6

Kent, K. M., Smith, E. R., Redwood, D. R., and Epstein, S. E. (1973). Electrical stability of acutely ischemic myocardium. Influences of heart rate and vagal stimulation. *Circulation* 47, 291–298. doi: 10.1161/01.CIR.47.2.291

Kleiger, R. E., Miller, J. P., Bigger, J. T., and Moss, A. J. (1987). Decreased heart rate variability and its association with increased mortality after acute myocardial infarction. *Am. J. Cardiol.* 59, 256–262. doi: 10.1016/0002-9149(87)90795-8

Kordalis, A., Tsiachris, D., Pietri, P., Tsioufis, C., and Stefanadis, C. (2018). Regression of organ damage following renal denervation in resistant hypertension: a meta-analysis. *J. Hypertens.* 36, 1614–1621. doi: 10.1097/HJH.0000000000001798

Kunze, D. L. (1972). Reflex discharge patterns of cardiac vagal efferent fibres. *J. Physiol.* 222, 1–15. doi: 10.1113/jphysiol.1972.sp009784

La Rovere, M. T., Bigger, J. T., Marcus, F. I., Mortara, A., and Schwartz, P. J. (1998). Baroreflex sensitivity and heart-rate variability in prediction of total cardiac mortality after myocardial infarction. *Lancet* 351, 478–484. doi: 10.1016/S0140-6736(97)11144-8

La Rovere, M. T., Maestri, R., Pinna, G. D., Sleight, P., and Febo, O. (2011). Clinical and haemodynamic correlates of heart rate turbulence as a non-invasive index of baroreflex sensitivity in chronic heart failure. *Clin. Sci.* 121, 279–284. doi: 10.1042/CS20110063

La Rovere, M. T., Pinna, G. D., Hohnloser, S. H., Marcus, F. I., Mortara, A., Nohara, R., et al. (2001). Baroreflex sensitivity and heart rate variability in the identification of patients at risk for life-threatening arrhythmias: implications for clinical trials. *Circulation* 103, 2072–2077. doi: 10.1161/01.CIR.103.16.2072

La Rovere, M. T., Pinna, G. D., Maestri, R., Mortara, A., Capomolla, S., Febo, O., et al. (2003). Short-term heart rate variability strongly predicts sudden cardiac death in chronic heart failure patients. *Circulation* 107, 565–570. doi: 10.1161/01.CIR.0000047275.25795.17

La Rovere, M. T., Pinna, G. D., and Raczak, G. (2008). Baroreflex sensitivity: measurement and clinical implications. *Ann. Noninvasive Electrocardiol.* 13, 191–207. doi: 10.1111/j.1542-474X.2008.00219.x

Landolina, M., Mantica, M., Pessano, P., Manfredini, R., Foresti, A., Schwartz, P. J., et al. (1997). Impaired baroreflex sensitivity is correlated with hemodynamic deterioration of sustained ventricular tachycardia. *J. Am. Coll. Cardiol.* 29, 568–575.

Levy, M. N., and Schwartz, P. J. (1994). *Vagal control of the heart: Experimental basis and clinical implications.* Armonk, NY: Futura Publishing Co.

Lewis, M. J., and Short, A. L. (2007). Sample entropy of electrocardiographic RR and QT time-series data during rest and exercise. *Physiol. Meas.* 28, 731–744. doi: 10.1088/0967-3334/28/6/011

Li, Y., Li, P., Karmakar, C., and Liu, C.-T. (2015). Distribution entropy for short-term QT interval variability analysis: a comparison between the heart failure and healthy control groups. *Comput. Cardiol.* 42, 1153–1156. doi: 10.1109/CIC.2015.7411120

Li, Y., Li, P., Wang, X., Karmakar, C., Liu, C., and Liu, C. (2019). Variability in patients with coronary artery disease and congestive heart failure: a comparison with healthy control subjects. *Med. Biol. Eng. Comput.* 57, 389–400. doi: 10.1007/s11517-018-1870-8

Lombardi, F., Sandrone, G., Porta, A., Torzillo, D., Terranova, G., Baselli, G., et al. (1996). Spectral analysis of short term R-Tapex interval variability during sinus rhythm and fixed atrial rate. *Eur. Heart J.* 17, 769–778. doi: 10.1093/oxfordjournals.eurheartj.a014945

Magnano, A. R., Holleran, S., Ramakrishnan, R., Reiffel, J. A., and Bloomfield, D. M. (2002). Autonomic nervous system influences on QT interval in normal subjects. *J. Am. Coll. Cardiol.* 39, 1820–1826. doi: 10.1016/s0735-1097(02)01852-1

Mahfoud, F., Lüscher, T. F., Andersson, B., Baumgartner, I., Cifkova, R., Dimario, C., et al. (2013). European Society of Cardiology. Expert consensus document from the European Society of Cardiology on catheter-based renal denervation. *Eur. Heart J.* 34, 2149–2157. doi: 10.1093/eurheartj/eht154

Malik, M. (2008). Beat-to-beat QT variability and cardiac autonomic regulation. *Am. J. Phys.* 295, H923–H925. doi: 10.1152/ajpheart.00709.2008

Malik, M., Hnatkova, K., Huikuri, H. V., Lombardi, F., Schmidt, G., and Zabel, M. (2019a). CrossTalk proposal: heart rate variability is a valid measure of cardiac autonomic responsiveness. *J. Physiol.* 597, 2595–2598. doi: 10.1113/JP277500

Malik, M., Hnatkova, K., Huikuri, H. V., Lombardi, F., Schmidt, G., and Zabel, M. (2019b). Rebuttal from Marek Malik, Katerina Hnatkova, Heikki V. Huikuri, Federico Lombardi, Georg Schmidt and Markus Zabel. *J. Physiol.* 597, 2603–2604. doi: 10.1113/JP277962

Malliani, A., Recordati, G., and Schwartz, P. J. (1973). Nervous activity of afferent cardiac sympathetic fibres with atrial and ventricular endings. *J. Physiol.* 229, 457–469. doi: 10.1113/jphysiol.1973.sp010147

Malliani, A., Schwartz, P. J., and Zanchetti, A. (1969). A sympathetic reflex elicited by experimental coronary occlusion. *Am. J. Phys.* 217, 703–709.

Mann, J. A., and Abraham, W. T. (2019). Cardiac contractility modulation and baroreflex activation therapy in heart failure patients. *Curr. Heart Fail. Rep.* 16, 38–46. doi: 10.1007/s11897-019-0422-3

Milan-Mattos, J. C., Porta, A., Perseguini, N. M., Minatel, V., Rehder-Santos, P., Takahashi, A. C. M., et al. (2018). Influence of age and gender on the phase and strength of the relation between heart period and systolic blood pressure spontaneous fluctuations. *J. Appl. Physiol.* 124, 791–804. doi: 10.1152/japplphysiol.00903.2017

Montano, N., Cogliati, C., Porta, A., Pagani, M., Malliani, A., Narkiewicz, K., et al. (1998). Central vagotonic effects of atropine modulate spectral oscillations of sympathetic nerve activity. *Circulation* 98, 1394–1399. doi: 10.1161/01.CIR.98.14.1394

Montano, N., Gnecchi-Ruscone, T., Porta, A., Lombardi, F., Pagani, M., and Malliani, A. (1994). Power spectrum analysis of heart rate variability to assess the changes in sympathovagal balance during graded orthostatic tilt. *Circulation* 90, 1826–1831. doi: 10.1161/01.CIR.90.4.1826

Mortara, A., La Rovere, M. T., Pinna, G. D., Prpa, A., Maestri, R., Febo, O., et al. (1997). Arterial baroreflex modulation of heart rate in chronic heart failure: clinical and hemodynamic correlates and prognostic implications. *Circulation* 96, 3450–3458. doi: 10.1161/01.CIR.96.10.3450

Nahshoni, E., Strasberg, B., Adler, E., Imbar, S., Sulkes, J., and Weizman, A. (2004). Complexity of the dynamic QT variability and RR variability in patients with acute anterior wall myocardial infarction: a novel technique using a non-linear method. *J. Electrocardiol.* 37, 173–179. doi: 10.1016/j.jelectrocard.2004.04.008

Negoescu, R., Dinca-Panaitescu, S., Filcescu, V., Ionescu, D., and Wolf, S. (1997). Mental stress enhances the sympathetic fraction of QT variability in an RR-independent way. *Integr. Physiol. Behav. Sci.* 32, 220–227. doi: 10.1007/BF02688620

Nollo, G., Faes, L., Porta, A., Antolini, R., and Ravelli, F. (2005). Exploring directionality in spontaneous heart period and systolic pressure variability interactions in humans: implications in the evaluation of baroreflex gain. *Am. J. Phys.* 288, H1777–H1785. doi: 10.1152/ajpheart.00594.2004

Oosterhoff, P., Tereshchenko, L. G., van der Heyden, M. A. G., Ghanem, R. N., Fetics, B. J., Berger, R. D., et al. (2011). Short-term variability of repolarization predicts ventricular tachycardia and sudden cardiac death in patients with structural heart disease: a comparison with QT variability index. *Heart Rhythm.* 8, 1584–1590. doi: 10.1016/j.hrthm.2011.04.033

Opthof, T., de Jonge, B., Schade, B., Jongsma, H. J., and Bouman, L. N. (1984). Cycle length dependence of the chronotropic effects of adrenaline, acetylcholine, Ca2+ and Mg2+ in the Guinea-pig sinoatrial node. *J. Auton. Nerv. Syst.* 11, 349–366.

Pagani, M., Montano, N., Porta, A., Malliani, A., Abboud, F. M., Birkett, C., et al. (1997). Relationship between spectral components of cardiovascular variabilities and direct measures of muscle sympathetic nerve activity in humans. *Circulation* 95, 1441–1448. doi: 10.1161/01.CIR.95.6.1441

Pagani, M., Schwartz, P. J., Banks, R., Lombardi, F., and Malliani, A. (1974). Reflex responses of sympathetic preganglionic neurons initiated by different cardiovascular receptors in spinal animals. *Brain Res.* 68, 215–225. doi: 10.1016/0006-8993(74)90391-6

Paintal, A. S. (1963). "Vagal afferent fibres" in *Ergebnisse Der Physiologie, Biologischen Chemie Und Experimentellen Pharmakologie*, Vol. 52, Springer-Verlag, 74–156.

Piccirillo, G., Cacciafesta, M., Lionetti, M., Nocco, M., Di Giuseppe, V., Moisè, A., et al. (2001). Influence of age, the autonomic nervous system and anxiety on QT-interval variability. *Clin. Sci.* 101, 429–438. doi: 10.1042/cs1010429

Piccirillo, G., Magnanti, M., Matera, S., Di Carlo, S., De Laurentis, T., Torrini, A., et al. (2006). Age and QT variability index during free breathing, controlled breathing and tilt in patients with chronic heart failure and healthy control subjects. *Transl. Res.* 148, 72–78. doi: 10.1016/j.trsl.2006.02.001

Piccirillo, G., Magrì, D., Matera, S., Magnanti, M., Torrini, A., Pasquazzi, E., et al. (2007). QT variability strongly predicts sudden cardiac death in asymptomatic subjects with mild or moderate left ventricular systolic dysfunction: a prospective study. *Eur. Heart J.* 28, 1344–1350. doi: 10.1093/eurheartj/ehl367

Pincus, S. M., and Goldberger, A. L. (1994). Physiological time-series analysis: what does regularity quantify? *Am. J. Phys.* 266, H1643–H1656. doi: 10.1152/ajpheart.1994.266.4.H1643

Pinna, G. D., Maestri, R., and La Rovere, M. T. (2015). Assessment of baroreflex sensitivity from spontaneous oscillations of blood pressure and heart rate: proven clinical value? *Physiol. Meas.* 36, 741–753. doi: 10.1088/0967-ss3334/36/4/741

Pinna, G. D., Maestri, R., Raczak, G., and La Rovere, M. T. (2002). Measuring baroreflex sensitivity from the gain function between arterial pressure and heart period. *Clin. Sci.* 103, 81–88. doi: 10.1042/cs1030081

Pinna, G. D., Porta, A., Maestri, R., De Maria, B., Dalla Vecchia, L. A., and La Rovere, M. T. (2017). Different estimation methods of spontaneous baroreflex sensitivity have different predictive value in heart failure patients. *J. Hypertens.* 35, 1666–1675. doi: 10.1097/HJH.0000000000001377

Pokushalov, E., Romanov, A., Katritsis, D. G., Artyomenko, S., Bayramova, S., Losik, D., et al. (2014). Renal denervation for improving outcomes of catheter ablation in patients with atrial fibrillation and hypertension: early experience. *Heart Rhythm.* 11, 1131–1138. doi: 10.1016/j.hrthm.2014.03.055

Pomeranz, B., Macaulay, R. J., Caudill, M. A., Kutz, I., Adam, D., Gordon, D., et al. (1985). Assessment of autonomic function in humans by heart rate spectral analysis. *Am. J. Phys.* 248, H151–H153. doi: 10.1152/ajpheart.1985.248.1.H151

Porta, A., Bari, V., Badilini, F., Tobaldini, E., Gnecchi-Ruscone, T., and Montano, N. (2011). Frequency domain assessment of the coupling strength between ventricular repolarization duration and heart period during graded head-up tilt. *J. Electrocardiol.* 44, 662–668. doi: 10.1016/j.jelectrocard.2011.08.002

Porta, A., Baselli, G., Caiani, E., Malliani, A., Lombardi, F., and Cerutti, S. (1998a). Quantifying electrocardiogram RT-RR variability interactions. *Med. Biol. Eng. Comput.* 36, 27–34.

Porta, A., Bari, V., De Maria, B., and Baumert, M. (2017). A network physiology approach to the assessment of the link between sinoatrial and ventricular cardiac controls. *Physiol. Meas.* 38, 1472–1489. doi: 10.1088/1361-6579/aa6e95

Porta, A., Baselli, G., Lombardi, F., Cerutti, S., Antolini, R., Del Greco, M., et al. (1998b). Performance assessment of standard algorithms for dynamic R-T interval measurement: comparison between R-Tapex and R-tend approach. *Med. Biol. Eng. Comput.* 36, 35–42.

Porta, A., Baselli, G., Rimoldi, O., Malliani, A., and Pagani, M. (2000). Assessing baroreflex gain from spontaneous variability in conscious dogs: role of causality and respiration. *Am. J. Phys.* 279, H2558–H2567. doi: 10.1152/ajpheart.2000.279.5.H2558

Porta, A., Castiglioni, P., Di Rienzo, M., Bari, V., Bassani, T., Marchi, A., et al. (2012). Short-term complexity indexes of heart period and systolic arterial pressure variabilities provide complementary information. *J. Appl. Physiol.* 113, 1810–1820. doi: 10.1152/japplphysiol.00755.2012

Porta, A., Di Rienzo, M., Wessel, N., and Kurths, J. (2009). Addressing the complexity of cardiovascular regulation. *Phil. Trans. R. Soc. A* 367, 1215–1218. doi: 10.1098/rsta.2008.0292

Porta, A., Girardengo, G., Bari, V., George, A. L., Brink, P. A., Goosen, A., et al. (2015). Autonomic control of heart rate and QT interval variability influences arrhythmic risk in long QT syndrome type 1. *J. Am. Coll. Cardiol.* 65, 367–374. doi: 10.1016/j.jacc.2014.11.015

Porta, A., Gnecchi-Ruscone, T., Tobaldini, E., Guzzetti, S., Furlan, R., and Montano, N. (2007). Progressive decrease of heart period variability entropy-based complexity during graded head-up tilt. *J. Appl. Physiol.* 103, 1143–1149. doi: 10.1152/japplphysiol.00293.2007

Porta, A., Tobaldini, E., Gnecchi-Ruscone, T., and Montano, N. (2010). RT variability unrelated to heart period and respiration progressively increases during graded head-up tilt. *Am. J. Phys.* 298, H1406–H1414. doi: 10.1152/ajpheart.01206.2009

Pueyo, E., Smetana, P., Caminal, P., Bayes de Luna, A., Malik, M., and Laguna, P. (2004). Characterization of QT interval adaptation to RR interval changes and its use as a risk-stratifier of arrhythmic mortality in amiodarone-treated survivors of acute myocardial infarction. *IEEE Trans. Biomed. Eng.* 51, 1511–1520. doi: 10.1109/TBME.2004.828050

Randall, W. C. (ed.) (1984). "Selective autonomic innervation of the heart" in *Nervous control of cardiovascular function* (New York: Oxford UP), 46–67.

Robbe, H. W., Mulder, L. J., Ruddel, H., Langewitz, W. A., Veldman, J. B., and Mulder, G. (1987). Assessment of baroreceptor reflex sensitivity by means of spectral analysis. *Hypertension* 10, 538–543. doi: 10.1161/01.HYP.10.5.538

Schmidt, G., Malik, M., Barthel, P., Schneider, R., Ulm, K., Rolnitzky, L., et al. (1999). Heart-rate turbulence after ventricular premature beats as a predictor of mortality after acute myocardial infarction. *Lancet* 353, 1390–1396. doi: 10.1016/S0140-6736(98)08428-1

Schwartz, P. J. (1985). Idiopathic long QT syndrome: progress and questions. *Am. Heart J.* 109, 399–411. doi: 10.1016/0002-8703(85)90626-X

Schwartz, P. J. (2014). Cardiac sympathetic denervation to prevent life-threatening arrhythmias. *Nat. Rev. Cardiol.* 11, 346–353. doi: 10.1038/nrcardio.2014.19

Schwartz, P. J. (2016). When the risk is sudden death, does quality of life matter? *Heart Rhythm.* 13, 70–71. doi: 10.1016/j.hrthm.2015.09.020

Schwartz, P. J., Billman, G. E., and Stone, H. L. (1984). Autonomic mechanisms in ventricular fibrillation induced by myocardial ischemia during exercise in dogs with healed myocardial infarction. An experimental preparation for sudden cardiac death. *Circulation* 69, 790–800. doi: 10.1161/01.CIR.69.4.790

Schwartz, P. J., De Ferrari, G. M., Sanzo, A., Landolina, M., Rordorf, R., Raineri, C., et al. (2008a). Long term vagal stimulation in patients with advanced heart failure. First experience in man. *Eur. J. Heart Fail.* 10, 884–891. doi: 10.1016/j.ejheart.2008.07.016

Schwartz, P. J., La Rovere, M. T., De Ferrari, G. M., and Mann, D. L. (2015). Autonomic modulation for the management of patients with chronic heart failure. *Circ. Heart Fail.* 8, 619–628. doi: 10.1161/CIRCHEARTFAILURE.114.001964

Schwartz, P. J., La Rovere, M. T., and Vanoli, E. (1992a). Autonomic nervous system and sudden cardiac death. Experimental basis and clinical observations for post-myocardial infarction risk stratification. *Circulation* 85, I77–I191.

Schwartz, P. J., Locati, E. H., Moss, A. J., Crampton, R. S., Trazzi, R., and Ruberti, U. (1991). Left cardiac sympathetic denervation in the therapy of congenital long QT syndrome: a worldwide report. *Circulation* 84, 503–511. doi: 10.1161/01.cir.84.2.503

Schwartz, P. J., Motolese, M., Pollavini, G., Lotto, A., Ruberti, U., Trazzi, R., et al. (1992b). Prevention of sudden cardiac death after a first myocardial infarction by pharmacologic or surgical antiadrenergic interventions. *J. Cardiovasc. Electrophysiol.* 3, 2–16. doi: 10.1111/j.1540-8167.1992.tb01090.x

Schwartz, P. J., Pagani, M., Lombardi, F., Malliani, A., and Brown, A. M. (1973). A cardiocardiac sympathovagal reflex in the cat. *Circ. Res.* 32, 215–220. doi: 10.1161/01.RES.32.2.215

Schwartz, P. J., Priori, S. G., Cerrone, M., Spazzolini, C., Odero, A., Napolitano, C., et al. (2004). Left cardiac sympathetic denervation in the management of high-risk patients affected by the long-QT syndrome. *Circulation* 109, 1826–1833. doi: 10.1161/01.CIR.0000125523.14403.1E

Schwartz, P. J., Priori, S. G., Spazzolini, C., Moss, A. J., Vincent, G. M., Napolitano, C., et al. (2001). Genotype-phenotype correlation in the long-QT syndrome: gene-specific triggers for life-threatening arrhythmias. *Circulation* 103, 89–95. doi: 10.1161/01.CIR.103.1.89

Schwartz, P. J., Snebold, N. G., and Brown, A. M. (1976a). Effects of unilateral cardiac sympathetic denervation on the ventricular fibrillation threshold. *Am. J. Cardiol.* 37, 1034–1040. doi: 10.1016/0002-9149(76)90420-3

Schwartz, P. J., and Stone, H. L. (1977). Tonic influence of the sympathetic nervous system on myocardial reactive hyperemia and on coronary blood flow distribution in dogs. *Circ. Res.* 41, 51–58. doi: 10.1161/01.RES.41.1.51

Schwartz, P. J., and Stone, H. L. (1979). Effects of unilateral stellectomy upon cardiac performance during exercise in dogs. *Circ. Res.* 44, 637–645. doi: 10.1161/01.RES.44.5.637

Schwartz, P. J., and Stone, H. L. (1980). Left stellectomy in the prevention of ventricular fibrillation caused by acute myocardial ischemia in conscious dogs with anterior myocardial infarction. *Circulation* 62, 1256–1265. doi: 10.1161/01.CIR.62.6.1256

Schwartz, P. J., and Stone, H. L. (1982). Left stellectomy and denervation supersensitivity in conscious dogs. *Am. J. Cardiol.* 49, 1185–1190. doi: 10.1016/0002-9149(82)90043-1

Schwartz, P. J., Stone, H. L., and Brown, A. M. (1976b). Effects of unilateral stellate ganglion blockade on the arrhythmias associated with coronary occlusion. *Am. Heart J.* 92, 589–599. doi: 10.1016/S0002-8703(76)80078-6

Schwartz, P. J., and Vanoli, E. (1981). Cardiac arrhythmias elicited by interaction between acute myocardial ischemia and sympathetic hyperactivity: a new experimental model for the study of antiarrhythmic drugs. *J. Cardiovasc. Pharmacol.* 3, 1251–1259. doi: 10.1097/00005344-198111000-00012

Schwartz, P. J., Vanoli, E., Crotti, L., Spazzolini, C., Ferrandi, C., Goosen, A., et al. (2008b). Neural control of heart rate is an arrhythmia risk modifier in long QT syndrome. *J. Am. Coll. Cardiol.* 51, 920–929. doi: 10.1016/j.jacc.2007.09.069

Schwartz, P. J., Vanoli, E., Stramba-Badiale, M., De Ferrari, G. M., Billman, G. E., and Foreman, R. D., (1988). Autonomic mechanisms and sudden death. New insights from analysis of baroreceptor reflexes in conscious dogs with and without a myocardial infarction. *Circulation* 78, 969–979. doi: 10.1161/01.CIR.78.4.969

Schwartz, P. J., Vanoli, E., Zaza, A., and Zuanetti, G. (1985). The effect of antiarrhythmic drugs on life-threatening arrhythmias induced by the interaction between acute myocardial ischemia and sympathetic hyperactivity. *Am. Heart J.* 109, 937–948. doi: 10.1016/0002-8703(85)90233-9

Segerson, N. M., Litwin, S. E., Daccarett, M., Wall, T. S., Hamdan, M. H., and Lux, R. L. (2008). Scatter in repolarization timing predicts clinical events in post-myocardial infarction patients. *Heart Rhythm.* 5, 208–214. doi: 10.1016/j.hrthm.2007.10.006

Sharp, T. E. 3rd, Polhemus, D. J., Li, Z., Spaletra, P., Jenkins, J. S., Reilly, J. P., et al. (2018). Renal denervation prevents heart failure progression via inhibition of the renin-angiotensin system. *J. Am. Coll. Cardiol.* 72, 2609–2621. doi: 10.1016/j.jacc.2018.08.2186

Shivkumar, K., Ajijola, O. A., Anand, I., Armour, J. A., Chen, P. S., Esler, M., et al. (2016). Clinical neurocardiology defining the value of neuroscience-based cardiovascular therapeutics. *J. Physiol.* 594, 3911–3954. doi: 10.1113/JP271870

Smyth, H. S., Sleight, P., and Pickering, G. W. (1969). Reflex regulation of the arterial pressure during sleep in man. A quantitative method of assessing baroreflex sensitivity. *Circ. Res.* 24, 109–121. doi: 10.1161/01.RES.24.1.109

Sosnowski, M., Czyz, Z., and Tendera, M. (2001). Scatterplots of RR and RT interval variability bring evidence for diverse non-linear dynamics of heart rate and ventricular repolarization duration in coronary heart disease. *Europace* 3, 39–45. doi: 10.1053/eupc.2000.0144

Steinberg, J. S., Shabanov, V., Ponomarev, D., Losik, D., Ivanickiy, E., Kropotkin, E., et al. (2020). Effect of renal denervation and catheter ablation vs catheter ablation alone on atrial fibrillation recurrence among patients with paroxysmal atrial fibrillation and hypertension: the ERADICATE-AF randomized clinical trial. *JAMA* 323, 248–255. doi: 10.1001/jama.2019.21187

Task Force of the European Society of Cardiology and the North American Society of Pacing and Electrophysiology (1996). Heart rate variability. Standards of measurement, physiological interpretation, and clinical use. *Eur. Heart J.* 17, 354–381. doi: 10.1093/oxfordjournals.eurheartj.a014868

Tereshchenko, L. G., Cygankiewicz, I., McNitt, S., Vazquez, R., Bayes-Genis, A., Han, L., et al. (2012). Predictive value of beat-to-beat QT variability index across the continuum of left ventricular dysfunction: competing risks of noncardiac or cardiovascular death and sudden or nonsudden cardiac death. *Circ. Arrhythm. Electrophysiol.* 5, 719–727. doi: 10.1161/CIRCEP.112.970541

Tobaldini, E., Toschi-Dias, E., Appratto de Souza, L., Rabello Casali, K., Vicenzi, M., Sandrone, G., et al. (2019). Cardiac and peripheral autonomic responses to orthostatic stress during transcutaneous vagus nerve stimulation in healthy subjects. *J. Clin. Med.* 8:496. doi: 10.3390/jcm8040496

Townsend, R. R., Mahfoud, F., Kandzari, D. E., Kario, K., Pocock, S., Weber, M. A., et al. (2017). Catheter-based renal denervation in patients with uncontrolled hypertension in the absence of antihypertensive medications (SPYRAL HTN-OFF MED): a randomised, sham-controlled, proof-of-concept trial. *Lancet* 390, 2160–2170. doi: 10.1016/S0140-6736(17)32281-X

Turianikova, Z., Javorka, K., Baumert, M., Calkovska, A., and Javorka, M. (2011). The effect of orthostatic stress on multiscale entropy of heart rate and blood pressure. *Physiol. Meas.* 32, 1425–1437. doi: 10.1088/0967-3334/32/9/006

Ukena, C., Bauer, A., Mahfoud, F., Schreieck, J., Neuberger, H.-R., Eick, C., et al. (2012). Renal sympathetic denervation for treatment of electrical storm:

first-in-man experience. *Clin. Res. Cardiol.* 101, 63–67. doi: 10.1007/s00392-011-0365-5

Vanoli, E., De Ferrari, G. M., Stramba-Badiale, M., Hull, S. S., Foreman, R. D., and Schwartz, P. J. (1991). Vagal stimulation and prevention of sudden death in conscious dogs with a healed myocardial infarction. *Circ. Res.* 68, 1471–1481. doi: 10.1161/01.RES.68.5.1471

Vaseghi, M., Gima, J., Kanaan, C., Ajijola, O. A., Marmureanu, A., Mahajan, A., et al. (2014). Cardiac sympathetic denervation in patients with refractory ventricular arrhythmias or electrical storm: intermediate and long-term follow-up. *Heart Rhythm.* 11, 360–366. doi: 10.1016/j.hrthm.2013.11.028

Wellens, H. J. J., Schwartz, P. J., Lindemans, F. W., Buxton, A. E., Goldberger, J. J., Hohnloser, S. H., et al. (2014). Risk stratification for sudden cardiac death: current status and challenges for the future. *Eur. Heart J.* 35, 1642–1651. doi: 10.1093/eurheartj/ehu176

Westerhof, B. E., Gisolf, J., Stok, W. J., Wesseling, K. H., and Karemaker, J. M. (2004). Time-domain cross-correlation baroreflex sensitivity: performance on the EUROBAVAR data set. *J. Hypertens.* 22, 1371–1380. doi: 10.1097/01.hjh.0000125439.28861.ed

Wurster, R. D. (1984). "Central nervous system regulation of the heart: an overview" in *Nervous control of cardiovascular function.* ed. W. C. Randall (New York: Oxford UP), 307–320.

Yeragani, V. K., Pohl, R., Jampala, V. C., Balon, R., Kay, J., and Igel, G. (2000a). Effect of posture and isoproterenol on beat-to-beat heart rate and QT variability. *Neuropsychobiology* 41, 113–123. doi: 10.1159/000026642

Yeragani, V. K., Pohl, R., Jampala, V. C., Balon, R., Ramesh, C., and Srinivasan, K. (2000b). Increased QT variability in patients with panic disorder and depression. *Psychiatry Res.* 93, 225–235. doi: 10.1016/S0165-1781(00)00119-0

Zannad, F., De Ferrari, G. M., Tuinenburg, A. E., Wright, D., Brugada, J., Butter, C., et al. (2015). Chronic vagal stimulation for the treatment of low ejection fraction heart failure: results of the NEural Cardiac TherApy foR Heart Failure (NECTAR-HF) randomized controlled trial. *Eur. Heart J.* 36, 425–433. doi: 10.1093/eurheartj/ehu345

Zaza, A., and Lombardi, F. (2001). Autonomic indexes based on the analysis of heart rate variability: a view from the sinus node. *Cardiovasc. Res.* 50, 434–442. doi: 10.1016/S0008-6363(01)00240-1

Zaza, A., Malfatto, G., and Schwartz, P. J. (1991). Sympathetic modulation of the relation between ventricular repolarization and cycle length. *Circ. Res.* 68, 1191–1203. doi: 10.1161/01.RES.68.5.1191

Zhu, C., Hanna, P., Rajendran, P. S., and Shivkumar, K. (2019). Neuromodulation for ventricular tachycardia and atrial fibrillation: a clinical scenario-based review. *JACC Clin. Electrophysiol.* 5, 881–896. doi: 10.1016/j.jacep.2019.06.009

9

Ankyrins and Spectrins in Cardiovascular Biology and Disease

Mona M. El Refaey[1,2*] *and Peter J. Mohler*[1,2,3]

[1] Dorothy M. Davis Heart and Lung Research Institute, Wexner Medical Center, The Ohio State University, Columbus, OH, United States, [2] Department of Physiology & Cell Biology, Wexner Medical Center, The Ohio State University, Columbus, OH, United States, [3] Department of Internal Medicine, Division of Cardiovascular Medicine, College of Medicine, Wexner Medical Center, The Ohio State University, Columbus, OH, United States

Correspondence:
Mona M. El Refaey
mona.elrefaey@osumc.edu

Ankyrins are adaptor proteins critical for the expression and targeting of cardiac membrane proteins, signaling molecules, and cytoskeletal elements. Findings in humans and animal models have highlighted the *in vivo* roles for ankyrins in normal physiology and in cardiovascular disease, most notably in cardiac arrhythmia. For example, human *ANK2* loss-of-function variants are associated with a complex array of electrical and structural phenotypes now termed "ankyrin-B syndrome," whereas alterations in the ankyrin-G pathway for Na_V channel targeting are associated with human Brugada syndrome. Further, both ankyrin-G and -B are now linked with acquired forms of cardiovascular disease including myocardial infarction and atrial fibrillation. Spectrins are ankyrin-associated proteins and recent studies support the critical role of ankyrin-spectrin interactions in normal cardiac physiology as well as regulation of key ion channel and signaling complexes. This review will highlight the roles of ankyrins and spectrins in cardiovascular physiology as well as illustrate the link between the dysfunction in ankyrin- and spectrin-based pathways and disease.

Keywords: ankyrin, spectrin, arrhythmia, heart disease, ion channel, signaling

INTRODUCTION

Cardiovascular disease is the leading cause of death in the United States (Rosamond et al., 2008). In 2013, the overall prevalence of death attributable to cardiovascular diseases (CVD) was 222.9 per 100,000 Americans. On the basis of 2013 data, more than 2,200 Americans die of CVD each day, representing an average of 1 death every 40 s. Arrhythmia is the direct cause of death in many cases. Nearly 80% of cases of sudden cardiac death are the result of ventricular arrhythmias (Mehra, 2007). Thus, understanding the molecular mechanisms underlying human arrhythmias has been an active area of cardiovascular research (Cunha and Mohler, 2006), with a major focus on ion channels, transporters and receptors that regulate the action potential at baseline and in disease. Ankyrins and spectrins are adaptor proteins now linked with both electrical and structural forms of heart disease. Here, we will review the roles of ankyrin and spectrin polypeptides as critical components of cardiac myocytes using findings from human and animal models.

ANKYRIN GENES

Ankyrins are a family of intracellular adaptor proteins that organize and anchor integral membrane protein complexes to the spectrin- and actin-based cytoskeleton (Bennett and Baines, 2001). In vertebrates, three genes (*ANK1*, *ANK2*, *ANK3*), encode ankyrin polypeptides. *ANK1* is located on human chromosome 8p11 and encodes ankyrin-R polypeptides (Lambert et al., 1990). *ANK2* is located on human chromosome 4q25-27 and encodes ankyrin-B polypeptides (Otto et al., 1991). *ANK3* is located on human chromosome 10q21 and encodes ankyrin-G polypeptides (Kordeli et al., 1995). Alternative splicing produces a series of ankyrin gene products with unique subcellular distributions and functional properties (Bennett and Baines, 2001; Cunha and Mohler, 2006; Cunha et al., 2008). For example, alternative splicing of *ANK2* results in 440 kDa and 220 kDa ankyrin-B (Kunimoto, 1995; Hashemi et al., 2009). Ankyrins R, B, and G polypeptides have been identified in ventricular myocytes (Li et al., 1993; Mohler et al., 2002, 2004a,b). However, the full extent of alternative splicing, expression, localization, and function is still under investigation.

ANKYRIN DOMAINS AND BINDING PARTNERS

Canonical ankyrins have four domains: a membrane-binding domain (MBD), a spectrin-binding domain (SBD), a death domain (DD) and a C-terminal domain (CTD) (Mohler, 2006). Together, DD and CTD encompass the "regulatory domain" (RD). Ankyrin-B and ankyrin-G are closely related in amino acid sequence with 67% amino acid identity between the MBD, SBD, and DD. Despite this homology and shared expression in cardiac myocytes, ankyrin-B and ankyrin-G maintain differential distributions and non-overlapping functions. For example, while ankyrin-B is required for the localization of the Na/K-ATPase and Na/Ca exchanger (NCX) (**Figure 1**) to transverse-tubule membranes, ankyrin-G is required for targeting $Na_V1.5$ to the intercalated disc (Mohler et al., 2004a; Makara et al., 2014; Wu et al., 2015).

The MBD is comprised of 24 consecutive *ANK* repeats. In heart, this domain is essential for the interaction with ion channels and transporters (**Figure 2**) including the Na/K-ATPase (Koob et al., 1988), NCX (Li et al., 1993), voltage-gated Na_V channel (Mohler et al., 2004a), the inward rectifier subunit (Kir6.2) (Li et al., 2010), voltage-gated Ca^{2+} channels ($Ca_V1.3$) (Cunha et al., 2011), and inositol trisphosphate receptor ($InsP_3$ receptor) (Bourguignon et al., 1993; Hortsch et al., 2009). MBD binds to a variety of cell adhesion molecules including members of the L1 family (Davis et al., 1993). The impact of these interactions in the heart is not well studied, but an important area for future research.

The SBD associates with high affinity to β spectrin polypeptides (Bennett and Stenbuck, 1979) via the N-terminal ZU5 (Zu5N) domain (Ipsaro and Mondragon, 2010). This interaction is critical for a number of physiological functions including maintenance of normal erythrocyte cell membrane stability (Bodine et al., 1984). As described later, human *ANK2* variants that alter spectrin-binding are now linked with potentially fatal forms of cardiac arrhythmia (Smith et al., 2015). The SBD also interacts with signaling molecules such as B56α, the regulatory subunit of protein phosphatase 2A (PP2A) (Bhasin et al., 2007; Little et al., 2015).

The ankyrin regulatory domain (RD) interacts with proteins including obscurin. Obscurin is a giant scaffolding protein with key roles in muscle myosin incorporation, A-band formation and lateral alignment of M-lines in adjacent myofibrils (Benian et al., 1996; Borisov et al., 2006; Cunha and Mohler, 2008). Cunha and colleagues demonstrated that ankyrin-B/obscurin interaction recruits PP2A to the cardiac M-line (Cunha and Mohler, 2008) (**Figure 1**). In addition to the intermolecular interactions, the regulatory domain regulates the intramolecular interactions with the ankyrin MBD (Abdi et al., 2006).

SPECTRIN POLYPEPTIDES IN CARDIAC PHYSIOLOGY

Spectrins are actin-associated proteins that provide structural support to the plasma membrane and play roles in the localization of membrane and signaling proteins in the heart (Hund and Mohler, 2010). Spectrin alpha (α) and beta (β) subunits are assembled laterally to form anti-parallel heterodimers, and these heterodimers are assembled to form a flexible hetero-tetramic molecule (Bennett and Baines, 2001). There are two α spectrin genes and five β spectrin genes that encode a diverse group of alternatively-spliced spectrin isoforms with specific functions (Bennett and Healy, 2009). In ventricular myocytes, αII and βII spectrin are found at transverse-tubule and sarcoplasmic reticulum (SR) membranes (Baines and Pinder, 2005), whereas βIV spectrin is located at the intercalated disc (Hund et al., 2010).

In heart, βII spectrin directly interacts with ankyrin-B at transverse-tubule membranes (Mohler et al., 2004c; Smith et al., 2015). In fact, βII spectrin is a critical element of the larger ankyrin-B complex that directly links membrane and signaling proteins including NCX, Na/K ATPase, and β56α with the underlying actin-based cytoskeleton. Loss of βII spectrin in adult ventricular myocytes directly impacts the expression and localization of ankyrin-B as well as ankyrin-B-associated proteins (Smith et al., 2015). Beyond loss of ankyrin-binding proteins, βII spectrin null myocytes unexpectedly showed abnormal localization of the cardiac ryanodine receptor. The relationship of βII spectrin and ryanodine receptor is currently unknown. At the animal level, loss of βII spectrin in mice is lethal in mid-gestation due to incomplete development of the heart (Tang et al., 2003). Conditional deletion of βII spectrin in ventricular myocytes results in sinus node dysfunction and ventricular arrhythmia. These mice also display cytoskeletal remodeling and accelerated heart failure following transverse aortic constriction. As described later, human *ANK2* variants that alter the interaction with βII spectrin are linked with congenital arrhythmia (Smith et al., 2015). Further, βII spectrin levels are altered in acquired forms of human heart failure and arrhythmia,

---

Abbreviations: MBD, Membrane-binding domain; CTD, C-terminal domain; SBD, Spectrin-binding domain; DD, Death domain; LQTS, Long QT syndrome; NCX, Sodium-Calcium exchanger; Na/K ATPase, Sodium-potassium ATPase; IP3R, Inositol trisphosphate receptor; cKO, Conditional knock-out; INa,L, Late component of Nav current; CaMKII, Calcium/calmodulin-dependent kinase; KATP, ATP-sensitive K+ channel; Cav1.3, Voltage gated L-type Ca2+ channel; PP2A, Protein phosphatase 2A; Nav1.5, Voltage-gated sodium channel; TREK-1, TWIK-related potassium channel-1.

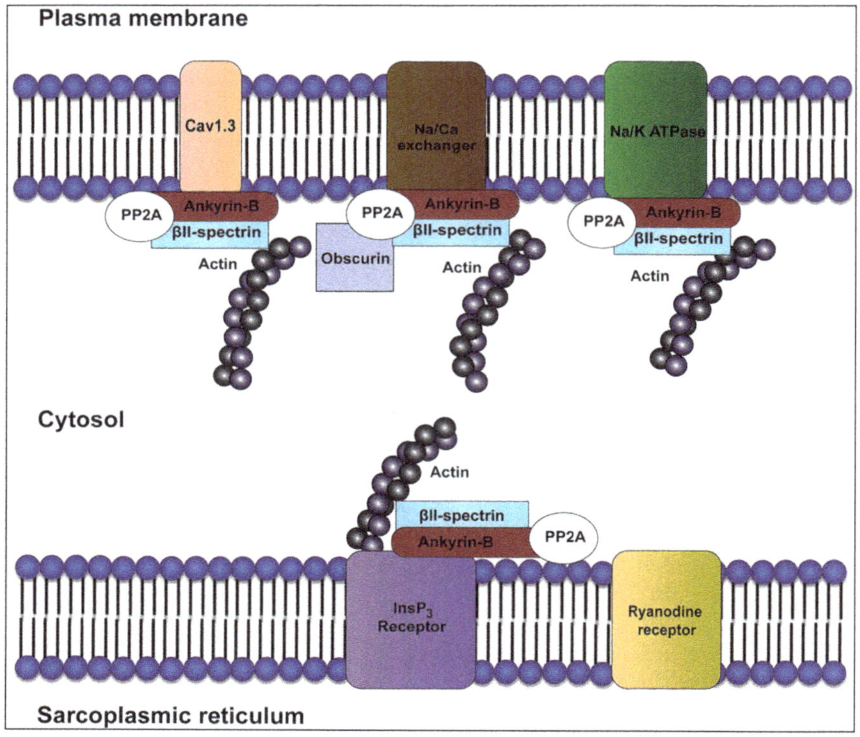

FIGURE 1 | Role of ankyrin-B in localization of the $InsP_3$ receptor, Na/K-ATPase, $Ca_V1.3$, and NCX. In heart, ankyrin-B targets and localizes ion channels and transporters such as inositol trisphosphate receptor ($InsP_3R$), sodium/potassium ATPase (Na/K-ATPase), $Ca_V1.3$, and Na/Ca exchanger (NCX). Ankyrin-B also targets protein phosphatase type 2A (PP2A) through its regulatory subunit B56α. Interaction between ankyrin-B and βII spectrin forms a complex that is important for the localization and stability of ion channels and transporters such as Na/K-ATPase, $Ca_V1.3$, $InsP_3R$, and NCX.

as well as in animal models of cardiovascular disease (Smith et al., 2016). Finally, individuals with Beckwith-Wiedemann syndrome (BWS) with a reduction in βII spectrin expression (Yao et al., 2010) show congenital heart failure and ventricular septal defects (Drut et al., 2006).

In heart, βIV spectrin directly associates with ankyrin-G and is required for the targeting of calcium/calmodulin-dependent kinase II (CaMKII) to the intercalated disc (Hund et al., 2010). Notably, this interaction is critical for the regulation of I_{Na} by modulating CaMKII-dependent phosphorylation of $Na_V1.5$ (Hund et al., 2010; Koval et al., 2012). Beyond, ankyrin-G and CaMKII, βIV spectrin regulates TREK-1, a mechano-sensitive K_{2P} channel (Heurteaux et al., 2004). More specifically, βIV spectrin and TREK-1 associate, and βIV spectrin is required for TREK-1 localization and function in ventricular myocytes (Hund et al., 2014). Mice lacking TREK-1 binding display delayed action potential repolarization and arrhythmia. These data support a broader role for βIV spectrin in cardiovascular electrophysiology by regulation of TREK-1 membrane localization and function. Like βII spectrin, βIV spectrin levels are altered in human heart failure as well as in animal models of cardiovascular disease (Hund et al., 2014).

Finally, αII spectrin-deficient embryos are embryonic lethal with abnormal cardiac shape, cardiac dilatation and changes in myocardium (Stankewich et al., 2011). Beyond ankyrins, Mena and VASP, important regulators of actin dynamics form a complex with αII spectrin in adult cardiomyocytes (Benz et al., 2013). The *in vivo* role(s) of αII spectrin in adult heart is currently unknown but an important area for future research.

IN VIVO ROLES FOR CARDIAC ANKYRINS

Ankyrin-G is Required for Targeting $Na_V1.5$

In neurons, the link between ankyrin-G and Na_V channel targeting is well established (Jenkins and Bennett, 2001; Saifetiarova et al., 2017). In heart, rat ventricular myocytes lacking ankyrin-G display a reduction in $Na_V1.5$ expression, localization, and I_{Na} (Lowe et al., 2008). In fact, in myocytes with reduced ankyrin-G expression, $Na_V1.5$ localization is limited in the perinuclear region of rat ventricular myocytes. Notably, this role is specific for ankyrin-G vs. ankyrin-B as ankyrin-B-null neonatal cardiomyocytes show no difference in $Na_V1.5$ expression or localization. Further, loss of ankyrin-G is specific for I_{Na} vs. other cardiac currents (e.g., $I_{Ca,L}$) (Lowe et al., 2008).

In animals, ankyrin-G expression is required for the targeting of $Na_V1.5$ and CaMKII to the intercalated disc (Makara et al., 2014). $Na_V1.5$ expression and I_{Na} is reduced in myocytes derived from mice with selective loss of cardiomyocyte ankyrin-G (cKO) (Makara et al., 2014). Further, βIV spectrin

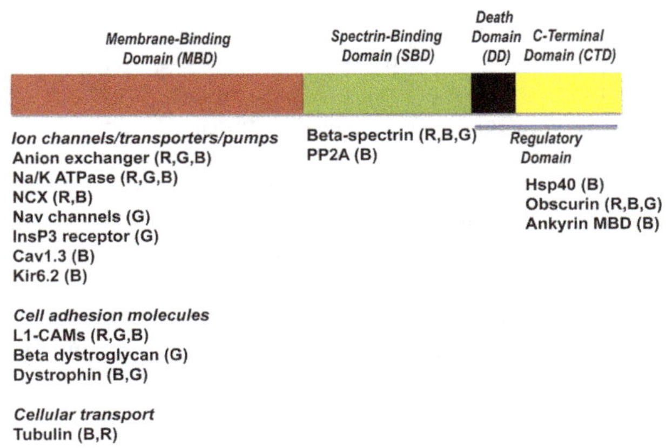

FIGURE 2 | Structure of ankyrins and ankyrin-binding partners. Ankyrins are formed of four distinct domains: a membrane-binding domain (MBD), a spectrin-binding domain (SBD), a death domain (DD) and a C-terminal domain (CTD). Each domain interacts with distinct ion channels, transporters and pumps. $Ca_V1.3$, calcium channel, voltage-dependent, L type, alpha 1D subunit; Na/K-ATPase, sodium/potassium ATPase; NCX, Na/Ca exchanger; $InsP_3R$, Inositol trisphosphate receptor; Kir6.2, Inward-rectifier potassium ion channel; Na_V channels, voltage-gated sodium channels; L1-CAMs, The L1 family of neural cell adhesion molecules; PP2A, protein phosphatase type 2A; Hsp40, Heat shock protein 40.

is absent in the intercalated disc of myocytes of ankyrin cKO mice. Electrocardiographic studies of these mice show significant reduction in heart rate, impaired atrioventricular conduction, and an increase in PR interval. Moreover, cKO mice display a significant increase in the QRS interval and delayed intraventricular conduction. Administration of flecainide or catecholamines (elevated adrenergic stimulation) induces arrhythmia in these mice.

Beyond animals, work in humans supports the link between ankyrin-G and Na_v channel targeting. Priori et al. (2000) identified an individual with Brugada syndrome harboring an *SCN5A* variant in the $Na_V1.5$ motif that interacts with ankyrin-G (Mohler et al., 2004a). The group identified the *SCN5A* variant in a 47-year-old female with a history of palpitations and an unexplained syncope at rest. Using *in vitro* binding assays, the p.E1053K variant was found to disrupt the interaction between $Na_V1.5$ and ankyrin-G resulting in abnormal targeting in myocytes.

A canine myocardial infarction (MI) model was used to study the role of ankyrin-G in acquired arrhythmic disease. At 5 days, there was a 42% reduction in $Na_V1.5$ protein expression and a 50% increase in ankyrin-G expression in the epicardial border zone. These data suggest that ankyrin-G levels increase to regulate $Na_V1.5$ recruitment to sarcolemmal membrane (Dun et al., 2013).

Ankyrin-B

First identified in brain, ankyrin-B has now been directly linked with a host of functions in the heart. Further, ankyrin-B dysfunction is now well documented in multiple forms of congenital and acquired cardiovascular disease. While ankyrin-B was known to directly associate with critical cardiac ion channels and transporters, an *in vivo* role for ankyrin-B in cardiac function was first illustrated using mice heterozygous for an ankyrin-B null mutation. While ankyrin-B null mice die shortly after birth, ankyrin-$B^{+/-}$ mice live to adulthood but display bradycardia, heart rate variability, prolonged QT intervals, and sudden cardiac death in response to exercise combined with catecholaminergic stimulation (Mohler et al., 2003). While adult ventricular myocytes from ankyrin-$B^{+/-}$ mice display normal action potential duration, these myocytes display early and delayed after-depolarizations in response to catecholamines. At the molecular level, ankyrin-$B^{+/-}$ ventricular myocytes display reduced expression and abnormal localization of ankyrin-B-binding partners including Na/K ATPase and NCX. As illustrated in computational models (Wolf et al., 2010), loss of Na/K ATPase and NCX results in increased SR calcium stores that result in an arrhythmogenic substrate in the ankyrin-$B^{+/-}$ animals (Mohler et al., 2004b). Subsequent work from Despa and colleagues revealed significant alterations in local $[Ca^{2+}]$ as well as hyper-phosphorylation of ryanodine receptors in ankyrin-$B^{+/-}$ ventricular myocytes (Camors et al., 2012; Popescu et al., 2016) potentially due to altered PP2A regulation (DeGrande et al., 2012). Further characterization of ankyrin-$B^{+/-}$ mice showed premature senescence and reduced longevity with mice showing loss of adiposity starting at 6 months of age (Mohler et al., 2007a).

Ankyrin-B dysfunction is directly linked with human cardiovascular disease. Over two decades ago, Schott and colleagues identified type 4 long QT syndrome in a large French kindred with sinus node dysfunction and episodes of atrial fibrillation (Schott et al., 1995). Prolonged QTc was observed among the 25 affected patients (21 adults and 4 children). Individuals in the family also displayed catecholaminergic polymorphic ventricular arrhythmia and sudden death. Sequencing of the gene encoding ankyrin-B *(ANK2)* revealed a positional transition (A to G) mutation at position 4,274 in exon 36, leading to the substitution of a glycine for a glutamic acid at amino acid residue 1,425 (p.E1425G) near the regulatory domain of ankyrin-B in forty-five family members (24 carriers and 21 non-carriers). The p.E1425G variant, subsequently identified as a loss-of-function variant in myocytes, showed prevalence in 22 out of 24 individuals with the LQT4 phenotype and was absent in non-affected individuals (Mohler et al., 2003). Since this initial discovery, a number of new ankyrin-B loss-of-function variants have been identified in individuals with ventricular arrhythmias. However, as discussed below, due to the diversity of non-ventricular phenotypes associated with the disease (including many lacking QTc prolongation), the term "ankyrin-B syndrome" has been adopted to describe individuals harboring *ANK2* loss-of-function variants (Mohler et al., 2004b, 2007b). As in the case of many cardiovascular disease genes, the penetrance of phenotypes in *ANK2* variant carriers is variable. As ankyrin-B polypeptide stability and function is directly impacted by physiological and pathological stress (e.g., inflammation, elevated reactive oxygen species), we predict that a "second hit" may be necessary for full disease penetrance.

Active areas of research in this field are currently focused on identifying the mechanisms underlying both congenital and acquired ankyrin-B loss in human disease as well as the discovery of new variants. For example, while loss-of-function variants were limited to the RD, new variants in the ankyrin-B MBD have shed light on new phenotypes associated with "ankyrin-B syndrome." Recently, a novel MBD variant in the *ANK2* gene (p.S646F) was identified in two Gitxan families with LQTS phenotypes by the Swayne and Arbour groups (Swayne et al., 2017). The first person identified was a 28-year old man with a clinical diagnosis of LQTS and recurrent syncope. Five of this patient's relatives were confirmed to harbor this variant. This variant was also identified in a second family with a clinical diagnosis of LQTS. Within these two families, a total of 13 adults and 5 children have been identified with this novel *ANK2* variant. *In vitro* evaluation illustrated that the expression of ankyrin MBD with p.S646F variant in bacteria was normal and MBD structural properties were intact. However, expression of ankyrin-B p.S646F variant in neonatal cardiomyocytes showed a reduction in ankyrin-B expression and alteration of expression of NCX (Swayne et al., 2017). Finally, beyond LQT and catecholaminergic polymorphic ventricular tachycardia, *ANK2* variants have been associated with other forms of ventricular arrhythmia including early repolarization syndrome (Krogh Broendberg et al., 2015).

ANK2 variants are not limited to MBD or RD. Smith et al. identified an *ANK2* arrhythmia variant (c.2969G>A) caused by the substitution of Arg to Gln at position 990 (p. R990Q). This variant is rare with a minor allele frequency of 0.007% and resides near the central ZU5 binding surface for βII spectrin. Using myocytes from ankyrin-B conditional knockout mice (cKO), exogenous expression of WT ankyrin-B, but not ankyrin-B p.R990Q was able to rescue the localization of NCX (Smith et al., 2015).

Ankyrin-B dysfunction is also linked with non-ventricular forms of human arrhythmia. Individuals with select *ANK2* loss-of-function variants display atrial fibrillation and/or sinus node dysfunction (Le Scouarnec et al., 2008; Cunha et al., 2011). Consistent with these data, ankyrin-B$^{+/-}$ mice also display both atrial and sinus node phenotypes. At the cellular level, primary atrial and sinus node myocytes from ankyrin-B$^{+/-}$ mice display shortened action potentials and loss of L-type Ca^{2+} current. In ankyrin-B$^{+/-}$ atrial myocytes, voltage-gated L-type Ca^{2+} channel $Ca_V1.3$ (but not $Ca_V1.2$) expression and function were reduced.

Until recently, *ANK2*-based disease was linked only to individuals with single "point mutations" (Mohler et al., 2004b, 2007b; Sherman et al., 2005; Krogh Broendberg et al., 2015; Swayne et al., 2017). However, recently a family was identified with an *ANK2* transection in chromosome 4 (Huq et al., 2017). The proband had a balanced translocation between the long arms of chromosomes 4 and 9. Five other family members were carriers of the same balanced translocation. The 16-week-old fetus of the proband from a terminated pregnancy was found to have multiple cardiac abnormalities. The proband showed normal echocardiography findings and only Holter monitor recorded few episodes of bradycardia at night. Isolated lymphoblasts from the proband demonstrated a significant reduction in ankyrin-B and binding partners, confirming a model of ankyrin-B haploinsufficiency. The mother of the proband was also a carrier of the translocation and displayed frequent ventricular ectopy and periods of bigeminy.

Beyond congenital disease, dysfunction in ankyrin-B-based pathways has been linked with acquired forms of cardiovascular disease. In a canine model of myocardial infarction, ankyrin-B mRNA levels were increased and protein levels were decreased in day 5-post infarction in the border zone (Hund et al., 2009). At the myocyte level, abnormal distribution of ankyrin-B was noted. The authors further showed changes in expression and/or distribution of downstream ankyrin-associated proteins Na/K ATPase, NCX, $InsP_3$ receptor and PP2A (Hund et al., 2009). In addition to its role in myocardial infarction, Li et al. identified the association of ATP-sensitive K^+ channel (K_{ATP}) with ankyrin-B as a cardio-protective mechanism against acute ischemia (Li et al., 2010). Ankyrin-B levels are now also known to be reduced in patients with atrial fibrillation (Cunha et al., 2011).

Ankyrin-R

To date, human variants in *ANK1* have not been directly linked with cardiac arrhythmia phenotypes. While not the focus on this review, it is of note that variants in *ANK1* are a primary cause for hereditary spherocytosis (Eber et al., 1996; Tse and Lux, 1999; Perrotta et al., 2008; Satchwell et al., 2016).

SUMMARY

Cardiac ankyrins and spectrins are key multifunctional molecules in the heart. In myocytes, ankyrins, and spectrins serve essential roles in targeting ion channels and transporters to critical membrane domains. However, beyond membrane proteins, these molecules serve as crucial cellular nodes to integrate membrane proteins with critical signaling and structural proteins in diverse cardiac cell types. While animals have served as important models to define ankyrin and spectrin function *in vivo*, more recent findings in patients have both solidified the importance of ankyrins and spectrin in human physiology and disease, and raised important questions related to unexpected roles of these polypeptides. Key future questions in the field remain the impact of environment or "second hit" gene variants on disease susceptibility/penetrance in *ANK2* variant carriers, as well as potential non-myocyte/non-cardiac phenotypes in patients with ankyrin gene variants.

AUTHOR CONTRIBUTIONS

All authors listed, have made substantial, direct and intellectual contribution to the work, and approved it for publication.

ACKNOWLEDGMENTS

This work was supported by National Heart, Lung and Blood Institute grants HL-135754, HL-134824, and HL-114383 (PM). ME is supported by Dorothy M. Davis Heart and Lung Research Institute Post-doctoral training fellowship in Congenital and Acquired Heart Diseases (5T32HL098039).

REFERENCES

Abdi, K. M., Mohler, P. J., Davis, J. Q., and Bennett, V. (2006). Isoform specificity of ankyrin-B: a site in the divergent C-terminal domain is required for intramolecular association. *J. Biol. Chem.* 281, 5741–5749. doi: 10.1074/jbc.M506697200

Baines, A. J., and Pinder, J. C. (2005). The spectrin-associated cytoskeleton in mammalian heart. *Front. Biosci.* 10, 3020–3033. doi: 10.2741/1759

Benian, G. M., Tinley, T. L., Tang, X., and Borodovsky, M. (1996). The Caenorhabditis elegans gene unc-89, required fpr muscle M-line assembly, encodes a giant modular protein composed of Ig and signal transduction domains. *J. Cell Biol.* 132, 835–848. doi: 10.1083/jcb.132.5.835

Bennett, V., and Baines, A. J. (2001). Spectrin and ankyrin-based pathways: metazoan inventions for integrating cells into tissues. *Physiol. Rev.* 81, 1353–1392. Available online at: http://physrev.physiology.org/content/81/3/1353.full-text.pdf+html

Bennett, V., and Healy, J. (2009). Membrane domains based on ankyrin and spectrin associated with cell-cell interactions. *Cold Spring Harb. Perspect. Biol.* 1:a003012. doi: 10.1101/cshperspect.a003012

Bennett, V., and Stenbuck, P. J. (1979). The membrane attachment protein for spectrin is associated with band 3 in human erythrocyte membranes. *Nature* 280, 468–473. doi: 10.1038/280468a0

Benz, P. M., Merkel, C. J., Offner, K., Abeßer, M., Ullrich, M., Fischer, T., et al. (2013). Mena/VASP and alphaII-spectrin complexes regulate cytoplasmic actin networks in cardiomyocytes and protect from conduction abnormalities and dilated cardiomyopathy. *Cell Commun. Signal* 11:56. doi: 10.1186/1478-811X-11-56

Bhasin, N., Cunha, S. R., Mudannayake, M., Gigena, M. S., Rogers, T. B., and Mohler, P. J. (2007). Molecular basis for PP2A regulatory subunit B56alpha targeting in cardiomyocytes. *Am. J. Physiol. Heart Circ. Physiol.* 293, H109–H119. doi: 10.1152/ajpheart.00059.2007

Bodine, D. M., Birkenmeier, C. S., and Barker, J. E. (1984). Spectrin deficient inherited hemolytic anemias in the mouse: characterization by spectrin synthesis and mRNA activity in reticulocytes. *Cell* 37, 721–729. doi: 10.1016/0092-8674(84)90408-2

Borisov, A. B., Sutter, S. B., Kontrogianni-Konstantopoulos, A., Bloch, R. J., Westfall, M. V., and Russell, M. W. (2006). Essential role of obscurin in cardiac myofibrillogenesis and hypertrophic response: evidence from small interfering RNA-mediated gene silencing. *Histochem. Cell Biol.* 125, 227–238. doi: 10.1007/s00418-005-0069-x

Bourguignon, L. Y., Jin, H., Iida, N., Brandt, N. R., and Zhang, S. H. (1993). The involvement of ankyrin in the regulation of inositol 1,4,5-trisphosphate receptor-mediated internal Ca2+ release from Ca2+ storage vesicles in mouse T-lymphoma cells. *J. Biol. Chem.* 268, 7290–7297.

Camors, E., Mohler, P. J., Bers, D. M., and Despa, S. (2012). Ankyrin-B reduction enhances Ca spark-mediated SR Ca release promoting cardiac myocyte arrhythmic activity. *J. Mol. Cell Cardiol.* 52, 1240–1248. doi: 10.1016/j.yjmcc.2012.02.010

Cunha, S. R., Hund, T. J., Hashemi, S., Voigt, N., Li, N., Wright, P., et al. (2011). Defects in ankyrin-based membrane protein targeting pathways underlie atrial fibrillation. *Circulation* 124, 1212–1222. doi: 10.1161/CIRCULATIONAHA.111.023986

Cunha, S. R., Le Scouarnec, S., Schott, J. J., and Mohler, P. J. (2008). Exon organization and novel alternative splicing of the human ANK2 gene: implications for cardiac function and human cardiac disease. *J. Mol. Cell Cardiol.* 45, 724–734. doi: 10.1016/j.yjmcc.2008.08.005

Cunha, S. R., and Mohler, P. J. (2006). Cardiac ankyrins: Essential components for development and maintenance of excitable membrane domains in heart. *Cardiovasc. Res.* 71, 22–29. doi: 10.1016/j.cardiores.2006.03.018

Cunha, S. R., and Mohler, P. J. (2008). Obscurin targets ankyrin-B and protein phosphatase 2A to the cardiac M-line. *J. Biol. Chem.* 283, 31968–31980. doi: 10.1074/jbc.M806050200

Davis, J. Q., McLaughlin, T., and Bennett, V. (1993). Ankyrin-binding proteins related to nervous system cell adhesion molecules: candidates to provide transmembrane and intercellular connections in adult brain. *J. Cell Biol.* 121, 121–133. doi: 10.1083/jcb.121.1.121

DeGrande, S., Nixon, D., Koval, O., Curran, J. W., Wright, P., Wang, Q., et al. (2012). CaMKII inhibition rescues proarrhythmic phenotypes in the model of human ankyrin-B syndrome. *Heart Rhythm* 9, 2034–2041. doi: 10.1016/j.hrthm.2012.08.026

Drut, R., Quijano, G., Altamirano, M. E., Jones, M. C., and Maffessoli, O. B. (2006). Vascular malformation and choroid plexus adrenal heterotopia: new findings in Beckwith-Wiedemann syndrome? *Fetal Pediatr. Pathol.* 25, 191–197. doi: 10.1080/15513810601015704

Dun, W., Lowe, J. S., Wright, P., Hund, T. J., Mohler, P. J., and Boyden, P. A. (2013). Ankyrin-G participates in INa remodeling in myocytes from the border zones of infarcted canine heart. *PLoS ONE* 8:e78087. doi: 10.1371/journal.pone.0078087

Eber, S. W., Gonzalez, J. M., Lux, M. L., Scarpa, A. L., Tse, W. T., Dornwell, M., et al. (1996). Ankyrin-1 mutations are a major cause of dominant and recessive hereditary spherocytosis. *Nat. Genet.* 13, 214–218. doi: 10.1038/ng0696-214

Hashemi, S. M., Hund, T. J., and Mohler, P. J. (2009). Cardiac ankyrins in health and disease. *J. Mol. Cell Cardiol.* 47, 203–209. doi: 10.1016/j.yjmcc.2009.04.010

Heurteaux, C., Guy, N., Laigle, C., Blondeau, N., Duprat, F., Mazzuca, M., et al. (2004). TREK-1, a K+ channel involved in neuroprotection and general anesthesia. *EMBO J.* 23, 2684–2695. doi: 10.1038/sj.emboj.7600234

Hortsch, M., Nagaraj, K., and Godenschwege, T. A. (2009). The interaction between L1-type proteins and ankyrins–a master switch for L1-type CAM function. *Cell Mol. Biol. Lett.* 14, 57–69. doi: 10.2478/s11658-008-0035-4

Hund, T. J., Koval, O. M., Li, J., Wright, P. J., Qian, L., Snyder, J. S., et al. (2010). A beta(IV)-spectrin/CaMKII signaling complex is essential for membrane excitability in mice. *J. Clin. Invest.* 120, 3508–3519. doi: 10.1172/JCI43621

Hund, T. J., and Mohler, P. J. (2010). Cardiac spectrins: alternative splicing encodes functional diversity. *J. Mol. Cell Cardiol.* 48, 1031–1032. doi: 10.1016/j.yjmcc.2010.02.002

Hund, T. J., Snyder, J. S., Wu, X., Glynn, P., Koval, O. M., Onal, B., et al. (2014). beta(IV)-Spectrin regulates TREK-1 membrane targeting in the heart. *Cardiovasc. Res.* 102, 166–175. doi: 10.1093/cvr/cvu008

Hund, T. J., Wright, P. J., Dun, W., Snyder, J. S., Boyden, P. A., and Mohler, P. J. (2009). Regulation of the ankyrin-B-based targeting pathway following myocardial infarction. *Cardiovasc. Res.* 81, 742–749.doi: 10.1093/cvr/cvn348

Huq, A. J., Pertile, M. D., Davis, A. M., Landon, H., James, P. A., Kline, C. F., et al. (2017). A novel mechanism for human cardiac Ankyrin-B syndrome due to reciprocal chromosomal translocation. *Heart Lung Circ.* 26, 612–618. doi: 10.1016/j.hlc.2016.09.013

Ipsaro, J. J., and Mondragón, A. (2010). Structural basis for spectrin recognition by ankyrin. *Blood* 115, 4093–4101. doi: 10.1182/blood-2009-11-255604

Jenkins, S. M., and Bennett, V. (2001). Ankyrin-G coordinates assembly of the spectrin-based membrane skeleton, voltage-gated sodium channels, and L1 CAMs at Purkinje neuron initial segments. *J. Cell Biol.* 155, 739–746. doi: 10.1083/jcb.200109026

Koob, R., Zimmermann, M., Schoner, W., and Drenckhahn, D. (1988). Colocalization and coprecipitation of ankyrin and Na+,K+-ATPase in kidney epithelial cells. *Eur. J. Cell Biol.* 45, 230–237.

Kordeli, E., Lambert, S., and Bennett, V. (1995). AnkyrinG. a new ankyrin gene with neural-specific isoforms localized at the axonal initial segment and node of ranvier. *J. Biol. Chem.* 270, 2352–2359. doi: 10.1074/jbc.270.5.2352

Koval, O. M., Snyder, J. S., Wolf, R. M., Pavlovicz, R. E., Glynn, P., Curran, J., et al. (2012). Ca2+/calmodulin-dependent protein kinase II-based regulation of voltage-gated Na+ channel in cardiac disease. *Circulation* 126, 2084–2094. doi: 10.1161/CIRCULATIONAHA.112.105320

Krogh Broendberg, A., Pedersen, L. N., Nielsen, J. C., and Jensen, H. K. (2015). Ankyrin-2 variants associated with idiopathic ventricular fibrillation storm in patients with intermittent early repolarization pattern. *HeartRhythm Case Rep.* 1, 337–341. doi: 10.1016/j.hrcr.2015.05.008

Kunimoto, M. (1995). A neuron-specific isoform of brain ankyrin, 440-kD ankyrinB, is targeted to the axons of rat cerebellar neurons. *J. Cell Biol.* 131(6 Pt 2), 1821–1829. doi: 10.1083/jcb.131.6.1821

Lambert, S., Yu, H., Prchal, J. T., Lawler, J., Ruff, P., Speicher, D., et al. (1990). cDNA sequence for human erythrocyte ankyrin. *Proc. Natl. Acad. Sci. U.S.A.* 87, 1730–1734. doi: 10.1073/pnas.87.5.1730

Le Scouarnec, S., Bhasin, N., Vieyres, C., Hund, T. J., Cunha, S. R., Koval, O., et al. (2008). Dysfunction in ankyrin-B-dependent ion channel and transporter targeting causes human sinus node disease. *Proc. Natl. Acad. Sci. U. S. A.* 105, 15617–15622. doi: 10.1073/pnas.0805500105

Li, J., Kline, C. F., Hund, T. J., Anderson, M. E., and Mohler, P. J. (2010). Ankyrin-B regulates Kir6.2 membrane expression and function in heart. *J. Biol. Chem.* 285, 28723–28730. doi: 10.1074/jbc.M110.147868

Li, Z. P., Burke, E. P., Frank, J. S., Bennett, V., and Philipson, K. D. (1993). The cardiac Na+-Ca2+ exchanger binds to the cytoskeletal protein ankyrin. *J. Biol. Chem.* 268, 11489–11491.

Little, S. C., Curran, J., Makara, M. A., Kline, C. F., Ho, H. T., Xu, Z., et al. (2015). Protein phosphatase 2A regulatory subunit B56alpha limits phosphatase activity in the heart. *Sci Signal* 8, ra72. doi: 10.1126/scisignal.aaa5876

Lowe, J. S., Palygin, O., Bhasin, N., Hund, T. J., Boyden, P. A., Shibata, E., et al. (2008). Voltage-gated Nav channel targeting in the heart requires an ankyrin-G dependent cellular pathway. *J. Cell Biol.* 180, 173–186. doi: 10.1083/jcb.200710107

Makara, M. A., Curran, J., Little, S. C., Musa, H., Polina, I., Smith, S. A., et al. (2014). Ankyrin-G coordinates intercalated disc signaling platform to regulate cardiac excitability *in vivo*. *Circ. Res.* 115, 929–938. doi: 10.1161/CIRCRESAHA.115.305154

Mehra, R. (2007). Global public health problem of sudden cardiac death. *J. Electrocardiol.* 40, S118–122. doi: 10.1016/j.jelectrocard.2007.06.023

Mohler, P. J. (2006). Ankyrins and human disease: what the electrophysiologist should know. *J. Cardiovasc. Electrophysiol.* 17, 1153–1159. doi: 10.1111/j.1540-8167.2006.00540.x

Mohler, P. J., Gramolini, A. O., and Bennett, V. (2002). The ankyrin-B C-terminal domain determines activity of ankyrin-B/G chimeras in rescue of abnormal inositol 1,4,5-trisphosphate and ryanodine receptor distribution in ankyrin-B (-/-) neonatal cardiomyocytes. *J. Biol. Chem.* 277, 10599–10607. doi: 10.1074/jbc.M110958200

Mohler, P. J., Healy, J. A., Xue, H., Puca, A. A., Kline, C. F., Allingham, R. R., et al. (2007a). Ankyrin-B syndrome: enhanced cardiac function balanced by risk of cardiac death and premature senescence. *PLoS ONE* 2:e1051. doi: 10.1371/journal.pone.0001051

Mohler, P. J., Le Scouarnec, S., Denjoy, I., Lowe, J. S., Guicheney, P., Caron, L., et al. (2007b). Defining the cellular phenotype of "ankyrin-B syndrome" variants: human ANK2 variants associated with clinical phenotypes display a spectrum of activities in cardiomyocytes. *Circulation* 115, 432–441. doi: 10.1161/CIRCULATIONAHA.106.656512

Mohler, P. J., Rivolta, I., Napolitano, C., LeMaillet, G., Lambert, S., Priori, S. G., et al. (2004a). Nav1.5 E1053K mutation causing Brugada syndrome blocks binding to ankyrin-G and expression of Nav1.5 on the surface of cardiomyocytes. *Proc. Natl. Acad. Sci. U.S.A.* 101, 17533–17538. doi: 10.1073/pnas.0403711101

Mohler, P. J., Schott, J. J., Gramolini, A. O., Dilly, K. W., Guatimosim, S., duBell, W. H., et al. (2003). Ankyrin-B mutation causes type 4 long-QT cardiac arrhythmia and sudden cardiac death. *Nature* 421, 634–639. doi: 10.1038/nature01335

Mohler, P. J., Splawski, I., Napolitano, C., Bottelli, G., Sharpe, L., Timothy, K., et al. (2004b). A cardiac arrhythmia syndrome caused by loss of ankyrin-B function. *Proc. Natl. Acad. Sci. U.S.A.* 101, 9137–9142. doi: 10.1073/pnas.0402546101

Mohler, P. J., Yoon, W., and Bennett, V. (2004c). Ankyrin-B targets beta2-spectrin to an intracellular compartment in neonatal cardiomyocytes. *J. Biol. Chem.* 279, 40185–40193. doi: 10.1074/jbc.M406018200

Otto, E., Kunimoto, M., McLaughlin, T., and Bennett, V. (1991). Isolation and characterization of cDNAs encoding human brain ankyrins reveal a family of alternatively spliced genes. *J. Cell Biol.* 114, 241–253. doi: 10.1083/jcb.114.2.241

Perrotta, S., Gallagher, P. G., and Mohandas, N. (2008). Hereditary spherocytosis. *Lancet* 372, 1411–1426. doi: 10.1016/S0140-6736(08)61588-3

Popescu, I., Galice, S., Mohler, P. J., and Despa, S. (2016). Elevated local [Ca2+] and CaMKII promote spontaneous Ca2+ release in ankyrin-B-deficient hearts. *Cardiovasc. Res.* 111, 287–294. doi: 10.1093/cvr/cvw093

Priori, S. G., Napolitano, C., Gasparini, M., Pappone, C., Della Bella, P., Brignole, M., et al. (2000). Clinical and genetic heterogeneity of right bundle branch block and ST-segment elevation syndrome: a prospective evaluation of 52 families. *Circulation* 102, 2509–2515. doi: 10.1161/01.CIR.102.20.2509

Rosamond, W., Flegal, K., Furie, K., Go, A., Greenlund, K., Haase, N., et al. (2008). Heart disease and stroke statistics—2008 update: a report from the American Heart Association Statistics Committee and Stroke Statistics Subcommittee. *Circulation* 117, e25–e146. doi: 10.1161/CIRCULATIONAHA.107.187998

Saifetiarova, J., Taylor, A. M., and Bhat, M. A. (2017). Early and late loss of the Cytoskeletal Scaffolding protein, Ankyrin G reveals its role in maturation and maintenance of nodes of Ranvier in Myelinated Axons. *J. Neurosci.* 37, 2524–2538. doi: 10.1523/JNEUROSCI.2661-16.2017

Satchwell, T. J., Bell, A. J., Hawley, B. R., Pellegrin, S., Mordue, K. E., van Deursen, C. T., et al. (2016). Severe Ankyrin-R deficiency results in impaired surface retention and lysosomal degradation of RhAG in human erythroblasts. *Haematologica* 101, 1018–1027. doi: 10.3324/haematol.2016.146209

Schott, J. J., Charpentier, F., Peltier, S., Foley, P., Drouin, E., Bouhour, J. B., et al. (1995). Mapping of a gene for long QT syndrome to chromosome 4q25-27. *Am. J. Hum. Genet.* 57, 1114–1122.

Sherman, J., Tester, D. J., and Ackerman, M. J. (2005). Targeted mutational analysis of ankyrin-B in 541 consecutive, unrelated patients referred for long QT syndrome genetic testing and 200 healthy subjects. *Heart Rhythm* 2, 1218–1223. doi: 10.1016/j.hrthm.2005.07.026

Smith, S. A., Hughes, L. D., Kline, C. F., Kempton, A. N., Dorn, L. E., Curran, J., et al. (2016). Dysfunction of the beta2-spectrin-based pathway in human heart failure. *Am. J. Physiol. Heart Circ. Physiol.* 310, H1583–H1591. doi: 10.1152/ajpheart.00875.2015

Smith, S. A., Sturm, A. C., Curran, J., Kline, C. F., Little, S. C., Bonilla, I. M., et al. (2015). Dysfunction in the betaII spectrin-dependent cytoskeleton underlies human arrhythmia. *Circulation* 131, 695–708. doi: 10.1161/CIRCULATIONAHA.114.013708

Stankewich, M. C., Cianci, C. D., Stabach, P. R., Ji, L., Nath, A., and Morrow, J. S. (2011). Cell organization, growth, and neural and cardiac development require alphaII-spectrin. *J. Cell Sci.* 124(Pt 23), 3956–3966. doi: 10.1242/jcs.080374

Swayne, L. A., Murphy, N. P., Asuri, S., Chen, L., Xu, X., McIntosh, S., et al. (2017). Novel variant in the ANK2 membrane-binding domain is associated with Ankyrin-B syndrome and structural heart disease in a first nations population with a high rate of long QT syndrome. *Circ. Cardiovasc. Genet.* 10:e001537. doi: 10.1161/CIRCGENETICS.116.001537

Tang, Y., Katuri, V., Dillner, A., Mishra, B., Deng, C. X., and Mishra, L. (2003). Disruption of transforming growth factor-beta signaling in ELF beta-spectrin-deficient mice. *Science* 299, 574–577. doi: 10.1126/science.1075994

Tse, W. T., and Lux, S. E. (1999). Red blood cell membrane disorders. *Br. J. Haematol.* 104, 2–13. doi: 10.1111/j.1365-2141.1999.01130.x

Wolf, R. M., Mitchell, C. C., Christensen, M. D., Mohler, P. J., and Hund, T. J. (2010). Defining new insight into atypical arrhythmia: a computational model of ankyrin-B syndrome. *Am. J. Physiol. Heart Circ. Physiol.* 299, H1505–H1514. doi: 10.1152/ajpheart.00503.2010

Wu, H. C., Yamankurt, G., Luo, J., Subramaniam, J., Hashmi, S. S., Hu, H., et al. (2015). Identification and characterization of two ankyrin-B isoforms in mammalian heart. *Cardiovasc. Res.* 107, 466–477. doi: 10.1093/cvr/cvv184

Yao, Z. X., Jogunoori, W., Choufani, S., Rashid, A., Blake, T., Yao, W., et al. (2010). Epigenetic silencing of beta-spectrin, a TGF-beta signaling/scaffolding protein in a human cancer stem cell disorder: Beckwith-Wiedemann syndrome. *J. Biol. Chem.* 285, 36112–36120. doi: 10.1074/jbc.M110.162347

10

Pro-Arrhythmic Ventricular Remodeling is Associated with Increased Respiratory and Low-Frequency Oscillations of Monophasic Action Potential Duration in the Chronic Atrioventricular Block Dog Model

David Jaap Sprenkeler*, Jet D. M. Beekman, Alexandre Bossu, Albert Dunnink and Marc A. Vos

Department of Medical Physiology, Division of Heart and Lungs, University Medical Center Utrecht, Utrecht, Netherlands

****Correspondence:***
David Jaap Sprenkeler
d.j.sprenkeler@umcutrecht.nl

In addition to beat-to-beat fluctuations, action potential duration (APD) oscillates at (1) a respiratory frequency and (2) a low frequency (LF) (<0.1 Hz), probably caused by bursts of sympathetic nervous system discharge. This study investigates whether ventricular remodeling in the chronic AV block (CAVB) dog alters these oscillations of APD and whether this has consequences for arrhythmogenesis. We performed a retrospective analysis of 39 dog experiments in sinus rhythm (SR), acute AV block (AAVB), and after 2 weeks of chronic AV block. Spectral analysis of left ventricular monophasic action potential duration (LV MAPD) was done to quantify respiratory frequency (RF) power and LF power. Dofetilide (0.025 mg/kg in 5 min) was infused to test for inducibility of Torsade de Pointes (TdP) arrhythmias. RF power was significantly increased at CAVB compared to AAVB and SR (log[RF] of −1.13 ± 1.62 at CAVB vs. log[RF] of −2.82 ± 1.24 and −3.29 ± 1.29 at SR and AAVB, respectively, $p < 0.001$). LF power was already significantly increased at AAVB and increased even further at CAVB (−3.91 ± 0.70 at SR vs. −2.52 ± 0.85 at AAVB and −1.14 ± 1.62 at CAVB, $p < 0.001$). In addition, LF power was significantly larger in inducible CAVB dogs (log[LF] −0.6 ± 1.54 in inducible dogs vs. −2.56 ± 0.43 in non-inducible dogs, $p < 0.001$). In conclusion, ventricular remodeling in the CAVB dog results in augmentation of respiratory and low-frequency (LF) oscillations of LV MAPD. Furthermore, TdP-inducible CAVB dogs show increased LF power.

Keywords: chronic AV block dog, electrical remodeling, respiration, action potential duration, low-frequency oscillations

INTRODUCTION

Repolarization lability, quantified as beat-to-beat fluctuations in action potential duration (APD), is known to contribute to arrhythmogenesis (Thomsen et al., 2004, 2007). An increased beat-to-beat repolarization variability has been found in patients with a high risk of ventricular arrhythmias, such as patients with heart failure (Berger et al., 1997; Hinterseer et al., 2010), ischemia (Murabayashi et al., 2002), long QT-syndrome (Hinterseer et al., 2008, 2009), hypertrophic cardiomyopathy (Atiga et al., 2000), or hypertension with left ventricular hypertrophy (Piccirillo et al., 2002). In these patients, adverse cardiac remodeling has led to heterogeneous downregulation of repolarizing ionic currents and a disruption of normal Ca^{2+} handling (Armoundas et al., 2001). As a result, the so called "repolarization reserve" is reduced, making the process of repolarization unstable and prone to arrhythmogenic challenges (Roden, 1998).

In addition to beat-to-beat variations in repolarization, the APD also oscillates at a broader range of frequencies. First, APD fluctuates with respiration, which appears to be independent of the respiratory effects on heart rate (Hanson et al., 2012). Second, APD oscillates at a LF of around 0.1 Hz, which has been attributed to LF bursts of sympathetic nerve terminals on the ventricular myocardium (Hanson et al., 2014). While a sympathetically mediated LF pattern of arterial blood pressure (known as Mayer waves) is well-known (Malpas, 2002), oscillations at 0.1 Hz have only recently been found in APD as well (Hanson et al., 2014; Porter et al., 2018). Moreover, these fluctuations have also been identified on the surface ECG as changes in T wave vector angle between consecutive beats, referred to as "periodic repolarization dynamics" (PRD; Rizas et al., 2014).

However, it is unknown whether APD oscillations at these frequency bands (i.e., respiratory and LF) reflect normal physiology or whether they are linked to the occurrence of ventricular arrhythmias. In this regard, a computational modeling study showed that during Ca^{2+} overload and reduction of repolarizing currents, APD oscillations could become arrhythmogenic and elicit afterdepolarizations (Pueyo et al., 2016). Furthermore, in clinical studies of post-myocardial infarction patients, PRD appears to be a strong independent predictor of all-cause mortality (Hamm et al., 2017; Rizas et al., 2017). Therefore, we could hypothesize that these oscillations are altered by ventricular remodeling, thereby further destabilizing repolarization and contributing to arrhythmogenesis.

In the present study, we evaluated both respiratory and low-frequency (LF) oscillations of APD in the chronic complete AV block dog model. In this arrhythmogenic animal model, creation of complete AV block results in cardiac remodeling and reduction of repolarization reserve. Administration of anesthesia and a pro-arrhythmic drug, i.e., the I_{Kr} blocker dofetilide, will act as the final "hit" on repolarization, resulting in electrical storm with multiple episodes of Torsades de Pointes arrhythmias (TdP) in approximately 75% of the dogs (Oros et al., 2008). This model has been widely used in our laboratory and by others to investigate the mechanisms of arrhythmogenesis in the remodeled heart (Thomsen et al., 2007; Zhou et al., 2008; Oosterhoff et al., 2010; Dunnink et al., 2012). Therefore, we could use this model to investigate whether ventricular remodeling alters respiratory and LF oscillations of APD.

The current study is a retrospective analysis of previously performed experiments in which we analyzed respiratory and LF oscillations under different conditions of remodeling, i.e., during sinus rhythm (SR), acutely after creation of AV block (AAVB) and after (at least 2 weeks) of remodeling at chronic AV block (CAVB). In addition, we compared inducible with non-inducible CAVB dogs, to evaluate the relevance of these oscillations for arrhythmogenesis.

MATERIALS AND METHODS

Animal handling was in accordance with the "Directive 2010/63/EU of the European Parliament and of the Council of 22 September 2010 on the protection of animals used for scientific purposes" and the Dutch law, laid down in the Experiments on Animals Act. All experiments were performed with approval of the Central Authority for Scientific Procedures on Animals (CCD).

We did a retrospective analysis on electrophysiological data in our database of dog experiments executed between 2014 and 2017, which were done to study the mechanisms of TdP arrhythmias or to test new anti-arrhythmic agents or interventions. In order to maintain a homogenous population, only dogs remodeled on their own idioventricular rhythm (IVR) were included, thereby excluding dogs that were chronically paced from the right ventricular apex (RVA), which has shown to influence the remodeling process. Furthermore, only baseline recordings before the administration of any anti-arrhythmic drugs were used for the analysis to exclude the effect of these interventions on the oscillatory pattern of APD. In addition, we excluded experiments that had a baseline recording shorter than 5 min or recordings that had too much ectopy or noise (approximately more than 10% of the recording).

Animal Experiments

Detailed description of the experimental set-up has been reported previously (Dunnink et al., 2010, 2012). In brief, all experiments were performed under general anesthesia with induction *via* pentobarbital sodium 25 mg/kg i.v. and maintained by isoflurane 1.5% in O_2 and N_2O, 1:2. Animals were ventilated with positive pressure ventilation at a rate of 12 breaths/min. Next, monophasic action potential catheters (Hugo Sachs Elektronik, March, Germany) were introduced *via* the femoral artery and vein into the heart to measure the left ventricular and right ventricular monophasic action potential duration (LV and RV MAPD). In the initial experiment, complete atrioventricular (AV) block was created by radiofrequency ablation of the proximal His bundle. Subsequently, the dogs remodeled for at least 2 up to 5 weeks on IVR.

In all experiments, after a baseline measurement of at least 5 min, inducibility of TdP arrhythmias was tested by infusing the I_{Kr} blocker dofetilide (0.025 mg/kg in 5 min or before the first TdP). TdP was defined as a run of five or more short-coupled (occurring before the end of the T wave) ectopic beats, with polymorphic twisting of the QRS-axis. When ≥3 TdP arrhythmias occurred in the first 10 min after the start of infusion, the dog was considered inducible. During baseline and dofetilide challenge, all subjects were paced from the RV-apex at 60 beats per minute.

Data Analysis

For this retrospective analysis, we used LV MAPD recordings at SR, AAVB, and CAVB conditions. The monophasic action potential was recorded with EP Tracer (Cardiotek, Maastricht,

The Netherlands) at a sampling frequency of 1,000 Hz. LV MAPD was measured offline semi-automatically from the initial peak to 80% of repolarization using custom-made software in MATLAB (MathWorks, Natick, USA). In addition, for analysis of LF oscillations, the absolute difference in LV MAPD between two consecutive beats was calculated. Any extrasystolic beats and the subsequent post-extrasystolic beats were removed. The 5-min time series of MAPD or MAPD difference was detrended and interpolated at 4 Hz *via* cubic spline interpolation to get evenly spaced samples. Data series were split into epochs of 512 samples with 50% overlap. Spectral analysis was performed in MATLAB with Welch's periodogram and a Hanning window to derive the power spectral density (PSD). The power of the frequency bands was calculated by integrating the area under the PSD plot for bandwidths of different frequencies. For the respiratory frequency (RF), we selected a frequency band between 0.19 and 0.21 Hz, since all dogs were ventilated at 12 breaths per minute (every 5 s, 0.2 Hz). For the LF oscillations, we used a frequency band between 0.04 and 0.15 Hz as has been used in previous studies (Hanson et al., 2014; Porter et al., 2018), since the frequency of sympathetic bursts can differ between individual subjects.

Measurement of RR-interval and QT-interval was performed in lead II of the surface ECG. QT-interval was corrected for heart rate (QT_c) with the van der Water formula (Van de Water et al., 1989). Short-term variability (STV) of LV MAPD was calculated over 31 consecutive beats using the formula: $STV = \sum |D_{n+1} - D_n| / 30 \times \sqrt{2}$, where D represents LV MAPD.

Statistical Analysis

Numerical values are expressed as mean ± standard deviation (SD). Logarithmic transformation of both RF and LF was used to correct for skewness of the data. Normality of the transformed data was checked with the Shapiro-Wilk test. Group comparison was done with an unpaired Students t-test. Group comparison of more than two groups was performed with a one-way analysis of variance (ANOVA) with Tukey's correction for multiple comparisons. p equal to or smaller than 0.05 was considered significant. GraphPad Prism 6 (GraphPad Software, Inc., La Jolla, CA, USA) was used for the statistical analysis.

RESULTS

A total of 39 experiments in 29 adult mongrel dogs (13 males, 16 females, weight 25 ± 2.5 kg) were used for the analysis. We included 10 dogs in SR, 10 dogs in AAVB, and 19 dogs in CAVB (14 inducible, 5 non-inducible). Of three dogs, data of both AAVB and CAVB experiment were used.

Baseline Electrophysiological Parameters

Baseline electrophysiological data at the three conditions (SR, AAVB, and CAVB) are depicted in **Table 1**. As expected, QT-interval increased acutely after the creation of AV block, due to the sudden drop in heart rate. In CAVB, electrical remodeling has occurred as seen by a significant increase in QT, QTc, and LV MAPD. Furthermore, STV is significantly increased, reflecting a reduced repolarization reserve. **Table 2** shows electrophysiological parameters separately for the non-inducible and inducible CAVB dogs. Only STV appears to be higher in the inducible dogs; however, this did not reach statistical significance ($p = 0.08$).

Respiratory Oscillations

Figure 1 shows an example of the respiratory fluctuations in MAPD of dogs in SR, AAVB, and CAVB in both, time domain and frequency domain. At SR and AAVB, low amplitude respiratory oscillations of LV MAPD were present, while at CAVB, larger oscillations are seen around the respiratory frequency. **Figure 2** displays the quantified logarithmic RF power (log[RF]) of the analyzed dogs. The remodeling process (**Figure 2A**) resulted in augmentation of the variability at the respiratory frequency, as seen by a significant increase in a log[RF] of −2.55 ± 1.48 and −2.99 ± 1.20 at SR and AAVB, respectively, to a log[RF] of −0.82 ± 1.53 ($p < 0.001$) at CAVB. When comparing inducible with non-inducible dogs, no significant difference could be found in RF power (**Figure 2B**).

Low-Frequency Oscillations

Next, we examined LF oscillations in MAPD difference in SR, AAVB, and CAVB. As depicted in **Figure 3A**, already a significant rise in LF power can be seen at AAVB compared to SR, which further increased after 2 weeks of remodeling (log[LF] of −3.91 ± 0.70 at SR, vs. −2.52 ± 0.85 at AAVB, and −1.14 ± 1.62 at CAVB, $p < 0.001$). Finally, we looked for differences of these oscillations between inducible and non-inducible CAVB dogs. A representative example of the MAPD during the 5-min recording of an inducible and a non-inducible dog is shown in **Figure 4A**. A clear oscillation can be observed in the

TABLE 1 | Baseline electrophysiological parameters.

	SR (n = 10)	AAVB (n = 10)	CAVB (n = 19)
RR (ms)	557 ± 32	1,000*	1,000
QT (ms)	267 ± 15	357 ± 19*	407 ± 56§
QTc (ms)	305 ± 15	357 ± 19	407 ± 56§
LV $MAPD_{80}$ (ms)	200 ± 11	243 ± 14*	275 ± 36§
STV LV $MAPD_{80}$ (ms)	0.31 ± 0.06	0.54 ± 0.30	1.20 ± 0.80§

*$p < 0.05$ vs. SR.
§$p < 0.05$ vs. AAVB.

TABLE 2 | Baseline electrophysiological parameters of inducible and non-inducible dogs.

	Inducible (n = 14)	Non-inducible (n = 5)
RR (ms)	1,000	1,000
QT (ms)	414 ± 60	388 ± 43
QTc (ms)	414 ± 60	388 ± 43
LV $MAPD_{80}$ (ms)	283 ± 34	260 ± 34
STV LV $MAPD_{80}$ (ms)	1.39 ± 0.83	0.64 ± 0.40

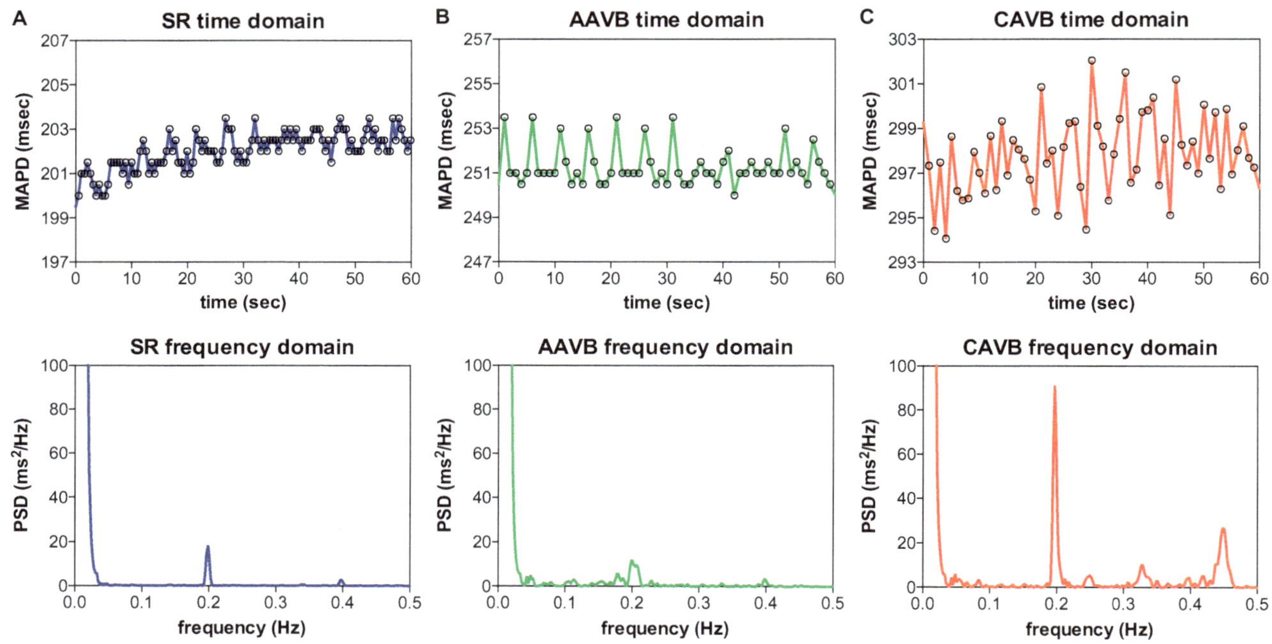

FIGURE 1 | Respiratory frequency oscillations in time and frequency domain. Representative examples of oscillations in monophasic action potential duration (MAPD) in the time domain (top) and frequency domain (bottom) during **(A)** sinus rhythm (SR), **(B)** acutely after creation of AV block (AAVB), and **(C)** after remodeling at chronic AV block (CAVB). A clear increase in a 0.2 Hz oscillation is seen at CAVB.

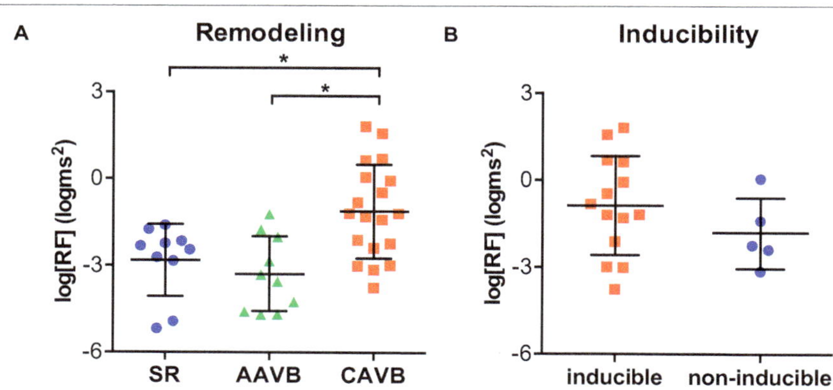

FIGURE 2 | Respiratory oscillations of monophasic action potential duration. **(A)** The logarithmic transformed power of respiratory oscillations of APD (log[RF]) at sinus rhythm (SR), acutely after AV block (AAVB), and at chronic AV block (CAVB). **(B)** log[RF] of the inducible vs. the non-inducible CAVB dogs. *$p < 0.05$.

inducible subject, with a rhythmic fluctuation in MAPD. This oscillatory behavior of MAPD can more clearly be discerned when the difference between consecutive beats is plotted against time (**Figure 4B**): approximately every 10–15 s, a clear increase in the variability between successive beats is seen. When this MAPD variability is visualized in the frequency domain by spectral analysis (**Figure 4C**), a prominent peak appears in the LF band (0.04–0.15 Hz). As depicted in **Figure 3B**, the inducible dogs demonstrated a significant higher LF power of MAPD difference when compared to non-inducible dogs (log[LF] −0.6 ± 1.54 vs. −2.56 ± 0.43, $p < 0.001$).

DISCUSSION

In this retrospective analysis of previously performed animal experiments, we demonstrated that (1) respiratory frequency oscillations of MAPD are increased after electrical remodeling, but they do not differ between inducible and non-inducible dogs and (2) LF oscillations of MAPD difference are already increased at AAVB and rise even further at CAVB. Furthermore, these 0.1 Hz oscillations are more pronounced in CAVB dogs that are susceptible to dofetilide-induced TdP arrhythmias.

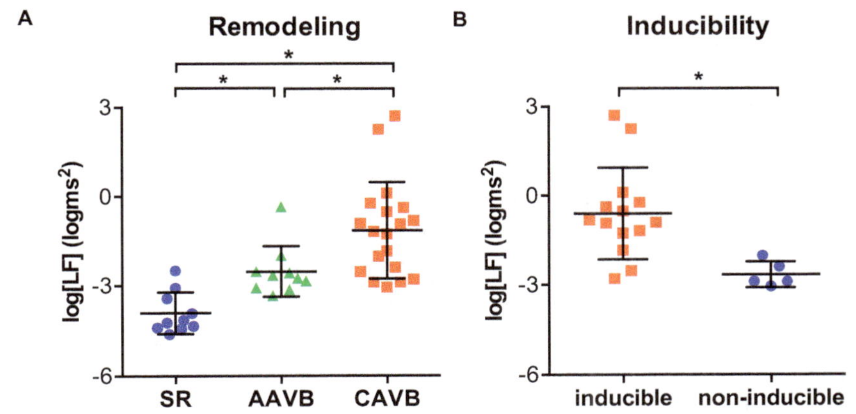

FIGURE 3 | Low-frequency (LF) oscillations of monophasic action potential duration. **(A)** The logarithmic transformed power of LF oscillations of APD (log[LF]) at sinus rhythm (SR), acutely after AV block (AAVB), and at chronic AV block (CAVB). **(B)** log[LF] of the inducible vs. the non-inducible CAVB dogs. $^*p < 0.05$.

The Chronic Atrioventricular Block Dog Model to Study the Effects of Electrical Remodeling on Arrhythmogenesis

A variety of structural heart diseases (e.g., myocardial infarction, pressure overload due to hypertension or aortic stenosis, volume overload as seen in valvular regurgitation) can lead to pathological cardiac remodeling, causing downregulation of potassium currents (I_{to}, I_{Ks}, I_{Kr}, and I_{K1}) (Long et al., 2015), enhanced late Na^+-current ($I_{Na\text{-}L}$) (Antzelevitch et al., 2014), and Ca^{2+} handling abnormalities (Sipido et al., 2002). As a result, repolarization reserve is reduced, making the heart prone to repolarization-dependent ventricular arrhythmias. The CAVB dog model, as used in this study, is a model of ventricular remodeling and reduced repolarization reserve that reflects the vulnerable patient at risk for these arrhythmias. In this model, it has been shown that beat-to-beat variability of APD, quantified as STV, is a better marker of reduced repolarization reserve and pro-arrhythmia than APD prolongation itself (Thomsen et al., 2004). STV is significantly increased at CAVB compared to AAVB and dogs susceptible to dofetilide-induced TdP arrhythmias show a further rise in STV prior to occurrence of arrhythmias (Thomsen et al., 2007).

In the current study, we have shown that not only successive beat-to-beat fluctuations of APD exists in the CAVB dog, but also that the APD oscillates at other frequency bands. This is in line with previous studies that have demonstrated important contributions of variation in heart rate (Hnatkova et al., 2013), respiration (Hanson et al., 2012), and autonomic nervous system activity (Baumert et al., 2011) on APD variability. Concerning heart rate, a complex and dynamic APD to heart rate relation exists that is highly individual-specific and contains significant hysteresis effects (Malik et al., 2008). In this study, we have eliminated important heart rate effects on APD by including only dogs that were paced during the experiments. Therefore, we could focus solely on the respiratory and autonomic influences on APD.

Respiratory Oscillations of Action Potential Duration in the Chronic Atrioventricular Block Dog

While heart rate is well-known to fluctuate with respiration, it was recently shown by Hanson et al. that APD, measured as activation recovery interval (ARI) from the intracardiac electrogram, also displays rhythmic fluctuations in synchrony with respiration, even when heart rate was controlled by pacing. The authors suggested multiple mechanisms for the respiratory oscillations of APD. One of these, mechano-electrical feedback, relates to the modulation of electrophysiology by changes in ventricular loading conditions. Both in animal models as in patient studies, a direct effect of altered mechanical load on APD have been found; increased ventricular load resulted in shortening of the APD, while reduction in load was associated with prolongation of the APD (Levine et al., 1988; Zabel et al., 1996). Stretch-activated ion-channels or alterations in Ca^{2+} handling have been suggested as the underlying molecular mechanism of load-dependent APD changes (Eckardt et al., 2001). Stretch-activated ion channels are non-specific cation (Na^+, K^+, and Ca^{2+}) channels that open in respond to changes in stretch instead of voltage (Zeng et al., 2000). In addition, mechanical stretch increases Ca^{2+} release from the sarcoplasmic reticulum, which can alter action potential duration *via* negative feedback on the L-type Ca^{2+}-channel or by exchange of Ca^{2+} for Na^+ *via* the Na^{2+}-Ca^{2+}-exchanger (Iribe et al., 2009). One important physiological mechanism that can alter ventricular loading conditions is the change in intrathoracic pressure difference during respiration. During spontaneous inspiration, intrathoracic pressure drops, causing an increased systemic venous return to the RV, which will shift the interventricular septum into the LV. As a result, left ventricular end-diastolic volume and left ventricular preload will decrease. The opposite will occur during positive pressure ventilation: in that situation, an increase in left ventricular preload will be seen during inspiration (Mitchell et al., 2005). Nevertheless, in either case,

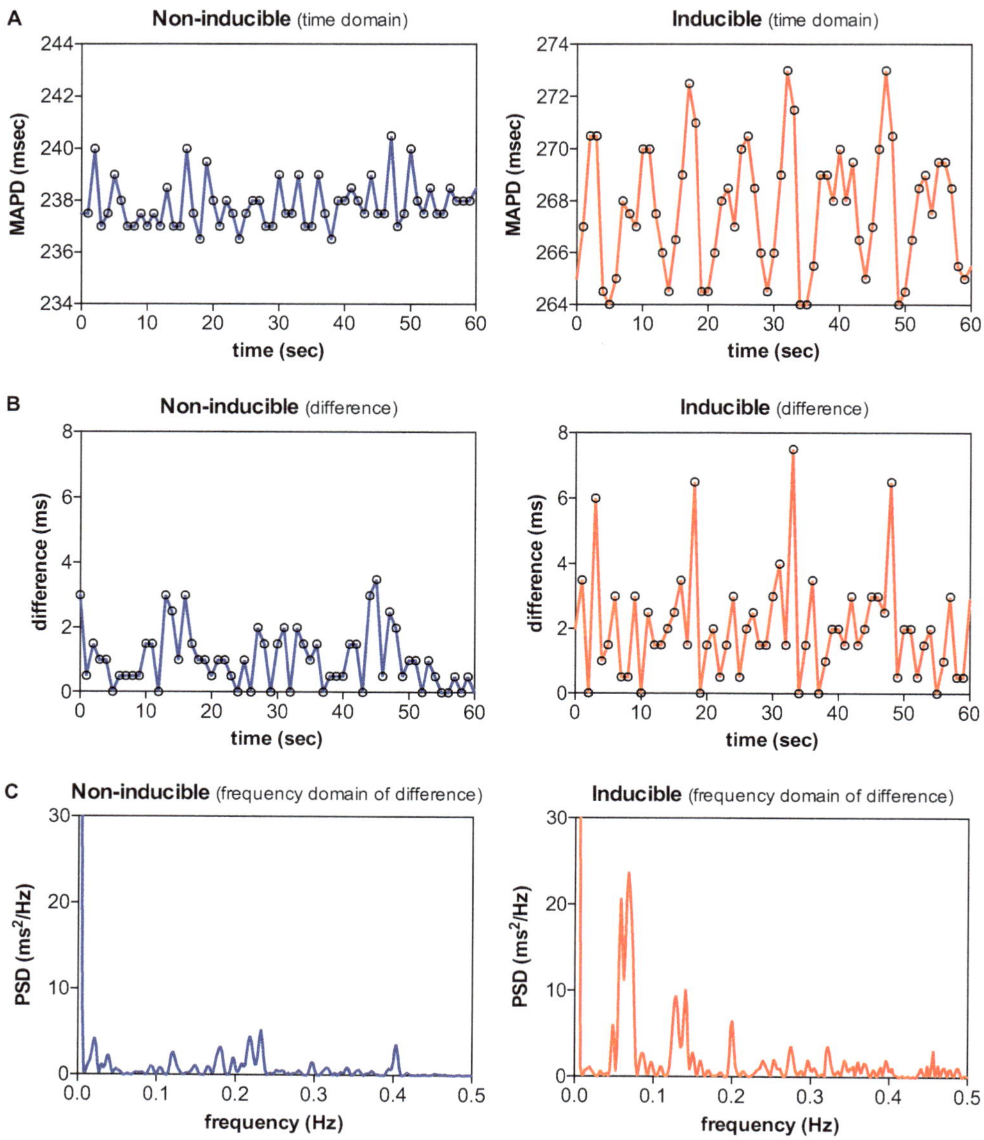

FIGURE 4 | Low-frequency (LF) oscillations in a non-inducible dog vs. an inducible dog. A representative example of MAPD **(A)**, MAPD difference in the time domain **(B)**, and MAPD difference in the frequency domain **(C)** of a non-inducible dog (left) and an inducible dog (right). A clear LF pattern in MAPD difference can be discerned in the inducible dog.

a respiratory oscillatory behavior of ventricular loading is present, which could therefore alter APD in a cyclical pattern.

In the present study, we showed that the modulating effect of respiration on APD is enhanced after cardiac remodeling. A possible explanation could be that alternating changes in ventricular loading have greater impact on repolarization, when repolarization reserve is already reduced. This is consistent with a study by Stams et al. in which the effect of preload changes on beat-to-beat variability of APD was studied in the CAVB dog (Stams et al., 2016). The authors used a pacing protocol with either a constant or alternating PQ interval to artificially control preload conditions. They observed that in AAVB, alternating preload had no effect on APD or STV. In contrast, in CAVB dogs pacing with an alternating PQ interval resulted in APD variability and a significantly higher STV compared to conditions of constant preload. Furthermore, blockade of stretch-activated ion current (I_{SAC}) by streptomycine prevented the increase of $STV_{LV\ MAPD}$ during alternating preload. Although streptomycine is not a selective (I_{SAC})-blocker and has affinity for other ion channels that could affect STV (like L-type Ca^{2+} channels), these results suggest that mechano-electrical feedback *via* specialized stretch-activated ion channels could have profound influence on repolarization during reduced repolarization reserve. This is further supported by a study of Kamkin et al., which showed that isolated cardiomyocytes from hypertrophied ventricles were more sensitive to stretch than control cardiomyocytes, resulting in prolongation of APD at smaller mechanical stimuli (Kamkin et al., 2000). Thus, we may hypothesize that after remodeling and downregulation of repolarizing K^+-currents, the relative contribution of I_{SAC} to the repolarization process is increased; therefore, we observed an augmentation of APD variability caused by changes in respiration-mediated loading conditions.

Interestingly, we did not find a difference in respiratory oscillations between inducible and non-inducible CAVB dogs. In both groups, electrical remodeling reduced repolarization reserve, as we observed by enhanced respiratory fluctuation of APD. A similar finding was reported by the study of Stams et al.: alternating preload, which led to an increase in APD variability, did not result in more TdP arrhythmias compared to conditions of constant preload. Thus, we could assume that an additional trigger is required to create the optimal environment for dofetilide-induced TdP arrhythmias.

Low-Frequency Oscillations of Action Potential Duration Difference in the Chronic Atrioventricular Block Dog

LF oscillations in the range from 0.04 to 0.15 Hz that are unrelated to respiration have long been observed in both heart rate and arterial blood pressure, and are referred to as Mayer waves (Julien, 2006). These oscillations have been linked to rhythmic bursts of sympathetic nervous system activity; however, the precise mechanism remains controversial. Two theories exist: (1) these oscillations are the effect of a central autonomous oscillator within the central nervous system that fires at a certain frequency and (2) they are the result of a time delay in the baroreflex loop, causing resonance in the feedback system (Malpas, 2002). Either way, states of increased sympathetic activation, such as during tilt test or when blood pressure was artificially lowered, resulted in an increase in the magnitude of Mayer waves (Pagani et al., 1997; Furlan et al., 2000). In addition, blockade of sympathetic drive resulted in a reduction of LF components of both RR interval and blood pressure (Pagani et al., 1997).

In addition to respiratory fluctuations, Hanson et al. also showed that APD displays an oscillatory pattern at Mayer wave frequency (Hanson et al., 2014). Moreover, these LF oscillations increased during autonomic challenge with Valsalva maneuver (Porter et al., 2018). A similar LF oscillatory pattern was found by Rizas et al. in T wave vector changes on the surface-ECG, called periodic repolarization dynamics (PRD; Rizas et al., 2014). These variations in T wave vector could also be increased with exercise and reduced by β-adrenergic blockade, suggesting a role for sympathetic input on the myocardium in the pathogenesis of these oscillations. Furthermore, increased PRD appeared to be a strong predictor of all-cause mortality in a cohort of more than 900 post-MI patients. Combined with a marker of vagal activity (i.e. deceleration capacity), PRD was able to accurately stratify mortality risk in these patients (Hamm et al., 2017). Nevertheless, the cause of death, whether arrhythmic or due to pump failure, was not further specified.

In this regard, the findings of the current study could be of great interest. In this study, we evaluated the effect of ventricular remodeling on LF oscillations, but, more importantly, whether these oscillations were different in dogs susceptible to arrhythmias. For this analysis, the MAPD difference between two consecutive beats was used, instead of MAPD itself. The reason for this is that in the previous study by Rizas et al., PRD was also measured on differences in T wave vector between beats. They observed that approximately every 10 s, the T wave vector changed markedly, while in the intermittent periods T wave vector remained relatively stable. We hypothesized that 0.1 Hz bursts of sympathetic discharge could also result in sudden changes in MAPD, which are more clearly visualized when spectral analysis is done of MAPD difference instead of MAPD.

Consequently, we could show that acutely after creation of AV block, LF power of APD difference is already significantly increased. The sudden drop in cardiac output and blood pressure that occur after creation of AV block will be sensed by baroreceptors in the aortic arch and carotid sinus, which will increase efferent sympathetic input on the heart, while simultaneously reducing parasympathetic firing. We observed this baroreflex-mediated increase in sympathetic tone by augmentation of LF APD oscillations acutely after AV block. More importantly, cardiac remodeling further increased the LF oscillatory behavior of APD difference, predominantly in CAVB dogs susceptible to drug-induced TdP arrhythmias. From the existing literature, it becomes clear that increased sympathetic nervous system activity is an important contributor to repolarization variability and arrhythmogenesis. A study by Johnson et al. in isolated cardiomyocytes showed that the addition of β-adrenergic stimulation to a state of reduced repolarization reserve (by blockade of I_{Ks}) led to a dramatically increase in beat-to-beat variability of repolarization (BVR; Johnson et al., 2010). In addition, sympathetic stimulation promoted Ca^{2+} overload, spontaneous Ca^{2+}-release and the formation of early and delayed afterdepolarizations (EADs/DADs; Johnson et al., 2013). Gallagher et al. found similar results in an *in vivo* canine model of drug-induced LQTS-1. Infusion of HMR1556, an I_{Ks} blocker, in combination with isoproterenol resulted in paradoxically increased APD, increased spatial and temporal dispersion of repolarization and reproducible TdP arrhythmias (Gallacher et al., 2007). The same was found in a study of Ter Bekke et al., who used direct left stellate ganglion stimulation instead of pharmacological adrenergic stimulation, combined with Iks blockade (Ter Bekke et al., 2019). A simulation study by Pueyo et al. evaluated the effect of phasic β-adrenergic stimulation on APD dynamics (Pueyo et al., 2016). They observed a LF oscillatory pattern of APD, whose magnitude increased with higher β-adrenergic strength. Interestingly, simulated pathological conditions of Ca^{2+}-overload and reduced repolarization reserve (comparable to the CAVB dog model) enhanced the APD oscillations caused by adrenergic stimulation. Therefore, the authors suggested an important role of these oscillations in arrhythmogenesis. In the present study, we could confirm these *in silico* results experimentally in an arrhythmogenic *in vivo* model.

The reason for the clear difference in LF oscillations of APD difference between inducible and non-inducible dogs remains speculative. Two mechanisms can be proposed: either repolarization reserve is even more reduced in the inducible dogs, therefore making the effect of β-adrenergic stimulation on repolarization more prominent and repolarization more vulnerable to arrhythmogenic challenges, or sympathetic output itself (either systematically or due to increased local density of sympathetic neurons) is further enhanced in the inducible dogs, causing increased repolarization instability, Ca^{2+} overload, and triggered activity. Concerning the latter, studies in dogs with chronic AV block and MI have shown that in addition to electrical remodeling, also neural remodeling takes place, as seen by denervation, hyperinnervation, and nerve sprouting (Cao et al., 2000a,b). Regional hyperinnervation, where some regions are more densely innervated than others, combined with heterogeneous electrical remodeling, further enhances spatial dispersion of repolarization; thereby, facilitating the initiation and perpetuation of ventricular arrhythmias.

Implications

In addition to beat-to-beat variation in APD or QT-interval, we have shown that fluctuations in other frequency bands are altered in subjects with pro-arrhythmic ventricular remodeling and an increased risk of ventricular arrhythmias. Therefore, these oscillations might eventually be used in risk stratification of patients at high risk of sudden cardiac death, who might benefit from implantation of an implantable cardioverter-defibrillator (ICD). While in the current study, MAP-catheters were used, Hanson et al. showed that respiratory and LF oscillations are also measurable on the ARI of intracardiac EGM, which could be obtained from implantable devices. Furthermore, PRD is a non-invasive parameter that can be measured from a converted 12-lead surface ECG, which would make it more suitable for risk stratification prior to ICD implantation. In this regard, PRD is currently being studied as a predictive marker in the multicentre, observational EU-CERT-ICD study (NCT02064192), which evaluates new risk stratification methods that could identify subgroups of patients with low or high risk of ICD-shocks or mortality.

Study Limitations

Since the CAVB dog is a specific model of ventricular remodeling caused by volume overload, extrapolation of these results to patients with other causes of remodeling (ischemia, infarction, and pressure overload) should be done with caution. Second, an important limitation of the study is its retrospective nature, which made it impossible to control for all, possible confounding, variables. By selecting only dogs remodeled on IVR without control of activation pattern, we tried to keep the analyzed group of dogs as homogeneous as possible. Third, all dogs were mechanically ventilated with positive pressures, which has an opposite effect on loading conditions of the heart compared to spontaneous breathing. Nevertheless, both ventilation techniques result in an oscillatory pattern, albeit with a shift in phase. Next, all experiments were done under general anesthesia, which has profound effects on the autonomic nervous system. In addition, no direct measurements of neural activity were done to confirm that the LF oscillations of APD we found were also caused by sympathetic discharge. Yet, preliminary data of our group shows that stellectomy results in significant reduction in TdP inducibility in the CAVB dog, which implies that, even under anesthetic conditions, the sympathetic nervous system contributes for a great part to arrhythmogenesis in this model [abstract presented at AHA 2017 (van Weperen et al., 2017, unpublished data)]. Finally, it would have been of great interest to measure PRD in the CAVB dog, so we could evaluate if the intracardiac MAP oscillations correlate with PRD on the surface ECG. Unfortunately, PRD measurement requires transformation of the ECG to Frank leads with either Kors or inverse Dower's matrix, which are not validated for the canine ECG. Furthermore, because of the complete AV-block, the T waves are often distorted by the interference of P waves, which impedes accurate measurement of beat-to-beat T wave changes.

CONCLUSION

In the chronic AV block dog model, we observed oscillations of LV MAPD at respiratory frequency, which are augmented after remodeling compared to non-remodeled conditions. In addition, LF oscillations of MAPD difference were already altered acutely after creation of AV block and increased even further at chronic AV block conditions. Furthermore, CAVB dogs, that are susceptible to drug-induced TdP, show increased LF oscillations compared to their non-inducible counterparts.

AUTHOR CONTRIBUTIONS

DS contributed in writing, data collection, and analysis. JB contributed in technical support. AB and AD conducted animal experiments. MV helped in supervision and review of manuscript.

REFERENCES

Antzelevitch, C., Nesterenko, V., Shryock, J. C., Rajamani, S., Song, Y., and Belardinelli, L. (2014). The role of late I Na in development of cardiac arrhythmias. *Handb. Exp. Pharmacol.* 221, 137–168. doi: 10.1007/978-3-642-41588-3_7

Armoundas, A. A., Wu, R., Juang, G., Marbán, E., and Tomaselli, G. F. (2001). Electrical and structural remodeling of the failing ventricle. *Pharmacol. Ther.* 92, 213–230. doi: 10.1016/S0163-7258(01)00171-1

Atiga, W. L., Fananapazir, L., McAreavey, D., Calkins, H., and Berger, R. D. (2000). Temporal repolarization lability in hypertrophic cardiomyopathy caused by beta-myosin heavy-chain gene mutations. *Circulation* 101, 1237–1242. doi: 10.1161/01.CIR.101.11.1237

Baumert, M., Schlaich, M. P., Nalivaiko, E., Lambert, E., Sari, C. I., Kaye, D. M., et al. (2011). Relation between QT interval variability and cardiac sympathetic activity in hypertension. *Am. J. Physiol. Circ. Physiol.* 300, H1412–H1417. doi: 10.1152/ajpheart.01184.2010

Berger, R. D., Kasper, E. K., Baughman, K. L., Marban, E., Calkins, H., and Tomaselli, G. F. (1997). Beat-to-beat QT interval variability: novel evidence for repolarization lability in ischemic and nonischemic dilated cardiomyopathy. *Circulation* 96, 1557–1565. doi: 10.1161/01.CIR.96.5.1557

Cao, J. M., Chen, L. S., Ken Knight, B. H., Ohara, T., Lee, M. H., Tsai, J., et al. (2000a). Nerve sprouting and sudden cardiac death. *Circ. Res.* 86, 816–821. doi: 10.1161/01.res.86.7.816

Cao, J. M., Fishbein, M. C., Han, J. B., Lai, W. W., Lai, A. C., Wu, T. J., et al. (2000b). Relationship between regional cardiac hyperinnervation and ventricular arrhythmia. *Circulation* 101, 1960–1969. doi: 10.1161/01.cir.101.16.1960

Dunnink, A., Sharif, S., Oosterhoff, P., Winckels, S., Montagne, D., Beekman, J., et al. (2010). Anesthesia and arrhythmogenesis in the chronic atrioventricular block dog model. *J. Cardiovasc. Pharmacol.* 55, 601–608. doi: 10.1097/FJC.0b013e3181da7768

Dunnink, A., van Opstal, J. M., Oosterhoff, P., Winckels, S. K. G., Beekman, J. D. M., van der Nagel, R., et al. (2012). Ventricular remodelling is a prerequisite for the induction of dofetilide-induced torsade de pointes arrhythmias in the anaesthetized, complete atrio-ventricular-block dog. *Europace* 14, 431–436. doi: 10.1093/europace/eur311

Eckardt, L., Kirchhof, P., Breithardt, G., and Haverkamp, W. (2001). Load-induced changes in repolarization: evidence from experimental and clinical data. *Basic Res. Cardiol.* 96, 369–380. doi: 10.1007/s003950170045

Furlan, R., Porta, A., Costa, F., Tank, J., Baker, L., Schiavi, R., et al. (2000). Oscillatory patterns in sympathetic neural discharge and cardiovascular variables during orthostatic stimulus. *Circulation* 101, 886–892. doi: 10.1161/01.CIR.101.8.886

Gallacher, D. J., Van de Water, A., van der Linde, H., Hermans, A. N., Lu, H. R., Towart, R., et al. (2007). In vivo mechanisms precipitating torsades de pointes in a canine model of drug-induced long-QT1 syndrome. *Cardiovasc. Res.* 76, 247–256. doi: 10.1016/j.cardiores.2007.06.019

Hamm, W., Stülpnagel, L., Vdovin, N., Schmidt, G., Rizas, K. D., and Bauer, A. (2017). Risk prediction in post-infarction patients with moderately reduced left ventricular ejection fraction by combined assessment of the sympathetic and vagal cardiac autonomic nervous system. *Int. J. Cardiol.* 249, 1–5. doi: 10.1016/j.ijcard.2017.06.091

Hanson, B., Gill, J., Western, D., Gilbey, M. P., Bostock, J., Boyett, M. R., et al. (2012). Cyclical modulation of human ventricular repolarization by respiration. *Front. Physiol.* 3:379. doi: 10.3389/fphys.2012.00379

Hanson, B., Child, N., Van Duijvenboden, S., Orini, M., Chen, Z., Coronel, R., et al. (2014). Oscillatory behavior of ventricular action potential duration in heart failure patients at respiratory rate and low frequency. *Front. Physiol.* 5:414. doi: 10.3389/fphys.2014.00414

Hinterseer, M., Thomsen, M. B., Beckmann, B.-M., Pfeufer, A., Schimpf, R., Wichmann, H.-E., et al. (2008). Beat-to-beat variability of QT intervals is increased in patients with drug-induced long-QT syndrome: a case control pilot study. *Eur. Heart J.* 29, 185–190. doi: 10.1093/eurheartj/ehm586

Hinterseer, M., Beckmann, B.-M., Thomsen, M. B., Pfeufer, A., Dalla Pozza, R., Loeff, M., et al. (2009). Relation of increased short-term variability of QT interval to congenital long-QT syndrome. *Am. J. Cardiol.* 103, 1244–1248. doi: 10.1016/j.amjcard.2009.01.011

Hinterseer, M., Beckmann, B.-M., Thomsen, M. B., Pfeufer, A., Ulbrich, M., Sinner, M. F., et al. (2010). Usefulness of short-term variability of QT intervals as a predictor for electrical remodeling and proarrhythmia in patients with nonischemic heart failure. *Am. J. Cardiol.* 106, 216–220. doi: 10.1016/j.amjcard.2010.02.033

Hnatkova, K., Kowalski, D., Keirns, J. J., van Gelderen, E. M., and Malik, M. (2013). Relationship of QT interval variability to heart rate and RR interval variability. *J. Electrocardiol.* 46, 591–596. doi: 10.1016/j.jelectrocard.2013.07.007

Iribe, G., Ward, C. W., Camelliti, P., Bollensdorff, C., Mason, F., Burton, R. A. B., et al. (2009). Axial stretch of rat single ventricular cardiomyocytes causes an acute and transient increase in Ca^{2+} spark rate. *Circ. Res.* 104, 787–795. doi: 10.1161/CIRCRESAHA.108.193334

Johnson, D. M., Heijman, J., Pollard, C. E., Valentin, J.-P., Crijns, H. J. G. M., Abi-Gerges, N., et al. (2010). IKs restricts excessive beat-to-beat variability of repolarization during beta-adrenergic receptor stimulation. *J. Mol. Cell. Cardiol.* 48, 122–130. doi: 10.1016/j.yjmcc.2009.08.033

Johnson, D. M., Heijman, J., Bode, E. F., Greensmith, D. J., van der Linde, H., Abi-Gerges, N., et al. (2013). Diastolic spontaneous calcium release from the sarcoplasmic reticulum increases beat-to-beat variability of repolarization in canine ventricular myocytes after β-adrenergic stimulation. *Circ. Res.* 112, 246–256. doi: 10.1161/CIRCRESAHA.112.275735

Julien, C. (2006). The enigma of Mayer waves: facts and models. *Cardiovasc. Res.* 70, 12–21. doi: 10.1016/j.cardiores.2005.11.008

Kamkin, A., Kiseleva, I., and Isenberg, G. (2000). Stretch-activated currents in ventricular myocytes: amplitude and arrhythmogenic effects increase with hypertrophy. *Cardiovasc. Res.* 48, 409–420. doi: 10.1016/S0008-6363(00)00208-X

Levine, J. H., Guarnieri, T., Kadish, A. H., White, R. I., Calkins, H., and Kan, J. S. (1988). Changes in myocardial repolarization in patients undergoing balloon valvuloplasty for congenital pulmonary stenosis: evidence for contraction-excitation feedback in humans. *Circulation* 77, 70–77. doi: 10.1161/01.CIR.77.1.70

Long, V. P., Bonilla, I. M., Vargas-Pinto, P., Nishijima, Y., Sridhar, A., Li, C., et al. (2015). Heart failure duration progressively modulates the arrhythmia substrate through structural and electrical remodeling. *Life Sci.* 123, 61–71. doi: 10.1016/j.lfs.2014.12.024

Malik, M., Hnatkova, K., Novotny, T., and Schmidt, G. (2008). Subject-specific profiles of QT/RR hysteresis. *Am. J. Physiol. Circ. Physiol.* 295, H2356–H2363. doi: 10.1152/ajpheart.00625.2008

Malpas, S. C. (2002). Neural influences on cardiovascular variability: possibilities and pitfalls. *Am. J. Physiol. Heart Circ. Physiol.* 282, H6–H20. doi: 10.1152/ajpheart.2002.282.1.H6

Mitchell, J. R., Whitelaw, W. A., Sas, R., Smith, E. R., Tyberg, J. V., and Belenkie, I. (2005). RV filling modulates LV function by direct ventricular interaction during mechanical ventilation. *Am. J. Physiol. Circ. Physiol.* 289, H549–H557. doi: 10.1152/ajpheart.01180.2004

Murabayashi, T., Fetics, B., Kass, D., Nevo, E., Gramatikov, B., and Berger, R. D. (2002). Beat-to-beat QT interval variability associated with acute myocardial ischemia. *J. Electrocardiol.* 35, 19–25. Available at: http://www.ncbi.nlm.nih.gov/pubmed/11786943 (Accessed December 29, 2017)

Oosterhoff, P., Thomsen, M. B., Maas, J. N., Atteveld, N. J. M., Beekman, J. D. M., VAN Rijen, H. V. M., et al. (2010). High-rate pacing reduces variability of repolarization and prevents repolarization-dependent arrhythmias in dogs with chronic AV block. *J. Cardiovasc. Electrophysiol.* 21, 1384–1391. doi: 10.1111/j.1540-8167.2010.01824.x

Oros, A., Beekman, J. D. M., and Vos, M. A. (2008). The canine model with chronic, complete atrio-ventricular block. *Pharmacol. Ther.* 119, 168–178. doi: 10.1016/j.pharmthera.2008.03.006

Pagani, M., Montano, N., Porta, A., Malliani, A., Abboud, F. M., Birkett, C., et al. (1997). Relationship between spectral components of cardiovascular variabilities and direct measures of muscle sympathetic nerve activity in humans. *Circulation* 95, 1441–1448. doi: 10.1161/01.CIR.95.6.1441

Piccirillo, G., Germanò, G., Quaglione, R., Nocco, M., Lintas, F., Lionetti, M., et al. (2002). QT-interval variability and autonomic control in hypertensive subjects with left ventricular hypertrophy. *Clin. Sci.* 102, 363–371. doi: 10.1042/cs1020363

Porter, B., van Duijvenboden, S., Bishop, M. J., Orini, M., Claridge, S., Gould, J., et al. (2018). Beat-to-beat variability of ventricular action potential duration oscillates at low frequency during sympathetic provocation in humans. *Front. Physiol.* 9:47. doi: 10.3389/fphys.2018.00147

Pueyo, E., Orini, M., Rodríguez, J. F., and Taggart, P. (2016). Interactive effect of beta-adrenergic stimulation and mechanical stretch on low-frequency oscillations of ventricular action potential duration in humans. *J. Mol. Cell. Cardiol.* 97, 93–105. doi: 10.1016/j.yjmcc.2016.05.003

Rizas, K. D., Nieminen, T., Barthel, P., Zürn, C. S., Kähönen, M., Viik, J., et al. (2014). Sympathetic activity-associated periodic repolarization dynamics predict mortality following myocardial infarction. *J. Clin. Invest.* 124, 1770–1780. doi: 10.1172/JCI70085

Rizas, K. D., McNitt, S., Hamm, W., Massberg, S., Kääb, S., Zareba, W., et al. (2017). Prediction of sudden and non-sudden cardiac death in post-infarction patients with reduced left ventricular ejection fraction by periodic repolarization dynamics: MADIT-II substudy. *Eur. Heart J.* 38, 2110–2118. doi: 10.1093/eurheartj/ehx161

Roden, D. M. (1998). Taking the "idio" out of "idiosyncratic": predicting torsades de pointes. *Pacing Clin. Electrophysiol.* 21, 1029–1034. doi: 10.1111/j.1540-8159.1998.tb00148.x

Sipido, K. R., Volders, P. G. A., Schoenmakers, M., De Groot, S. H. M., Verdonck, F., and Vos, M. A. (2002). Role of the Na/Ca exchanger in arrhythmias in compensated hypertrophy. *Ann. N. Y. Acad. Sci.* 976, 438–445. doi: 10.1111/j.1749-6632.2002.tb04773.x

Stams, T. R., Oosterhoff, P., Heijdel, A., Dunnink, A., Beekman, J. D., van der Nagel, R., et al. (2016). Beat-to-beat variability in preload unmasks latent risk of torsade de pointes in anesthetized chronic atrioventricular block dogs. *Circ. J.* 80, 1336–1345. doi: 10.1253/circj.CJ-15-1335

Ter Bekke, R. M. A., Moers, A. M. E., de Jong, M. M. J., Johnson, D. M., Schwartz, P. J., Vanoli, E., et al. (2019). Proarrhythmic proclivity of left-stellate ganglion stimulation in a canine model of drug-induced long-QT syndrome type 1. *Int. J. Cardiol.* 286, 66–72. doi: 10.1016/j.ijcard.2019.01.098

Thomsen, M., Oros, A., Schoenmakers, M., van Opstal, J., Maas, J., Beekman, J., et al. (2007). Proarrhythmic electrical remodelling is associated with increased beat-to-beat variability of repolarisation. *Cardiovasc. Res.* 73, 521–530. doi: 10.1016/j.cardiores.2006.11.025

Thomsen, M. B., Verduyn, S. C., Stengl, M., Beekman, J. D. M., de Pater, G., van Opstal, J., et al. (2004). Increased short-term variability of repolarization predicts d-sotalol-induced torsades de pointes in dogs. *Circulation* 110, 2453–2459. doi: 10.1161/01.CIR.0000145162.64183.C8

Van de Water, A., Verheyen, J., Xhonneux, R., and Reneman, R. S. (1989). An improved method to correct the QT interval of the electrocardiogram for changes in heart rate. *J. Pharmacol. Methods* 22, 207–217. Available at: http://www.ncbi.nlm.nih.gov/pubmed/2586115 (Accessed August 30, 2016)

Zabel, M., Portnoy, S., and Franz, M. R. (1996). Effect of sustained load on dispersion of ventricular repolarization and conduction time in the isolated intact rabbit heart. *J. Cardiovasc. Electrophysiol.* 7, 9–16. doi: 10.1111/j.1540-8167.1996.tb00455.x

Zeng, T., Bett, G. C. L., and Sachs, F. (2000). Stretch-activated whole cell currents in adult rat cardiac myocytes. *Am. J. Physiol. Circ. Physiol.* 278, H548–H557. doi: 10.1152/ajpheart.2000.278.2.H548

Zhou, S., Jung, B.-C., Tan, A. Y., Trang, V. Q., Gholmieh, G., Han, S.-W., et al. (2008). Spontaneous stellate ganglion nerve activity and ventricular arrhythmia in a canine model of sudden death. *Heart Rhythm.* 5, 131–139. doi: 10.1016/j.hrthm.2007.09.007

11

Kir2.1-Nav1.5 Channel Complexes are Differently Regulated than Kir2.1 and Nav1.5 Channels Alone

Raquel G. Utrilla[1,2†], Paloma Nieto-Marín[1,2†], Silvia Alfayate[1,2], David Tinaquero[1,2], Marcos Matamoros[1,2], Marta Pérez-Hernández[1,2], Sandra Sacristán[2], Lorena Ondo[1,2], Raquel de Andrés[3], F. Javier Díez-Guerra[3], Juan Tamargo[1,2], Eva Delpón[1,2‡] and Ricardo Caballero[1,2‡]*

[1] Department of Pharmacology, School of Medicine, Instituto de Investigación Sanitaria Gregorio Marañón, Universidad Complutense, Madrid, Spain, [2] CIBERCV, Madrid, Spain, [3] Departamento de Biología Molecular and Centro de Biología Molecular "Severo Ochoa" (UAM-CSIC), Universidad Autónoma de Madrid, Madrid, Spain

***Correspondence:**
Eva Delpón
edelpon@med.ucm.es

[†] These authors have contributed equally to this work.
[‡] Co-senior authors.*

Cardiac Kir2.1 and Nav1.5 channels generate the inward rectifier K^+ (I_{K1}) and the Na^+ (I_{Na}) currents, respectively. There is a mutual interplay between the ventricular I_{Na} and I_{K1} densities, because Nav1.5 and Kir2.1 channels exhibit positive reciprocal modulation. Here we compared some of the biological properties of Nav1.5 and Kir2.1 channels when they are expressed together or separately to get further insights regarding their putative interaction. First we demonstrated by proximity ligation assays (PLAs) that in the membrane of ventricular myocytes Nav1.5 and Kir2.1 proteins are in close proximity to each other (<40 nm apart). Furthermore, intracellular dialysis with anti-Nav1.5 and anti-Kir2.1 antibodies suggested that these channels form complexes. Patch-clamp experiments in heterologous transfection systems demonstrated that the inhibition of the Ca^{2+}/calmodulin-dependent protein kinase II (CaMKII) decreased the I_{Na} and the I_{K1} generated by Nav1.5 and Kir2.1 channels when they were coexpressed, but not the I_{K1} generated by Kir2.1 channels alone, suggesting that complexes, but not Kir2.1 channels, are a substrate of CaMKII. Furthermore, inhibition of CaMKII precluded the interaction between Nav1.5 and Kir2.1 channels. Inhibition of 14-3-3 proteins did not modify the I_{Na} and I_{K1} densities generated by each channel separately, whereas it decreased the I_{Na} and I_{K1} generated when they were coexpressed. However, inhibition of 14-3-3 proteins did not abolish the Nav1.5-Kir2.1 interaction. Inhibition of dynamin-dependent endocytosis reduced the internalization of Kir2.1 but not of Nav1.5 or Kir2.1-Nav1.5 complexes. Inhibition of cytoskeleton-dependent vesicular trafficking via the dynein/dynactin motor increased the I_{K1}, but reduced the I_{Na}, thus suggesting that the dynein/dynactin motor is preferentially involved in the backward and forward traffic of Kir2.1 and Nav1.5, respectively. Conversely, the dynein/dynactin motor participated in the forward movement of Kir2.1-Nav1.5 complexes. Ubiquitination by Nedd4-2 ubiquitin-protein ligase promoted the Nav1.5 degradation by the proteasome, but not that of Kir2.1 channels. Importantly, the Kir2.1-Nav1.5 complexes were degraded following this route as demonstrated by the overexpression of Nedd4-2 and the inhibition of the proteasome with MG132. These results suggested that Kir2.1 and Nav1.5 channels closely interact with each other leading to the formation of a pool of complexed channels whose biology is similar to that of the Nav1.5 channels.

Keywords: Nav1.5, Kir2.1, heart, ion channel biology, patch-clamp

INTRODUCTION

Kir2.1 channels generate the inward rectifier K^+ current (I_{K1}) that plays a key role in the control of the resting membrane potential and the duration of the late-phase of repolarization in human cardiac cells (Anumonwo and Lopatin, 2010; de Boer et al., 2010). On the other hand, Nav1.5 channels carry the inward Na^+ current (I_{Na}), which determines the Na^+ influx that depolarizes the membrane potential during the upstroke of the action potential (Abriel, 2010; Wilde and Brugada, 2011). It has been recently demonstrated that there is a positive reciprocal modulation between Kir2.1 and Nav1.5 channels, in such a way that an increase in Kir2.1 channels expression leads to the increase of the I_{Na} density in cardiac ventricular myocytes and *vice versa* (Milstein et al., 2012; Matamoros et al., 2016). The reciprocal modulation is mediated by the binding of both channel types to α1-syntrophin, a scaffolding protein containing a PDZ domain (Matamoros et al., 2016). Indeed Nav1.5 channels interact with α1-syntrophin via two different PDZ-binding domains, one the canonical, constituted by the three last C-terminal residues (SIV) and another "PDZ-like" domain, determined by the presence of Ser20 and located "internally" at the N-terminus of the channel (Matamoros et al., 2016). Conversely, Kir2.1 channels exhibit a unique α1-syntrophin binding site within its C-terminal PDZ-binding domain (Matamoros et al., 2016), suggesting that Nav1.5, but not Kir2.1, could bind two molecules of α1-syntrophin at a time (Matamoros et al., 2016). These results suggested that at least some Nav1.5 and Kir2.1 channels form a multiprotein complex in which they interact directly or indirectly. The aims of the present work are to explore whether these complexes, if any, are formed just at the plasma membrane or at early stages of the protein assembly, as well as to characterize some of their biological properties (such as their anterograde or retrograde trafficking routes). The existence of such complexes would allow a dynamic and delicate control of the expression of these cardiac ion channels whose balanced function is critical for an adequate control of the excitability and cardiac impulse propagation. The results obtained demonstrate that at least a pool of Kir2.1 and Nav1.5 channels are in close proximity and interact at the membrane of cardiac cells forming complexes with anterograde and retrograde trafficking routes similar to those of the Nav1.5 channels alone.

METHODS

Kir2.x and Nav1.5 Constructs and Chinese Hamster Ovary (CHO) Cell Transfection

Human Kir2.1 (kindly provided by Dr. José Jalife; University of Michigan, USA) was subcloned into pcDNA3.1 plasmid (Invitrogen, USA). Human cardiac Nav1.5 (hH1) and Navβ1 cDNA subcloned in pCGI vector were kindly gifted by Dr. Connie R. Bezzina (University of Amsterdam, The Netherlands). CHO cells were cultured as previously described (Caballero et al., 2010b, 2017; Núñez et al., 2013; Matamoros et al., 2016) and transiently transfected with the cDNA encoding Nav1.5 channels (1.6 μg) and hNavβ1 (1.6 μg; Nav1.5-β) alone or together with Kir2.1 (1.6 μg) plus the cDNA encoding the CD8 antigen (0.5 μg) by using FUGENE XtremeGENE (Roche Diagnostics, Switzerland) following manufacturer instructions. Forty-eight hours after transfection, cells were incubated with polystyrene microbeads precoated with anti-CD8 antibody (Dynabeads M450; Life Technologies, USA). Most of the cells that were beaded also had channel expression. Coexpression of Nav1.5 and Kir2.1 channels was always tested electrophysiologically and only cells coexpressing both channels were patched.

Human Nedd4-2 (KIAA0439), p.K44A dynamin-2 mutant, and p.R56,60A 14-3-3 (14-3-3DN) mutant cDNAs subcloned in pcDNA3.1 were kindly gifted by Prof. Dr. Hugues Abriel (University of Bern, Switzerland), Dr. Federico Sesti (Rutgers University, USA), and Dr. Isabelle Baro (INSERM, France), respectively. In some experiments, Kir2.1 and Nav1.5 channels were cotransfected with the p50 subunit of the dynein/dynactin complex (1.6 μg, Origene, USA), p.K44A dynamin-2 (1.6 μg), 14-3-3DN (1.6 μg), or Nedd4-2 (1.6 μg).

Patch-Clamping

Kir2.1 ($I_{Kir2.1}$) and Nav1.5 ($I_{Nav1.5}$) currents were recorded at room temperature (21-23°C) using the whole-cell patch-clamp technique using an Axopatch-200B amplifier (Molecular Devices, USA) (Caballero et al., 2010a,b, 2017; Núñez et al., 2013; Matamoros et al., 2016). Recording pipettes were pulled from 1.0 mm o.d. borosilicate capillary tubes (GD1, Narishige Co., Ltd, Japan) using a programmable patch micropipette puller (Model P-2000 Brown-Flaming, Sutter Instruments Co., USA) and were heat-polished with a microforge (Model MF-83, Narishige). Micropipette resistance was kept below 3.5 and 1.5 MΩ for $I_{Kir2.1}$ and $I_{Nav1.5}$ recordings, respectively, when filled with the internal solution and immersed in the external solution. In all experiments, series resistance was compensated

Abbreviations: AIP, autocamtide-2-related inhibitory peptide; BFA, Brefeldin-A; CAF, chronic atrial fibrillation; CaMKII, Ca^{2+}/calmodulin-dependent protein kinase II; CHO, Chinese Hamster Ovary; COPI, coat-associated protein I; DAPI, 4',6-diamidino-2-phenylindole; ER, Endoplasmic reticulum; HEK-293, Human Embryonic Kidney-293; I_{K1}, Inward rectifier potassium current; $I_{Kir2.1}$, Current generated by Kir2.1 channels; I_{Na}, Inward sodium current; I_{NaL}, late sodium current; $I_{Nav1.5}$, Current generated by Nav1.5 channels; I-V, current-voltage; LJP, Liquid junction potential; PBS, Phosphate buffered saline; PKA, protein kinase A; PLA, proximity ligand assay; TRITC, Tetramethylrhodamine.

manually by using the series resistance compensation unit of the Axopatch amplifier, and ≥80% compensation was achieved. Uncompensated access resistance and CHO cell capacitance were 1.6 ± 0.3 MΩ and 12.8 ± 0.2 pF (n = 663), respectively. Peak $I_{Kir2.1}$ and $I_{Nav1.5}$ amplitudes were −2.3 ± 0.1 and −2.9 ± 0.2 nA, respectively. Therefore, under our experimental conditions no significant voltage errors (<5 mV) due to series resistance were expected with the micropipettes used.

To record $I_{Kir2.1}$ and $I_{Nav1.5}$, CHO cells were perfused with an external solution containing (mM): NaCl 136, KCl 4, $CaCl_2$ 1.8, $MgCl_2$ 1, HEPES 10, and glucose 10 (pH 7.4 with NaOH). Recording pipettes were filled with an internal solution containing (mM): K-aspartate 80, KCl 42, KH_2PO_4 10, MgATP 5, phosphocreatine 3, HEPES 5, and EGTA 5 (pH 7.2 with KOH) to record $I_{Kir2.1}$ (liquid junction potential-LJP = −13.2 mV) or NaF 10, CsF 110, CsCl 20, HEPES 10, and EGTA 10 (pH 7.35 with CsOH) to record $I_{Nav1.5}$. $I_{Kir2.1}$ current-voltage (I-V) curves were corrected according to the calculated LJP between the pipette and external solution (Caballero et al., 2010b, 2017; Matamoros et al., 2016). To minimize the contribution of time-dependent shifts of channel availability during sodium current recordings, all data were collected 20 min after establishing the whole-cell configuration. Under these conditions current amplitudes and voltage dependence of activation and inactivation were stable during the time of recordings (Matamoros et al., 2016; Caballero et al., 2017).

In some experiments, $I_{Kir2.1}$ and $I_{Nav1.5}$ were recorded in transiently transfected CHO cells dialyzed with anti-Kir2.1 or anti-Nav1.5 antibodies added to the internal solution (Archer et al., 1998). For the experiments conducted to determine the effect of the presence of both Nav1.5 and Kir2.1 on channel internalization kinetics, $I_{Nav1.5}$ and $I_{Kir2.1}$ were recorded at different time points after addition of 50 ng/mL brefeldin-A (BFA) to the culture medium (Rougier et al., 2005). In some experiments, cells were incubated with the Ca^{2+}/calmodulin-dependent protein kinase II (CaMKII) inhibitor KN93 (1 μM, 24 h; Wagner et al., 2006) or with the proteasome inhibitor MG132 (20 μM, 2 h; Shy et al., 2014). In another group of patch-clamp experiments the CaMKII inhibitor autocamtide-2-related inhibitory peptide (AIP) was added to the internal solution (1 nM) that dialyzes the cells.

Pulse Protocols and Analysis

The protocol to record $I_{Nav1.5}$ consisted of 50-ms pulses in 5 mV increments from −120 mV to potentials between −80 and +50 mV. $I_{Nav1.5}$ amplitude was measured at the peak of the current traces. For $I_{Kir2.1}$, the protocol to obtain I-V curves consisted of 250-ms pulses in 10 mV increments from −60 mV to potentials between −120 and +20 mV (Caballero et al., 2010b, 2017; Matamoros et al., 2016). $I_{Kir2.1}$ amplitude was measured at the end of the pulse. $I_{Kir2.1}$ and $I_{Nav1.5}$ recordings were sampled at 4 and 50 kHz, respectively, filtered at half the sampling frequency, and stored on the hard disk of a computer for subsequent analysis. Data were analyzed using pCLAMP software (Molecular Devices). In each experiment, current amplitudes were normalized to membrane capacitance to obtain current densities.

Rat Ventricular Myocyte Isolation

Single ventricular myocytes were isolated from hearts of male Sprague–Dawley rats (225–250 g) by enzymatic dissociation with collagenase type II (Worthington) following previously described methods (Matamoros et al., 2016; Caballero et al., 2017). Rats were heparinized (1.000 U/kg i.p.) and anesthetized with sodium pentobarbital (50 mg/kg i.p.). Animal studies were approved by the University Committee on the Use and Care of animals at the Complutense University and conformed to the Guidelines from Directive 2010/63/EU of the European Parliament on the protection of animals used for scientific purposes.

Proximity Ligation Assay

The Duolink® (Sigma, USA) proximity ligation assay (PLA) was conducted by using previously described methods (Söderberg et al., 2006; Shy et al., 2014) in non-permeabilized rat ventricular myocytes. This assay allows for the *in situ* detection of proteins that are located in close proximity to each other (<40 nm apart). Experiments were performed according to the manufacturer's recommendations and using all incubation buffers without detergents in order to avoid cell membrane permeabilization. Isolated ventricular myocytes were fixed and incubated in blocking solution and then, incubated with primary antibodies as specified in previously described methods (Núñez et al., 2013). Subsequent incubation steps were performed at 37°C and the appropriate washing buffers were used after each incubation, as specified in the manufacturer's protocol. After washing three times in phosphate buffered saline (PBS) to remove the primary antibody, Duolink secondary antibodies, conjugated to PLA probes, were added to the myocytes for a 1 h incubation. These PLA probes consist of oligonucleotides which were subsequently joined together in a circle after addition of ligation solution (containing ligase enzyme) and incubation for 30 min. Next, rolling circle amplification of this circular template was achieved by addition of amplification solution, containing polymerase and fluorescently labeled oligonucleotides which hybridized to the circular template during 100 min of incubation. Samples were then mounted with Duolink *in situ* mounting medium with 4′,6-diamidino-2-phenylindole (DAPI) and viewed with a confocal microscope. Cell images and fluorescent signals were acquired on a Leica TCS-SP5 AOBS confocal microscope (Mannheim, Germany) with a 40x and 63x oil objectives, using a tetramethylrhodamine (TRITC) filter to visualize fluorescently labeled oligonucleotides (λ_{ex} = 554 nm; λ_{em} = 579 nm). Laser lines at 561 and 358 nm for excitation of fluorescently labeled oligonucleotides and DAPI were provided by a diode-pumped solid-state laser and a UV laser, respectively. Samples without primary antibodies were used as negative controls. Images were analyzed with ImageJ software (National Institutes of Health, USA) assigning green color to images taken under TRITC channel.

Cell Imaging

Cell surface labeling of Kir2.1 channels cotransfected or not with Nav1.5 in Human Embryonic Kidney-293 (HEK-293) cells was performed by confocal microscopy (Núñez et al., 2013;

Confocal Microscope Zeiss LSM710 with objective 63X/1.4 Plan-Apochromat Oil DIC M27). Kir2.1 channels were fused to the circularly permuted Venus 173 (Kir2.1-CpVenus) fluorescent protein and images were acquired by exciting Venus at 500 nm and monitoring its emission at 535/22 nm. The capture conditions of the confocal microscope were optimized to obtain very thin optical sections (<300 nm, <1 Airy unit) as stated by the Nyquist sampling criterium (Pawley, 2006). ImageJ software was used to process the images and measure signal intensity (Núñez et al., 2013).

Co-immunoprecipitation and Western Blot Analysis

Co-immunoprecipitation was performed in CHO cells as previously described (Matamoros et al., 2016). Forty-eight hours after transfection with the plasmids encoding Kir2.1-CpVenus and/or Nav1.5 channel, CHO cells were washed with cold PBS and lysed in RIPA buffer to extract proteins and, thereafter, incubated for 30 min at 4°C. Precleared supernatant was incubated with 2 μg anti-Kir2.1 (N112B/14; Neuromab), 4 μg anti-CaMKIIδ (A010-56AP; Badrilla) or 3.2 μg anti-Nav1.5 (S0819, Sigma) antibodies for 3 h at 4°C, after which 20 μl of protein A/G-Sepharose beads (Santa Cruz Biotechnology Inc, USA) were added overnight at 4°C in rotation. Protein-antibody complexes were centrifuged and washed four times with cold PBS buffer. After the last centrifugation, 30 μl of loading dye with β-mercaptoethanol were added to the protein–antibody complexes and lysates and supernatants were prepared adding 20 μl of protein plus 30 μl of loading dye with β-mercaptoethanol. Thereafter, all samples were heated at 95°C for 5 min and then separated by SDS/PAGE and immunoblotted following described methods (Matamoros et al., 2016; Caballero et al., 2017). Briefly, samples were run on 10% Mini-PROTEAN® TGX™ gels (Bio-Rad, USA) and transferred to nitrocellulose membranes (Bio-Rad). Non-specific binding sites were blocked with 5% non-fat dry milk in PBS with Tween-20 (0.5%) for 1 h at room temperature. Membranes were then incubated with anti-GFP or anti-CaMKIIδ specific primary antibodies diluted in 5% non-fat dry milk overnight at 4°C. After washing, membranes were incubated with peroxidase-conjugated secondary antibodies or HRP-protein A. Antigen complexes were detected using enhanced chemiluminescence (Supersignal West Femto, Thermofisher, UK) and visualized using the Chemidoc MP System and Image Lab 5.2.1. software (Bio-Rad). Original blots are shown in Supplemental Figures 3–5.

Antibodies

In the PLA, mouse monoclonal anti-Nav1.5 (1:50; ab62388, Abcam, UK) and rabbit monoclonal anti-Kir2.1 (1:100, ab109750, Abcam) primary antibodies were used. These antibodies bind to extracellular domains of Nav1.5 (residues 59-72 of human Nav1.5) and Kir2.1 (residues 107-122 of human Kir2.1 channels), respectively. Duolink secondary antibodies conjugated to PLA probes were also used. For electrophysiological experiments, rabbit anti-Nav1.5 (1.2 μg/mL, S0819, Sigma) and rabbit anti-Kir2.1 (1:1,000, ab65796, Abcam) were used. Both Nav1.5 (residues 493–511 located at the cytoplasmic loop between Domain I and II) and Kir2.1 (residues 1–81) antibodies bind to intracellular domains of the channels. For co-immunoprecipitation and western blot analysis rabbit polyclonal anti-CAMKIIδ (1:5,000 A010-56AP, Badrilla, UK) and rabbit polyclonal anti-GFP (1:1,000 ab290; Abcam) primary antibodies were used for detection of the C-terminal domain of CAMKIIδ and Kir2.1-CpVenus, respectively. Peroxidase-conjugated secondary antibodies (Jackson ImmunoResearch, USA) were used for detection of the proteins in lysates and HRP-protein A (Life Technologies) was used for detection of the immunoprecipitated proteins. Non-immune antibodies (IgG from rabbit or mouse serum) used as negative controls for co-immunoprecipitation experiments were obtained from Sigma-Aldrich.

Statistical Analysis

Results are expressed as mean ± SEM. Unpaired t-test or one-way ANOVA followed by Newman–Keuls test were used where appropriate. In small-size samples ($n < 15$), statistical significance was confirmed by using non-parametric tests. To take into account repeated sample assessments, data were analyzed with multilevel mixed-effects models. A value of $P < 0.05$ was considered significant.

RESULTS

The positive reciprocal modulation between Kir2.1 and Nav1.5 channels is not due to a change of the biophysical properties, such as single channel conductance or open probability of the channels (Milstein et al., 2012). These results led to propose that it is due to an increase of their expression at the cell membrane. To test this hypothesis, we conducted immunofluorescence analyses in HEK-293 cells transfected with Kir2.1 alone or together with Nav1.5 channels. **Figure 1A** left shows representative z-stack confocal images obtained in a cell expressing Kir2.1-CpVenus alone. The intensity of the signal emitted by CpVenus throughout the cell region selected (yellow line) has been represented as an inset (top left). The maximum signal, which corresponds to the cell membrane, is represented by the two discrete peaks. As can be observed in the right panel of **Figure 1A** and **Figure 1B**, coexpression with Nav1.5 channels significantly increased the intensity of the maximum signal emitted by CpVenus. Even though considering the limitations of the experimental approach, these results suggested that the amount of Kir2.1 channels at the cell membrane increases ($P < 0.05$).

Next, we measured the putative association between Nav1.5 and Kir2.1 channels using PLA in rat ventricular myocytes by means of the Duolink® technology. In PLA, a fluorescent signal is only generated when the plus and minus probes attached to each antibody are bound together, allowing for the *in situ* detection of proteins that are located in close proximity to each other (<40 nm apart; Söderberg et al., 2006; Shy et al., 2014). Importantly, to conduct these experiments myocytes were not permeabilized and, thus, the antibodies, which bind to extracellular domains of Nav1.5 and Kir2.1 channels (see section Methods), only detected the Nav1.5 and Kir2.1 channels present at the cell membrane. **Figure 1C** (bottom middle) shows

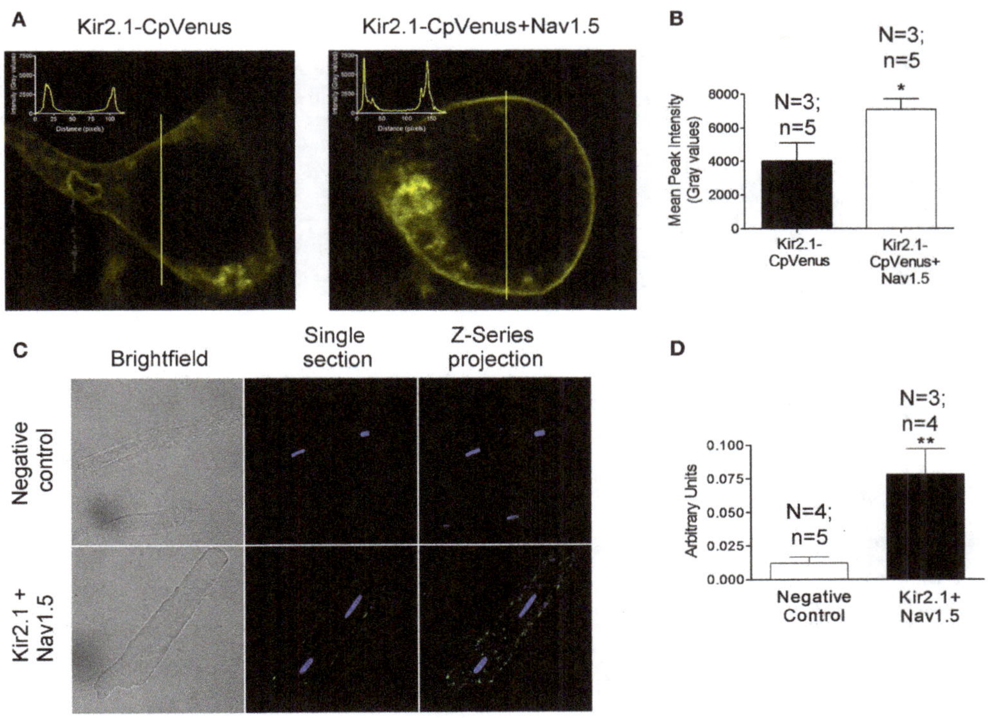

FIGURE 1 | Kir2.1 and Nav1.5 channels are in close proximity at the membrane of cardiac myocytes. **(A)** Confocal microscopy images of HEK293 cells expressing Kir2.1-CpVenus alone (left) or in the presence of Nav1.5 (right). The insets show the intensity of the signal emitted by CpVenus throughout the cell region selected (yellow line). **(B)** Peak mean signal corresponding to the cell membrane in cells expressing Kir2.1-CpVenus with or without Nav1.5 channels. **(C)** Confocal microscopy images of rat ventricular myocytes processed using Duolink® PLA. The green signal demonstrates a physical interaction between Nav1.5 and Kir2.1. Cell nuclei were visible by DAPI staining (blue). **(D)** Mean intensity of the green signal in the negative control and in the presence of Nav1.5+Kir2.1 antibodies. In **(B,D)**, each bar represents the mean ± SEM of "*n*" cells of "*N*" preparations. $^{*}P < 0.05$ vs. Kir2.1-CpVenus alone. $^{**}P < 0.01$ vs. negative control.

a single section image from the center of a rat ventricular myocyte showing a sparse fluorescent signal distributed along the cell membrane. The Z-series projection (bottom right) shows more abundant fluorescent spots corresponding to the top of the membrane. Comparison of the mean intensity data demonstrated a ≈6.5-fold increase in the fluorescence signal (**Figure 1D**) compared to the negative controls (**Figure 1C** top panels) consisting of myocytes assayed with Duolink® technology but without incubating with the primary Nav1.5 and Kir2.1 antibodies ($P < 0.01$). Further negative controls were developed in human atrial myocytes in which PLA was developed after extracellular treatment with either anti-Kir2.1 or anti-Nav1.5 antibodies alone. Supplemental Figure 1 confirms that in the absence of one of the antibodies the Duolink assay did not produce any fluorescent signal. These data demonstrated that at the cardiomyocyte membrane at least a pool of Nav1.5 and Kir2.1 channels physically interacts with each other.

To further elucidate the degree of proximity of Kir2.1 and Nav1.5 channels at the cell membrane, the $I_{Kir2.1}$ and $I_{Nav1.5}$ were recorded in CHO cells transfected with Kir2.1, Nav1.5 channels or both and dialyzed with an internal solution supplemented with either anti-Kir2.1 or anti-Nav1.5 antibodies. In these experiments, the tip of the pipette was filled with antibody-free internal solution, in order to obtain "control" current records. Importantly, the epitope of the anti-Nav1.5 and anti-Kir2.1 antibodies used in these experiments (see section Methods) were intracellular domains of Nav1.5 and Kir2.1 channels, respectively. **Figures 2E,F** show the normalized density of $I_{Kir2.1}$ recorded at −120 mV and of peak $I_{Nav1.5}$ as a function of time elapsed after seal breaking and, thus of time in the presence of their corresponding antibodies. As expected, neither $I_{Kir2.1}$ (**Figures 2A,E**) nor $I_{Nav1.5}$ (**Figures 2B,F**) decreased in cells dialyzed with anti-Nav1.5 or anti-Kir2.1 antibodies (squares), respectively (**Figure 2H**). Conversely, and also as expected, both $I_{Kir2.1}$ (**Figure 2E**) and $I_{Nav1.5}$ (**Figure 2F**) progressively decreased in cells dialyzed with anti-Kir2.1 and anti-Nav1.5 antibodies (circles), respectively ($P < 0.05$; **Figure 2H**). **Figures 2C,D** show superimposed $I_{Kir2.1}$ (**Figure 2C**) and $I_{Nav1.5}$ (**Figure 2D**) traces recorded in cells cotransfected with Kir2.1+Nav1.5 channels and dialyzed with anti-Nav1.5 and anti-Kir2.1 antibodies, respectively, while **Figure 2G** shows the normalized density of $I_{Kir2.1}$ and of peak $I_{Nav1.5}$ as a function of dialyzing time. Surprisingly, $I_{Kir2.1}$ density decreased in cells dialyzed with anti-Nav1.5 antibodies and $I_{Nav1.5}$ also diminished in cells dialyzed with anti-Kir2.1 antibodies (**Figures 2C,D,G,H**; $P < 0.05$). These results would suggest that

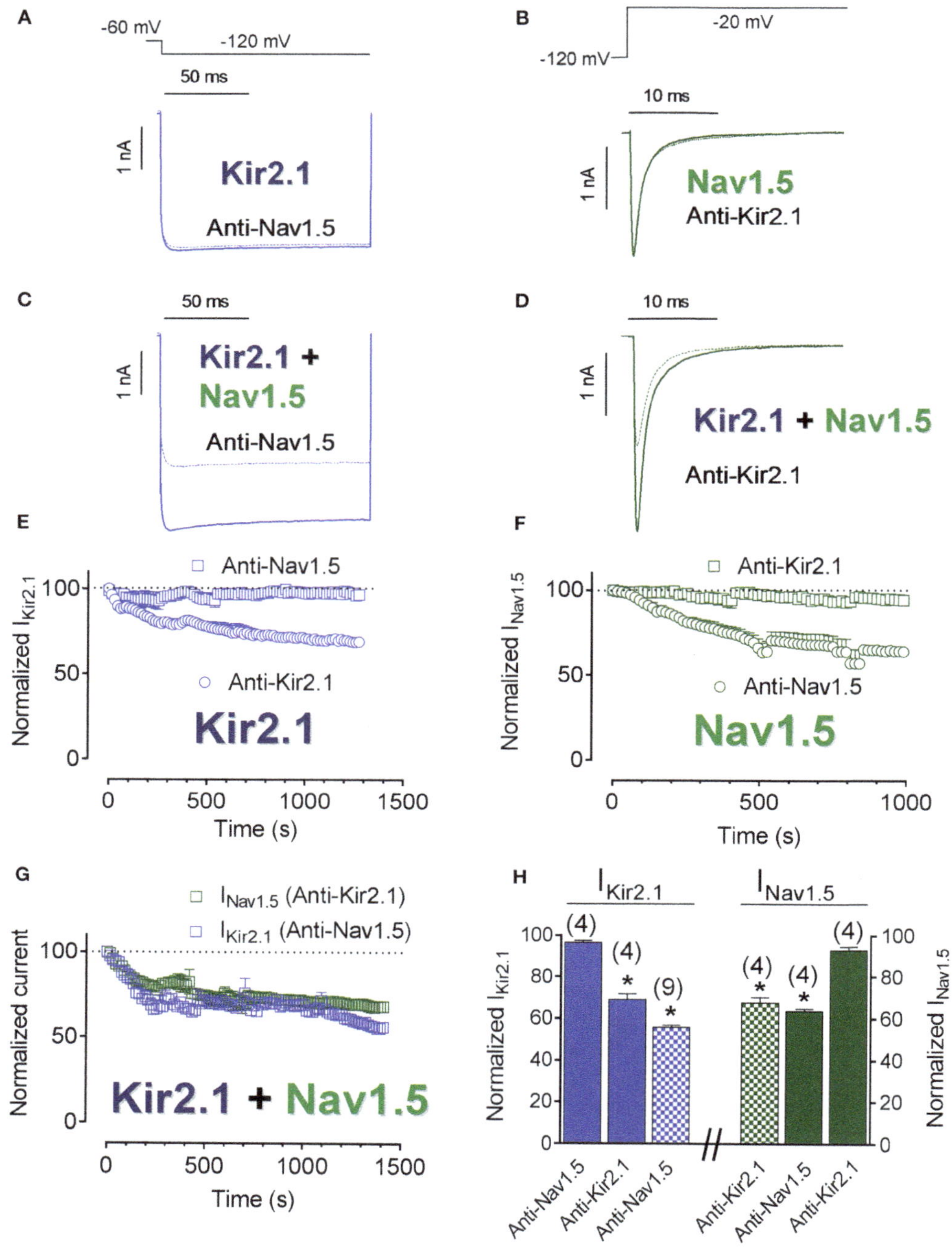

FIGURE 2 | Kir2.1 and Nav1.5 channels closely interact at the cell membrane. **(A–D)** $I_{Kir2.1}$ **(A,C)** and $I_{Nav1.5}$ **(B,D)** traces recorded by applying the protocols shown at the top in CHO cells expressing Kir2.1 or Nav1.5 channels alone **(A,B)** or together **(C,D)** in control conditions (solid lines) or after dialyzing the cell with the antibodies indicated (dashed lines). **(E–G)** Normalized $I_{Kir2.1}$ (measured at −120 mV) **(E,G)** and peak $I_{Nav1.5}$ **(F,G)** measured in the absence and presence of anti-Kir2.1 or anti-Nav1.5 antibodies in cells transfected with Kir2.1 or Nav1.5 channels alone **(E,F)** or cotransfected with both **(G)** plotted as a function of time. **(H)** Bar graphs showing the mean normalized current density values measured in each experimental group at the end of the recordings. Each point/bar represents the mean ± SEM of (*n*) cells of ≥ 3 preparations. In **(H)**, $^{*}P < 0.05$ vs. $I_{Kir2.1}$ or $I_{Nav1.5}$ generated by Kir2.1 or Nav1.5 channels alone in the presence of anti-Nav1.5 or anti-Kir2.1 antibodies. For clarity the results of other statistical comparisons were not shown.

the distance between both channels is narrow enough to allow Kir2.1 channels to be "silenced" when the Nav1.5 antibody interacts with the Nav1.5 channels present in the Kir2.1-Nav1.5 complexes and *vice versa* and further supported the hypothesis that at least a pool of Kir2.1 and Nav1.5 channels interact at the cell membrane forming complexes.

Effects of CaMKII on Kir2.1 and Nav1.5 Channels and Kir2.1-Nav1.5 Complexes

It is well-established that Nav1.5 channels are one of the most important targets of CaMKII in cardiac myocytes (Wagner et al., 2006; Ashpole et al., 2012; Herren et al., 2015). Electrophysiological studies in HEK-293 cells have demonstrated that the kinase phosphorylates residues located in the cytoplasmic loop between domains I and II of the channel leading to an increase of the late I_{Na} (I_{NaL}) and to a shift of the voltage-dependence of Nav1.5 channel inactivation to hyperpolarized potentials (Ashpole et al., 2012). To analyze the modulatory role of CaMKII on the channels expressed separately or together, we recorded the $I_{Kir2.1}$ and $I_{Nav1.5}$ in cells transfected with the channels and incubated or not with the CaMKII inhibitor KN93 (1 μM) for 24 h. Under our experimental conditions, inhibition of CaMKII did not modify $I_{Kir2.1}$ in cells transfected with Kir2.1 alone ($n \geq 10$; $P > 0.05$; **Figure 3A**) whereas it significantly decreased the $I_{Nav1.5}$ in cells transfected with Nav1.5 channels alone ($P < 0.05$; **Figure 3B**). Furthermore, inhibition of the CaMKII-dependent phosphorylation significantly decreased the I_{NaL} recorded at the end of 500 ms pulses and shifted the inactivation curve to depolarized potentials (Supplemental Figure 2). Coexpression of Nav1.5 and Kir2.1 channels markedly and significantly increased both $I_{Kir2.1}$ (**Figure 3A**) and $I_{Nav1.5}$ (**Figure 3B**) (gray bars) as a consequence of the reciprocal positive modulation (Milstein et al., 2012; Matamoros et al., 2016), and the I_{NaL} (Supplemental Figure 2). Interestingly, in cells cotransfected with Kir2.1 and Nav1.5 channels simultaneously, incubation with KN93 significantly reduced the $I_{Nav1.5}$ (**Figure 3B**) and I_{NaL} as expected (Supplemental Figure 2), and, unexpectedly, it also reduced the $I_{Kir2.1}$ compared to that generated in cotransfected cells in which CaMKII was not inhibited (**Figure 3A**). In another group of experiments CaMKII was

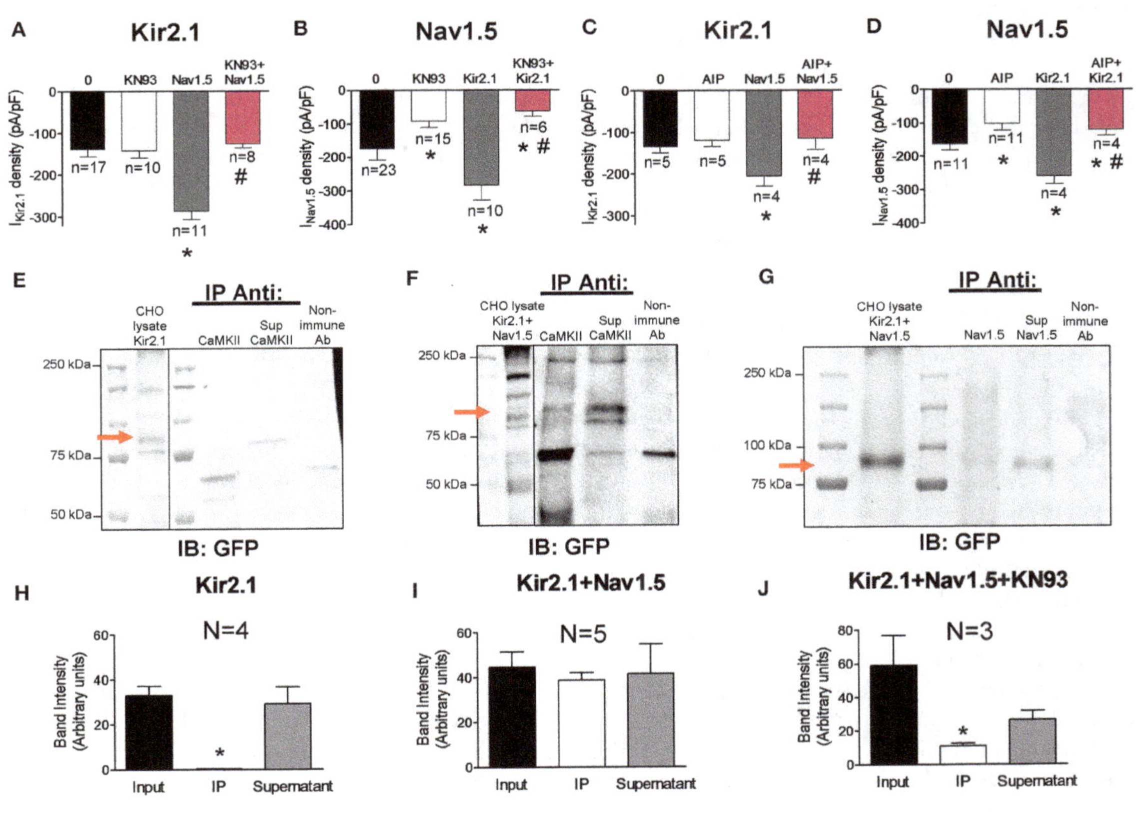

FIGURE 3 | Effects of CaMKII inhibition on Kir2.1 and Nav1.5 channel complexes. **(A,B)** $I_{Kir2.1}$ density at −120 mV **(A)** and peak $I_{Nav1.5}$ **(B)** recorded in CHO cells expressing the constructs indicated, incubated or not with KN93 (1 μM-24 h). **(C,D)** $I_{Kir2.1}$ density at−120 mV **(C)** and peak $I_{Nav1.5}$ **(D)** recorded in CHO cells expressing the constructs indicated, dialyzed or not with AIP (1 nM). **(E–G)** Kir2.1 did not immunoprecipitate with CaMKII in the lysates obtained from CHO cells transfected with Kir2.1-CpVenus alone **(E)**, while partially immunoprecipitated in cells cotransfected with Nav1.5 channels **(F)**. In the presence of KN93 (1 μM-24 h incubation), Kir2.1 did not immunoprecipitate with Nav1.5 **(G)**. CpVenus was detected by western blot in the lysates by using an anti-GFP antibody. Also shown is the supernatant (Sup) recovered after centrifugation of the immunoprecipitant (IP). All immunoprecipitation reactions used membrane-enriched preparations. As a negative control, lysate treated with non-specific IgG (and Protein A/G) was used ("Non-immune Ab" lane). IB, antibody used for immunoblotting; IP Anti, antibody used for immunoprecipitation. **(H–J)** Densitometric analysis of the co-immunoprecipitation experiments depicted in **(E–G)** showing the mean intensity of the bands of the inputs, immunoprecipitants (IP) and supernatants. In **(A–D)** and **(H–J)**, each bar represents the mean ± SEM of "*n*" cells of ≥2 preparations **(A–D)** or "*N*" preparations **(H–J)**. In **(A–D)**, $^*P < 0.05$ vs. cells transfected with Kir2.1 or Nav1.5 channels alone; $^{\#}P < 0.05$ vs. cells transfected with Kir2.1+Nav1.5. For clarity the results of other statistical comparisons were not shown. In **(H,J)**, $^*P < 0.05$ vs. input and supernatant.

inhibited with autocamtide-2-related inhibitory peptide (AIP) which was added to the "internal" solution that dialyzes the cells after the patch rupture (1 nM). Data presented in **Figures 3C,D** and Supplemental Figure 2 confirmed that CaMKII inhibition significantly decreased the $I_{Nav1.5}$ and the I_{NaL} in cells expressing Nav1.5 channels either alone or in the presence of Kir2.1 channels. Conversely, CaMKII inhibition only decreased the $I_{Kir2.1}$ generated in cells cotransfected with Kir2.1 and Nav1.5 channels. Overall the results suggest that when both Kir2.1 and Nav1.5 channels are expressed together, a pool of Kir2.1 channels, probably those that are interacting with Nav1.5 channels, becomes a target for CaMKII (**Figures 3B,D**). To test this hypothesis co-immunoprecipitation experiments with Kir2.1-CpVenus channels cotransfected or not with Nav1.5 were conducted. As can be observed in **Figures 3E,H**, and consistently with the electrophysiological results, in cells expressing Kir2.1-CpVenus alone CaMKII did not co-immunoprecipitate with Kir2.1 channels, that were detected in the supernatant fraction by means of anti-GFP antibody which recognizes CpVenus. Conversely, CaMKII partially co-immunoprecipitated with Kir2.1 in cells cotransfected with both Kir2.1 and Nav1.5 channels (**Figures 3F,I**). The results pointed to a relevant role of CaMKII in the reciprocal positive modulation between Kir2.1 and Nav1.5 channels. Thus, we conducted co-immunoprecipitation experiments in cells cotransfected with Nav1.5 and Kir2.1 and incubated with KN93. Under these conditions Kir2.1-CpVenus channels did not co-immunoprecipitate with Nav1.5 channels (**Figures 3G,J**).

Regulation of Kir2.1-Nav1.5 Complexes by 14-3-3 Proteins

14-3-3 is a family of 30-kDa cytosolic acidic proteins with multiple effects including regulation of ion channel trafficking (Obsil and Obsilova, 2011). Furthermore, it has been demonstrated that 14-3-3 could prevent phosphatase action on phosphorylated residues (Tutor et al., 2006; Obsil and Obsilova, 2011). It has been shown that 14-3-3η can interact with Nav1.5 channels at the intercalated discs of cardiac myocytes. Moreover, 14-3-3 in COS7 cells modify the voltage dependence of inactivation and recovery from inactivation kinetics, but not the $I_{Nav1.5}$ density (Allouis et al., 2006). To test whether 14-3-3 regulate somehow Kir2.1, Nav1.5, and Kir2.1-Nav1.5 complexes we used a double mutant (p.R56A,60A) of 14-3-3 which acts as a dominant negative (14-3-3DN; Allouis et al., 2006). Cotransfection of 14-3-3DN in cells expressing Kir2.1 or Nav1.5 alone did not significantly modify either $I_{Kir2.1}$ or $I_{Nav1.5}$ densities (**Figures 4A,B**; $P>0.05$). Interestingly, 14-3-3DN abolished the positive reciprocal modulation thus inhibiting both the $I_{Kir2.1}$ and $I_{Nav1.5}$ in cells cotransfected with both channels (**Figures 4A,B**; $P < 0.05$). These results would suggest that 14-3-3 proteins may target Kir2.1 and Nav1.5 channel complexes in a different way that each channel separately. However, these results could also be explained considering that 14-3-3 proteins are responsible for the positive reciprocal modulation. Therefore, we analyzed whether the inhibition of the 14-3-3 proteins precludes the interaction between Nav1.5 and Kir2.1 channels. To this end, we recorded the $I_{Kir2.1}$ and $I_{Nav1.5}$ in cells expressing both channels, cotransfected with 14-3-3DN, and dialyzed with an internal solution containing anti-Nav1.5 or anti-Kir2.1 antibodies, respectively. As can be observed in **Figures 4C,D**, when 14-3-3 proteins are inhibited, intracellular dialysis with anti-Nav1.5 and anti-Kir2.1 antibodies significantly decreased the $I_{Kir2.1}$ and $I_{Nav1.5}$, respectively. These results strongly suggested that inhibition of 14-3-3 proteins did not preclude the formation of Nav1.5-Kir2.1 complexes.

Trafficking of Nav1.5 and Kir2.1 Complexes

In the next groups of experiments we further analyzed the biological properties of the Kir2.1-Nav1.5 complexes by comparing the trafficking of Kir2.1 and Nav1.5 channels when they are expressed alone or together in CHO cells. It has been proposed that the dynein/dynactin complex plays a role in normal vesicular traffic of ion channels toward and from the sarcolemma (Balse et al., 2012). Overexpression of dynamitin (the p50 subunit of dynactin) has been routinely used to block the dynein function since it dissociates the dynactin complex, decoupling the dynein motor from its cargo (**Figure 5A**; Burkhardt et al., 1997; Balse et al., 2012). **Figures 5B,C** show the current-density voltage curves for $I_{Kir2.1}$ and $I_{Nav1.5}$ recorded in cells cotransfected or not with p50. Cotransfection of p50 increased the $I_{Kir2.1}$ at potentials between −120 and −90 mV and between −70 and −50 mV (**Figures 5B,D**; $P < 0.05$), suggesting that the dynein/dynactin complex is involved in the retrograde trafficking of Kir2.1 channels. Conversely, p50 reduced the $I_{Nav1.5}$ at potentials ranging −40 and +30 mV in cells expressing Nav1.5 channels alone (**Figures 5C,E**; $P < 0.05$), thus confirming previous results that demonstrate the role of the dynein/dynactin complex in the anterograde trafficking of Nav1.5 channels (Chatin et al., 2014). When Kir2.1 and Nav1.5 channels were expressed together, both $I_{Kir2.1}$ and $I_{Nav1.5}$ were significantly increased as expected (**Figures 5B–E**). Conversely, overexpression of p50 abolished the reciprocal modulation between Kir2.1 and Nav1.5 (**Figures 5B–E**). In fact, in cells expressing Kir2.1+Nav1.5 channels in which the dynein function was blocked the $I_{Kir2.1}$ was not increased (**Figures 5B,D**; $P >$ 0.05). On the other hand, the density of the $I_{Nav1.5}$ recorded in cells expressing Nav1.5, Kir2.1, and p50 was smaller than that recorded in cells expressing either Nav1.5 channels alone or Kir2.1+Nav1.5 (**Figures 5C,E**; $P > 0.05$). These results indicate that Kir2.1 channels are affected differently by the blockade of the dynein/dynactin complex when they are expressed alone or in combination with Nav1.5 channels and suggest that the dynein/dynactin complex is involved in the anterograde trafficking of Nav1.5 channels alone and of the Kir2.1-Nav1.5 channel complexes.

Internalization and Retrograde Trafficking of Nav1.5 and Kir2.1 Complexes

BFA is a fungal metabolite commonly used to block protein trafficking to cell membrane through the classical secretory pathway involving the endoplasmic reticulum (ER) and the Golgi apparatus (Rougier et al., 2005; Mercier et al., 2015). To test whether the Nav1.5 and Kir2.1 internalization kinetics are

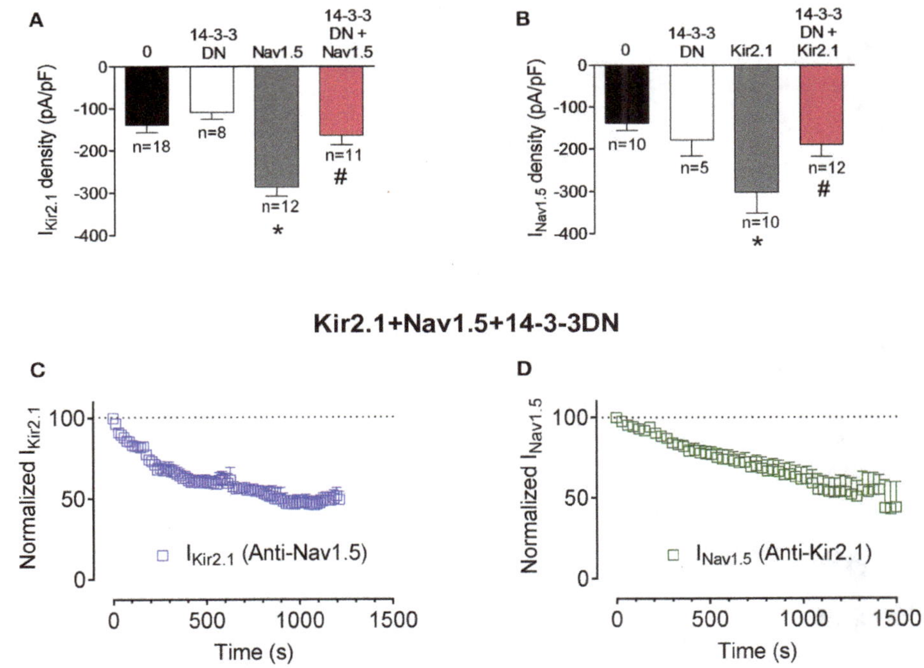

FIGURE 4 | Effects of 14-3-3 inhibition on Kir2.1-Nav1.5 channel complexes. **(A,B)** $I_{Kir2.1}$ density at −120 mV **(A)** and peak $I_{Nav1.5}$ **(B)** recorded in CHO cells expressing the constructs indicated, cotransfected or not with 14-3-3DN. Each bar represents the mean±SEM of "n" cells of ≥ 4 preparations. *$P < 0.05$ vs. cells transfected with Kir2.1 or Nav1.5 channels alone; #$P < 0.05$ vs. cells transfected with Kir2.1+Nav1.5. For clarity the results of other statistical comparisons were not shown. **(C,D)** Normalized $I_{Kir2.1}$ measured at −120 mV **(C)** and peak $I_{Nav1.5}$ **(D)** measured in the absence and presence of anti-Nav1.5 and anti-Kir2.1 antibodies, respectively, in cells cotransfected with Kir2.1, Nav1.5, and 14-3-3DN plotted as a function of time. Each point represents the mean ± SEM of 4 experiments of ≥3 preparations in each group.

affected by the presence of both channels together, $I_{Nav1.5}$ and $I_{Kir2.1}$ were recorded after incubation with BFA (50 ng/mL) for progressively increasing periods of time. Using this approach, it would be expected that most of the trafficking of newly synthesized channels to the cell membrane is blocked, and thus, the time course of internalization of the channels located in the membrane can be assessed. **Figures 6A–D** show the normalized mean density of $I_{Kir2.1}$ and $I_{Nav1.5}$ recorded in CHO cells as a function of the duration of the incubation with BFA and, as can be observed, both $I_{Kir2.1}$ and $I_{Nav1.5}$ densities gradually decreased to a residual value upon incubation with BFA. In contrast, $I_{Kir2.1}$ and $I_{Nav1.5}$ densities did not change when cells were incubated with 1% ethanol, the BFA vehicle, for 6 or 24 h (**Figures 6A–D**). The fit of a monoexponential function to the data obtained in the presence of BFA yielded the half-time constants (τ) which for Kir2.1 and Nav1.5 channel internalization averaged 5.1 and 4.9 h, respectively (**Figures 6A,B**). In cells cotransfected with Kir2.1 and Nav1.5 channels the time course of Kir2.1 and Nav1.5 channel internalization was not significantly modified (**Figures 6C,D**; $n \geq 4$; $P > 0.05$).

It has been demonstrated that dynamin-2 has an important role in the endocytosis of different ion channels including Kir2.1 (Tong et al., 2001; Boyer et al., 2009). To test whether the Kir2.1 channel internalization is modified in the presence of Nav1.5 channels we took advantage of a dynamin-2 mutant (p.K44A; **Figure 7A**), which functions as a dominant negative and inhibits the activity of the endogenous dynamin-2 (Hinshaw and Schmid, 1995). In **Figures 7B,C** $I_{Kir2.1}$ and $I_{Nav1.5}$ traces recorded in CHO cells transfected with Kir2.1, Nav1.5 alone or together and cotransfected with p.K44A dynamin-2 are presented. In cells expressing Kir2.1 (**Figures 7B,D**) or Nav1.5 (**Figures 7C,E**) channels separately, overexpression of p.K44A dynamin-2 significantly increased the $I_{Kir2.1}$ but did not modify the $I_{Nav1.5}$ density, confirming that internalization of Kir2.1, but not that of Nav1.5, channels is dynamin-dependent. Again, coexpression of Nav1.5 and Kir2.1 channels reciprocally and positively modulated the $I_{Kir2.1}$ and the $I_{Nav1.5}$ densities (**Figures 7D,E**). Interestingly, in cells expressing Kir2.1 and Nav1.5 channels, p.K44A dynamin-2 expression did not further increase either the $I_{Kir2.1}$ or the $I_{Nav1.5}$ densities ($P > 0.05$), suggesting that, as Nav1.5 channels alone, the Kir2.1-Nav1.5 complexes are resistant to the dynamin-2 inhibition (**Figures 7D,E**).

It has been extensively demonstrated that the ubiquitin-protein ligase Nedd4-2 ubiquitinates Nav1.5 by binding to the PY motif located at the C-terminus of the channel and promotes its degradation by the proteasome (van Bemmelen et al., 2004; Rougier et al., 2005; Xu et al., 2009). On the other hand, it was demonstrated that Nedd4-2 reduces the $I_{Kir2.1}$ density in *Xenopus* oocytes, although the molecular determinants were not identified (Alesutan et al., 2011). The degradation route of

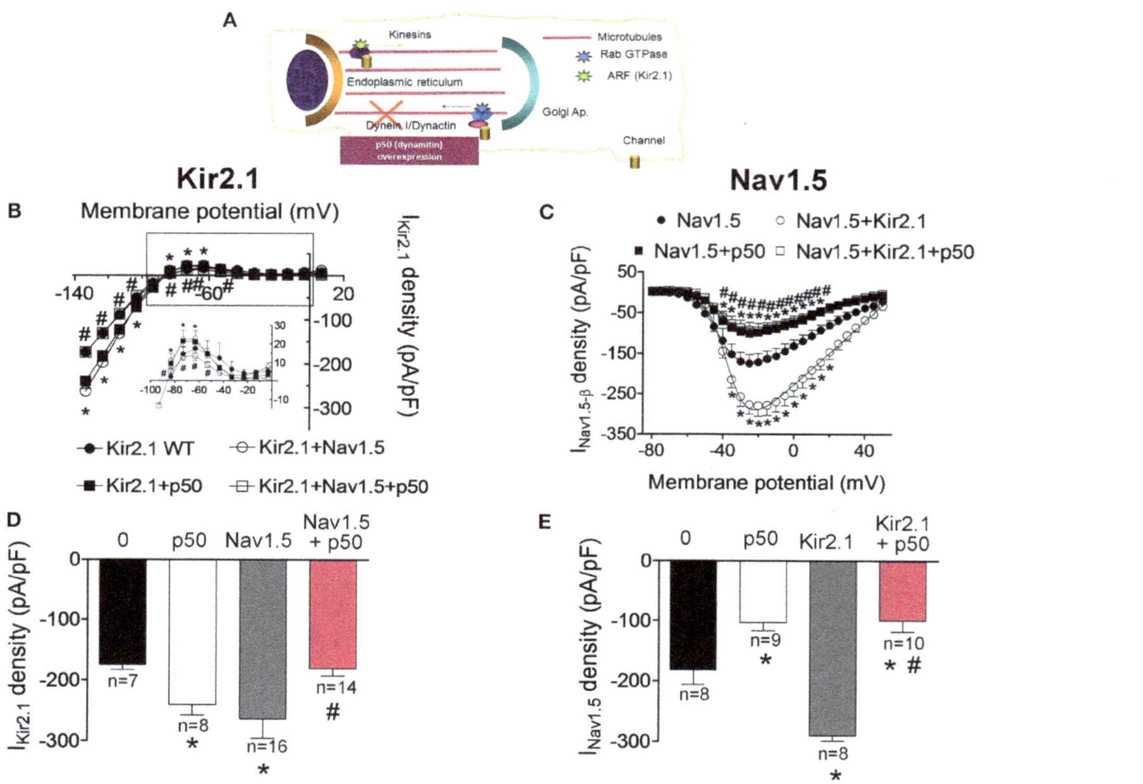

FIGURE 5 | Effects of the dynein/dynactin complex inhibition on Kir2.1 and Nav1.5 channels trafficking. **(A)** Schematic representation of a cell highlighting the role of the dynein/dynactin complex on ion channel trafficking. **(B,C)** Current-density voltage relationships for $I_{Kir2.1}$ **(B)** and $I_{Nav1.5}$ **(C)** recorded in CHO cells expressing the constructs indicated together or not with dynamitin (the p50 subunit of dynactin) to inhibit the dynein/dynactin complex. **(D,E)** $I_{Kir2.1}$ density at −120 mV **(D)** and peak $I_{Nav1.5}$ **(E)** recorded in cells expressing the constructs indicated alone or together with p50. Each point/bar represents the mean ± SEM of "*n*" cells of ≥4 preparations. *$P < 0.05$ vs. cells transfected with Kir2.1 or Nav1.5 channels alone; #$P < 0.05$ vs. cells transfected with Kir2.1+Nav1.5 without p50. For clarity the results of other statistical comparisons were not shown.

the putative Kir2.1-Nav1.5 complexes was further analyzed by cotransfecting the cells with Nedd4-2. Under our conditions, Nedd4-2 did not significantly modify the $I_{Kir2.1}$ in cells expressing Kir2.1 alone (**Figure 8A**; $P > 0.05$) but, as expected (van Bemmelen et al., 2004), it significantly decreased the $I_{Nav1.5}$ in cells expressing Nav1.5 channels alone ($P < 0.05$; **Figure 8B**), confirming that Nav1.5, but not Kir2.1 channels, are targeted by Nedd4-2. Importantly, both $I_{Kir2.1}$ and $I_{Nav1.5}$ densities recorded in cells coexpressing Kir2.1, Nav1.5, and Nedd4-2 were significantly reduced ($P < 0.05$). These results indicated that Kir2.1-Nav1.5 complexes were targeted by Nedd4-2 as Nav1.5 channels were and suggested that these complexes are degraded by the proteasome. To test this hypothesis, $I_{Kir2.1}$ (**Figure 8C**) and $I_{Nav1.5}$ (**Figure 8D**) were recorded in cells incubated with the proteasome inhibitor MG132 (20 μM) for 2 h (Shy et al., 2014). MG132 treatment increased the $I_{Nav1.5}$ in cells expressing Nav1.5 channels alone (**Figure 8D**; $P < 0.05$) without modifying the $I_{Kir2.1}$ in cells expressing Kir2.1 channels alone (**Figure 8C**; $P > 0.05$). It could be possible that the absence of effects of MG132 on $I_{Kir2.1}$ is due to the fact that degradation of Kir2.1 channels by the proteasome takes more time than that of Nav1.5 channels. To analyze this possibility, $I_{Kir2.1}$ was recorded in cells incubated with MG132 for a longer period of time (4 h). Under these conditions, $I_{Kir2.1}$ density was not significantly modified either (−159 ± 14 vs. −155 ± 18 pA/pF at −120 mV; $P > 0.05$). All these results are in agreement with the selective role of the proteosome in the degradation of Nav1.5 channels but not of Kir2.1 channels. In cells coexpressing Kir2.1 and Nav1.5 channels, incubation with MG132 produced a further increase of $I_{Kir2.1}$ and $I_{Nav1.5}$ densities compared to those generated by the positive reciprocal modulation (**Figures 8C,D**; $n \geq 6$; $P < 0.05$). These results would confirm that Nav1.5 channels and Kir2.1-Nav1.5 complexes are degraded by the proteasome.

DISCUSSION

The present results suggest that there is a pool of Nav1.5 and Kir2.1 channels that form complexes that exhibit biological properties similar to those of Nav1.5 channels.

Previous data have shown that in ventricular myocytes there is a positive reciprocal modulation between Kir2.1 and Nav1.5 channels (Milstein et al., 2012; Matamoros et al., 2016) which is due to their interaction with α1-syntrophin (Matamoros et al., 2016). The results here obtained with immunofluorescence

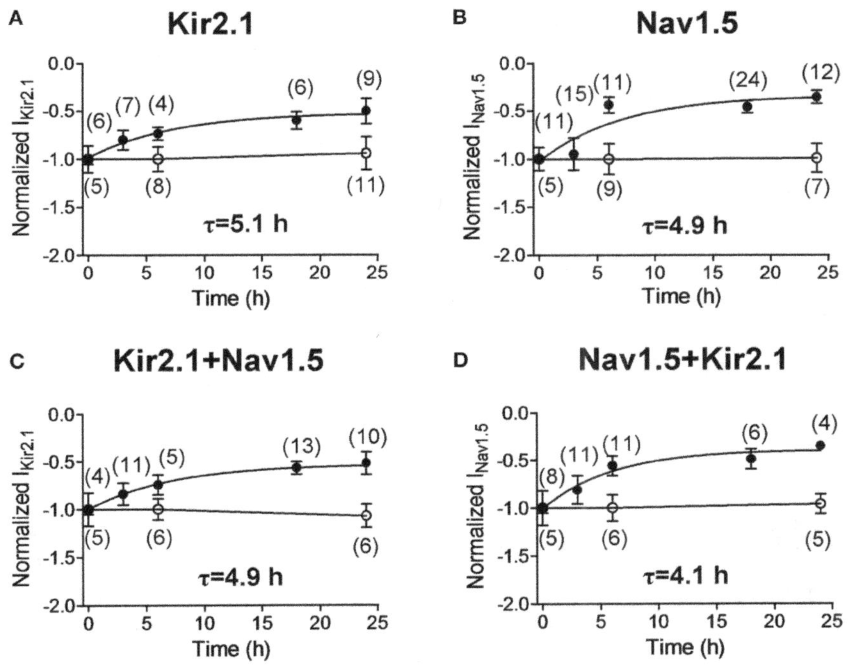

FIGURE 6 | Time course of internalization of Kir2.1 and Nav1.5 channels. **(A–D)** Mean normalized density of the currents recorded in CHO cells expressing the constructs indicated and incubated with BFA (50 ng/mL) (solid circles) for 0 (Control), 3, 6, 18, and 24 h or with 1% ethanol (open circles) for 0, 6, and 24 h. Half-time constants (τ) yielded by the monoexponential fit to the BFA data are also shown. Each point represents the mean ± SEM of (*n*) cells of ≥4 preparations.

experiments in heterologous expression systems suggested that cotransfection with Nav1.5 channels markedly increased the expression of Kir2.1. Therefore, these results seem to add further support to the hypothesis that the Kir2.1-Nav1.5 reciprocal modulation relies on the increase in the expression of the channels in the cell membrane. On the other hand, the PLA here conducted demonstrated that Kir2.1 and Nav1.5 channels are in close proximity to each other at the membrane of cardiac cells (<40 nm). Moreover, when both channels are expressed together, intracellular targeting Kir2.1 with a specific antibody reduces the $I_{Nav1.5}$ and *vice versa*. Therefore, we propose that there is a pool of Kir2.1 and Nav1.5 channels that form complexes (Milstein et al., 2012; Matamoros et al., 2016). Similarly, it has been shown that two voltage-dependent K^+ channels, Kv11.1 (hERG) and Kv7.1 (KvLQT1), may interact in such a way that expression of Kv7.1 increases Kv11.1 currents without major biophysical changes (Ehrlich et al., 2004). Recently it has been shown that this modulation is not due to the formation of heterotetrameric Kv11.1-Kv7.1 channels, suggesting that the positive modulation was due to the interaction between both subunits (Biliczki et al., 2015) in a similar way as we propose for Nav1.5 and Kir2.1.

It has been demonstrated that CaMKII co-immunoprecipitates with and phosphorylates Nav1.5 (Wagner et al., 2006; Herren et al., 2015). This modulation acutely affects the channel gating increasing the I_{NaL} without a noticeable effect over the peak current in HEK-293 cells (Ashpole et al., 2012). In our hands inhibition of CaMKII decreased the I_{NaL} and shifted the voltage dependence of $I_{Nav1.5}$ inactivation toward more positive potentials, results that are in agreement with those observed previously (Wagner et al., 2006). Additionally, here we demonstrated that long lasting CaMKII inhibition with KN93 or intracellular dialysis with AIP (two CaMKII inhibitors) decreased somehow the peak $I_{Nav1.5}$. On the other hand, Wagner et al. (2009) demonstrated that CaMKII can produce dual effects on Kir2.1 channels, downregulating the mRNA and protein expression, but acutely increasing the I_{K1} density in rabbit and mouse myocytes. Our co-immunoprecipitation experiments showed that Kir2.1 channels alone did not co-immunoprecipitate with CaMKII, conversely, in cells expressing both Kir2.1+Nav1.5 channels they did. In agreement with these results, KN93 significantly reduced the $I_{Kir2.1}$ when Kir2.1 and Nav1.5 channels are expressed together. Of note, in cardiac myocytes Nav1.5 and Kir2.1 channels are always expressed simultaneously, thus our results in transfection systems are in agreement with those obtained in native cells, i.e., CaMKII acutely increases $I_{Kir2.1}$ and its inhibition diminishes the current density. It can be speculated that the presence of Nav1.5 together with Kir2.1 promotes a conformation of Kir2.1 channels that allows their interaction with the kinase (Wagner et al., 2006, 2009). Alternatively, it is possible that CaMKII-induced phosphorylation of Nav1.5 affects Kir2.1 when both channels form complexes. Furthermore, the coexpression with Kir2.1 channels significantly increased the I_{NaL} which, in turn, was diminished by the inhibition of CamKII. Moreover, when the CaMKII is inhibited, Kir2.1 channels did not co-immunoprecipitate with Nav1.5 channels anymore. Therefore, we propose that formation of Nav1.5-Kir2.1

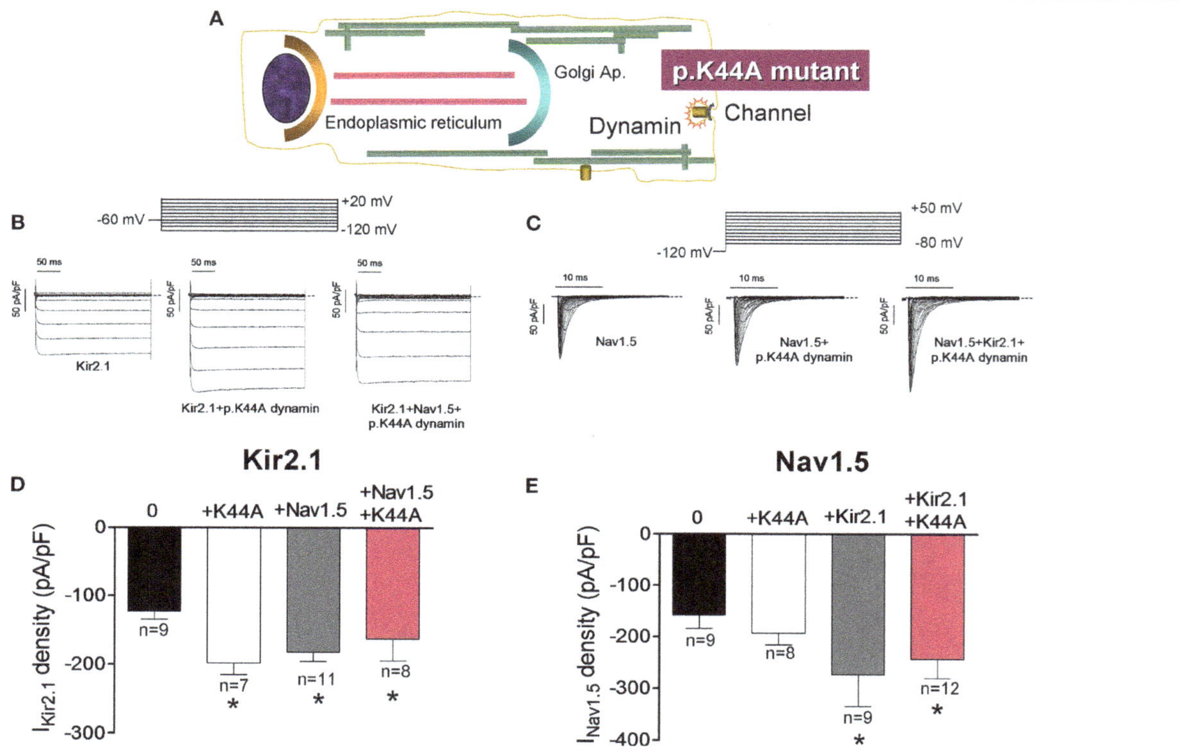

FIGURE 7 | Effects of the dynamin-2 inhibition on Kir2.1 and Nav1.5 channels internalization. **(A)** Schematic representation of a cell highlighting the role of dynamin-2 in ion channel endocytosis. **(B,C)** $I_{Kir2.1}$ **(B)** and $I_{Nav1.5}$ **(C)** traces recorded by applying the protocols shown at the top in CHO cells transfected with the constructs indicated. The dashed lines represent the zero current level. **(D,E)** Bar graphs depicting $I_{Kir2.1}$ density at −120 mV **(D)** and peak $I_{Nav1.5}$ **(E)** in cells expressing Kir2.1 and Nav1.5 channels, respectively in the absence or presence of the constructs indicated cotransfected or not with p.K44A dynamin-2. Each bar represents the mean ± SEM of "n" experiments of ≥3 preparations. $^{*}P < 0.01$ vs. cells transfected with Kir2.1 or Nav1.5 channels alone. For clarity the results of other statistical comparisons were not shown.

complexes strengthens the interaction of CaMKII with both Kir2.1 and Nav1.5 channels, and, importantly, that CaMKII plays a role in the positive reciprocal modulation between Nav1.5 and Kir2.1 channels that merits to be elucidated.

It has been proposed that binding of 14-3-3 to ER retention motifs (RXR) decreases channel affinity for coat-associated protein I (COPI), an essential component for the recycling of membrane proteins from the Golgi to the ER, promoting surface expression of properly folded channels (Balse et al., 2012). In our hands, 14-3-3DN did not modify $I_{Kir2.1}$ and $I_{Nav1.5}$ densities in cells expressing the individual channels but inhibited both currents in cells expressing Kir2.1+Nav1.5 channels. These results would mean that the presence of both channels together promotes the existence of a structural conformation that allows the ER retention motifs (RXR) of the channel proteins to be accessible for 14-3-3 preventing their binding to COPI (**Figure 9**). It is also possible that the effects observed upon 14-3-3 inhibition could be the consequence of the disruption of the interaction between Kir2.1 and Nav1.5 channels, avoiding the formation of the complexes. However, the results obtained with the intracellular application of anti-Kir2.1 and anti-Nav1.5 antibodies suggested that 14-3-3 inhibition did not preclude the formation of Nav1.5-Kir2.1 complexes. It has been demonstrated that protein kinase A (PKA)-dependent phosphorylation of Nav1.5 channels enhances Nav1.5-trafficking from the ER toward the membrane in rat cardiomyocytes (Zhou et al., 2002). This effect seems to be mediated by the PKA phosphorylation of sites (S525 and S528) that are proximally-located to an ER retention signal (Zhou et al., 2002). On the other hand, 14-3-3 proteins preferentially bind to phosphorylated proteins and protect them from dephosphorylation, thus enhancing the effects derived from phosphorylation (Kagan et al., 2002; Tutor et al., 2006). Allouis and co-workers demonstrated that 14-3-3 proteins bind to the intracellular I to II linker of Nav1.5 channels, i.e., close to the PKA phosphorylation site (Allouis et al., 2006) and, thus, also probably protect Nav1.5 channels from dephosphorylation. Should this occur, binding of 14-3-3 proteins to Nav1.5 channels would increase the I_{Na} by enhancing the Nav1.5 trafficking from the ER toward the plasma membrane. Conversely, 14-3-3 binding to Nav1.5 channels does not increase the I_{Na} density (Allouis et al., 2006) as demonstrated in experiments conducted in hetereologous expression systems in which only Nav1.5 channels were transfected (Allouis et al., 2006 and the present results). It can be hypothesized that 14-3-3 proteins enhance the anterograde traffic of Nav1.5-Kir2.1 channel complexes, but not that of Nav1.5 channels alone. This would explain why

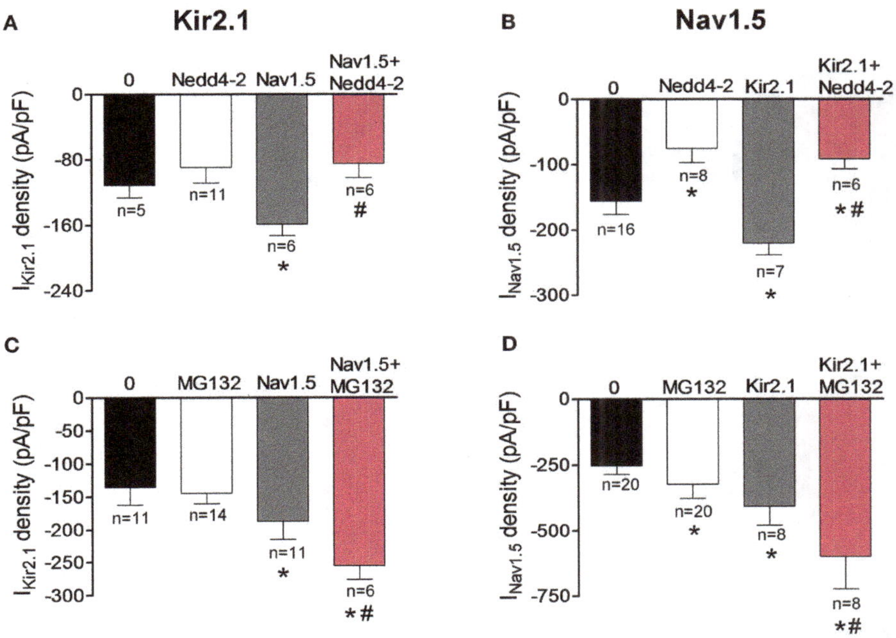

FIGURE 8 | Kir2.1 and Nav1.5 channel complexes are ubyquitinated and degraded by the proteasome. **(A,B)** $I_{Kir2.1}$ density at −120 mV **(A)** and peak $I_{Nav1.5}$ **(B)** recorded in cells expressing Kir2.1 and Nav1.5 channels cotransfected or not with the ubiquitin ligase Nedd4-2. **(C,D)** $I_{Kir2.1}$ density at −120 mV **(C)** and peak $I_{Nav1.5}$ **(D)** recorded in cells expressing Kir2.1 and Nav1.5 channels incubated or not with the proteasome inhibitor MG132 (2 μM for 2 h). Each bar represents the mean ± SEM of "n" experiments of ≥4 preparations. $^*P < 0.05$ vs. cells transfected with Kir2.1 or Nav1.5 channels alone; $^\#P < 0.05$ vs. cells transfected with Kir2.1+Nav1.5. For clarity the results of other statistical comparisons were not shown.

inhibition of 14-3-3 proteins decreased the $I_{Nav1.5}$ density in cells cotransfected with Nav1.5+Kir2.1 channels but not in cells transfected with Nav1.5 channels alone. Similarly, this would explain the $I_{Kir2.1}$ increase observed in cells cotransfected with Nav1.5 and Kir2.1 channels. Further experiments are needed to test this hypothesis.

Overall, data here presented support the contention that at least a pool of Nav1.5 and Kir2.1 channels form complexes whose behavior is not identical to each channel separately (**Figure 9**). It has been described that in the brain Kir2.1 can form complexes with several anchoring and regulatory proteins such as SAP97 and Veli (Leonoudakis et al., 2004). However, the existence of such complexes in the heart has not been described thus far. Therefore, to further characterize the biology of the complexes, we analyzed how some of the mechanisms involved in anterograde and retrograde trafficking of the individual channels are affected when they are expressed together. Microtubule cytoskeleton is involved in ion channel trafficking by means of the dynein and kinesin motors that track along microtubules (Balse et al., 2012). The experiments conducted in cells overexpressing the p50 subunit to inhibit the dynein/dynamitin motor complex showed that it is involved in the retrograde and anterograde trafficking of Kir2.1 and Nav1.5 channels, respectively. Our results confirm previous data showing that p50 interacts with Nav1.5 channels reducing their expression at the cell surface and the $I_{Nav1.5}$ density (Chatin et al., 2014). Importantly, our results also suggested that the dynein/dynamitin motor complex is critical for the anterograde trafficking of the pool of Kir2.1 and Nav1.5 channels that form the complexes, supporting the hypothesis that their biology may be similar to that of Nav1.5 channels (**Figure 9**).

The experiments conducted in cells incubated with BFA, demonstrated that internalization kinetics of Kir2.1-Nav1.5 complexes is similar to that of Kir2.1 and Nav1.5 channels alone. However, our results suggest that the internalization process of Kir2.1 channels is qualitatively different to that of the Kir2.1-Nav1.5 complexes. We demonstrated that dynamin-2 inhibition by overexpression of the p.K44A mutant increased the $I_{Kir2.1}$, but not the $I_{Nav1.5}$, confirming that Kir2.1 channel endocytosis is dynamin-dependent (Tong et al., 2001; Boyer et al., 2009), whereas that of Nav1.5 is not (Laedermann et al., 2014). Interestingly, p.K44A did not modify $I_{Kir2.1}$ and $I_{Nav1.5}$ generated in cells expressing both channels, suggesting that the internalization of Kir2.1-Nav1.5 complexes is not dynamin-dependent either (**Figure 9**). It has been shown that Nav1.5 channels internalization relies on ubiquitination by Nedd4-2 (van Bemmelen et al., 2004; Rougier et al., 2005; Laedermann et al., 2014). Data on Kir2.1 ubiquitination are scarce, although it was proposed that Nedd4-2 may reduce $I_{Kir2.1}$ density in *Xenopus* oocytes (Alesutan et al., 2011). Our results confirmed that overexpression of Nedd4-2 reduces the $I_{Nav1.5}$ but not the $I_{Kir2.1}$ in cells expressing Nav1.5 and Kir2.1 channels alone, respectively. Interestingly, both $I_{Kir2.1}$ and $I_{Nav1.5}$ were reduced in cells expressing both Kir2.1 and Nav1.5 channels suggesting that the putative Kir2.1-Nav1.5 complexes are ubiquitinated by Nedd4-2 (**Figure 9**). It has been proposed that the fate of the ubiquitinated

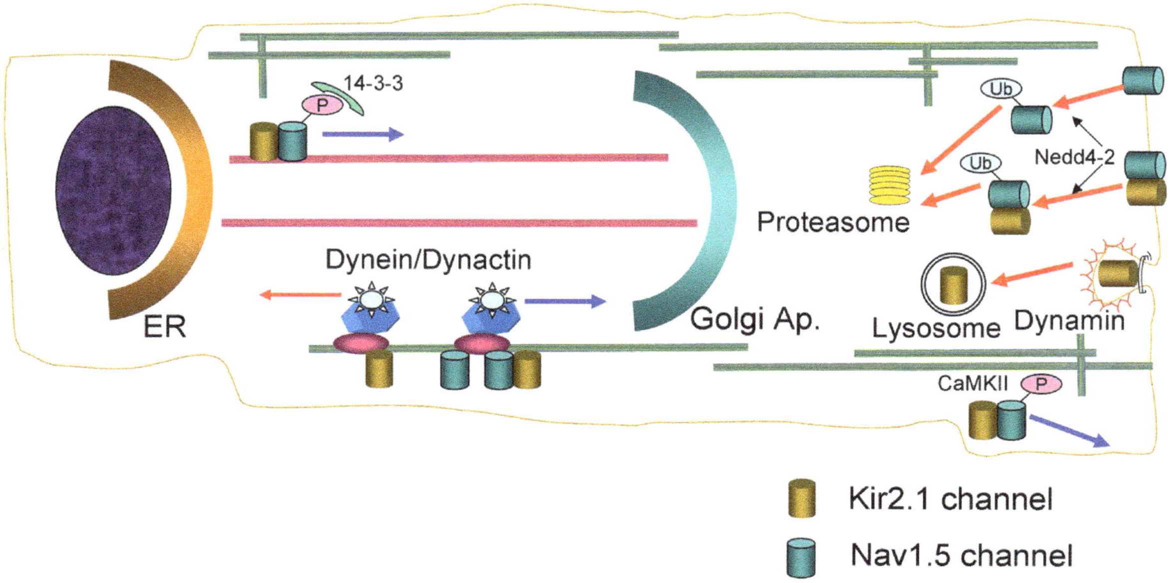

FIGURE 9 | Schematic diagram summarizing the main findings of the present study. Nav1.5 and Kir2.1 channels are represented by green and golden cylinders, respectively. ER, endoplasmic reticulum; P, phosphate; Ub, ubiquitin chains.

channels is different depending on whether they are mono- or polyubiquitinated. Monoubiquitinated proteins are more prone to enter a recycling pathway, whereas polyubiquitinated ones are preferentially degraded by the proteasome (Laedermann et al., 2014). Rougier et al. (2005) demonstrated that in HEK293 cells Nav1.5 channels are polyubiquitinated suggesting that they are subject to proteasomal degradation. Other studies, however, suggested that *in vivo* Nav1.5 could be mono- or polyubiquitinated (Laedermann et al., 2014). Our results suggested that Nav1.5 and Kir2.1-Nav1.5 complexes are polyubiquitinated and degraded by the proteasome (**Figure 9**).

Physiological Relevance

I_{K1} and I_{Na} play a key role in regulating cardiac excitability under physiological conditions and in the control of the frequency of the rotors that are responsible for fibrillating arrhythmias (Jalife, 2016). The classical paradigm considered that these currents were functionally coupled. Our results provide new evidences demonstrating that there is also a physical interaction between a pool of Nav1.5 and Kir2.1 channels that allows the formation of complexes, which probably are formed at early stages of protein assembly. By means of such a mechanism, the membrane expression of these ion channels in the ventricles can be strictly and simultaneously regulated, allowing a tighter control of the resting membrane potential and excitability and thus, preventing the ocurrence of fibrillating arrhythmias. Therefore, it can be speculated that changes in the expression of one of the channels, such as those produced by disease-associated remodeling or mutations, could concomitantly alter the expression of the other channel. We recently demonstrated that in human atrial myocytes obtained from patients in sinus rhythm and chronic atrial fibrillation (CAF) the CAF-induced I_{K1} increase was not accompanied by an I_{Na} increase. This result was explained considering that the presence of Kir2.3 subunits precludes the reciprocal positive modulation between Nav1.5 and Kir2.x channels (Matamoros et al., 2016) and that in the human atria Kir2.3 channels are preferentially expressed (Gaborit et al., 2007). Further studies are needed to analyze whether changes in the expression of Kir2.1 or Nav1.5 produced by disease-associated remodeling process (for instance the Kir2.1 decrease produced by heart failure) might be accompanied by reciprocal decreases of either the I_{Na} or the I_{K1} in the human ventricle. On the other hand, the consequences of the presence of mutated Nav1.5 or Kir2.1 channels on the ventricular I_{K1} and the I_{Na}, respectively, must also be elucidated.

Limitations of the Study

Most of the results were obtained in heterologous expression systems and not in cardiac myocytes. This allowed us to compare separately the effects of each experimental maneuver on Nav1.5 and Kir2.1 channels as well as on the Kir2.1-Nav1.5 complexes. It is important to note that the vast majority of the information on cardiac ion channel biology has been obtained in expression systems (Balse et al., 2012). This could be accounted for considering the limited survival of cultured cardiac myocytes, since for the analysis of the channel biology the transfection with the cDNA encoding several proteins or the incubation with some reagents with high toxicity is needed. Our results stress the fact that results obtained in heterologous expression systems with isolated channels could be different to what actually occurs in cardiac myocytes where the rest of the channels are also present.

CONCLUSION

Overall our results suggest that there is a pool of Nav1.5 and Kir2.1 channels that form complexes with anterograde and retrograde trafficking routes similar to those of Nav1.5 channels alone. These complexes allow a tight control of the current densities that determine cardiac excitability and action potential propagation. Therefore, the formation of the complexes would have an important physiological and/or pathological relevance that merits further investigation.

AUTHOR CONTRIBUTIONS

Conducting experiments, acquiring and analyzing data, RGU, PN-M, SA, DT, MM, MP-H, SS, LO, RdA, and FJD-G. Designing research, analyzing data, and writing MS: JT, ED, and RC.

ACKNOWLEDGMENTS

We thank Paloma Vaquero for her invaluable technical assistance.

REFERENCES

Abriel, H. (2010). Cardiac sodium channel Na(v)1.5 and interacting proteins: physiology and pathophysiology. *J. Mol. Cell. Cardiol.* 48, 2–11. doi: 10.1016/j.yjmcc.2009.08.025

Alesutan, I., Munoz, C., Sopjani, M., Dërmaku-Sopjani, M., Michael, D., Fraser, S., et al. (2011). Inhibition of Kir2.1 (KCNJ2) by the AMP-activated protein kinase. *Biochem. Biophys. Res. Commun.* 408, 505–510. doi: 10.1016/j.bbrc.2011.04.015

Allouis, M., Le Bouffant, F., Wilders, R., Péroz, D., Schott, J. J., Noireaud, J., et al. (2006). 14-3-3 is a regulator of the cardiac voltage-gated sodium channel Nav1.5. *Circ. Res.* 98, 1538–1546. doi: 10.1161/01.RES.0000229244.97497.2c

Anumonwo, J. M., and Lopatin, A. N. (2010). Cardiac strong inward rectifier potassium channels. *J. Mol. Cell. Cardiol.* 48, 45–54. doi: 10.1016/j.yjmcc.2009.08.013

Archer, S. L., Souil, E., Dinh-Xuan, A. T., Schremmer, B., Mercier, J. C., El Yaagoubi, A., et al. (1998). Molecular identification of the role of voltage-gated K^+ channels, Kv1.5 and Kv2.1, in hypoxic pulmonary vasoconstriction and control of resting membrane potential in rat pulmonary artery myocytes. *J. Clin. Invest.* 101, 2319–2330. doi: 10.1172/JCI333

Ashpole, N. M., Herren, A. W., Ginsburg, K. S., Brogan, J. D., Johnson, D. E., Cummins, T. R., et al. (2012). Ca^{2+}/calmodulin-dependent protein kinase II (CaMKII) regulates cardiac sodium channel $Na_V1.5$ gating by multiple phosphorylation sites. *J. Biol. Chem.* 287, 19856–19869. doi: 10.1074/jbc.M111.322537

Balse, E., Steele, D. F., Abriel, H., Coulombe, A., Fedida, D., and Hatem, S. N. (2012). Dynamic of ion channel expression at the plasma membrane of cardiomyocytes. *Physiol. Rev.* 92, 1317–1358. doi: 10.1152/physrev.00041.2011

Biliczki, P., Rüdiger, A., Girmatsion, Z., Pourrier, M., Mamarbachi, A. M., Hébert, T. E., et al. (2015). The interaction between delayed rectifier channel alpha-subunits does not involve hetero-tetramer formation. *Naunyn Schmiedebergs Arch. Pharmacol.* 388, 973–981. doi: 10.1007/s00210-015-1108-3

Boyer, S. B., Slesinger, P. A., and Jones, S. V. (2009). Regulation of Kir2.1 channels by the Rho-GTPase, Rac1. *J. Cell Physiol.* 218, 385–393. doi: 10.1002/jcp.21610

Burkhardt, J. K., Echeverri, C. J., Nilsson, T., and Vallee, R. B. (1997). Overexpression of the dynamitin (p50) subunit of the dynactin complex disrupts dynein-dependent maintenance of membrane organelle distribution. *J. Cell Biol.* 139, 469–484. doi: 10.1083/jcb.139.2.469

Caballero, R., de la Fuente, M. G., Gómez, R., Barana, A., Amorós, I., Dolz-Gaitón, P., et al. (2010a). In humans, chronic atrial fibrillation decreases the transient outward current and ultrarapid component of the delayed rectifier current differentially on each atria and increases the slow component of the delayed rectifier current in both. *J. Am. Coll. Cardiol.* 55, 2346–2354. doi: 10.1016/j.jacc.2010.02.028

Caballero, R., Dolz-Gaitón, P., Gómez, R., Amorós, I., Barana, A., González de la Fuente, M., et al. (2010b). Flecainide increases Kir2.1 currents by interacting with cysteine 311, decreasing the polyamine-induced rectification. *Proc. Natl. Acad. Sci. U.S.A.* 107, 15631–15636. doi: 10.1073/pnas.1004021107

Caballero, R., Utrilla, R. G., Amorós, I., Matamoros, M., Pérez-Hernández, M., Tinaquero, D., et al. (2017). Tbx20 controls the expression of the KCNH2 gene and of hERG channels. *Proc. Natl. Acad. Sci. U.S.A.* 114, E416–E425. doi: 10.1073/pnas.1612383114

Chatin, B., Colombier, P., Gamblin, A. L., Allouis, M., and Le Bouffant, F. (2014). Dynamitin affects cell-surface expression of voltage-gated sodium channel Nav1.5. *Biochem. J.* 463, 339–349. doi: 10.1042/BJ20140604

de Boer, T. P., Houtman, M. J., Compier, M., and van der Heyden, M. A. (2010). The mammalian K(IR)2.x inward rectifier ion channel family: expression pattern and pathophysiology. *Acta Physiol.* 199, 243–256. doi: 10.1111/j.1748-1716.2010.02108.x

Ehrlich, J. R., Pourrier, M., Weerapura, M., Ethier, N., Marmabachi, A. M., Hébert, T. E., et al. (2004). KvLQT1 modulates the distribution and biophysical properties of HERG. A novel alpha-subunit interaction between delayed rectifier currents. *J. Biol. Chem.* 279, 1233–1241. doi: 10.1074/jbc.M309087200

Gaborit, N., Le Bouter, S., Szuts, V., Varro, A., Escande, D., Nattel, S., et al. (2007). Regional and tissue specific transcript signatures of ion channel genes in the non-diseased human heart. *J. Physiol.* 582, 675–693. doi: 10.1113/jphysiol.2006.126714

Herren, A. W., Weber, D. M., Rigor, R. R., Margulies, K. B., Phinney, B. S., and Bers, D. M. (2015). CaMKII phosphorylation of Na(v)1.5: novel *in vitro* sites identified by mass spectrometry and reduced S516 phosphorylation in human heart failure. *J. Proteome Res.* 14, 2298–2311. doi: 10.1021/acs.jproteome.5b00107

Hinshaw, J. E., and Schmid, S. L. (1995). Dynamin self-assembles into rings suggesting a mechanism for coated vesicle budding. *Nature* 374, 190–192. doi: 10.1038/374190a0

Jalife, J. (2016). Dynamics and molecular mechanisms of ventricular fibrillation in structurally normal hearts. *Card. Electrophysiol. Clin.* 8, 601–612. doi: 10.1016/j.ccep.2016.04.009

Kagan, A., Melman, Y. F., Krumerman, A., and McDonald, T. V. (2002). 14-3-3 amplifies and prolongs adrenergic stimulation of HERG K^+ channel activity. *EMBO J.* 21, 1889–1898. doi: 10.1093/emboj/21.8.1889

Laedermann, C. J., Decosterd, I., and Abriel, H. (2014). Ubiquitylation of voltage-gated sodium channels. *Handb. Exp. Pharmacol.* 221, 231–250. doi: 10.1007/978-3-642-41588-3_11

Leonoudakis, D., Conti, L. R., Radeke, C. M., McGuire, L. M., and Vandenberg, C. A. (2004). A multiprotein trafficking complex composed of SAP97, CASK, Veli, and Mint1 is associated with inward rectifier Kir2 potassium channels. *J. Biol. Chem.* 279, 19051–19063. doi: 10.1074/jbc.M400284200

Matamoros, M., Pérez-Hernández, M., Guerrero-Serna, G., Amorós, I., Barana, A., Núñez, M., et al. (2016). Nav1.5 N-terminal domain binding to α1-syntrophin increases membrane density of human Kir2.1, Kir2.2 and Nav1.5 channels. *Cardiovasc. Res.* 110, 279–290. doi: 10.1093/cvr/cvw009

Mercier, A., Clément, R., Harnois, T., Bourmeyster, N., Bois, P., and Chatelier, A. (2015). Nav1.5 channels can reach the plasma membrane through distinct N-glycosylation states. *Biochim. Biophys. Acta* 1850, 1215–1223. doi: 10.1016/j.bbagen.2015.02.009

Milstein, M. L., Musa, H., Balbuena, D. P., Anumonwo, J. M., Auerbach, D. S., Furspan, P. B., et al. (2012). Dynamic reciprocity of sodium and potassium channel expression in a macromolecular complex controls cardiac excitability and arrhythmia. *Proc. Natl. Acad. Sci. U.S.A.* 109, E2134–E2143. doi: 10.1073/pnas.1109370109

Núñez, L., Barana, A., Amorós, I., de la Fuente, M. G., Dolz-Gaitón, P., Gómez, R., et al. (2013). p.D1690N Nav1.5 rescues p.G1748D mutation gating defects in a compound heterozygous Brugada syndrome patient. *Heart Rhythm* 10, 264–272. doi: 10.1016/j.hrthm.2012.10.025

Obsil, T., and Obsilova, V. (2011). Structural basis of 14-3-3 protein functions. *Semin. Cell Dev. Biol.* 22, 663–672. doi: 10.1016/j.semcdb.2011.09.001

Pawley, J. B. (2006). "Points, pixels, and gray levels: digitizing image data," in *Handbook of Biological Confocal Microscopy, 3rd Edn.*, ed B. J. Pawley (New York, NY: Springer Science+Business Media, LLC), 64–68.

Rougier, J. S., van Bemmelen, M. X., Bruce, M. C., Jespersen, T., Gavillet, B., Apothéloz, F., et al. (2005). Molecular determinants of voltage-gated sodium channel regulation by the Nedd4/Nedd4-like proteins. *Am. J. Physiol. Cell Physiol.* 288, C692–C701. doi: 10.1152/ajpcell.00460.2004

Shy, D., Gillet, L., Ogrodnik, J., Albesa, M., Verkerk, A. O., Wolswinkel, R., et al. (2014). PDZ domain-binding motif regulates cardiomyocyte compartment-specific Nav1.5 channel expression and function. *Circulation* 130, 147–160. doi: 10.1161/CIRCULATIONAHA.113.007852

Söderberg, O., Gullberg, M., Jarvius, M., Ridderstråle, K., Leuchowius, K. J., Jarvius, J., et al. (2006). Direct observation of individual endogenous protein complexes *in situ* by proximity ligation. *Nat. Methods* 3, 995–1000. doi: 10.1038/nmeth947

Tong, Y., Brandt, G. S., Li, M., Shapovalov, G., Slimko, E., Karschin, A., et al. (2001). Tyrosine decaging leads to substantial membrane trafficking during modulation of an inward rectifier potassium channel. *J. Gen. Physiol.* 117, 103–118. doi: 10.1085/jgp.117.2.103

Tutor, A. S., Delpón, E., Caballero, R., Gómez, R., Núñez, L., Vaquero, M., et al. (2006). Association of 14-3-3 proteins to β1-adrenergic receptors modulates Kv11.1 K^+ channel activity in recombinant systems. *Mol. Biol. Cell* 17, 4666–4674. doi: 10.1091/mbc.E06-05-0422

van Bemmelen, M. X., Rougier, J. S., Gavillet, B., Apothéloz, F., Daidié, D., Tateyama, M., et al. (2004). Cardiac voltage-gated sodium channel Nav1.5 is regulated by Nedd4-2 mediated ubiquitination. *Circ. Res.* 95, 284–291. doi: 10.1161/01.RES.0000136816.05109.89

Wagner, S., Dybkova, N., Rasenack, E. C., Jacobshagen, C., Fabritz, L., Kirchhof, P., et al. (2006). Ca^{2+}/calmodulin-dependent protein kinase II regulates cardiac Na^+ channels. *J. Clin. Invest.* 116, 3127–3138. doi: 10.1172/JCI26620

Wagner, S., Hacker, E., Grandi, E., Weber, S. L., Dybkova, N., Sossalla, S., et al. (2009). Ca/calmodulin kinase II differentially modulates potassium currents. *Circ. Arrhythm. Electrophysiol.* 2, 285–294. doi: 10.1161/CIRCEP.108.842799

Wilde, A. A., and Brugada, R. (2011). Phenotypical manifestations of mutations in the genes encoding subunits of the cardiac sodium channel. *Circ. Res.* 108, 884–897. doi: 10.1161/CIRCRESAHA.110.238469

Xu, P., Duong, D. M., Seyfried, N. T., Cheng, D., Xie, Y., Robert, J., et al. (2009). Quantitative proteomics reveals the function of unconventional ubiquitin chains in proteasomal degradation. *Cell* 137, 133–145. doi: 10.1016/j.cell.2009.01.041

Zhou, J., Shin, H. G., Yi, J., Shen, W., Williams, C. P., and Murray, K. T. (2002). Phosphorylation and putative ER retention signals are required for protein kinase A-mediated potentiation of cardiac sodium current. *Circ. Res.* 91, 540–546. doi: 10.1161/01.RES.0000033598.00903.27

12

The Effect of Emotional Valence on Ventricular Repolarization Dynamics is Mediated by Heart Rate Variability: A Study of QT Variability and Music-Induced Emotions

Michele Orini[1,2], Faez Al-Amodi[1], Stefan Koelsch[3] and Raquel Bailón[4,5]*

[1] Institute of Cardiovascular Sciences, University College London, London, United Kingdom, [2] The William Harvey Research Institute, Queen Mary University of London, London, United Kingdom, [3] Department of Biological and Medical Psychology, University of Bergen, Bergen, Norway, [4] Aragon Institute for Engineering Research, University of Zaragoza, Zaragoza, Spain, [5] Center for Biomedical Research in the Network in Bioengineering, Biomaterials and Nanomedicine (CIBER-BBN), Madrid, Spain

***Correspondence:**
Michele Orini
m.orini@ucl.ac.uk;
michele.orini.maculotti@gmail.com

Background: Emotions can affect cardiac activity, but their impact on ventricular repolarization variability, an important parameter providing information about cardiac risk and autonomic nervous system activity, is unknown. The beat-to-beat variability of the QT interval (QTV) from the body surface ECG is a non-invasive marker of repolarization variability, which can be decomposed into QTV related to RR variability (QTVrRRV) and QTV unrelated to RRV (QTVuRRV), with the latter thought to be a marker of intrinsic repolarization variability.

Aim: To determine the effect of emotional valence (pleasant and unpleasant) on repolarization variability in healthy volunteers by means of QTV analysis.

Methods: 75 individuals (24.5 ± 3.2 years, 36 females) without a history of cardiovascular disease listened to music-excerpts that were either felt as pleasant ($n = 6$) or unpleasant ($n = 6$). Excerpts lasted about 90 s and were presented in a random order along with silent intervals ($n = 6$). QTV and RRV were derived from the ECG and the time-frequency spectrum of RRV, QTV, QTVuRRV and QTVrRRV as well as time-frequency coherence between QTV and RRV were estimated. Analysis was performed in low-frequency (LF), high frequency (HF) and total spectral bands.

Results: The heart rate-corrected QTV showed a small but significant increase from silence (median 347/interquartile range 31 ms) to listening to music felt as unpleasant (351/30 ms) and pleasant (355/32 ms). The dynamic response of QTV to emotional valence showed a transient phase lasting about 20 s after the onset of each musical excerpt. QTV and RRV were highly correlated in both HF and LF (mean coherence ranging 0.76–0.85). QTV and QTVrRRV decreased during listening to music felt as pleasant and unpleasant with respect to silence and further decreased during listening to music felt as pleasant. QTVuRRV was small and not affected by emotional valence.

Conclusion: Emotional valence, as evoked by music, has a small but significant effect on QTV and QTVrRRV, but not on QTVuRRV. This suggests that the interaction between emotional valence and ventricular repolarization variability is mediated by cycle length dynamics and not due to intrinsic repolarization variability.

Keywords: QT variability, heart rate variability, repolarization, music-induced emotions, emotional valence, time-frequency

INTRODUCTION

The beat to beat variability of the QT interval (QTV) of the electrocardiogram is an established measure of ventricular repolarization dynamics and a marker of both cardiovascular risk and cardiac autonomic modulation (Baumert et al., 2016). Since the QTV correlates with the cardiac cycle length through cardiac restitution properties (Orini et al., 2016), QTV is largely affected by RR variability (RRV), which reflects supra-ventricular as opposed to ventricular dynamics. A methodology that separates QTV into two components, one related to RRV and the other unrelated to RRV and thought to represent intrinsic repolarization variability, has been recently proposed (Orini et al., 2018).

Emotions are known to be associated with changes in cardiac function, mediated by the autonomic nervous system. These changes include parameters such as heart rate, heart rate variability and respiration (Steptoe and Brydon, 2009; Steptoe and Kivimäki, 2012). In some studies, emotions have been linked to increased risk of malignant arrhythmias and cardiovascular diseases (Taggart et al., 2011a,b), in particular when related to stress (Steptoe and Kivimäki, 2012). Emotions can be measured along two dimensions: intensity (arousal) and valence (attractiveness versus averseness), with the former exerting a stronger effect on physiological parameters (Hilz et al., 2014). The impact of emotional valence on cardiac repolarization is unknown.

This study investigates for the first time the dynamic interactions between emotional valence and QTV in healthy volunteers, and sought to determine whether the QTV response reflects intrinsic ventricular repolarization dynamics or is mediated by RRV. As in previous studies (Orini et al., 2010; Krabs et al., 2015), emotional states with opposite valence (pleasantness and unpleasantness) were induced by listening to pleasant or noise-like unpleasant music, while silence was used as a baseline control.

MATERIALS AND METHODS

Experimental Set-Up

The experimental set-up was described in details in previous studies (Orini et al., 2010; Krabs et al., 2015) and examples of the acoustic stimuli can be found in Krabs et al. (2015). Briefly, 75 volunteers (age 24.5 ± 3.2 years, 36 female) listened to acoustic stimuli through headphones at a comfortable loudness of around 60 dB in supine position with closed eyes. Participants were exposed to: (1) Six excerpts of pleasant joyful instrumental music (pleasant condition). (2) Six excerpts of isochronous Shepard tones. (3) Six excerpts of isochronous Shepard tones overlaid with unpleasant dissonant music-like noise (unpleasant condition). These were electronically created by recording backward a modified version of the pleasant excerpts, previously simultaneously recorded one semitone above and a tritone below the original pitch. (4) Six intervals of silence (resting condition). All excerpts and intervals of silence lasted about 90 s and were presented in the same randomized order (an example will be described in the "Results" section). All excerpts were matched by tempo and volume in an attempt to control for emotional arousal. Successive excerpts were separated by a 20 s pause during which participants were requested to rate how they felt by pressing response buttons (participants were asked to rate their own emotional state on a six point scale from 1, "very pleasant" to 6, "very unpleasant"). To ensure that participants paid equal attention to all excerpts, they were instructed to listen carefully and to tap the meter of the stimuli with their right index finger. No tapping was required during the resting condition. The study was approved by the ethics committee of the University of Leipzig. Written informed consent was obtained from all participants.

ECG Analysis

Standard 12 lead electrocardiograms were measured using a 32 MREFA amplifier (Twente Medical Systems, Enschede, Netherlands) and digitized with a sampling rate of 1000 Hz. For the sake of this study, lead V4 was analyzed to derive the main results while lead II was used to assess intra-lead reproducibility. This was chosen because lead V4 usually shows tall R- and T-waves and was therefore assumed to be characterized by high signal-to-noise ratio (Baumert et al., 2016), whereas lead II is one of the most clinically relevant and most widely used lead. The data were analyzed off-line using MATLAB, MathWorks. The peak of the R-wave and the end of the T-wave were detected, with the latter measured using the tangent method (**Figure 1**). The RT interval was used as a robust estimate of the QTV, which is particularly suitable for analysis of beat to beat variability. In fact, QT and RT variabilities are expected to be very similar, because the beat-to-beat variability of the QRS duration in sinus rhythm in healthy volunteers is negligible, and RT measurement is more robust than QT measurement as the identification of the R-wave peak is easier than the identification of QRS onset. All recordings were revised. Artifacts and ectopic beats were rare and were corrected using a bespoke graphical user interface as in previous studies (Orini et al., 2016, 2017b).

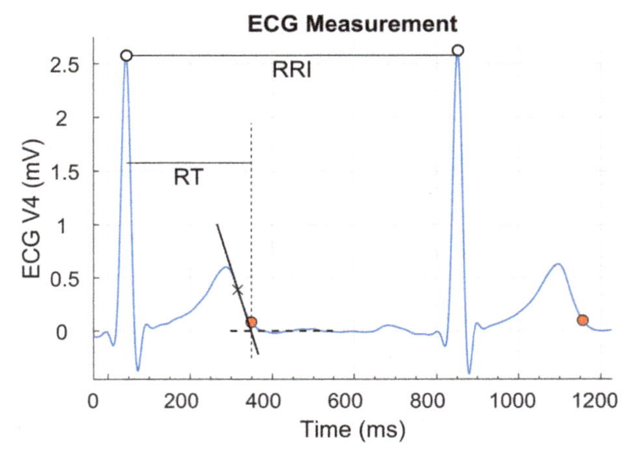

FIGURE 1 | Measurement of RR and QT intervals. White and red circles identify the R-wave and the end of the T-wave, respectively. The RT interval variability was used as robust surrogate for QT variability.

QTV and HRV Analysis

Time series were evenly resampled at 4 Hz. Time-frequency distributions were used to study the time course of the signals' spectral components and overcome the limitations of traditional spectral analysis in non-stationary conditions (Cohen, 1989; Hlawatsch and Boudreaux-Bartels, 1992). The Wigner-Ville distribution of RRV and QTV signals were filtered using a kernel designed to provide the minimum amount of time-frequency smoothing while achieving complete elimination of crossterms and time-frequency coherence bounded between zero and one (Orini et al., 2012c,d). Temporal and spectral resolutions were 12.5 s and 0.039 Hz, respectively. The time-frequency coherence between QTV and RRV was computed using previously described algorithms (Orini et al., 2012c). This time-frequency representation provides an assessment of the local linear coupling between the signals' spectral components in both time and frequency. It ranges from zero to one, and it is equal to one for a given time, t_0, and frequency, f_0, if at time t_0 the two signals show an oscillation with same instantaneous frequency f_0. The time-frequency spectrum of QTV was separated into two components, one representing QTV related to RRV (QTVrRRV) and the other representing QTV unrelated to RRV (QTVuRRV). This was achieved by modulating the time-frequency spectrum of QTV, $S_{QT}(t, f)$, by the time-frequency coherence between QTV and RRV, $\gamma_{QTV,RV}(t, f)$ as demonstrated in Orini et al. (2018):

$$S_{QTVuRR}(t, f) = S_{QTV}(t, f) - S_{QTVrRRV}(t, f) =$$

$$\left(1 - \left|\gamma_{QTV,RRV}(t, f)\right|^2\right) S_{QTV}(t, f)$$

The time course of the magnitude of low frequency (LF) and high frequency (HF) oscillations were obtained by averaging the time-frequency distributions in the LF (0.04–0.15 Hz) and HF (0.15–0.4) spectral bands. The time course of the total signals' magnitude was obtained by averaging the time-frequency distributions in the spectral band (0.04–0.4 Hz).

Statistical Analysis

ECG recordings from five individuals were discarded due to insufficient signal quality.

To assess physiological changes between different conditions, pair-wise comparisons were performed using the Wilcoxon signed-rank test for related samples. 18 physiological indices were considered (see **Table 1**). For each one of them, the temporal mean was obtained in 50 s long temporal windows starting 20 s after the onset of a given condition to exclude the transient occurring immediately after the condition's onset (Orini et al., 2010). This provided a single value for each one of the 24 epochs (6 different excerpts × 4 conditions). Values corresponding to the same condition (i.e., pleasant, unpleasant, rest, and Shepard tones) were grouped and averaged to provide a single value per condition per individual. Mathematically, this is described as:

$$X_i^C = \frac{1}{T \times R} \sum_{j=1}^{6} \overline{X_i^{C,j}}$$

where X_i^C is a scalar representing a given physiological index X for the individual $i = \{1 : N\}$ during condition $C = \{Pleasant, Unpleasant, Rest, Shepard\}$ obtained by averaging the tempotal mean $\overline{X_i^{C,j}}$ across epochs j.

For the sake of this study, the condition characterized by Shepard tones was not considered and comparisons were performed between pleasant, unpleasant and resting conditions. In total, 54 pairwise tests were performed (5 time-frequency indices × 3 spectral bands × 3 comparisons + 3 time invariant indices × 3 comparisons). Threshold for significance was set at $P < 9.26 \times 10^{-4}$ after Bonferroni correction.

RESULTS

There was agreement between the participants' ratings, with all participants rating the consonant excerpts as more pleasant than the dissonant ones (see **Supplementary Figure S1**). On a scale from 1 (very pleasant) to 6 (very unpleasant), ratings were equal to (median, 1st–3rd quartiles): 2.4, 1.9–2.9 for silence, 1.8, 1.7–2.2 for pleasant music, 4.7, 4.2–5.2 for noise-like unpleasant music and 4.1, 3.54.5 for Shepard's tones. All comparisons were highly significant after Bonferroni correction ($P < 5 \times 10^{-6}$, Wilcoxon signed-rank test).

A representative example of temporal fluctuations in QT and RR intervals during the entire procedure is shown in **Figure 2**, where vertical dashed lines represent different epochs. As shown in the inset at the bottom of the figure, QT and RR exhibit similar oscillations and they were therefore characterized by a high level of time-frequency coherence.

Detailed results, including median and interquartile range of all physiological parameters as well as P-values for all 54 pair-wise comparisons, are shown in **Table 1**.

TABLE 1 | Median (interquartile range) of cardiac parameters during rest, pleasant, and unpleasant conditions evaluated within the stable phase (20–70 s after the onset of excerpts) are shown on the left.

	Rest	Pleasant	Unpleasant	Rest vs. pleasant	Rest vs. unpleasant	Pleasant vs. unpleasant
RR	878 (163)	835 (182)	864 (179)	**2.11E-10**	**8.00E-10**	**3.62E-04**
QT	333 (37)	328 (36)	329 (35)	**5.30E-08**	**4.31E-09**	9.80E-01
QTc	347 (31)	355 (32)	351 (30)	**9.02E-11**	**8.76E-10**	**5.24E-07**
QTV-LF	0.73 (0.62)	0.56 (0.50)	0.56 (0.47)	**1.28E-05**	6.28E-03	6.28E-03
QTV-HF	0.95 (1.04)	0.67 (0.87)	0.74 (0.89)	**9.27E-08**	**3.80E-06**	**8.92E-05**
QTV-TOT	1.88 (1.72)	1.31 (1.20)	1.45 (1.28)	**2.98E-07**	**2.02E-05**	**1.80E-04**
RRV-LF	577 (583)	289 (371)	363 (357)	**3.99E-08**	**4.36E-06**	**2.22E-05**
RRV-HF	558 (684)	224 (326)	345 (419)	**3.45E-11**	**8.76E-10**	**5.08E-10**
RRV-TOT	1226 (1235)	518 (801)	763 (842)	**2.01E-10**	**1.75E-08**	**1.31E-08**
QTVuRRV-LF	0.11 (0.08)	0.10 (0.10)	0.11 (0.09)	4.78E-02	1.95E-01	9.63E-02
QTVuRRV-HF	0.17 (0.14)	0.17 (0.17)	0.17 (0.17)	3.09E-01	2.70E-01	9.97E-01
QTVuRRV-TOT	0.31 (0.20)	0.28 (0.25)	0.27 (0.25)	7.17E-01	7.11E-01	5.98E-01
QTVrRRV-LF	0.59 (0.50)	0.42 (0.32)	0.48 (0.36)	**9.13E-07**	1.07E-02	3.05E-03
QTVrRRV-HF	0.68 (0.97)	0.46 (0.61)	0.58 (0.67)	**5.08E-10**	**1.13E-07**	**2.50E-06**
QTVrRRV-TOT	1.54 (1.49)	1.04 (0.94)	1.16 (1.11)	**6.35E-09**	**6.35E-06**	**2.22E-05**
Cohe-LF	0.87 (0.10)	0.84 (0.11)	0.85 (0.07)	9.82E-03	4.84E-01	3.82E-02
Cohe-HF	0.80 (0.13)	0.76 (0.17)	0.77 (0.14)	**1.61E-07**	**2.19E-04**	**1.65E-04**
Cohe-TOT	0.81 (0.11)	0.78 (0.14)	0.79 (0.11)	**3.60E-07**	1.07E-03	**1.70E-04**

P-values of pairwise tests (signed rank Wilcoxon test) are shown on the right, with P-values lower than the Bonferroni-corrected threshold reported in bold. RR: R-R interval; QT: QT interval; QTc: heart rate corrected QT; LF, HF, and TOT: low-frequency, high-frequency, and total spectral bands; QTV and RRV: QT and RR variability, respectively; QTVrRRV and QTVuRRV: QTV related and unrelated to RRV, respectively. Cohe: time-frequency coherence.

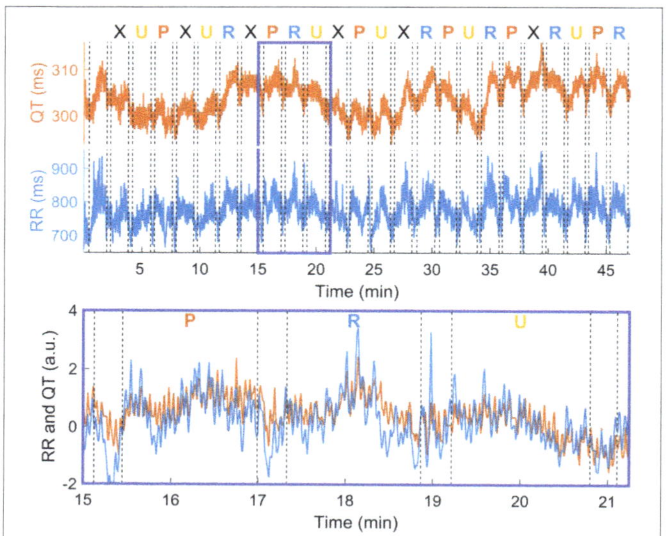

FIGURE 2 | QT and RR interval oscillations in one individual during the entire recording **(top)** and during three consecutive conditions **(bottom)**. Dashed vertical lines represent the beginning and the end of each condition, which are separated by about 20 s pause. The type of condition is reported above the **top panel**. R: rest; P: pleasant music; U: unpleasant music; X: sequence of Shepard tones (not considered in statistical analysis).

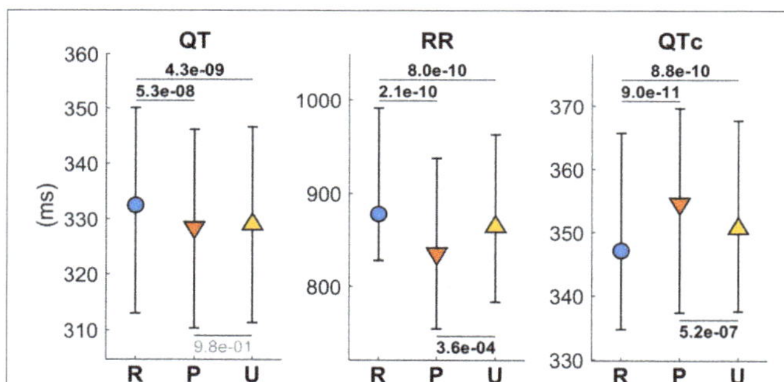

FIGURE 3 | QT, RR, and QTc (QT corrected for heart rate) during listening to pleasant music (P), unpleasant music (U), and rest (R). Markers represent the median values and bars span from the first to the third quartile. *P*-values measuring pair-wise differences are reported in bold if significant and in light gray if not significant.

QT Interval

Changes in the QTV during different conditions are shown in **Figure 3**. The QTV was significantly shorter during both unpleasant (329/35 ms, median/interquartile range) and pleasant (328/36 ms) than during resting (333/37 ms) condition ($P < 5.3 \times 10^{-8}$). After correcting for heart rate using the Bazett's formula, this pattern changed, with corrected QTV increasing from resting (347/41 ms) to unpleasant (351/30 ms) to pleasant (355/32 ms) ($P < 5 \times 10^{-7}$) (**Figure 3**).

QTV Related and Unrelated to RRV

A representative example of time-frequency representations during three consecutive epochs (resting, pleasant and unpleasant) is shown in **Figure 4**. These include the time-frequency spectra of QTV and RRV, $S_{QT}(t,f)$ and $S_{RRV}(t,f)$ respectively, the time-frequency coherence between QTV

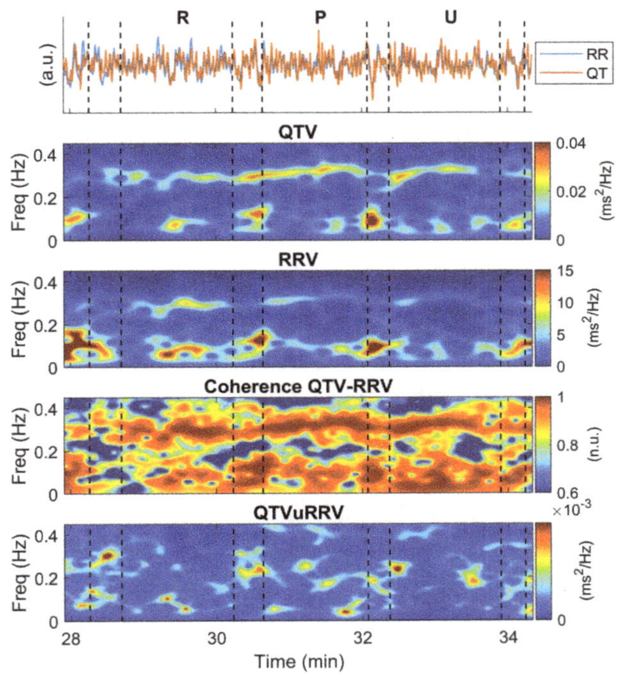

FIGURE 4 | Example of time-frequency representations in a representative individual. The same interval including three consecutive epochs (resting, pleasant and unpleasant conditions) shown in **Figure 2** is analyzed. From **top** to **bottom**: QTV and RRV superimposed and normalized to show same amplitude, QTV and RRV time-frequency spectra, time-frequency coherence between QTV and RRV and time-frequency spectrum of QTV unrelated to RRV. R: Rest; P: Pleasant condition; U: Unpleasant condition.

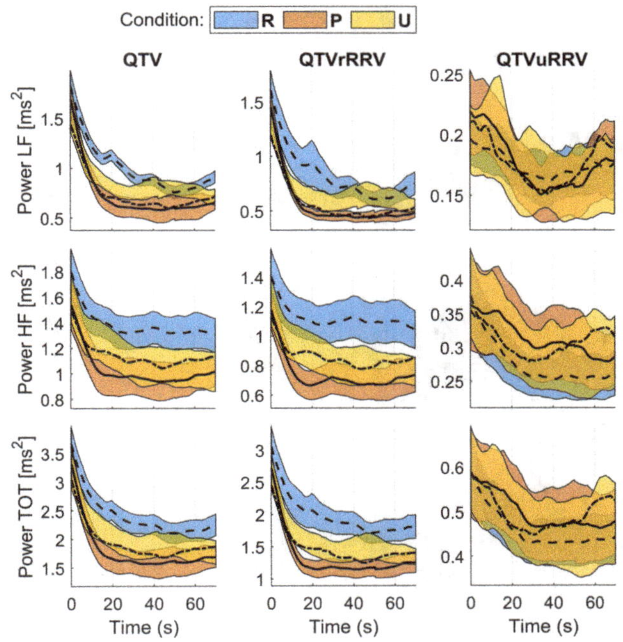

FIGURE 5 | QTV trends. From **left** to **right**: QTV, QTV related to RRV (QTVrRRV), and QTV unrelated to RRV (QTVrRRV). From **top** to **bottom**: instantaneous power of LF, HF, and total spectral band. Solid lines represent the mean trend across all individuals and shaded areas represent standard error. R: rest; P: pleasant condition; U: unpleasant condition.

and RRV, $\gamma_{QTV,RV}(t,f)$and the time-frequency spectrum of QTVuRRV, $S_{QTVuRRV}(t,f)$ Changes in the patterns of color in these time-frequency representations indicate changes in the magnitude and frequency of the signals' spectral components typical of non-stationary conditions. QTV and RRV showed similar time-frequency structures and high coherence. This implies that most of the spectral content of QTV was related to RRV and QTVuRRV was much smaller than QTV (note the different scale of the color bars in **Figure 4**).

The time course of the QTV's spectral components (instantaneous power) presented two phases (**Figure 5**): A sharp decrease with respect to the preceding interval (the pause between two consecutive epochs during which the individuals were asked to rate how they felt) during the first 20 s with subsequent stabilization during the remaining 50–60 s until the end of the epoch. QTVrRRV showed the biggest intra-condition changes (**Figure 5**, middle panel) whereas QTVuRRV showed little intra-condition changes as demonstrated by overlapping trends in the right hand side of **Figure 5**.

Figure 6 shows the distribution of mean QTV, QTV related and unrelated to RRV during the stable phase of the recordings (from 20 to 50 s after the onset of each epoch). QTV and QTVrRRV show similar patterns, with oscillations of higher magnitude in all spectral band during rest than during pleasant and unpleasant conditions, and with lower magnitude for HF oscillations and total power during pleasant than unpleasant condition. The time-frequency coherence between QTV and RRV was high (0.76–0.85) in all spectral bands for all conditions. In HF, a small but significant decrease in coherence was observed from rest (0.80/0.13) to unpleasant (0.77/0.14) to pleasant (0.76/0.17) conditions (**Table 1**). QTVuRRV was much smaller than QTVrRRV and did not show any significant change in any spectral band (**Table 1**).

Intra-Lead Reproducibility

The entire analysis was repeated using beat to beat QTVs obtained from lead II for assessment of intra-lead reproducibility. Correlation between the time series of QTVs from lead V4 and lead II was high, with Spearman's correlation coefficient equal to 0.95/0.09. However, the correlation between QTV was lower at 0.59/0.26. A lower intra-lead correlation for QTV than for the QTV is expected as QTV has a much lower magnitude than the QTV series, which show very slow oscillations (i.e., very low frequency components with frequency <0.03 Hz) that are removed from QTV. The standard deviation of the QTV signals (entire recording) across all patients was slightly higher in lead II than V4

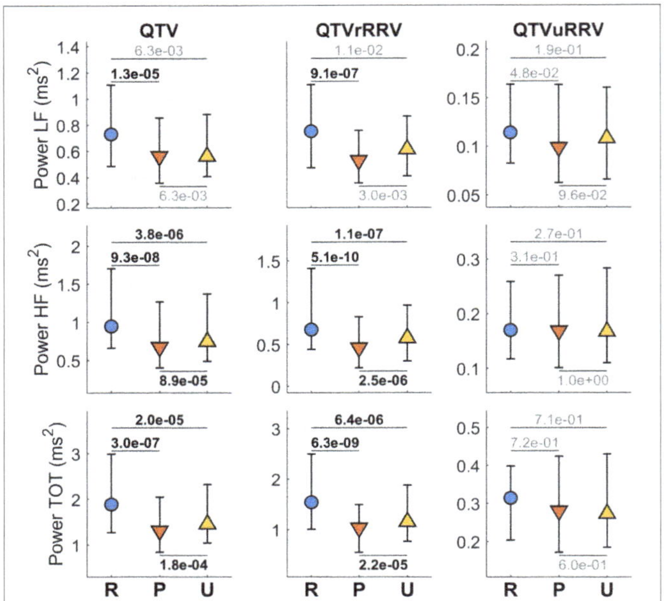

FIGURE 6 | QTV and QTV related and unrelated to RRV during listening to pleasant music (P), unpleasant music (U), and rest (R). From **left** to **right**: QTV, QTV related to RRV (QTVrRRV), and QTV unrelated to RRV (QTVrRRV). From **top** to **bottom**: mean power of LF, HF and total spectral band. Markers represent the median values and bars span from the first to the third quartile. *P*-values measuring pair-wise differences are reported in bold if significant and in light gray if not significant.

at 1.8/0.7 ms versus 1.7/0.6 ms, $P < 0.001$, and their correlation was equal to $cc = 0.78$. There was no difference in the SNR of the leads V4 and II ($P = 0.60$). The correlation coefficient between the standard deviation of QTV and SNR was equal to -0.49 ($P = 8.1 \times 10^{-5}$) in lead V4 and -0.60 in lead II ($P = 3.6 \times 10^{-7}$). This suggests that QTV in lead V4 was less affected by noise than QTV in lead II.

During the different conditions (silence, pleasant and unpleasant), changes in the QTV and QTc from lead II (**Supplementary Figure S2**) mirrored those from lead V4. Changes in QTV, QTVrRRV, and QTVuRRV followed a similar pattern in both leads. However, in lead II some differences were no longer significant after Bonferroni's correction (**Supplementary Figure S3**).

DISCUSSION

This study investigated the effect of emotional valence on cardiac repolarization and repolarization dynamics by analyzing the QTV response to music. The main findings are: (1) The QTV decreases during both unpleasant and pleasant emotional states, mirroring similar changes in the RR interval. This pattern is reversed after correction for heart rate, with QTc showing small but significant increase during listening to both pleasant and unpleasant music compared to silence, and during pleasant compared to unpleasant music. (2) The dynamic response of QTV to emotional valence showed a transient phase of about 20 s. (3) Because of the strong coupling between QTV and RRV, both QTV and QTVrRRV followed a similar pattern showing a decrease in variability during both pleasant and unpleasant conditions with respect to the resting condition and a further decrease during pleasant condition with respect to unpleasant condition in HF and in the total spectral components. (4) QTVuRRV was small and not affected by emotional valence.

The existence of a link between emotions or psychological stress and cardiovascular mortality has been demonstrated by many studies (Steptoe and Brydon, 2009). Strong emotions, i.e., characterized by a high level of arousal, have an acute impact on the cardiovascular function and can serve as triggers for arrhythmias and cardiovascular disease, mainly through a complex interaction with the autonomic nervous system (Kreibig, 2010; Taggart et al., 2011b). While it is accepted that emotional arousal (activating versus deactivating) has a stronger effect on human physiology than emotional valence (positive versus negative feeling), the latter has been less investigated and its effect on cardiac repolarization remained undetermined. This is the first study to investigate the simultaneous interaction between emotional valence and QT dynamics. A unique feature of this study is that the experimental set-up was designed to control for arousal by matching excerpts by tempo and volume with the intent of focusing on the effect of felt pleasantness with respect to unpleasantness.

Previous studies have demonstrated a link between intense emotions and potentially pro-arrhythmic repolarization changes (Ziegelstein, 2007; Lampert, 2016). In patients with a history of ventricular arrhythmia, psychological stress induces autonomically mediated repolarization changes (Lampert et al., 2005), while anger-induced T-wave alternans, a marker of repolarization variability (Orini et al., 2019), predicts future ventricular arrhythmias (Lampert et al., 2009). In patients with structurally normal hearts, mental stress altered repolarization inhomogeneity balance (Taggart et al., 2005) and dispersion of repolarization (Child et al., 2014; Finlay et al., 2016). A recent study has shown that not only acute and strong emotions, but also subtle everyday fluctuations in emotional arousal can affect repolarization, with a more noticeable impact in patients with Long QT syndrome and ischemic heart disease (Lane et al., 2018). In the same study, similar QT changes were observed as a response of emotions characterized by both positive and negative valence, which may suggest that the effect of everyday emotions could be primarily a function of arousal.

Music-induced emotions affect several cerebrovascular and cardiovascular parameters, especially heart rate and heart rate variability (Koelsch and Jancke, 2015). Although music-induced emotions may have a smaller impact on cardiac activity as compared to other types of emotions, evidence shows that music can reduce pain and anxiety, and that relaxing music is associated with lower heart rate and blood pressure (Koelsch and Jancke, 2015), which could be beneficial in particular in patients with cardiovascular disease.

The interest in the QTV response to music-induced emotions is motivated by the fact that QTV, and in particular QTVuRRV, provides an indirect assessment of ventricular repolarization variability, which is believed to be modulated by sympathetic drive directed to the ventricles (Porta et al., 2010; El-Hamad et al., 2015). Recent studies have demonstrated the existence of respiratory and LF oscillations in the ventricular action potential of the intact human heart during steady state ventricular pacing and therefore unrelated to cycle length variations (Hanson et al., 2014; Van Duijvenboden et al., 2016; Porter et al., 2019). Several studies have shown that indices of ventricular repolarization, mainly based on QTV, are associated with cardiac risk (Tereshchenko et al., 2009; Oosterhoff et al., 2011; Baumert et al., 2016), with periodic repolarization dynamics being affected by music (Cerruto et al., 2017). The mechanisms promoting intrinsic ventricular repolarization variability are still under investigation, but may imply both the autonomic nervous system (adrenergic stimulation) and mechano-electric feedback (Pueyo et al., 2016; Orini et al., 2017a).

One of the main results of this study is that in young healthy individuals listening to pleasant and unpleasant music, QTV dynamics are largely determined by RRV, whereas QTVuRRV remains stable. This highlights the importance of separating RRV-related and unrelated components to reveal intrinsic repolarization variability (Orini et al., 2018).

In this cohort of young healthy volunteers, the effect of emotional valence on QT and QTV was significant but relatively small, whereas its effect on QTVuRRV was not significant. Although these findings may not have an immediate impact on clinical practice, they provide valuable information to advance our understanding of the interplay between emotions and cardiac disease. Further research is needed to test the effect of emotional valence in the context of preexisting cardiac disorders and to better understand how to translate these findings in strategies that can impact patients' health. The observation that valance and not only arousal affects the QTV is interesting, because it suggests that potentially clinically relevant changes in arrhythmogenic substrates may be triggered by emotions unrelated to dramatic events. For instance, a small but significant increase in QTc associated with pleasant emotions may be relevant for arrhythmogenesis in the context of repolarization disorders such as long QT syndrome. A recent study analyzing the effect of everyday emotions on the QTV has suggested that in patients with heart conditions (long QT syndrome and ischemic heart disease), but not in healthy individuals, these can affect arrhythmia susceptibility (Lane et al., 2018). Interestingly, although the authors concluded that emotional arousal had a predominant effect with respect to valance, they observed a prolongation of QTc with positive and low-arousal emotions, which, despite important methodological differences between the two studies, is in agreement with our findings. Of note, silence has been previously reported to have a strong relaxing effect on the respiratory rate, heart rate and blood pressure (Bernardi et al., 2006; Orini et al., 2010). The finding that QTc decreases while QTV increases during silence provides further support to the protective effect of relaxation that could be used in specific cohorts to reduce cardiovascular risk (Schneider et al., 2005).

Limitations and Future Directions

Although this study is based on a relatively large cohort, it only includes young healthy individuals. The presentence of heart disease may amplify the effect of emotions (Lampert, 2016; Lane et al., 2018) and future studies should include patients with a pre-existing arrhythmogenic substrate. Emotions were induced using musical excerpts. Functional neuroimaging studies using similar stimuli have demonstrated that music can modulate activity in brain structures that are known to be crucially involved in emotion (Koelsch et al., 2006; Koelsch, 2014). Future studies are needed to determine if the effect of music-induced emotions can be generalized to other types of emotions and psychological stress. Inter-subject variability in the emotional predisposition to and elaboration of the stimuli were not controlled during the study and may have played a role in the physiological response. For instance, interoceptive awareness has been shown to modulate the heart rate response to emotional pictures (Pollatos et al., 2007) and may also play a role in the modulation cardiac repolarization. This may be assessed in future studies. Although the tangent method is a standard method for identifying the end of the T-wave, it has some limitations (Baumert et al., 2016). Although results obtained from the analysis of lead V4 (main text) generally correlated with those obtained from lead II (**Supplementary Material**), the statistical significance of some differences differ, especially in the LF band of QTV. Intra-lead differences in QTV have been previously reported and linked to T-wave amplitude, with QTV increasing in leads showing smaller T-waves (Hasan et al., 2012). This is in agreement with our finding that QTV in lead V4, which shows taller T-waves than lead II, was less affected by noise than QTV in lead II. Thus, results obtained from the analysis of V4 are more robust. Although these intra-lead differences are partially due to the technical challenge of measuring small amplitude oscillations of the order of few ms, ECG leads capture repolarization dynamics of different cardiac segments (Srinivasan et al., 2019) and small intra-leads differences may also partially reflect a spatially heterogeneous response of ventricular repolarization.

Finally, although the time-frequency approach implemented in this study is built upon a robust framework that has been tested in several studies (Orini et al., 2012a,b,c,d, 2018), other approaches to decompose QT variability in its different component exist (Porta et al., 2010, 2017; El-Hamad et al., 2015) and future studies may investigate the reproducibility of these findings.

CONCLUSION

Emotional valence, as evoked by music, has a small but significant effect on beat-to-beat repolarization variability and this effect is principally mediated by heart rate variability.

AUTHOR CONTRIBUTIONS

MO contributed to the design of the analysis. MO and FA-A contributed to the data and statistical analysis. MO and RB contributed to the methodological development. SK contributed to the experimental set-up. MO contributed to the drafting of the work. MO, FA-A, SK, and RB contributed to the critical revision and proofreading.

REFERENCES

Baumert, M., Porta, A., Vos, M. A., Malik, M., Couderc, J. P., Laguna, P., et al. (2016). QT interval variability in body surface ECG: measurement, physiological basis, and clinical value: position statement and consensus guidance endorsed by the European Heart Rhythm Association jointly with the ESC Working Group on cardiac cellular electroph. *Europace* 18, 925–944. doi: 10.1093/europace/euv405

Bernardi, L., Porta, C., and Sleight, P. (2006). Cardiovascular, cerebrovascular, and respiratory changes induced by different types of music in musicians and non-musicians: the importance of silence. *Heart* 92, 445–452. doi: 10.1136/hrt.2005.064600

Cerruto, G., Mainardi, L., Koelsch, S., and Orini, M. (2017). The periodic repolarization dynamics index identifies changes in ventricular repolarization oscillations associated with musicinduced emotions. *Comput. Cardiol.* 44, 2–5. doi: 10.22489/CinC.2017.259-372

Child, N., Hanson, B., Bishop, M., Rinaldi, C. A., Bostock, J., Western, D., et al. (2014). Effect of mental challenge induced by movie clips on action potential duration in normal human subjects independent of heart rate. *Circ. Arrhythmia Electrophysiol.* 7, 518–523. doi: 10.1161/CIRCEP.113.000909

Cohen, L. (1989). Time-frequency distributions-a review. *Proc. IEEE* 77, 941–981. doi: 10.1109/5.30749

El-Hamad, F., Lambert, E., Abbott, D., and Baumert, M. (2015). Relation between QT interval variability and muscle sympathetic nerve activity in normal subjects. *Am. J. Physiol. Hear. Circ. Physiol.* 309, H1218–H1224. doi: 10.1152/ajpheart.00230.2015

Finlay, M. C., Lambiase, P. D., Ben-Simon, R., and Taggart, P. (2016). Effect of mental stress on dynamic electrophysiological properties of the endocardium and epicardium in humans. *Heart Rhythm* 13, 175–182. doi: 10.1016/j.hrthm.2015.08.011

Hanson, B., Child, N., Van Duijvenboden, S., Orini, M., Chen, Z., Coronel, R., et al. (2014). Oscillatory behavior of ventricular action potential duration in heart failure patients at respiratory rate and low frequency. *Front. Physiol.* 5:414. doi: 10.3389/fphys.2014.00414

Hasan, M. A., Abbott, D., and Baumert, M. (2012). Relation between beat-to-beat QT interval variability and t-wave amplitude in healthy subjects. *Ann. Noninvasive Electrocardiol.* 17, 195–203. doi: 10.1111/j.1542-474X.2012.00508.x

Hilz, M. J., Stadler, P., Gryc, T., Nath, J., Habib-Romstoeck, L., Stemper, B., et al. (2014). Music induces different cardiac autonomic arousal effects in young and older persons. *Auton. Neurosci. Basic Clin.* 183, 83–93. doi: 10.1016/j.autneu.2014.02.004

Hlawatsch, F., and Boudreaux-Bartels, G. F. F. (1992). Linear and quadratic time-frequency signal representations. *IEEE Signal. Process. Mag.* 9, 21–67. doi: 10.1109/79.127284

Koelsch, S. (2014). Brain correlates of music-evoked emotions. *Nat. Rev. Neurosci.* 15, 170–180. doi: 10.1038/nrn3666

Koelsch, S., Fritz, T., Cramon, D. Y. V., Müller, K., and Friederici, A. D. (2006). Investigating emotion with music: an fMRI study. *Hum. Brain Mapp.* 27, 239–250. doi: 10.1002/hbm.20180

Koelsch, S., and Jancke, L. (2015). Music and the heart. *Eur. Heart J.* 36, 3043–3048. doi: 10.1093/eurheartj/ehv430

Krabs, R. U., Enk, R., Teich, N., and Koelsch, S. (2015). Autonomic effects of music in health and Crohn's disease: the impact of isochronicity, emotional valence, and tempo. *PLoS One* 10:e0126224. doi: 10.1371/journal.pone.0126224

Kreibig, S. D. (2010). Autonomic nervous system activity in emotion: a review. *Biol. Psychol.* 84, 394–421. doi: 10.1016/j.biopsycho.2010.03.010

Lampert, R. (2016). Mental stress and ventricular arrhythmias. *Curr. Cardiol. Rep.* 18:118. doi: 10.1007/s11886-016-0798-796

Lampert, R., Shusterman, V., Burg, M., McPherson, C., Batsford, W., Goldberg, A., et al. (2009). Anger-induced T-Wave alternans predicts future ventricular arrhythmias in patients with implantable cardioverter-defibrillators. *J. Am. Coll. Cardiol.* 53, 774–778. doi: 10.1016/j.jacc.2008.10.053

Lampert, R., Shusterman, V., Burg, M. M., Lee, F. A., Earley, C., Goldberg, A., et al. (2005). Effects of psychologic stress on repolarization and relationship to autonomic and hemodynamic factors. *J. Cardiovasc. Electrophysiol.* 16, 372–377. doi: 10.1046/j.1540-8167.2005.40580.x

Lane, R. D., Reis, H. T., Hsu, C.-H., Kern, K. B., Couderc, J. P., Moss, A. J., et al. (2018). Abnormal repolarization duration during everyday emotional arousal in long QT syndrome and Coronary Artery disease. *Am. J. Med.* 131:565-572.e2. doi: 10.1016/j.amjmed.2017.12.017

Oosterhoff, P., Tereshchenko, L. G., Van Der Heyden, M. A. G., Ghanem, R. N., Fetics, B. J., Berger, R. D., et al. (2011). Short-term variability of repolarization predicts ventricular tachycardia and sudden cardiac death in patients with structural heart disease: a comparison with QT variability index. *Heart Rhythm* 8, 1584–1590. doi: 10.1016/j.hrthm.2011.04.033

Orini, M., Bailón, R., Enk, R., Koelsch, S., Mainardi, L., and Laguna, P. (2010). A method for continuously assessing the autonomic response to music-induced emotions through HRV analysis. *Med. Biol. Eng. Comput.* 48, 423–433. doi: 10.1007/s11517-010-0592-3

Orini, M., Bailón, R., Laguna, P., Mainardi, L. T., and Barbieri, R. (2012a). A multivariate timefrequency method to characterize the influence of respiration over heart period and arterial pressure. *EURASIP J. Adv. Signal Process.* 2012:214. doi: 10.1186/1687-6180-2012-2214

Orini, M., Bailón, R., Mainardi, L., and Laguna, P. (2012b). Synthesis of HRV signals characterized by predetermined time-frequency structure by means of time-varying ARMA models. *Biomed. Signal. Process. Control* 7, 141–150. doi: 10.1016/j.bspc.2011.05.003

Orini, M., Bailon, R., Mainardi, L. T., Laguna, P., and Flandrin, P. (2012c). Characterization of dynamic interactions between cardiovascular signals by time-frequency coherence. *IEEE Trans. Biomed. Eng.* 59, 663–673. doi: 10.1109/TBME.2011.2171959

Orini, M., Laguna, P., Mainardi, L. T. T., and Bailón, R. (2012d). Assessment of the dynamic interactions between heart rate and arterial pressure by the cross time–frequency analysis. *Physiol. Meas.* 33, 315–331. doi: 10.1088/0967-3334/33/3/315

Orini, M., Nanda, A., Yates, M., Di Salvo, C., Roberts, N., Lambiase, P. D., et al. (2017a). Mechanoelectrical feedback in the clinical setting: current perspectives. *Prog. Biophys. Mol. Biol.* 130(Pt B), 365–375. doi: 10.1016/j.pbiomolbio.2017.06.001

Orini, M., Tinker, A., Munroe, P. B., and Lambiase, P. D. (2017b). Long-term intra-individual reproducibility of heart rate dynamics during exercise and recovery in the UK Biobank cohort. *PLoS One* 12:e0183732. doi: 10.1371/journal.pone.0183732

Orini, M., Pueyo, E., Laguna, P., and Bailon, R. (2018). A time-varying nonparametric methodology for assessing changes in QT variability unrelated to heart rate variability. *IEEE Trans. Biomed. Eng.* 65, 1443–1451. doi: 10.1109/TBME.2017.2758925

Orini, M., Taggart, P., Srinivasan, N., Hayward, M., and Lambiase, P. D. (2016). Interactions between activation and repolarization restitution properties in the intact human heart: in-vivo whole-heart data and mathematical description. *PLoS One* 11:e0161765. doi: 10.1371/journal.pone.0161765

Orini, M., Yanni, J., Taggart, P., Hanson, B., Hayward, M., Smith, A., et al. (2019). Mechanistic insights from targeted molecular profiling of repolarization alternans in the intact human heart. *Europace* 21, 981–989. doi: 10.1093/europace/euz007

Pollatos, O., Herbert, B. M., Matthias, E., and Schandry, R. (2007). Heart rate response after emotional picture presentation is modulated by interoceptive awareness. *Int. J. Psychophysiol.* 63, 117–124. doi: 10.1016/j.ijpsycho.2006.09.003

Porta, A., Bari, V., De Maria, B., and Baumert, M. (2017). A network physiology approach to the assessment of the link between sinoatrial and ventricular cardiac controls. *Physiol. Meas.* 38, 1472–1489. doi: 10.1088/1361-6579/aa6e95

Porta, A., Tobaldini, E., Gnecchi-Ruscone, T., and Montano, N. (2010). RT variability unrelated to heart period and respiration progressively increases during graded head-up tilt. *Am. J. Physiol. Heart Circ. Physiol.* 298, H1406–H1414. doi: 10.1152/ajpheart.01206.2009

Porter, B., Bishop, M. J., Claridge, S., Child, N., Van Duijvenboden, S., Bostock, J., et al. (2019). Left ventricular activation-recovery interval variability predicts spontaneous ventricular tachyarrhythmia in patients with heart failure. *Heart Rhythm* 16, 702–709. doi: 10.1016/j.hrthm.2018.11.013

Pueyo, E., Orini, M., Rodríguez, J. F. J. F., and Taggart, P. (2016). Interactive effect of betaadrenergic stimulation and mechanical stretch on low-frequency oscillations of ventricular action potential duration in humans. *J. Mol. Cell. Cardiol.* 97, 93–105. doi: 10.1016/j.yjmcc.2016.05.003

Schneider, R. H., Alexander, C. N., Staggers, F., Rainforth, M., Salerno, J. W., Hartz, A., et al. (2005). Long-term effects of stress reduction on mortality in persons =55 years of age with systemic hypertension. *Am. J. Cardiol.* 95, 1060–1064. doi: 10.1016/j.amjcard.2004.12.058

Srinivasan, N. T., Orini, M., Providencia, R., Simon, R., Lowe, M., Segal, O. R., et al. (2019). Differences in the upslope of the precordial body surface ECG T wave reflect right to left dispersion of repolarization in the intact human heart. *Heart Rhythm* 16, 943–951. doi: 10.1016/j.hrthm.2018.12.006

Steptoe, A., and Brydon, L. (2009). Emotional triggering of cardiac events. *Neurosci. Biobehav. Rev.* 33, 63–70. doi: 10.1016/j.neubiorev.2008.04.010

Steptoe, A., and Kivimäki, M. (2012). Stress and cardiovascular disease. *Nat. Rev. Cardiol.* 9, 360–370. doi: 10.1038/nrcardio.2012.45

Taggart, P., Boyett, M. R., Logantha, S. J. R. J., and Lambaise, P. D. (2011a). Anger, emotion, and arrythimias: from brain to heart. *Front Physiol.* 2:67. doi: 10.3389/fphys.2011.00067

Taggart, P., Critchley, H., and Lambiase, P. D. (2011b). Heart-brain interactions in cardiac arrhythmia. *Heart* 97, 698–708. doi: 10.1136/hrt.2010.209304

Taggart, P., Sutton, P., Redfern, C., Batchvarov, V. N., Hnatkova, K., Malik, M., et al. (2005). The effect of mental stress on the non-dipolar components of the T wave: modulation by hypnosis. *Psychosom. Med.* 67, 376–383. doi: 10.1097/01.psy.0000160463.10583.88

Tereshchenko, L. G., Fetics, B. J., Domitrovich, P. P., Lindsay, B. D., and Berger, R. D. (2009). Prediction of ventricular tachyarrhythmias by intracardiac repolarization variability analysis. *Circ. Arrhythmia Electrophysiol.* 2, 276–284. doi: 10.1161/CIRCEP.108.829440

Van Duijvenboden, S., Orini, M., Child, N., Gill, J. S., Taggart, P., and Hanson, B. (2016). Investigation of causal interactions between ventricular action potential duration, blood pressure and respiration. *Comput. Cardiol.* 42, 621–624. doi: 10.1109/CIC.2015.7410987

Ziegelstein, R. C. (2007). Acute emotional stress and cardiac arrhythmias. *J. Am. Med. Assoc.* 298, 324–329. doi: 10.1001/jama.298.3.324

13

Four TRPM4 Cation Channel Mutations Found in Cardiac Conduction Diseases Lead to Altered Protein Stability

Beatrice Bianchi[1], *Lijo Cherian Ozhathil*[1], *Argelia Medeiros-Domingo*[2], *Michael H. Gollob*[3] *and Hugues Abriel*[1*]

[1] Swiss National Centre of Competence in Research (NCCR) TransCure, Institute of Biochemistry and Molecular Medicine, University of Bern, Bern, Switzerland, [2] Department of Cardiology, Inselspital, University Hospital Bern, Bern, Switzerland, [3] Department of Medicine, Peter Munk Cardiac Centre, Toronto General Hospital, University of Toronto, Toronto, ON, Canada

***Correspondence:**
Hugues Abriel
hugues.abriel@ibmm.unibe.ch*

Transient receptor potential melastatin member 4 (TRPM4), a non-selective cation channel, mediates cell membrane depolarization in immune response, insulin secretion, neurological disorders, and cancer. Pathological variants in *TRPM4* gene have been linked to several cardiac phenotypes such as complete heart block (CHB), ventricular tachycardia, and Brugada syndrome (BrS). Despite recent findings regarding the functional implications of TRPM4 in cardiac diseases, the molecular and cellular mechanisms leading to altered conduction are poorly understood. In the present study, we identify and characterize four novel *TRPM4* variants found in patients with CHB or ventricular fibrillation. Three of them, p.A101T, p.S1044C and a double variant p.A101T/P1204L, led to a decreased expression and function of the channel. On the contrary, the variant p.Q854R showed an increase in TRPM4 current. Recent evidence indicates that altered degradation rate of mutant proteins represents a pathogenic mechanism underlying genetic diseases. In consequence, protein turnover of WT-TRPM4 and TRPM4 variants overexpressed in HEK293 cells was analyzed using cycloheximide, an inhibitor of protein biosynthesis. Upon addition of cycloheximide, WT-TRPM4 decayed with a half-life of ~20 h, while loss-of-expression variants showed a ~30% increase in degradation rate, with a half-life close to 12 h. Together, the gain-of-expression variant showed a higher stability and a doubled half-life compared to WT-TRPM4. In conclusion, decreased or increased protein expression of several TRPM4 variants linked to cardiac conduction disorders or ventricular arrhythmias were found to be caused by altered TRPM4 half-life compared to the WT form.

Keywords: TRPM4, protein trafficking, cycloheximide, cardiac disorders, protein stability, ion channels, mutations

INTRODUCTION

The transient receptor potential melastatin 4 (TRPM4) protein is an intracellular Ca^{2+}-activated non-selective cation channel, which is impermeable to Ca^{2+}. TRPM4 exhibits a voltage dependence, which has not been previously described for any TRP channel, indicating that TRPM4 is both a Ca^{2+}-activated and voltage-modulated cation channel (Nilius et al., 2005). At negative membrane potentials, TRPM4 allows Na^{+} entry into the cell, leading to cellular membrane depolarization. At positive membrane potentials, TRPM4 channels permit cellular K^+ efflux, leading to membrane repolarization (Launay et al., 2002; Ramsey et al., 2006). TRPM4 is widely expressed in several tissues and is involved in a variety of physiological processes, including modulation of immune cells activity, such as T-cells (Launay et al., 2004), mast cells (Shimizu et al., 2009) and dendritic cells (Barbet et al., 2010), insulin secretion by pancreatic β cells (Cheng et al., 2007), mechanotransduction in cerebral arteries (Vennekens and Nilius, 2007), and Ca^{2+} signaling in cancer (Sozucan et al., 2015; Ceylan et al., 2016; Sagredo et al., 2017). In addition, TRPM4 has been linked to several neurological disorders such as experimental autoimmune encephalomyelitis and multiple sclerosis (Schattling et al., 2012), spinal cord injuries (Gerzanich et al., 2009), and traumatic brain injuries (Simard et al., 2010). TRPM4 was reported to participate in electrical perturbations following cardiac ischemia and reperfusion episodes because of its sensitivity to Ca^{2+} and ATP (Kalogeris et al., 2012). It has been shown that in a model of hypoxia-reoxygenation using isolated mouse interventricular septum, TRPM4 inhibitors 9-phenantrol and flufenamic acid reduced $[Ca^{2+}]_i$ overload, thus reducing the so called early afterdepolarization (EAD) (Simard et al., 2012). However, the physiological role for this channel in cardiac function remains unclear. Recent studies have linked genetic variants of *TRPM4* gene to progressive familial heart block type 1 (PFHB1) (Kruse et al., 2009; Daumy et al., 2016), isolated cardiac conduction disease (ICCD) (Liu et al., 2010), atrio-ventricular block (AVB) (Stallmeyer et al., 2012; Syam et al., 2016), right bundle branch block (RBBB) (Stallmeyer et al., 2012) and Brugada syndrome (BrS) (Liu et al., 2013; Gualandi et al., 2017). Several TRPM4 variants linked to inherited cardiac diseases were shown to cause either gain- or loss-of-function of the channel activity. However, the molecular details of these alterations, and how both gain- and loss-of-function variants may lead to conduction defects remains poorly understood.

In the present study, we identified four novel *TRPM4* genetic variants found in patients with either complete heart block (CHB) or idiopathic ventricular fibrillation (IVF). Biochemical and functional characterizations of these variants identified three with loss-of-function and one with gain-of-function. We further examined the possible mechanisms leading to altered protein stability using cycloheximide, an inhibitor of protein synthesis. Our results revealed an altered protein turnover in loss- and gain-of-expression mutant compared to the WT form of TRPM4, showing that altered half-life of TRPM4 is one of the mechanisms leading to several cardiac conduction disorders.

MATERIALS AND METHODS

Patient Genetic Screening

The study was conducted according to the Swiss and Canadian guidelines for genetic research and approved by the ethics committees of University Hospital Bern and the University of Ottawa Heart Institute respectively. All subjects gave written informed consent in accordance with the Declaration of Helsinki. Genomic DNA was isolated from peripheral macrophages by standard procedures using Gentra Puregene Blood kit (Qiagen, Hilden, Germany). A targeted exome panel sequencing was performed by Next Generation Sequencing using the TrueSight One Sequencing Panel (Illumina, San Diego, CA, USA). Sequence data were compared with the reference sequence of the human *TRPM4* gene (MIM# 606936; RefSeq NM_017636.3; Ensembl gene reference: ENSG00000130529, referring to isoform *TRPM4b*).

Generation of TRPM4 Mutants

The complete human wild-type HA-tagged *TRPM4* cDNA was cloned in a pcDNA4/TO vector. Mutants were obtained by *in vitro* mutagenesis using Q5 Site-Directed Mutagenesis kit (New England Biolabs, Ipswich, MA, USA). Mutant cDNA clones were then sequenced before using them in experiments.

Cell Culture and Transfection

Human embryonic kidney (HEK293) cells were cultured with Dulbecco's modified Eagle's culture medium supplemented with 4 mM Glutamine, 10% FBS and a cocktail of streptomycin-penicillin antibiotics. For the electrophysiological studies, the cells were transiently transfected with 240 ng of HA-TRPM4 WT or HA-TRPM4 p.A101T, HA-TRPM4 p.Q854R, HA-TRPM4 p.S1044C, HA-TRPM4 p.P1204L, and double variant HA-TRPM4 p.A101T/P1204L in a 35 mm dish (BD Falcon, Durham, North Carolina, USA) mixed with 4 μL of JetPEI (Polyplus transfection, Illkirch, France) and 46 μL of 150 mM NaCl. The cells were incubated for 24 h at 37°C with 5% CO_2. All transfections included 100 ng of eGFP as a reporter gene. Expression of GFP was used to identify transfected cells, for patch clamp experiments.

For the biochemical experiments, HEK293 cells were transiently transfected with 240 ng of either HA-TRPM4 WT, or HA-TRPM4 p.A101T, HA-TRPM4 p.Q854R, HA-TRPM4 p.S1044C, HA-TRPM4 p.P1204L, and double variant HA-TRPM4 p.A101T/P1204L, or empty vector (pcDNA4TO) in a P100 dish (BD Falcon, Durham, North Carolina, USA) mixed with 30 μL of JetPEI (Polyplus transfection, Illkirch, France) and 250 μL of 150 mM NaCl. The cells were incubated for 48 h at 37°C with 5% CO_2.

Cell Surface Biotinylation Assay

Following 48 h of incubation, transiently transfected HEK293 cells, previously washed twice with cold 1X PBS, were treated with EZlinkTM Sulfo-NHS-SS-Biotin (Thermo Scientific, Waltham, MA, USA) 0.5 mg/mL in cold 1X PBS for 15 min at 4°C. Subsequently, the cells were washed twice with 200 mM Glycine in cold 1X PBS and twice with cold 1X PBS to inactivate and remove the excess biotin, respectively. The cells were then lysed with 1X lysis buffer [50 mM HEPES pH 7.4; 150 mM NaCl; 1.5 mM $MgCl_2$; 1 mM EGTA pH 8.0; 10% Glycerol; 1% Triton X-100; 1X Complete Protease Inhibitor Cocktail (Roche, Mannheim, Germany)] for 1 h at 4°C. Cell lysates were centrifuged at 16,000 g at 4°C for 15 min. Two milligrams of the supernatant were incubated with 50 μL Streptavidin Sepharose High Performance beads (GE Healthcare, Uppsala, Sweden) for 2 h at 4°C, and the remaining supernatant was kept as the input. The beads were subsequently washed five times with 1X lysis buffer before elution with 50 μL of 2X NuPAGE sample buffer (Invitrogen, Carlsbad, CA, USA) plus 100 mM DTT at 37°C for

30 min. These biotinylated fractions were analyzed as TRPM4 expressed at the cell surface. The input fractions, analyzed as total expression of TRPM4, were resuspended with 4X NuPAGE Sample Buffer plus 100 mM DTT to give a concentration of 1 mg/mL and incubated at 37°C for 30 min.

Western Blot Experiments

Protein samples were analyzed on 9% polyacrylamide gels, transferred with the TurboBlot dry blot system (Biorad, Hercules, CA, USA) and detected with anti-TRPM4 (generated by Pineda, Berlin, Germany), anti α-actin A2066 (Sigma-Aldrich, St. Louis, MO, USA), anti-alpha Na^+/K^+ ATPase α1 ab7671 (Abcam, Cambridge, UK) antibodies using SNAP i.d. (Millipore, Billerica, MA, USA). The anti-TRPM4 antibody was generated by Pineda (Berlin, Germany) using the following peptide sequence: NH2-CRDKRESDSERLKRTSQKV-CONH2. A fraction of the antisera, which was subsequently used in this study, was affinity purified. Actin and alpha-Na^+/K^+ ATPase were used to normalize TRPM4 protein band intensity in total fraction and surface fraction respectively. Original Western blot pictures of the three replicates for total and surface fractions were shown in **Supplementary Figures 1**, **9**, and **11** for total expression, and **Supplementary Figures 2**, **10** and **12** for surface expression. A summary of raw WB picture was also submitted as **Supplementary Figure 13**. All the Western Blots have been quantified using Image Studio Lite software from LI-COR Biosciences (Lincoln, NE, USA).

Immunoprecipitation and Protein Half-Life Determination Experiments

For half-life experiments, HEK 293 transiently transfected cells were treated with 100 μg/mL cycloheximide (Millipore, Billerica, MA, USA) or 0,3% DMSO as control and lysed at various time points using 1X UBI buffer [50 mM HEPES pH 7.4, 150 mM NaCl, 1 mM EGTA pH 8.0, 10% Glycerol, 1% Triton X-100, 1X Complete Protease Inhibitor Cocktail EDTA-free (Roche, Mannheim, Germany)]. Two milligrams of protein lysate were incubated overnight with 20 μg of anti-TRPM4 antibody in a final volume of 1 mL. The lysate-antibody was then transferred on Protein G Sepharose 4 Fast Flow beads (GE Healthcare, Uppsala, Sweden) and rotated overnight at 4°C. Beads were washed 5 times with 1X UBI buffer with 0.5% Triton before elution with 50 μL of 2X NuPAGE sample buffer (Invitrogen, Carlsbad, CA, USA) plus 100 mM DTT at 37°C for 30 min. Samples were loaded on a 9% polyacrylamide gel and TRPM4 expression was revealed using anti-HA antibody (Enzo Life Sciences, Lausen, Switzerland). Original Western blot pictures are shown in Supplementary data (**Supplementary Figures 3–8**). To extrapolate the half-life of WT-TRPM4 and TRPM4 variants, the relative protein band intensity was fitted with mono-exponential function, and time for 50% decay of intensity was estimated.

Quantitative Real Time PCR

Total RNA isolation was performed using TRIzol Reagent (Applied Biosystems, Foster City, CA, USA) as described by the manufacturer. Concentration and purity of total RNA was determined by optical density measurement using a NanoDrop 2000 spectrophotometer (Thermo Scientific, Waltham, MA, USA). cDNA was synthesized using High Capacity cDNA Reverse Transcription kit (Applied Biosystems, Foster City, CA, USA) and quantitative expression analysis was performed with 7500 Fast Real-Time PCR System (Applied Biosystems, Foster City, CA, USA). Quantification of mRNA expression levels was investigated with TaqMan gene expression assay Hs00214167_m1 for human *TRPM4*, using *GAPDH* TaqMan gene expression assay Hs02758991_g1 as a control. Relative expression of the studied gene was calculated with the $2^{-\Delta\Delta Ct}$ method.

Cellular Electrophysiology

Electrophysiological recordings were performed in the inside-out patch clamp configuration with patch pipettes (1–2 μm tip opening) pulled from 1.5 mm borosilicate glass capillaries (Zeitz-Instruments, GmbH, München, Germany) using micropipette puller P 97 (Sutter Instruments, Novato, CA, USA). The tips were polished to have a pipette resistance of 2–4 MΩ in the bath solution. The pipette solution contained (in mM) 150 NaCl, 10 HEPES, and 2 $CaCl_2$ (pH 7.4 with NaOH). The bath solution contained (in mM) 150 NaCl 10 HEPES, 2 HEDTA (pH 7.4 with NaOH) as 0 Ca^{2+} solution. Solutions containing 300 μM Ca^{2+} were made by adding the appropriate concentration of $CaCl_2$ without buffer to a solution containing (in mM) 150 NaCl, 10 HEPES (pH 7.4 with NaOH) as reported previously (Zhang et al., 2005). Bath solution with 0 and 300 μM Ca^{2+} concentrations were applied to cells by a modified rapid solution exchanger (Perfusion Fast-Step SF-77B; Warner Instruments Corp., CT, USA). Membrane currents were recorded with a Multiclamp 700B amplifier (Molecular Devices, Sunnyvale CA, USA) controlled by Clampex 10 via a Digidata 1332A (Molecular Devices, Sunnyvale, CA, USA). Data were low-pass filtered at 5 kHz and sampled at 10 kHz. Experiments were performed at room temperature (20–25°C). For measuring steady state currents, stimulation protocol consisted of a single 200 ms voltage step to −100 and then to +100 mV.

Statistical Analysis

Data are represented as the mean ± s.e.m. One-way ANOVA followed by Sidak's multiple comparison test was used to compare the samples, with a $p < 0.05$ considered as significant. Electrophysiology data were exported and analyzed using IGOR PRO 6 (Wavematrix, London, UK).

RESULTS

Patients Information

In the present study, we performed genetic analysis of the *TRPM4* gene in patients to elucidate its role in various types of cardiac conduction disorders or ventricular arrhythmias. The clinical details of the variant carriers are presented in **Table 1** and the electrocardiogram (ECG) recordings are shown in **Figure 1**. In Ottawa Heart Institute, 26 patients with premature heart block (age <60 years) were screened. Together, 100 patients from an elderly (age > 70 years) control population were screened for the identified rare variants. In Bern, the *TRPM4* gene is

TABLE 1 | Patients characteristics.

Patient ID	Protein	Sex	Age at diagnosis (years)	Circumstances of discovery	Family history	Phenotype
1	p.A101T	Male	54	Dizziness	No	CHB
1A	p.A101T	Male	71	Asymptomatic	No	cRBBB
2	p.Q854R	Female	53	Syncope	Unknown	CHB
3	p.S1044C	Female	48	Syncope	Mother had PM (deceased)	CHB
4	p.A101T/P1204L	Female	17	Resuscitated SCD	Yes	IVF

CHB, complete heart block; cRBBB, complete right bundle branch block; PM, pacemaker; SCD, sudden cardiac death; IVF, idiopathic ventricular fibrillation.

screened routinely in cases with suspected channelopathies. In these cohorts, four novel *TRPM4* variants leading to cardiac disorders were identified (**Figure 1A**). The p.A101T variant was found in a 54 years old male with dizziness, who was diagnosed with CHB (**Figure 1B**). The same variant was also found in an asymptomatic control patient who was subsequently identified to have a complete RBBB on ECG. Other variants in the control patient were absent (**Table 1**). The p.Q854R and p.S1044C variants were found in two female patients with syncope and an ECG presentation of CHB at 53 and 48 years of age respectively. The mother of the 48 years old patient also had a pacemaker (**Table 1**). The missense p.A101T mutation was also found, together with a p.P1204L mutation, in a 17 years old patient from the University Hospital Bern who had sudden cardiac death. This patient had exhibited frequent monomorphic premature ventricular beats during exercise prior to her sudden cardiac death (SCD) event (**Figures 1C,D**). She had history of recurrent syncope since she was 14 years old. ECG and magnetic resonance imaging (MRI) were normal. This patient had also a novel homozygous mutation in ryanodine receptor 2 (RYR2) in position c.365G>A (p.R122H), but no clear Catecholaminergic Polymorphic Ventricular Tachycardia (CPVT) was observed. Relatives have been tested for the three mutations: both parents are heterozygous for RYR2-R122H, and the mother is carrier of both TRPM4 mutations. Both parents are asymptomatic and exhibit no obvious cardiac pathological phenotype. Given the uncertainty of the causative genotype, p.P1204L has been also investigated as a single variant, but was already reported to be implicated in cardiac conduction disturbances and/or BrS (Stallmeyer et al., 2012; Liu et al., 2013). To predict the impact of the amino acid substitution, exome variant server (http://evs.gs.washington.edu/EVS/), as well as Polyphen2, SIFT and Mutation Taster were used (**Table 2**). For data interpretation, human gene mutation database (HGMD, Biobase), 1000 genoms and ExAC browser were used.

TRPM4 Variants Expression Pattern

To understand the consequences of the four novel mutations on the TRPM4 channel, we analyzed total expression of TRPM4 after transient transfection of HEK293 cells and its expression at the cell surface by Western Blot and cell surface biotinylation experiments. As previously reported (Syam et al., 2014), we observed that the TRPM4 channel is expressed in fully and core glycosylated forms. As shown in **Figure 2**, we observed a 50% reduction in the total expression of p.A101T and p.S1044C, when compared to the WT TRPM4, both in fully and in core glycosylated bands (**Figures 2A–C**). p.P1204L and the double variant p.A101T/P1204L showed a more severe reduction in the total expression, in both fully and core glycosylated bands (70 and 75% respectively), when compared to WT TRPM4 (**Figures 2A–C**). The decrease in TRPM4 expression was more pronounced at the cell surface for all the loss-of-expression variants (70% loss for p.A101T and p.A101T/P1204L, 60% loss for p.S1044C, 80% loss for p.P1204L), for both fully and core glycosylated bands (**Figures 2B–D**). On the other hand, p.Q854R showed an increased protein expression in both fully and core glycosylated bands of total and surface expression (130 and 110% respectively) (**Figures 2B–D**). However, these increases were not statistically significant. We then performed quantitative Real-Time PCR experiments to determine whether these differences in protein expression may have been due to variable mRNA levels after transient transfection. No significant differences were observed in mRNA expression among the variants when compared to WT *TRPM4* gene (**Figure 3**).

Functional Analysis

To determine possible functional alterations caused by these variants, macro-patch current recordings were performed using inside-out patch clamp on HEK293 cells expressing WT TRPM4 or p.A101T, p.Q854R, p.S1044C, p.P1204L, and p.A101T/P1204L. **Figure 4** shows that a 200 ms voltage step from −100 to +100 mV from a holding voltage of 0 mV elicited small outward Na^+ currents when exposed to nominally 0 Ca^{2+} bath solution (39.6 ± 9.5 pA), whereas it induced large outward currents in presence of 300 μM Ca^{2+} (4768.7 ± 574.6 pA). The amplitude of outward current measured at the end of voltage step to +100 mV varied among the variants. In line with the western blot data (**Figure 2**), variants p.A101T (249.7 ± 44.5 pA, $n = 7$), p.S1044C (314 ± 95.4 pA, $n = 6$), p.P1204L (248.7 ± 82.9 pA, $n = 7$), and double variant p.A101T/P1204L (142.6 ± 27.7 pA, $n = 11$) showed reduced current while the variant p.Q854R (8735 ± 637.7 pA, $n = 7$) showed increased outward current when compared to WT (4768.7 ± 574.6 pA, $n = 13$; **Figure 4B**).

Half-Life of WT-TRPM4 and TRPM4 Variants

To understand the cellular mechanism leading to loss- or gain-of-expression in TRPM4 variants, the half-life of WT and mutated TRPM4 was analyzed using the protein synthesis blocker cycloheximide. Approximately 24 h after transfection, transiently transfected HEK293 cells were incubated with 100 μg/mL cycloheximide and harvested prior to inhibition (0 h)

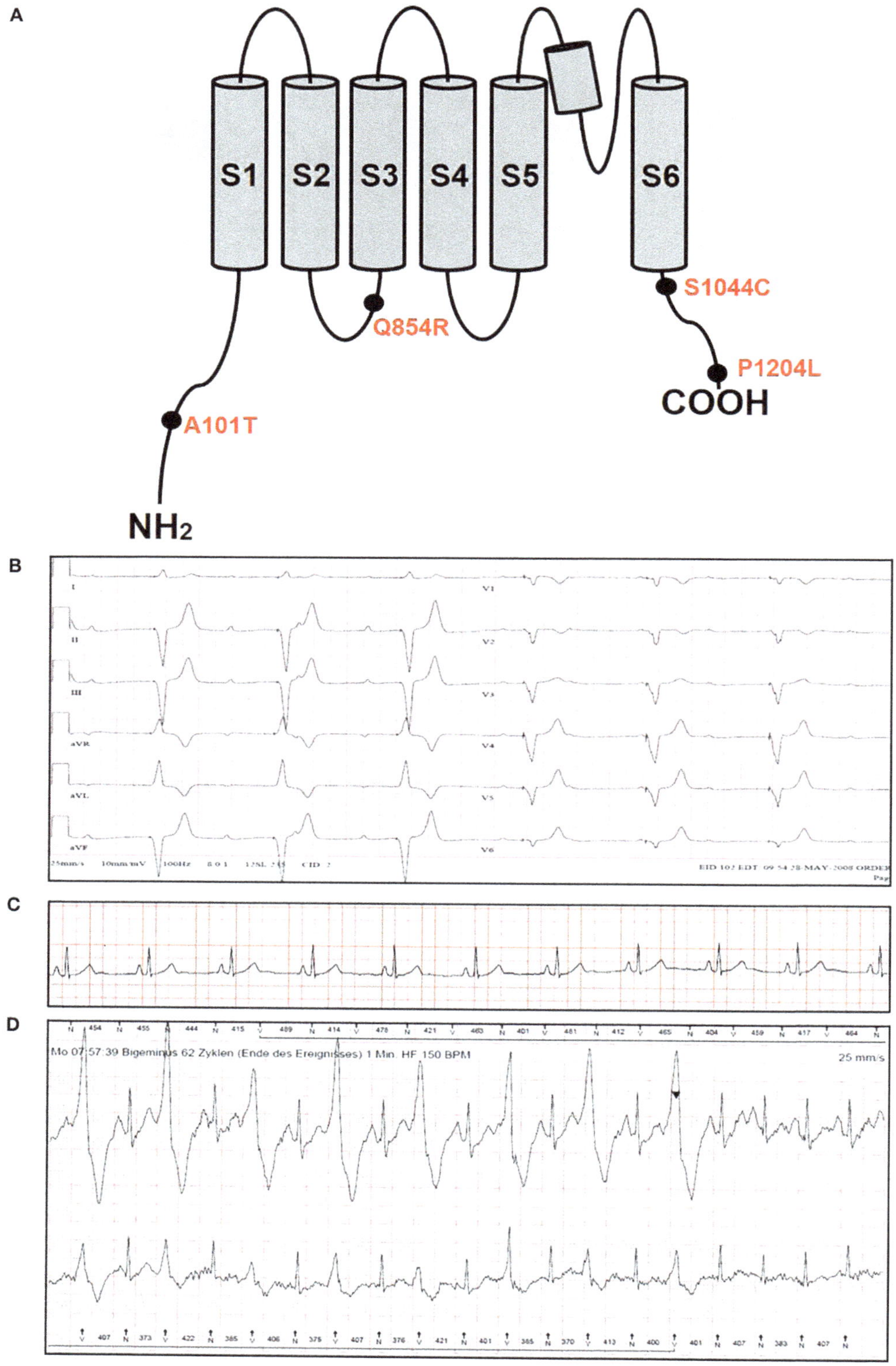

FIGURE 1 | ECG recordings and variants information. **(A)** Variants location in the TRPM4 protein. **(B)** ECG from patient 1 carrying p.A101T variant and showing a complete heart block phenotype. **(C,D)** ECG from patient 5 carrying p.A101T/P1204L variant at rest **(C)** and under physical exercise showing IVF phenotype **(D)**. The arrowhead shows the administration of beta-blockers.

TABLE 2 | Variants characteristics.

Patient ID	cDNA	Exon	Protein	Predicted protein localization	GVS function	EVS Eur-Am	PolyPhen-2 analysis
1	c.301G>A	3	p.A101T	N-terminal, cytoplasmic	Missense	A = 161/G = 8439	Benign (Score:0.000)
2	c.2561A>G	17	p.Q854R	Cytoplasmic	Missense	G = 10/A = 8550	Benign (Score:0.008)
3	c.3130A>T	20	p.S1044C	Helical	n.d.	N.P	n.d.
4	c.3611C>T	23	p.P1204L	C-terminal, cytoplasmic	Missense	T = 28/C = 8542	Possibly damaging (Score:0.008)
4	c.301G>A; c.3611C>T	3;23	p.A101T/P1204L	N-terminal, C-terminal, cytoplasmic	n.d.	N.P	n.d.

EVS Eur-Am, Exome Variant Server European-American Population; GVS, Genome Variation Server; N.P., not present in Exome Variant Server; n.d., not determined.

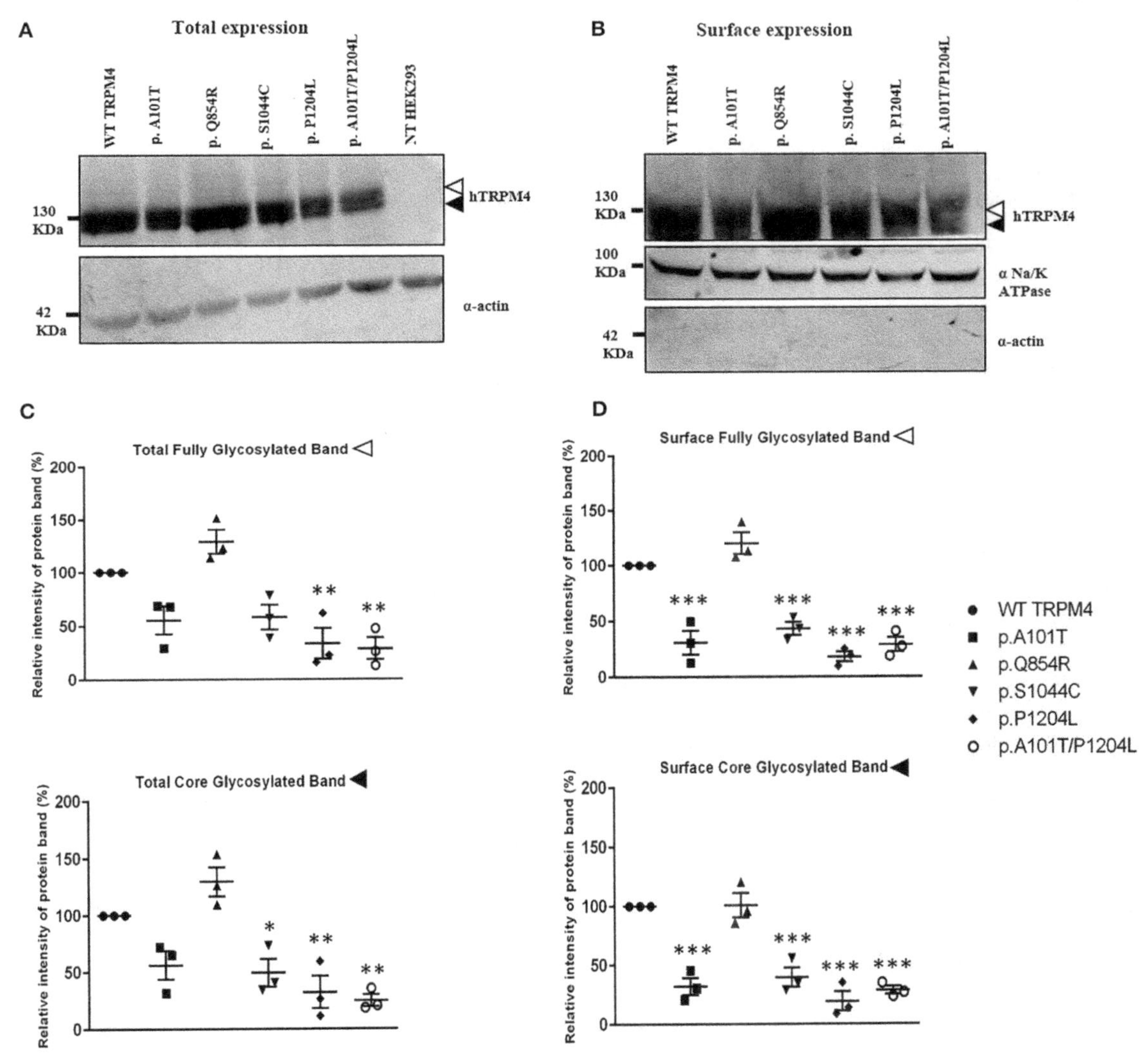

FIGURE 2 | Western Blot analysis of HEK293 cells transiently expressing WT-TRPM4 and TRPM4 variants. Representative immunoblots of human TRPM4 expression at the total **(A)** and surface expression **(B)**. Actin and alpha Na^{+}/K^{+} ATPase were used for normalization of the total and the surface expression respectively. White and black arrowheads represent fully and core glycosylated band respectively. Quantification of the total expression **(C)** and surface expression **(D)** is shown as relative intensity of protein band for both full and core glycosylated forms of TRPM4 in each fraction. Data are represented as mean ± s.e.m. of $n = 3$; $^{*}P < 0.05$; $^{**}P < 0.005$; $^{***}P < 0.001$.

and at 4, 16, 24, and 36 h post-treatment using a TRPM4 immunoprecipitation protocol. For each time point, a 0.3% DMSO control was used to normalize TRPM4 expression. The observed pattern of WT-TRPM4 protein expressed over time following cycloheximide treatment (**Figure 5**) provided a half-life of ~18 h for the fully glycosylated form, and

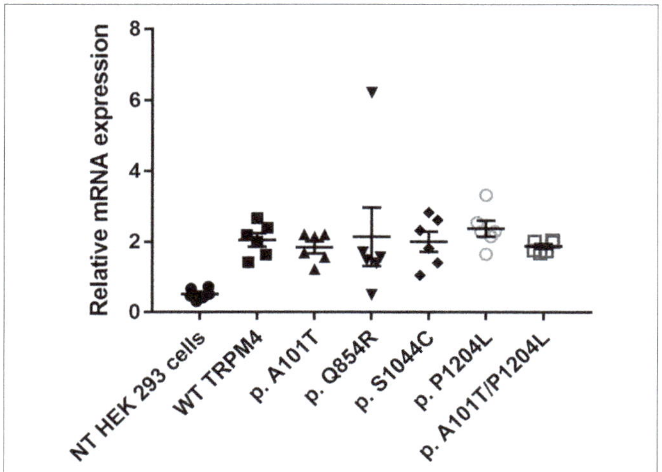

FIGURE 3 | mRNA TRPM4 expression of WT and variants. qPCR analysis on *TRPM4* gene expression in HEK 293 cells transiently transfected with WT-TRPM4 and TRPM4 variants. Data are represented as relative mRNA expression. The expression of *GAPDH* is used as reference (mean ± s.e.m. of $n = 6$). No significant differences are observed between WT and variants.

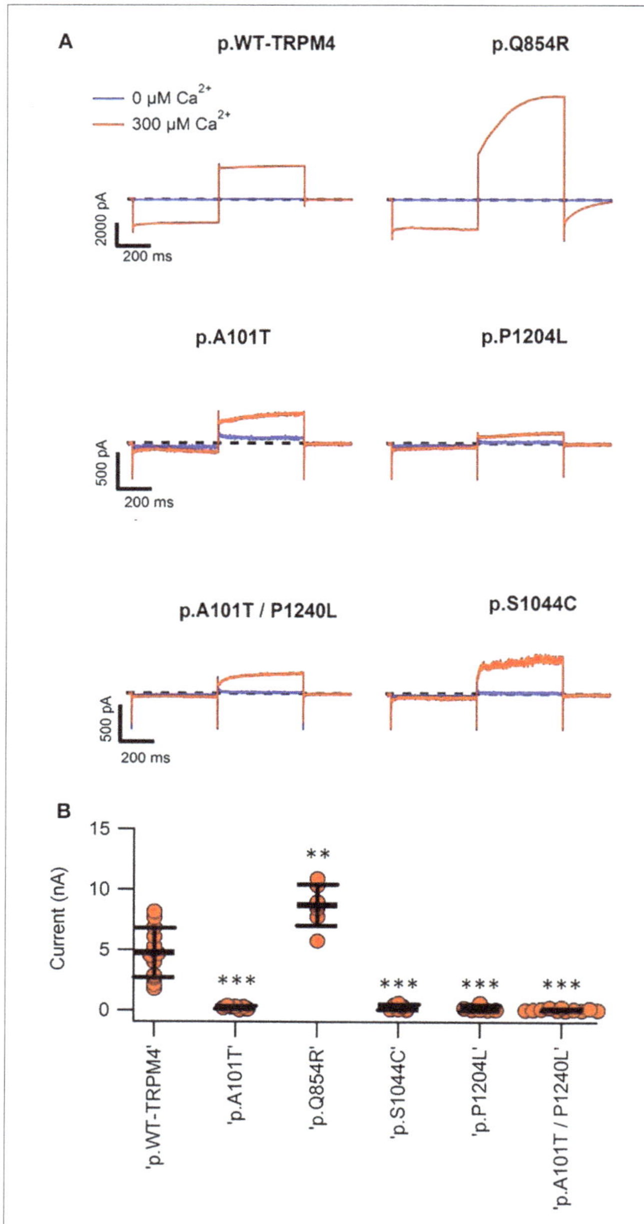

FIGURE 4 | Inside-out patch clamp recordings of WT and TRPM4 variants. **(A)** Individual current traces of WT TRPM4 and TRPM4 variants after applying 300 μM Ca^{2+}. **(B)** Quantification of currents of WT and cardiac conduction disorders variants. **$P < 0.005$; ***$P < 0.001$ (WT, $n = 13$; A101T, $n = 7$; Q854R, $n = 7$; S1044C, $n = 6$; P1204L, $n = 7$; A101T/P1204L, $n = 11$).

30 h for the core glycosylated form (**Figure 6** and **Table 3**). Interestingly, in presence of cycloheximide we observed a more rapid decay in TRPM4 expression of all loss-of-expression variants, with a half-life of ~12 h for p.A101T, p.S1044C and the double variant p.A101T/P1204L, for both fully and core glycosylated fractions (**Figures 5, 6** and **Table 3**). p.P1204L was even more rapidly degraded, and the signal was only partially detectable after 10 h incubation, leading to a half-life of both fully and core glycosylated band of ~8 h (**Figure 6** and **Table 3**). Under the same conditions, gain-of-expression p.Q854R variant half-life has been estimated, resulting to exceed 24 h, and reaching 50 h in both fully and core glycosylated band (**Figure 6** and **Table 3**). Taken together, these experiments indicate that the difference in plasma membrane expression of WT-TRPM4 and TRPM4 variants reflects different degradation kinetics, which causes variations in protein expression.

DISCUSSION

In the present study, four novel *TRPM4* variants have been identified in patients with CHB and IVF. Biochemical and electrophysiological studies revealed a reduced protein expression and function for p.A101T, p.S1044C, and p.A101T/P1204L compared to WT, while p.Q854R showed an increased TRPM4-mediated current. Furthermore, we observed that, when expressed in HEK293 cells, these variant TRPM4 proteins had either increased or decreased degradation rates when compared to WT protein.

The underlying mechanisms leading to conduction defects caused by TRPM4 mutations are not yet understood. Moreover, in this work, both gain and loss of function variants led to the same pathology. A similar observation was made in a series of Brugada cases with mutations in the TRPM4 channel (Liu et al., 2013) and in another series of patients with congenital or childhood atrioventricular block (Syam et al., 2016). While it may seem paradoxical that both gain- and loss-of-function can lead to similar phenotype, one may propose that, if TRPM4 is influencing the resting membrane potential of conduction system cells, both membrane hyperpolarization and depolarization will cause conduction slowing (Abriel et al., 2012), in analogy to

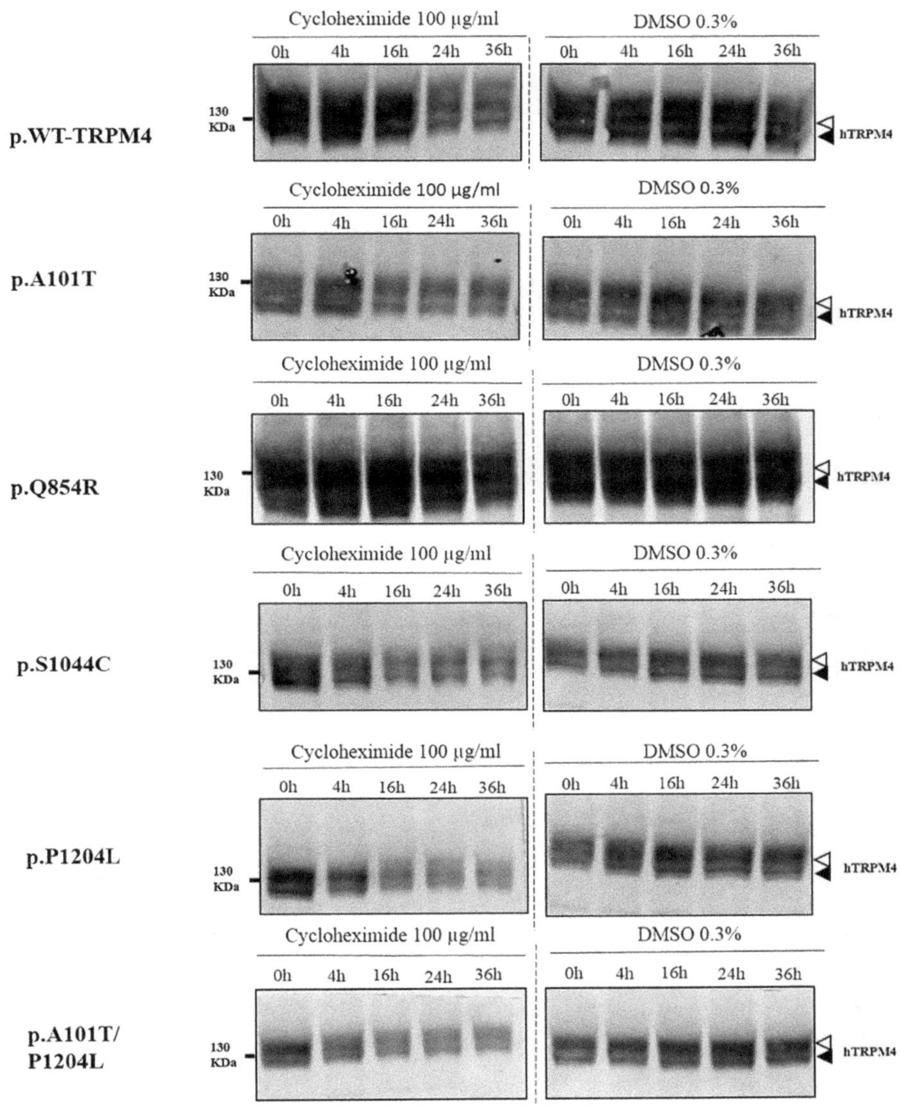

FIGURE 5 | Half-life of WT and TRPM4 variants. Immunoblots showing immunoprecipitation with anti-TRPM4 antibody. Cells were harvested prior to treatment (0 h) and 4, 16, 24, and 36 h after treatment with 100 μg/ml cycloheximide. TRPM4 is detected using anti-HA antibody in presence of 100 μg/ml cycloheximide (left panel), or 0.3% DMSO (right panel). White and black arrowheads represent fully and core glycosylated band respectively. Data are representative of three independent experiments.

the supernormal conduction phenomenon which has been described in atrioventricular conduction (Moore et al., 1993). However, to date, there is no report demonstrating a direct role of TRPM4 in this phenomenon, hence motivating further investigation on the role of TRPM4 in the conduction pathway (Mathar et al., 2014). The presence of a TRPM4 loss-of-function variant in a case with IVF is intriguing and we can thus far only speculate that its possible consequences on impulse propagation may exacerbate the arrhythmogenic potential of the observed RYR2 mutation. It is however impossible to exclude that this presents a variant with no direct functional consequences *in vivo*. A recent report investigated the involvement of TRPM4 in conduction block and arrhythmic phenomena associated with cardiac remodeling and injury, showing that TRPM4 channel is activated by a physiological range of Ca^{2+} concentrations and that its excessive activity can cause arrhythmic changes (Hu et al., 2017). In mouse ventricles, a negative impact of TRPM4 channel activity on cardiac contractility despite action potential prolongation has been proposed, and this mechanism was found to be suppressed in TRPM4 KO mice (Mathar et al., 2014). Further improvement of action potential models may help to understand more complex mechanisms underlying arrhythmias and conduction failures associated with TRPM4 genetic mutations.

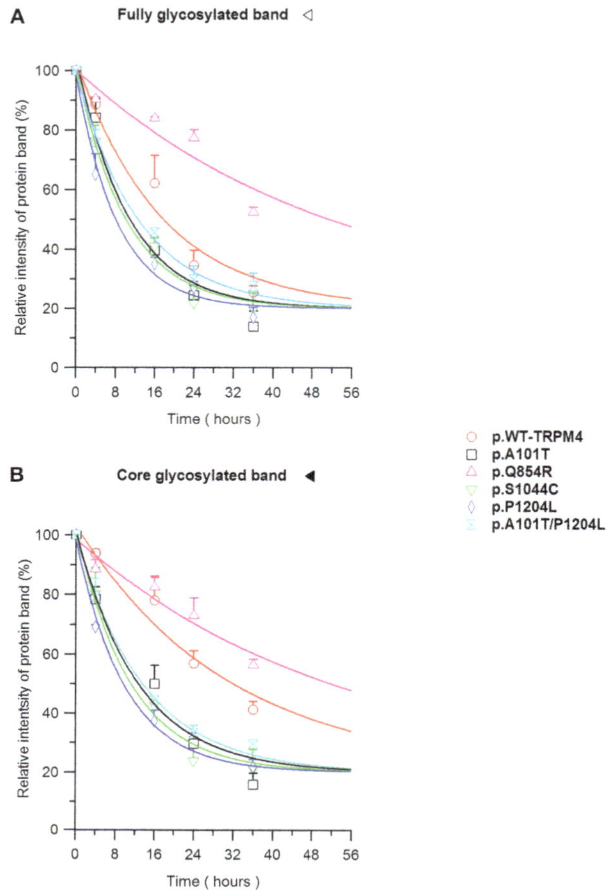

FIGURE 6 | TRPM4 protein expression decay. Immunoblots from **Figure 5** are quantified as relative intensity of protein band of the fully **(A)** and the core **(B)** glycosylated band. 0.3% DMSO values are used at each time point for normalization. Statistical analysis has been performed using one-way ANOVA and results are shown in **Supplementary Table 1**.

Using cycloheximide, we investigated whether the variant-induced altered expression of TRPM4 in HEK293 cells may result from modified protein stability. TRPM4 half-lives of the core and fully glycosylated fractions have been determined for the WT and variant proteins causing conduction defects. Our findings revealed that the fully and the core glycosylated fractions of WT channels had half-lives of ~20 and ~30 h, respectively. These values are in line with Woo and colleagues' study, where they observed a half-life of ~24 h for WT mouse TRPM4 (Woo et al., 2013). Together, loss-of-expression mutants undergo a more rapid degradation rate, resulting in reduced half-life compared to WT. Interestingly, the mutation leading to gain-of-expression significantly decreased the degradation rate of the fully and core glycosylated fractions, with a half-life of ~50 h. In contrast, the loss-of-expression variant half-life alterations were mainly seen in the core glycosylated fractions. These observation are consistent with a model where the decrease and increase of TRPM4 currents are due to changes in TRPM4 channel

TABLE 3 | Variants half-life values.

Variant	Fully glycosylated band half-life values (hours ± s.e.m.)	Core glycosylated band half-life values (hours ± s.e.m.)
WT-TRPM4	17.4 ± 1.6	31.4 ± 2.6
p.A101T	10.5 ± 1.1	12.7 ± 1.2
p.Q854R	52.3 ± 6.8	53.8 ± 4.7
p.S1044C	10.1 ± 0.7	11.0 ± 0.6
p.P1204L	8.3 ± 0.6	9.9 ± 0.4
p.A101T/P1204L	13.0 ± 0.6	13.8 ± 0.4

densities at the plasma membrane caused by variant-induced trafficking alterations. However, it is likely that the mechanisms leading to the loss of expression are not the same as the one underlying the gain of expression. It can be hypothesized that the increased degradation rates of the core-glycosylated fractions reflect misfolding of the nascent proteins and subsequent ER-associated protein degradation (ERAD) (Meusser et al., 2005). In a recent study (Syam et al., 2016), two loss-of-expression TRPM4 variants found in patients with congenital AVB were rescued upon decreased incubation temperature for 24 h suggesting that variant-induced misfolding of TRPM4 may be a common molecular mechanism similar to the case of human ether-a-go-go-related gene voltage-gated potassium channel Kv11.1 (Zhou et al., 1999). On the other hand, assuming that the fully glycosylated TRPM4 fraction is predominant at the plasma membrane, it can be speculated that the reduced degradation of the p.Q854R variant reflects a decreased internalization rate as proposed for other gain of function variants (Kruse et al., 2009). Future experiments will have to be performed to assess this hypothesis.

Ion channels, including many TRP channels, are subjected to post-translational modifications which regulate their trafficking and stability at the cell membrane. It has been reported that human and mouse TRPM4 are N-linked glycosylated at a unique residue, Asn^{992} and Asn^{988} respectively (Woo et al., 2013; Syam et al., 2014). N-glycosylation has been found to be crucial for surface expression of several TRP channels, but most studies have been performed on heterologous systems, with induced ion channels overexpression; therefore, native and recombinant proteins may act differently due to differences in *in vivo* glycosylation. Recent reports suggested the role of SUMOylation as a possible post-translational modification implicated in TRPM4 trafficking. Kruse and colleagues proposed that the p.E7K TRPM4 mutation leading to a gain-of-function and expression was subjected to an increased SUMOylation which augments its membrane expression (Kruse et al., 2009). In contrast, Syam et al. showed immunoprecipitation experiments with WT TRPM4 and the gain-of-expression variant p.G582S, where no direct SUMOylation of TRPM4 seemed to be observed (Syam et al., 2016). Ubiquitination is another frequent post-translational modification of ion channels. In our previous work (Syam et al., 2016), we performed GST-S5a pull down experiments to address whether ubiquitination was involved in differences in expression and degradation between WT and variants. Our findings revealed that the difference in degradation rate of WT and mutants does not depend on a different rate of ubiquitination. Based on these contrasting results, the involvement of SUMOylation and/or ubiquitination leading to increased TRPM4 expression in patients with cardiac conduction disorders still remains to be elucidated.

Recently, the electron cryo-microscopy structure of the human TRPM4 has been reported (Winkler et al., 2017). It is shown there that TRPM4 is composed by four cytosolic C-terminal domains which form an umbrella-like structure, with a coil domain for the "pole" and four N-terminal helical "ribs." p.A101T and p.P1204L are found in well conserved N-terminal and C-terminal residues respectively, while p.Q854R is located in the S2-S3 linker and does not seem to play a crucial role in TRPM4 structure. Interestingly, p.S1044C has been identified to be located in the intracellular gate and might play a role in TRPM4 permeability to Na^+ (Winkler et al., 2017). Further studies would be required to assess S1044 specific role in the channel function.

LIMITATIONS OF THE STUDY

The novel TRPM4 variants described in this work were not assessed in terms of their intrinsic biophysical properties. Further studies using cardiac cells instead of HEK 293 cells may give additional information regarding their relevance in action potential conduction and could lead to a better understanding of the role of TRPM4 in cardiac conduction disorders. In conclusion, although the molecular mechanism underlying protein degradation dysfunctions and their role in cardiac diseases are only beginning to be revealed, it has become clear that altered protein degradation affecting protein half-life may play an important role in a variety of genetic cardiac disorders, including cardiac conduction defects in presence of TRPM4 mutations. Further studies, using knock-in mice or CRISPR/Cas9-dependent editing of human iPS-derived cardiomyocytes, may help to develop clinically relevant strategies to correct protein trafficking abnormalities, including misfolded TRPM4 mutants in cardiac conduction phenotypes.

AUTHOR CONTRIBUTIONS

BB and HA: conceived the study and wrote the manuscript; LO and BB: contributed to the biochemical and functional analyses; MG and AM-D: recruited the patients and provided expert clinical advice. All authors interpreted the data, contributed and commented on drafts of the article, and approved the final version.

ACKNOWLEDGMENTS

We thank Dr. Jean-Sébastien Rougier for his help and useful comments on the manuscript.

SUPPLEMENTARY MATERIAL

Supplementary Figure 1 | Raw WB picture 1 of total expression.

Supplementary Figure 2 | Raw WB picture 1 of surface expression.

Supplementary Figure 3 | Raw WB picture of WT-TRPM4 half-life.

Supplementary Figure 4 | Raw WB picture of p.A101T half-life.

Supplementary Figure 5 | Raw WB picture of p.Q854R half-life.

Supplementary Figure 6 | Raw WB picture of p.S1044C half-life.

Supplementary Figure 7 | Raw WB picture of p.P1204L half-life.

Supplementary Figure 8 | Raw WB picture of p.A101T/P1204L half-life

Supplementary Figure 9 | Raw WB picture 2 of total expression.

Supplementary Figure 10 | Raw WB picture 2 of surface expression.

Supplementary Figure 11 | Raw WB picture 3 of total expression.

Supplementary Figure 12 | Raw WB picture 3 of surface expression.

Supplementary Figure 13 | Summary of raw WB used for **Figures 2A,B**.

Supplementary Table 1 | Half-lives statistical values.

REFERENCES

Abriel, H., Syam, N., Sottas, V., Amarouch, M. Y., and Rougier, J. S. (2012). TRPM4 channels in the cardiovascular system: physiology, pathophysiology, and pharmacology. *Biochem. Pharmacol.* 84, 873–881. doi: 10.1016/j.bcp.2012.06.021

Barbet, G., Demion, M., Moura, I. C., Serafini, N., Vrtovsnik, F., Monteiro, R. C., et al. (2010). *Nature Immunol.* 9, 1148–1156. doi: 10.1038/ni.1648.

Ceylan, G. G., Önalan, E. E., Kuloglu, T., Aydog, G., Keleş, I., Tonyali, S., et al. (2016). Potential role of melastatin-related transient receptor potential cation channel subfamily M gene expression in the pathogenesis of urinary bladder cancer. *Oncol. Lett.* 12, 5235–5239. doi: 10.3892/ol.2016.5359

Cheng, H., Beck, A., Launay, P., Gross, S. A., Stokes, A. J., Kinet, J. P., et al. (2007). TRPM4 controls insulin secretion in pancreatic beta-cells. *Cell Calcium* 41, 51–61. doi: 10.1016/j.ceca.2006.04.032

Daumy, X., Amarouch, M. Y., Lindenbaum, P., Bonnaud, S., Charpentier, E., Bianchi, B., et al. (2016). Targeted resequencing identifies TRPM4 as a major gene predisposing to progressive familial heart block type i. *Int. J. Cardiol.* 207, 349–358. doi: 10.1016/j.ijcard.2016.01.052

Gerzanich, V., Woo, S. K., Vennekens, R., Tsymbalyuk, O., Ivanova, S., Ivanov, A., et al. (2009). De novo expression of Trpm4 initiates secondary hemorrhage in spinal cord injury. *Nat. Med.* 15, 185–191. doi: 10.1038/nm.1899

Gualandi, F., Zaraket, F., Malagù, M., Parmeggiani, G., Trabanelli, C., Fini, S., et al. (2017). Mutation load of multiple ion channel gene mutations in brugada syndrome. *Cardiology* 137, 256–260. doi: 10.1159/000471792

Hu, Y., Duan, Y., Takeuchi, A., Hai-Kurahara, L., Ichikawa, J., Hiraishi, K., et al. (2017). Uncovering the arrhythmogenic potential of TRPM4 activation in atrial-derived HL-1 cells using novel recording and numerical approaches. *Cardiovasc. Res.* 113, 1243–1255. doi: 10.1093/cvr/cvx117

Kalogeris, T., Baines, C. P., Krenz, M., and Korthuis, R. J. (2012). Cell biology of ischemia/reperfusion injury. *Int. Rev. Cell Mol. Biol.* 298, 229–317. doi: 10.1016/B978-0-12-394309-5.00006-7

Kruse, M., Schulze-Bahr, E., Corfield, V., Beckmann, A., Stallmeyer, B., Kurtbay, G., et al. (2009). Impaired endocytosis of the ion channel TRPM4 is associated with human progressive familial heart block type I. *J. Clin. Invest.* 119, 2737–2744. doi: 10.1172/JCI38292

Launay, P., Cheng, H., Srivatsan, S., Penner, R., Fleig, A., and Kinet, J. P. (2004). TRPM4 regulates calcium oscillations after T cell activation. *Science* 306, 1374–1377. doi: 10.1126/science.1098845

Launay, P., Fleig, A., Perraud, A. L., Scharenberg, A. M., Penner, R., and Kinet, J. P. (2002). TRPM4 is a Ca^{2+}-activated nonselective cation channel mediating cell membrane depolarization. *Cell* 109, 397–407. doi: 10.1016/S0092-8674(02)00719-5

Liu, H., Chatel, S., Simard, C., Syam, N., Salle, L., Probst, V., et al. (2013). Molecular genetics and functional anomalies in a series of 248 brugada cases with 11 mutations in the TRPM4 channel. *PLoS ONE* 8:e54131. doi: 10.1371/journal.pone.0054131

Liu, H., El Zein, L., Kruse, M., Guinamard, R., Beckmann, A., Bozio, A., et al. (2010). Gain-of-function mutations in TRPM4 cause autosomal dominant isolated cardiac conduction disease. *Circ. Cardiovasc. Genet.* 3, 374–385. doi: 10.1161/CIRCGENETICS.109.930867

Mathar, I., Kecskes, M., Van der Mieren, G., Jacobs, G., Camacho Londoño, J. E., Uhl, S., et al. (2014). Increased β-adrenergic inotropy in ventricular myocardium from Trpm4-/- mice. *Circ. Res.* 114, 283–294. doi: 10.1161/CIRCRESAHA.114.302835

Meusser, B., Hirsch, C., Jarosch, E., and Sommer, T. (2005). ERAD: the long road to destruction. *Nat. Cell Biol.* 7, 766–772. doi: 10.1038/ncb0805-766

Moore, E. N., Spear, J. F., and Fisch, C. (1993). "Supernormal" conduction and excitability. *J. Cardiovasc. Electrophysiol.* 4, 320–337. doi: 10.1111/j.1540-8167.1993.tb01234.x

Nilius, B., Prenen, J., Tang, J., Wang, C., Owsianik, G., Jannssens, A., et al. (2005). Regulation of the Ca2+ sensitivity of the nonselective cation channel TRPM4. *J. Biol. Chem.* 280, 6423–6433. doi: 10.1074/jbc.M4110 89200

Ramsey, I. S., Delling, M., and Clapham, D. E. (2006). An introduction to TRP channels. *Annu. Rev. Physiol.* 68, 619–647. doi: 10.1146/annurev.physiol.68. 040204.100431

Sagredo, A. I., Sagredo, E. A., Cappelli, C., Báez, P., Rodrigo, A. M., Blanco, C., et al. (2017). TRPM4 regulates Akt/GSK3-β activity and enhances β-catenin signaling and cell proliferation in prostate cancer cells. *Mol. Oncol.* 12, 151–165. doi: 10.1002/1878-0261.12100

Schattling, B., Steinbach, K., Thies, E., Kruse, M., Menigoz, A., Ufer, F., et al. (2012). TRPM4 cation channel mediates axonal and neuronal degeneration in experimental autoimmune encephalomyelitis and multiple sclerosis. *Nat. Med.* 18, 1805–1811. doi: 10.1038/nm.3015

Shimizu, T., Owsianik, G., Freichel, M., Flockerzi, V., Nilius, B., and Vennekens, R. (2009). TRPM4 regulates migration of mast cells in mice. *Cell Calcium* 45, 226–232. doi: 10.1016/j.ceca.2008.10.005

Simard, C., Sallè, L., Rouet, R., and Guinamard, R. (2012). Transient receptor potential melastatin 4 inhibitor 9-phenanthrol abolishes arrhythmias indiced by hypoxia and reoxigenation in mouse ventricle. *Br. J. Pharmacol.* 165, 2354–2364. doi: 10.1111/j.1476-5381.2011.01715.x

Simard, J. M., Kahle, K. T., and Gerzanich, V. (2010). Molecular mechanisms of microvascular failure in central nervous system injury–synergistic roles of NKCC1 and SUR1/TRPM4. *J. Neurosurg.* 113, 622–629. doi: 10.3171/2009.11.JNS081052

Sozucan, Y., Kalender, M. E., Sari, I., Suner, A., Oztuzcu, S., Arman, K., et al. (2015). TRP genes family expression in colorectal cancer. *Exp. Oncol.* 37, 208–212.

Stallmeyer, B., Zumhagen, S., Denjoy, I., Duthoit, G., Hébert, J.-L., Ferrer, X., et al. (2012). Mutational spectrum in the Ca^{2+}-activated cation channel gene TRPM4 in patients with cardiac conductance disturbances. *Hum. Mutat.* 33, 109–117. doi: 10.1002/humu.21599

Syam, N., Chatel, S., Ozhathil, L. C., Sottas, V., Baruteau, A., Rougier, J. S., Amarouch, M., et al. (2016). Variants of transient receptor potential melastatin member 4 in childhood atrioventricular block. *J. Am. Heart Assoc.* 5:e001625. doi: 10.1161/JAHA.114.001625

Syam, N., Rougier, J. S., and Abriel, H. (2014). Glycosylation of TRPM4 and TRPM5 channels: molecular determinants and functional aspects. *Front. Cell. Neurosci.* 8:52. doi: 10.3389/fncel.2014.00052

Vennekens, R., and Nilius, B. (2007). Insights into TRPM4 function, regulation and physiological role. *Handb. Exp. Pharmacol.* 179, 269–285. doi: 10.1007/978-3-540-34891-7_16

Winkler, P. A., Huang, Y., Sun, W., Du, J., and Lü, W. (2017). Electron cryo-microscopy structure of a human TRPM4 channel. *Nature* 552, 200–204. doi: 10.1038/nature24674

Woo, S. K., Kwon, M. S., Ivanov, A., Geng, Z., Gerzanich, V., and Simard, J. M. (2013). Complex n-Glycosylation stabilizes surface expression of transient receptor potential melastatin 4b protein. *J. Biol. Chem.* 288, 36409–36417. doi: 10.1074/jbc.M113.530584

Zhang, Z., Okawa, H., Wang, Y., and Liman, E. R. (2005). Phosphatidylinositol 4, 5-Bisphosphate rescues TRPM4 channels from desensitization. *J. Biol. Chem.* 280, 39185–39192. doi: 10.1074/jbc.M506965200

Zhou, Z., Gong, Q., and January, C. T. (1999). Correction of defective protein trafficking of a mutant HERG potassium channel in human long QT syndrome. *J. Biol. Chem.* 274, 31123–31126. doi: 10.1074/jbc.274.44.31123

14

Low-Frequency Oscillations in Cardiac Sympathetic Neuronal Activity

Richard Ang[1] and Nephtali Marina[1,2]**

[1] Centre for Cardiovascular and Metabolic Neuroscience, Neuroscience, Physiology and Pharmacology, University College London, London, United Kingdom, [2] Division of Medicine, University College London, London, United Kingdom

***Correspondence:**
Richard Ang
r.ang@nhs.net
Nephtali Marina
n.marina@ucl.ac.uk

Sudden cardiac death caused by ventricular arrhythmias is among the leading causes of mortality, with approximately half of all deaths attributed to heart disease worldwide. Periodic repolarization dynamics (PRD) is a novel marker of repolarization instability and strong predictor of death in patients post-myocardial infarction that is believed to occur in association with low-frequency oscillations in sympathetic nerve activity. However, this hypothesis is based on associations of PRD with indices of sympathetic activity that are not directly linked to cardiac function, such as muscle vasoconstrictor activity and the variability of cardiovascular autospectra. In this review article, we critically evaluate existing scientific evidence obtained primarily in experimental animal models, with the aim of identifying the neuronal networks responsible for the generation of low-frequency sympathetic rhythms along the neurocardiac axis. We discuss the functional significance of rhythmic sympathetic activity on neurotransmission efficacy and explore its role in the pathogenesis of ventricular repolarization instability. Most importantly, we discuss important gaps in our knowledge that require further investigation in order to confirm the hypothesis that low frequency cardiac sympathetic oscillations play a causative role in the generation of PRD.

Keywords: sympathetic, arrhythmia, oscillations, cardiac repolarization, cardiac innervation

INTRODUCTION

Sudden cardiac death caused by ventricular arrhythmias is a leading cause of mortality globally, resulting in approximately 50% of all cardiovascular-related deaths each year (Wong et al., 2019). Excessive sympathetic activity is a crucial factor known to promote myocardial repolarization abnormalities that increase the vulnerability of developing ventricular fibrillation and fatal cardiac arrhythmias (Maling and Moran, 1957; Cao et al., 2000). Recent studies have shown that ventricular repolarization instability after an acute myocardial infarction (MI) exhibits a pronounced rhythmic pattern that is believed to mimic the characteristic low-frequency (LF) oscillations in sympathetic efferent activity (Rizas et al., 2014, 2017; Pueyo et al., 2016). This electrophysiological phenomenon has been termed periodic repolarization dynamics (PRD) and it can be measured non-invasively from the vector angle of the electrocardiogram (ECG) T wave (Rizas et al., 2014).

This article aims to review the available evidence in support of the hypothesis that rhythmic sympathetic nerve traffic to the myocardium underlies the origin of PRD. We first focus on how excessive adrenergic signaling affects myocardial repolarization. We then present a comprehensive review of published data obtained in rodent brain tissue *in vitro* and in whole animal preparations *in vivo* that prove that sympathetic neuronal networks most likely involved in the control of cardiac function can exhibit LF oscillatory activity under some experimental conditions. We then discuss the mechanisms involved in the generation of rhythmic sympathetic discharges and explore the physiological role of patterned activity in the sympathetic system and its impact on neurotransmission efficacy. In doing so, we identify important gaps in our knowledge that need to be addressed in future studies.

Cardiac Ventricular Repolarization and the Surface ECG T Wave

Cardiomyocyte repolarization represents a complex sequence of electrical events that occur during phases 1 to 3 of the action potential in which the net outward current exceeds the net inward current, causing the return of the membrane potential to its baseline resting state prior to the next depolarization. Cardiac ventricular repolarization is a significant determinant of the QT interval, represented on the surface ECG by the interval between the start of the QRS complex and the end of the T wave (Yan et al., 2003).

There is general agreement that the T wave is the result of voltage gradients that exist within the ventricular myocardium during cardiac repolarization although the precise mechanism appears to differ depending on the species studied and the experimental preparation used. Using arterially perfused canine right ventricular wedge preparations, Antzelevitch found three layers of electrically and functionally distinct cell types of the ventricular myocardium: the epicardial cells, the M cells and the endocardial cells (Antzelevitch, 2006). These studies demonstrated that the T wave arises due to transmural voltage gradients across the ventricular myocardium which develop as a result of the difference in the time course of repolarization of the three layers, with the M cells having the longest action potential duration (APD) followed by the endocardial layer and the epicardial layer. However, mapping studies using arterially perfused left ventricular wedge preparations and intact hearts suggest that transmural repolarization differences do not fully explain T wave genesis (Opthof et al., 2007; Boukens et al., 2015). By comparing electrical and optical mapping of both intact and left ventricular wedge preparation of canine hearts, Boukens et al. (2017) demonstrated that electrical gradients from wedge preparations differed from those of intact hearts, implying that findings from wedge preparations may not extrapolate to the whole heart.

In addition to the transmural electrical gradient, there is also evidence of electrical heterogeneity between the apex to base (Autenrieth et al., 1975; Watanabe et al., 1985; Franz et al., 1987) and left to right ventricles of the heart (Durrer et al., 1970; Srinivasan et al., 2016). Indeed, whole heart studies have shown that the T wave is an index of dispersion of repolarization across the whole heart and not due to transmural electrical gradients (Meijborg et al., 2014; Opthof et al., 2017; Srinivasan et al., 2019).

Effects of Sympathoexcitation on Cardiac Repolarization and Ventricular Arrhythmia

Sympathoexcitation leads to norepinephrine release which activates β-adrenoceptors (β-AR) to modulate myocardial repolarization and contractility. β-AR stimulation increases L-type Ca^{2+} current which leads to an increase in APD but this is counterbalanced by the concomitant increase in outwards K^+ currents via the rapidly (I_{Kr}) and slowly (I_{Ks}) activating delayed rectifier potassium channels (Hartzell, 1988). Sympathoexcitation can lead to both APD shortening or prolongation depending on the net effect of the inwards and outwards currents (Priori and Corr, 1990). This effect is species-dependent and in humans it has been shown to lead to APD prolongation (Jakob et al., 1988; Veldkamp et al., 2001).

The arrhythmogenic effects of excessive noradrenergic tone are exerted at different levels. At the cellular level, β-AR activation leads to cyclic AMP (cAMP) dependent phosphorylation of proteins involved in excitation–contraction coupling which includes L-type Ca^{2+} channels, ryanodine receptors (RyR) and phospholamban, with concomitant increase in sarcoplasmic reticulum (SR) Ca^{2+}-ATPase (SERCA) activity (Hartzell, 1988). This results in an increase in cytosolic and SR Ca^{2+} levels which can result in a triggered action potential via Na^+/Ca^{2+} exchanger (NCX) and membrane depolarizations during phase 4 of the action potential. This process is also known as delayed after depolarizations (DADs) (Pogwizd and Bers, 2004) and pathological processes such as MI and subsequent heart failure are believed to increase the likelihood of DADs by inducing an increase in the expression of NCX (Pogwizd et al., 1999) and by promoting SR Ca^{2+} leak via RyR (Shannon et al., 2003) and a decreased I_{Kr} current (Pogwizd et al., 2001). At the tissue level, a further requirement for arrhythmogenesis is electrical coupling between the focus of origin and the surrounding tissue (Kumar et al., 1996). Electrical coupling through gap junctions silences "unstable" tissue by the surrounding "stable" cells (also described as "source-sink" effect) (Xie et al., 2010). DADs occurring simultaneously in several thousand cells is hence required to generate enough depolarizing current to produce a propagating action potential, which is manifested clinically as premature ventricular complexes (PVCs) (Myles et al., 2012). Adverse remodeling secondary to disease processes can lead to decreased gap junction coupling which results in a lower number of cells with DADs required to generate an abnormal impulse (Poelzing and Rosenbaum, 2004). On a macro level, overt tissue fibrosis can also result in areas of electrically unexcitable tissue which creates the condition for re-entrant arrhythmias to occur (Vaquero et al., 2008). Finally, at the whole heart level, the heterogeneous distribution of sympathetic nerves across the heart may also play an important role in the generation of ventricular arrhythmias. The density of sympathetic nerve terminals appears to be more abundant at the ventricular base compared to the apex and these regional differences may have a profound effect on the APD gradient from endocardial to epicardial layers (Nabauer et al., 1996; Brunet et al., 2004; Ieda et al., 2007; Lorentz et al., 2010). As a result, even under non-pathological conditions, sympathetic activation would lead to non-uniform changes in APD across the ventricles, increasing the dispersion of repolarization and the potential for re-entrant arrhythmias. In pathological conditions (i.e., diabetes, obesity, MI, and heart failure), where maladaptive cardiac sympathetic innervation remodeling occurs, heterogeneity of APD and repolarization may become even more pronounced (Gardner et al., 2016).

In summary, sympathoexcitation leads to both an increase in triggered activity, and dispersion of repolarization. This leads to abnormalities in activation and propagation of electrical activity in the ventricular myocardium that have been shown in experimental and clinical studies to be pro-arrhythmic (Maling and Moran, 1957; Cao et al., 2000).

Low Frequency Oscillation T Wave Dynamics as a Marker of Sympathoexcitation and Susceptibility to Ventricular Arrhythmia

An area of intense clinical research has been the search for a reliable biomarker of increased susceptibility to potentially fatal ventricular arrhythmia which would help direct clinical intervention such as prophylactic implantation of an implantable cardioverter defibrillator device (ICD). Various non-invasive methods have been studied, including assessments of increased/altered sympathetic tone [heart rate variability (Schmidt et al., 1999) and baroreflex sensitivity (Billman et al., 1982)] and measurements of abnormalities in cardiac repolarization [QT interval (Zhang et al., 2011), QT dispersion (Day et al., 1990), Tpeak to Tend (Panikkath et al., 2011) and microvolt T wave alternans (Verrier et al., 2011)]. However, these methods are not accurate as they only provide an indirect probe of the sympathetic effect on cardiac repolarization. For example, the effect of autonomic tone on sinus node activity is not excluded when studying QT interval as the heart rate is not kept constant and changes in heart rate in itself may affect the QT interval. Furthermore, there may also be concomitant influences of the sympathovagal tone on the vasculatures and on the renin-angiotensin-aldosterone system which may confound the interpretation of the results.

Periodic repolarization dynamics has been proposed as a promising risk marker for susceptibility to ventricular arrhythmia. PRD is assessed using a high resolution ECG recorded in 'Frank lead configuration' with three orthogonal axes X-, Y-, and Z-. Low frequency ($\leq$0.1 Hz) periodic changes of the T wave vector provide an index to measure both sympathetic activity and its effects on ventricular repolarization. In a cohort of 908 patients, increased PRD predicted total and cardiovascular mortality in survivors of MI and was independent of underlying heart rate and respiratory activity. Furthermore, in multivariate analysis PRD provided incremental prognostic value in addition to established risk markers such as LV ejection fraction and measure of T wave alternans (Rizas et al., 2014). A recent 5-year prospective multicenter study (EUropean Comparative Effectiveness Research to Assess the Use of Primary ProphylacTic Implantable Cardioverter Defibrillators, EU-CERT-ICD) showed a strong correlation between the magnitude of the oscillations of ventricular repolarization with both arrhythmia and sudden death in patients with ischemic and non-ischemic cardiomyopathy. Thus, PRD has great potential as a clinical tool for risk stratification of patients who would benefit from implantation of implantable cardioverter defibrillators (Bauer et al., 2019).

The link between PRD and the level of sympathetic activity was demonstrated in clinical studies showing that manipulations that trigger sympathoexcitatory responses (i.e., exercise or the tilt test) enhance the magnitude of PRD whilst pharmacological blockade of β-adrenergic antagonists have the opposite effect (Rizas et al., 2014). The periodicity of the oscillations in ventricular repolarization appears to be in the same frequency range of the LF oscillatory patterns detected in muscle sympathetic nerve activity recordings (MSNA) (Furlan et al., 2000) and in the spontaneous beat-to-beat oscillations in the R–R interval (RRi) (Pagani et al., 1986; Malliani et al., 1991). Other studies have also demonstrated similar rhythmic patterns of APD in patients with heart failure which are coherent with the 0.1 Hz oscillatory frequency of arterial blood pressure Mayer waves (Hanson et al., 2014). Similarly, a recent study has shown that LF oscillations in APD were reduced following β-ADR blockade and were correlated with changes in RRi (Duijvenboden et al., 2019). Together, this evidence has led to the suggestion that LF oscillatory patterns in APD and PRD represent the effect of sympathetic nerve activity on the myocardium (Rizas et al., 2014, 2016). However, this hypothesis is based on associations of PRD with indirect measurements of sympathetic activity which are not anatomically or functionally involved in the regulation of ventricular excitability and repolarization: first, RRi is believed to represent sympathetic influences on the sino-atrial node (Malliani et al., 1991) which explains why PRD is not affected when heart rate variability is eliminated in subjects with fixed atrial pacing (Rizas et al., 2014). Second, arterial blood pressure Mayer waves are believed to result from rhythmic oscillations of muscle vasoconstrictor activity (Julien, 2006). Third, MSNA is a direct measurement of sympathetic vasomotor tone that is usually recorded at the peroneal nerve (Macefield, 2013). Thus, in the following sections we have sought to identify experimental evidence of the existence of oscillatory activity in neuronal networks and peripheral nerves along the neurocardiac axis which might have a more direct role in the regulation of ventricular myocardial excitability.

Rhythmic Sympathetic Activity

One of the most remarkable characteristics of sympathetic neuronal discharges is their rhythmic nature. Autonomic neuroscientists have applied power spectral analysis methods based on fast Fourier transform (FFT) algorithms to detect rhythmic patterns in sympathetic neurons and peripheral nerves both in experimental laboratory animals and in human subjects (Montano et al., 2009).

Rhythmic sympathetic oscillations occur over a wide spectrum of distinct frequencies, ranging from 0.1 to 10 Hz, depending on the sympathetic outflow being measured (Malpas, 1998). In humans, a LF rhythm ($\leq$0.1 Hz) is often found in direct recordings of MSNA (Furlan et al., 2000) and in the variability of heart rate (HR) and systolic arterial blood pressure (SAP) (Pagani et al., 1986; Malliani et al., 1991). However, these sympathetic outflows are unlikely to have a direct role in the control of cardiac excitability since they are not anatomically linked with the innervation of ventricular cardiomyocytes and their control mechanisms may differ from the systems that control cardiac sympathetic outflow. Since direct measurements of cardiac sympathetic outflows cannot be investigated in human subjects, we will primarily discuss evidence obtained in experimental laboratory animals using invasive techniques for the direct assessment of cardiac sympathetic neuronal activity (CSNA).

Low-frequency oscillations in sympathetic outflows appear to be less ubiquitous than cardiac-related (2–6 Hz) and respiratory-related (1–3 Hz) rhythms. Nevertheless, numerous studies have found that LF rhythms are a robust feature of sympathetic neuronal networks involved in the control of cardiac function. Although none of the studies discussed in the following sections have investigated rhythmic sympathetic oscillations in the context of ventricular repolarization instability, the mechanisms described herein are likely to contribute, at least in part, to the origin, regulation and synchronization of PRD.

LF Oscillations in Brainstem Neuronal Circuits

Sympathetic activity originates in a lower brainstem region known as the rostral ventrolateral medulla (RVLM). The RVLM contains a group of C1 catecholaminergic neurons and a group of non-catecholaminergic neurons believed to produce glutamate (Brown and Guyenet, 1985; Schreihofer and Guyenet, 1997; Guyenet, 2006). RVLM neurons send monosynaptic excitatory inputs to sympathetic preganglionic neurons (spns) within the thoraco-lumbar spinal cord (Amendt et al., 1979; Ross et al., 1981) that are crucial for the maintenance of resting vascular tone and heart rate (Marina et al., 2011).

Low-frequency oscillatory patterns have been identified in single RVLM neurons in experiments conducted in unanesthetized, decerebrated, vagotomised and artificially ventilated cats with denervated baroreceptors (Montano et al., 1995, 1996) and in rats anesthetized with urethane with either intact or denervated baroreceptors (Tseng et al., 2009). RVLM neuronal LF oscillations were shown to be correlated with the LF component of the systolic arterial pressure variability (Montano et al., 1995) and were found to be involved in the generation of coherent LF oscillations in renal sympathetic nerve outflows (Tseng et al., 2009). Although the identity of the target organ innervated by these neurons was not identified in these studies, these data strongly suggest that LF sympathetic oscillations have a central origin as they were detected in the absence of cardio-respiratory and baroreceptor inputs. Experiments conducted in adult decerebrated cats have also identified the presence of 0.1 Hz oscillatory activity in pontine neurons involved in respiratory pattern generation and in medullary raphé neurons that modulate both, sympathetic nerve activity and the activity of brainstem respiratory networks (Morris et al., 2010). LF oscillations in pontine and raphé neurons were coordinated with arterial blood pressure Mayer waves and became synchronized with the central respiratory rhythm after elimination of pulmonary stretch receptor inputs (Morris et al., 2010). Together, these results suggest that LF oscillatory activity originates in a dispersed supraspinal neuronal network that participates in the integration of vasomotor, cardiac-related and respiratory rhythms.

Little is known about the cellular mechanisms that contribute to the origin of LF oscillations in supraspinal neuronal networks. At the single cell level, *in vitro* studies have demonstrated that RVLM neurons have the capability of displaying intrinsic pacemaker activity in conditions of reduced synaptic activity, which suggests that synaptic inputs are only involved in the modulation of rhythmic patterns (Sun et al., 1988a,b). Intracellular recordings conducted in retrogradely identified cells in isolated neonatal spinal cord preparations confirmed that a population of non-adrenergic reticulospinal neurons in the RVLM possess pacemaker-like properties such as an after-hyperpolarization at the end of the spike followed by a slow depolarization with no evidence of excitatory postsynaptic potentials (EPSPs) between action potentials (Sun et al., 1988b). However, single cell recordings in intact preparations (anesthetized rats) failed to support this "pacemaker hypothesis," arguing that pacemaker-like activity recorded in RVLM neurons results from the anatomical or functional elimination of synaptic inputs (Lipski et al., 1996). Thus, a "network" hypothesis has been suggested which proposes that 2- to 6-Hz and 10-Hz oscillatory activities in medullary neurons originate from the influence of synaptic influences from neighboring brainstem oscillators located in the lateral tegmental field (LTF) which can be entrained by baroreceptor inputs (Barman and Gebber, 1987, 1993). Although these results illustrate some general mechanisms underlying the generation of rhythmic activity in bulbospinal neurons, they highlight the lack of evidence that might explain how cardiac presympathetic neurons generate LF oscillatory patterns, in particular in conditions of enhanced sympathetic drive.

LF Oscillations in Sympathetic Preganglionic Neurons of the Spinal Cord

Neurons located across four distinct regions of the thoracolumbar spinal cord integrate descending excitatory inputs from the RVLM and other sympathoexcitatory areas in the hypothalamus. These centers include the intermediolateral cell column (IML), nucleus intermediolateralis thoracolumbalis pars funicularis, intercalated nucleus (IN), and central autonomic area (CA). The axon from the spns exit the spinal cord through the ventral root to make synaptic contact with cardiac sympathetic ganglia via white rami communicans. Anatomical tracing studies in guinea pigs (Dalsgaard and Elfvin, 1981) and cats (Chung et al., 1975, 1979) have shown that spns that control cardiac function are mainly distributed along lower cervical and upper thoracic spinal segments (C8-T11).

Most of the evidence showing LF oscillatory activity in preganglionic neuronal networks comes primarily from *in vivo* studies conducted in whole animal preparations. Neuronal recordings from thoracic preganglionic axons in anesthetized cats with high spinal transection at the C1 level showed neuronal discharge variability in the range of 0.1 Hz that were temporally synchronized with the oscillations in systemic arterial pressure (Fernandez de Molina and Perl, 1965). Similar recordings conducted in decerebrated, unanesthetized cats confirmed the presence of rhythmic neuronal discharges in the LF range at the level of the third thoracic (T3) white ramus communicans that correlated with the LF component of the R–R interval (Lombardi et al., 1990; Montano et al., 1992). The power of LF oscillations was increased in response to a fall in systemic blood pressure and conversely, was decreased in response to elevations in arterial blood pressure (Montano et al., 1992). In a subsequent study Montano et al. (2000) found that LF preganglionic neuronal oscillations were preserved following acute spinal transection at the C1 level and the rhythmic discharges remained synchronized with the variability of the R–R interval and systolic blood pressure (Montano et al., 2000). In these conditions, the power of LF sympathetic discharges in preganglionic fibers innervating the stellate ganglion was found to increase in response to increases in arterial blood pressure and this effect was abolished when cardiovascular afferent inputs to the spinal cord were physically interrupted by a dorsal rhizotomy (Montano et al., 2000). Together, these data suggest that LF oscillations are generated locally within preganglionic sympathetic neuronal circuits and that positive-feedback spinal reflexes play an important role in the potentiation of LF oscillatory activity in cardiac-related spns.

The rhythmic properties of spns neuronal discharge have been studied primarily *in vitro* using acute spinal cord slices and isolated spinal cord preparations from neonatal rats. These studies have shown that the mechanisms underlying the generation of this rhythmic pattern result from a complex interaction between intrinsic membrane properties in individual neurons, synaptic inputs and network interactions within the spinal cord. At the single cell level, patch-clamp recordings in neonatal rat spinal cord slices revealed the presence of spontaneous membrane potential oscillations in spns independent of excitatory or inhibitory synaptic inputs, which suggests that oscillatory activity arises from intrinsic membrane properties in spns (Spanswick and Logan, 1990; Shen et al., 1994). At the network level, synchronized sympathetic activity is believed to emerge as a consequence of transmission of spontaneous membrane potential oscillations between gap-junction-coupled spns (Logan et al., 1996; Nolan et al., 1999). In support of this network hypothesis, our immunohistochemical studies have revealed that thoracic spns express connexin-36 proteins along somato-dendritic sites of close apposition (Marina et al., 2008) and pharmacological studies in spinal cord slices have shown that blockade of gap junctions attenuates and in some cases abolishes rhythmic activity in spns (Pierce et al., 2010).

Synaptic mechanisms have also been implicated in the generation of rhythmic activity in spns. Several studies have shown that rhythmic oscillations can be induced pharmacologically by activation of 5-HT receptors in spinal cord preparations *in vitro* (Pickering et al., 1994; Lewis and Coote, 1996; Pierce et al., 2010) and in *in situ* "isolated spinal cord preparations" in anesthetized rats (Marina et al., 2006). This suggests that oscillatory activity in preganglionic neuronal networks is generated in response to direct descending serotonergic excitatory inputs from the medulla oblongata (Smith et al., 1998).

Although rhythmic sympathetic activity in the spinal cord has received significant research attention, very little information is available about the putative mechanisms that give rise to the generation of LF oscillations in spns (Su, 2001; Sourioux et al., 2018). Electrophysiological recordings of preganglionic fibers innervating the celiac ganglion revealed the presence of spontaneous bursting activity in the range of <0.1 Hz that was abolished in the presence of a high Mg^{+} solution and was attenuated by application of non-NMDA receptor blockers (Su, 2001). A recent study showed that activation of muscarinic cholinergic receptors (mAchRs) trigger LF oscillatory activity in spns in coordination with somatomotor neuronal activity (Sourioux et al., 2018). These studies have thus identified cholinergic and glutamatergic neurotransmission mechanisms that play an important role in the generation of LF oscillations in spns that innervate visceral organs. Future studies should determine whether similar mechanisms operate in upper thoracic spinal segments which may facilitate the generation of LF oscillatory activity in sympathetic preganglionic networks that control the electrical activity of the heart.

LF Oscillations in Cardiac Sympathetic Postganglionic Fibers

Extra-cardiac sympathetic neurons are located across numerous thoracic ganglia in particular in the stellate, middle cervical, superior cervical and mediastinal ganglia (Janes et al., 1986; Ardell and Armour, 2016). The electrophysiological properties of neurons located within the stellate ganglion and postganglionic axons traveling along the cardiac sympathetic nerve (CSN) have been studied extensively in several animal models *in vivo*, including ambulatory cats (Tsuchimochi et al., 2002), dogs (Han et al., 2012; Chan et al., 2015) sheep (Jardine et al., 2002, 2005, 2007; Charles et al., 2018) and anesthetized cats (Nishikawa et al., 1994). Experiments conducted in conscious and anesthetized cats with either intact or denervated baroreceptors have been the model of choice to study periodic oscillations in CSNA. However, the frequency of rhythmic neuronal oscillations reported so far appears to be dominated by cardiac-related rhythms in the 2-to 6-Hz range (Ninomiya et al., 1989, 1990, 1993; Kocsis et al., 1990; Hedman et al., 1994; Kocsis, 1994; Hedman and Ninomiya, 1995; Kocsis and Gyimesi-Pelczer, 1998; Larsen et al., 2000) or by respiratory-related rhythms in synchrony with the discharge frequency of the phrenic nerve (Kollai and Koizumi, 1980). The presence of LF oscillations in cardiac postganglionic fibers has not been documented yet, which appears to be counterintuitive, since the final synaptic relay in the neurocardiac axis would be expected to follow the same oscillatory pattern generated by either bulbar presympathetic or spinal preganglionic neuronal networks. However, this apparent lack of scientific evidence does not preclude the existence of LF oscillations in cardiac postganglionic fibers, as this might be the consequence of the experimental conditions used to obtain the data. As mentioned previously, LF oscillations in preganglionic axons have only been detected in decerebrated cats in the absence of general anesthesia (Montano et al., 1992, 2000). Previous studies have shown that anesthetic drugs produce a profound suppression of cardiac sympathetic nerve activity in cats (Matsukawa et al., 1993). This suggests that LF oscillations might have been suppressed and therefore were probably not detected in the studies where animals were anesthetized with chloralose (Kollai and Koizumi, 1980; Kocsis et al., 1990; Kocsis, 1994), sodium pentobarbital (Hedman et al., 1994) or urethane (Kocsis, 1994; Larsen et al., 2000). Another factor that might have interfered with the detection of LF oscillations in cardiac postganglionic fibers is the signal processing methods used for the discrimination of rhythmic components. In the decerebrated cat, cardiac preganglionic fiber power spectra are primarily dominated by a 3.3 Hz component which relates to the rhythm synchronous with the cardiac cycle. In contrast, the power spectral density of LF components in the 0–0.5 Hz range in these preparations is only minor (Lombardi et al., 1990). In order to better identify synchronized preganglionic activity in the LF range, cardiac synchronous rhythmicity needs to be eliminated by filtering the signal with low pass filters with a cut-off frequency of 1 Hz. This allows sampling of the neural signal once per-heart beat and application of autoregressive modeling analysis of sympathetic nerve discharges and R–R interval duration (Lombardi et al., 1990; Montano et al., 1992, 2000). In contrast, the studies assessing cardiac postganglionic nerve discharges cited above did not take measurements to eliminate cardiac-related synchronous activity which may have prevented the detection of LF oscillations (Kocsis et al., 1990; Kocsis, 1994; Kocsis and Gyimesi-Pelczer, 1998; Larsen et al., 2000).

LF Oscillations in Intrinsic Ganglionated Cardiac Plexus

The intrinsic innervation of the heart includes a heterogeneous collection of sympathetic (Moravec and Moravec, 1989; Moravec et al., 1990) and parasympathetic (Yuan et al., 1993) cardiac ganglia collectively termed ganglionated plexus (GP). According to the classification proposed by Beaumont et al. (2013), intracardiac local circuit neurons (LCNs) fall into three main categories: (a) secondary afferent LCNs that detect mechanical and chemical stress signals from different regions of the heart, (b) secondary efferent LCNs that respond to sympathetic and/or parasympathetic neuronal inputs from higher brain centers, medullary networks, spinal preganglionic neurons and thoracic extracardiac ganglia, and (c) convergent LCNs that integrate afferent sensory information with efferent autonomic inputs. LCNs are believed to generate coordinated responses that control chronotropic, dromotropic, inotropic, and lusotropic properties of the heart (Armour, 1997, 2004; Armour et al., 1998).

In vivo studies conducted in anesthetized dogs showed that GP neurons residing in the ventral ventricular GP display spontaneous activity in synchrony to the cardiac cycle and the respiratory rhythm and are exquisitely sensitive to stimulation of β-adrenergic receptors and mechanical stimulation (Ardell et al., 1991). A subsequent study also found that epicardial application of voltage-gated sodium channel agonist veratridine induced robust bursting discharges in the range of 0.1 Hz in both, intrinsic ventricular GP neurons and extrinsic cardiac neurons. However, neuronal discharges were frequently found to be out of synchrony (Armour et al., 1998). In some experiments, transection of sympathetic and vagal neuronal connections also resulted in the generation of bursting activity in intrinsic and middle cervical ganglia neurons (Armour et al., 1998). However, manipulations to produce mechanical activation of carotid sinus baroreceptors failed to produce a significant activation of intrinsic cardiac neurons. These data suggest that LF bursting patterns are primarily displayed by ventricular secondary afferent intracardiac LCNs in response to the detection of chemical clues that are normally released in situations of myocardial damage. Future studies should aim to determine whether LF rhythmic activity generated by intracardiac LCNs is mechanistically linked to the facilitation of LF repolarization instability as observed in PRD.

Cardiac Sympathetic Oscillations Post-MI

Clinical studies have shown that LF oscillations in the variability of muscle sympathetic nerve activity (MSNA) are significantly increased in patients after MI (Martinez et al., 2011). However, sympathetic vasoconstrictor fibers innervate arterioles that determine peripheral resistance which have no anatomical connection with regional cardiac targets. MSNA might be different to CSNA in terms of the regulation of central mechanisms underlying the generation of oscillatory patterns. Thus, increased MSNA is unlikely to be directly linked to the periodic fluctuations in cardiac repolarization observed in patients post-MI (Rizas et al., 2014).

To our best knowledge, there are no studies in experimental animals models of MI that have investigated changes in the power of the LF component in the variability of neuronal discharges of bulbospinal RVLM neurons, spns in the IML and postganglionic sympathetic neurons of the CSN. Electrophysiological studies conducted to investigate the neuronal response properties to MI in anesthetized cats have shown that interruption of the left coronary artery blood flow produced a substantial increase in the discharge of afferent sympathetic fibers that supply the ventricular myocardium and this effect was mimicked by intracoronary administration of bradykinin (Lombardi et al., 1981). Functional changes in sympathetic innervation are thus likely to contribute to post-MI hypersensitivity and may eventually lead to the loss of sympathetic fibers within the infarcted myocardium.

Mi triggers a cardio-cardiac reflex which results in increased activity of preganglionic fibers of the third thoracic white ramus communicans and these responses were found to be preserved in animals with spinal cord transection (Malliani et al., 1969). Experiments in conscious cats (Ninomiya et al., 1986) sheep (Jardine et al., 2005) and dogs (Han et al., 2012) have shown that neuronal discharges of the cardiac postganglionic neurons in the stellate ganglion and CSN increase significantly immediately after MI. Chronic stellate ganglion nerve activity (SGNA) recordings in ambulatory dogs revealed that increased neuronal excitability was observed in viable recordings for as long as 2 months and these changes were associated with increased nerve density at the stellate ganglion (Han et al., 2012).

A recent study using a porcine model of MI revealed that the spontaneous LF rhythmic firing rate of intracardiac GP neurons in the left ventricle are preserved at the same level following a MI, however, with a significant reduction in the detection of afferent inputs. These functional changes were associated with a significant increase in intracardiac neuron cell size and an upregulation in the expression of the sympathetic neuronal marker Tyrosine Hydroxylase (Rajendran et al., 2016). Future preclinical studies should investigate further whether periodic oscillations in ventricular repolarization in subjects post- MI are related to the function of intracardiac PG neurons.

Functional Significance of Cardiac Sympathetic Oscillatory Activity

The physiological meaning of sympathetic oscillatory activity remains unclear. Many studies support the notion that rhythmic activity promotes the coordination of neuronal firing of individual sympathetic neurons which may lead to a highly coordinated and more efficient release of neurotransmitter at the nerve terminal (Nilsson et al., 1985; Ando et al., 1993; Janssen et al., 1997; Lisman, 1997; Dibona and Sawin, 1999). Also, rhythmicity is believed to allow the coordination of nerve discharges between different sympathetic outflows which may help to generate integrated responses that help maintain homeostasis (Barman and Kenney, 2007).

At present, the physiological mechanisms underlying the genesis of PRD are unknown. In this review article we worked under the unverified assumption that recurrent periods of ventricular repolarization instability follow the LF rhythm of cardiac sympathetic postganglionic activity. In support of this hypothesis, *in vitro* studies conducted in fully innervated isolated rabbit hearts have shown that electrical stimulation of CSN (with a stimulation frequency of 15 Hz for 50 s) changed the spatial dispersion of repolarization (DOR) from apex toward the base to base toward the apex within 15 s following the start of the stimulation (Mantravadi et al., 2007). When sympathetic nerve stimulation was interrupted, DOR returned slowly to baseline levels and to its original direction (i.e., apex to base) after approximately 2 min. Although the dynamics of the responses obtained under these experimental conditions (50 s stimulation) make it difficult to extrapolate these results with the periodicity of PRD reported to occur every 10 s (Rizas et al., 2014, 2016), these data provide important clues about the transfer function between neurotransmitter release from the cardiac sympathetic terminals and the concomitant changes in cardiomyocyte repolarization (Mantravadi et al., 2007). Further work needs to be done using similar experimental models but providing rhythmic bursts of sympathetic stimulation to conclusively determine whether LF oscillatory cardiac sympathetic activity translates into periodic oscillations of ventricular repolarization instability.

CONCLUSION

Since Adrian et al. (1932) published their seminal study on rhythmic spontaneous bursting activity in sympathetic nerves of anesthetized animals, a considerable amount of literature has been generated describing the features, mechanisms and possible physiological implications of sympathetic rhythmic activity. However, the translational potential of this mechanism has remained obscure for almost a century.

The discovery of PRD as a novel marker of CSN traffic and strong predictor of death has recently reignited the interest in the phenomenon of sympathetic rhythmicity. The experimental evidence reviewed here identified sympathetic circuitries contained in the brainstem and in the spinal cord which may have direct connections with the ventricular myocardium and that are capable of generating LF oscillatory activity. However, the hypothesis that PRD is directly driven by sympathetic neuronal oscillations (Rizas et al., 2014, 2016) is still missing crucial pieces of evidence, specifically: (i) can postganglionic sympathetic fibers to the heart exhibit LF oscillations, in particular in conditions associated with increased cardiac sympathetic tone?, (ii) are LF sympathetic oscillations themselves pro-arrhythmogenic?, and (iii) is it the amplitude of PRD oscillations what determines its arrhythmogenic potential? The latter is particular relevant since PRD oscillations can be detected in healthy individuals and their amplitude can be increased in response to pharmacological and physiological sympathoexcitatory interventions (Rizas et al., 2014). However, physiological increases in cardiac sympathetic tone and therefore increases in the amplitude of PRD oscillations in healthy subjects do not appear to have arrhythmogenic effects. In contrast, in a cohort of post-MI patients who did not survive the 5-year follow up period, the amplitude of PRD oscillations appears to be much greater than in surviving patients (Rizas et al., 2014). This suggests that the myocardium in non-survivors is more vulnerable to the arrhythmogenic effects of sympathetic oscillatory activity. Alternatively, we speculate that in post-MI subjects with high mortality risk, increased amplitude of PRD oscillations might reflect a higher degree of synchronization among cardiac presympathetic and preganglionic neurons which would allow the recruitment of previously silent postganglionic fibers that innervate specific targets within the heart, such as the myocardium. This would result in the release of copious amounts of norepinephrine from the sympathetic terminals and perhaps the release of arrhythmogenic co-transmitters such as Neuropeptide Y (Kalla et al., 2019) which may ultimately precipitate profound periodic changes in ventricular repolarization.

AUTHOR CONTRIBUTIONS

NM designed the review and drafted the manuscript. RA contributed to the writing of the final version of the manuscript. Percentage contributions are NM 70% and RA 30%. All authors read and approved the final manuscript.

REFERENCES

Adrian, E. D., Bronk, D. W., and Phillips, G. (1932). Discharges in mammalian sympathetic nerves. *J. Physiol.* 74, 115–133. doi: 10.1113/jphysiol.1932.sp002832

Amendt, K., Czachurski, J., Dembowsky, K., and Seller, H. (1979). Bulbospinal projections to the intermediolateral cell column: a neuroanatomical study. *J. Auton. Nerv. Syst.* 1, 103–107.

Ando, S., Imaizumi, T., and Takeshita, A. (1993). Effects of patterns of sympathetic nerve stimulation on vasoconstricting responses in the hindquarter of rabbits. *J. Auton. Nerv. Syst.* 45, 225–233. doi: 10.1016/0165-1838(93)90054-x

Antzelevitch, C. (2006). Cellular basis for the repolarization waves of the ECG. *Ann. N. Y. Acad. Sci.* 1080, 268–281. doi: 10.1196/annals.1380.021

Ardell, J. L., and Armour, J. A. (2016). Neurocardiology: structure-based function. *Compr. Physiol.* 6, 1635–1653. doi: 10.1002/cphy.c150046

Ardell, J. L., Butler, C. K., Smith, F. M., Hopkins, D. A., and Armour, J. A. (1991). Activity of in vivo atrial and ventricular neurons in chronically decentralized canine hearts. *Am. J. Physiol.* 260(3 Pt 2), H713–H721. doi: 10.1152/ajpheart.1991.260.3.H713

Armour, J. A. (1997). Intrinsic cardiac neurons involved in cardiac regulation possess alpha 1-, alpha 2-, beta 1- and beta 2-adrenoceptors. *Can. J. Cardiol.* 13, 277–284.

Armour, J. A. (2004). Cardiac neuronal hierarchy in health and disease. *Am. J. Physiol. Regul. Integr. Comp. Physiol.* 287, R262–R271. doi: 10.1152/ajpregu.00183.2004

Armour, J. A., Collier, K., Kember, G., and Ardell, J. L. (1998). Differential selectivity of cardiac neurons in separate intrathoracic autonomic ganglia. *Am. J. Physiol.* 274, R939–R949. doi: 10.1152/ajpregu.1998.274.4.R939

Autenrieth, G., Surawicz, B., and Kuo, C. S. (1975). Sequence of repolarization on the ventricular surface in the dog. *Am. Heart J.* 89, 463–469. doi: 10.1016/0002-8703(75)90152-0

Barman, S. M., and Gebber, G. L. (1987). Lateral tegmental field neurons of cat medulla: a source of basal activity of ventrolateral medullospinal sympathoexcitatory neurons. *J. Neurophysiol.* 57, 1410–1424. doi: 10.1152/jn.1987.57.5.1410

Barman, S. M., and Gebber, G. L. (1993). Lateral tegmental field neurons play a permissive role in governing the 10-Hz rhythm in sympathetic nerve discharge. *Am. J. Physiol.* 265(5 Pt 2), R1006–R1013. doi: 10.1152/ajpregu.1993.265.5.R1006

Barman, S. M., and Kenney, M. J. (2007). Methods of analysis and physiological relevance of rhythms in sympathetic nerve discharge. *Clin. Exp. Pharmacol. Physiol.* 34, 350–355. doi: 10.1111/j.1440-1681.2007.04586.x

Bauer, A., Klemm, M., Rizas, K. D., Hamm, W., von Stulpnagel, L., Dommasch, M., et al. (2019). Prediction of mortality benefit based on periodic repolarisation dynamics in patients undergoing prophylactic implantation of a defibrillator: a prospective, controlled, multicentre cohort study. *Lancet* 394, 1344–1351. doi: 10.1016/S0140-6736(19)31996-8

Beaumont, E., Salavatian, S., Southerland, E. M., Vinet, A., Jacquemet, V., Armour, J. A., et al. (2013). Network interactions within the canine intrinsic cardiac nervous system: implications for reflex control of regional cardiac function. *J. Physiol.* 591, 4515–4533. doi: 10.1113/jphysiol.2013.259382

Billman, G. E., Schwartz, P. J., and Stone, H. L. (1982). Baroreceptor reflex control of heart rate: a predictor of sudden cardiac death. *Circulation* 66, 874–880. doi: 10.1161/01.cir.66.4.874

Boukens, B. J., Meijborg, V. M. F., Belterman, C. N., Opthof, T., Janse, M. J., Schuessler, R. B., et al. (2017). Local transmural action potential gradients are absent in the isolated, intact dog heart but present in the corresponding coronary-perfused wedge. *Physiol. Rep.* 5:e13251. doi: 10.14814/phy2.13251

Boukens, B. J., Sulkin, M. S., Gloschat, C. R., Ng, F. S., Vigmond, E. J., and Efimov, I. R. (2015). Transmural APD gradient synchronizes repolarization in the human left ventricular wall. *Cardiovasc. Res.* 108, 188–196. doi: 10.1093/cvr/cvv202

Brown, D. L., and Guyenet, P. G. (1985). Electrophysiological study of cardiovascular neurons in the rostral ventrolateral medulla in rats. *Circ. Res.* 56, 359–369. doi: 10.1161/01.res.56.3.359

Brunet, S., Aimond, F., Li, H., Guo, W., Eldstrom, J., Fedida, D., et al. (2004). Heterogeneous expression of repolarizing, voltage-gated K+ currents in adult mouse ventricles. *J. Physiol.* 559(Pt 1), 103–120. doi: 10.1113/jphysiol.2004.063347

Cao, J. M., Fishbein, M. C., Han, J. B., Lai, W. W., Lai, A. C., Wu, T. J., et al. (2000). Relationship between regional cardiac hyperinnervation and ventricular arrhythmia. *Circulation* 101, 1960–1969. doi: 10.1161/01.cir.101.16.1960

Chan, Y. H., Tsai, W. C., Shen, C., Han, S., Chen, L. S., Lin, S. F., et al. (2015). Subcutaneous nerve activity is more accurate than heart rate variability in estimating cardiac sympathetic tone in ambulatory dogs with myocardial infarction. *Heart Rhythm* 12, 1619–1627. doi: 10.1016/j.hrthm.2015.03.025

Charles, C. J., Jardine, D. L., Rademaker, M. T., and Richards, A. M. (2018). Systemic angiotensin II does not increase cardiac sympathetic nerve activity in normal conscious sheep. *Biosci. Rep.* 38:BSR20180513. doi: 10.1042/BSR20180513

Chung, J. M., Chung, K., and Wurster, R. D. (1975). Sympathetic preganglionic neurons of the cat spinal cord: horseradish peroxidase study. *Brain Res.* 91, 126–131. doi: 10.1016/0006-8993(75)90471-0

Chung, K., Chung, J. M., LaVelle, F. W., and Wurster, R. D. (1979). Sympathetic neurons in the cat spinal cord projecting to the stellate ganglion. *J. Comp. Neurol.* 185, 23–29. doi: 10.1002/cne.901850103

Dalsgaard, C. J., and Elfvin, L. G. (1981). The distribution of the sympathetic preganglionic neurons projecting onto the stellate ganglion of the guinea pig. A horseradish peroxidase study. *J. Auton. Nerv. Syst.* 4, 327–337. doi: 10.1016/0165-1838(81)90036-9

Day, C. P., McComb, J. M., and Campbell, R. W. (1990). QT dispersion: an indication of arrhythmia risk in patients with long QT intervals. *Br. Heart J.* 63, 342–344. doi: 10.1136/hrt.63.6.342

Dibona, G. F., and Sawin, L. L. (1999). Functional significance of the pattern of renal sympathetic nerve activation. *Am. J. Physiol.* 277, R346–R353. doi: 10.1152/ajpregu.1999.277.2.R346

Duijvenboden, S. V., Porter, B., Pueyo, E., Sampedro-Puente, D. A., Fernandez-Bes, J., Sidhu, B., et al. (2019). Complex interaction between low-frequency APD oscillations and beat-to-beat APD variability in humans is governed by the sympathetic nervous system. *Front. Physiol.* 10:1582. doi: 10.3389/fphys.2019.01582

Durrer, D., van Dam, R. T., Freud, G. E., Janse, M. J., Meijler, F. L., and Arzbaecher, R. C. (1970). Total excitation of the isolated human heart. *Circulation* 41, 899–912. doi: 10.1161/01.cir.41.6.899

Fernandez de Molina, A., and Perl, E. R. (1965). Sympathetic activity and the systemic circulation in the spinal cat. *J. Physiol.* 181, 82–102. doi: 10.1113/jphysiol.1965.sp007747

Franz, M. R., Bargheer, K., Rafflenbeul, W., Haverich, A., and Lichtlen, P. R. (1987). Monophasic action potential mapping in human subjects with normal electrocardiograms: direct evidence for the genesis of the T wave. *Circulation* 75, 379–386. doi: 10.1161/01.cir.75.2.379

Furlan, R., Porta, A., Costa, F., Tank, J., Baker, L., Schiavi, R., et al. (2000). Oscillatory patterns in sympathetic neural discharge and cardiovascular variables during orthostatic stimulus. *Circulation* 101, 886–892. doi: 10.1161/01.cir.101.8.886

Gardner, R. T., Ripplinger, C. M., Myles, R. C., and Habecker, B. A. (2016). Molecular mechanisms of sympathetic remodeling and arrhythmias. *Circ. Arrhythm. Electrophysiol.* 9:e001359. doi: 10.1161/CIRCEP.115.001359

Guyenet, P. G. (2006). The sympathetic control of blood pressure. *Nat. Rev. Neurosci.* 7, 335–346. doi: 10.1038/nrn1902

Han, S., Kobayashi, K., Joung, B., Piccirillo, G., Maruyama, M., Vinters, H. V., et al. (2012). Electroanatomic remodeling of the left stellate ganglion after myocardial infarction. *J. Am. Coll. Cardiol.* 59, 954–961. doi: 10.1016/j.jacc.2011.11.030

Hanson, B., Child, N., Van Duijvenboden, S., Orini, M., Chen, Z., Coronel, R., et al. (2014). Oscillatory behavior of ventricular action potential duration in heart failure patients at respiratory rate and low frequency. *Front. Physiol.* 5:414. doi: 10.3389/fphys.2014.00414

Hartzell, H. C. (1988). Regulation of cardiac ion channels by catecholamines, acetylcholine and second messenger systems. *Prog. Biophys. Mol. Biol.* 52, 165–247. doi: 10.1016/0079-6107(88)90014-4

Hedman, A. E., Matsukawa, K., and Ninomiya, I. (1994). Origin of cardiac-related synchronized cardiac sympathetic nerve activity in anaesthetized cats. *J. Auton. Nerv. Syst.* 47, 131–140. doi: 10.1016/0165-1838(94)90074-4

Hedman, A. E., and Ninomiya, I. (1995). Periodicity, amplitude and width of synchronized cardiac sympathetic nerve activity in anaesthetized cats. *J. Auton. Nerv. Syst.* 55, 81–91. doi: 10.1016/0165-1838(95)00031-r

Ieda, M., Kanazawa, H., Kimura, K., Hattori, F., Ieda, Y., Taniguchi, M., et al. (2007). Sema3a maintains normal heart rhythm through sympathetic innervation patterning. *Nat. Med.* 13, 604–612. doi: 10.1038/nm1570

Jakob, H., Nawrath, H., and Rupp, J. (1988). Adrenoceptor-mediated changes of action potential and force of contraction in human isolated ventricular heart muscle. *Br. J. Pharmacol.* 94, 584–590. doi: 10.1111/j.1476-5381.1988.tb11564.x

Janes, R. D., Brandys, J. C., Hopkins, D. A., Johnstone, D. E., Murphy, D. A., and Armour, J. A. (1986). Anatomy of human extrinsic cardiac nerves and ganglia. *Am. J. Cardiol.* 57, 299–309. doi: 10.1016/0002-9149(86)90908-2

Janssen, B. J., Malpas, S. C., Burke, S. L., and Head, G. A. (1997). Frequency-dependent modulation of renal blood flow by renal nerve activity in conscious rabbits. *Am. J. Physiol.* 273(2 Pt 2), R597–R608. doi: 10.1152/ajpregu.1997.273.2.R597

Jardine, D. L., Charles, C. J., Ashton, R. K., Bennett, S. I., Whitehead, M., Frampton, C. M., et al. (2005). Increased cardiac sympathetic nerve activity following acute myocardial infarction in a sheep model. *J. Physiol.* 565(Pt 1), 325–333. doi: 10.1113/jphysiol.2004.082198

Jardine, D. L., Charles, C. J., Frampton, C. M., and Richards, A. M. (2007). Cardiac sympathetic nerve activity and ventricular fibrillation during acute myocardial infarction in a conscious sheep model. *Am. J. Physiol. Heart Circ. Physiol.* 293, H433–H439. doi: 10.1152/ajpheart.01262.2006

Jardine, D. L., Charles, C. J., Melton, I. C., May, C. N., Forrester, M. D., Frampton, C. M., et al. (2002). Continual recordings of cardiac sympathetic nerve activity in conscious sheep. *Am. J. Physiol. Heart Circ. Physiol.* 282, H93–H99. doi: 10.1152/ajpheart.2002.282.1.H93

Julien, C. (2006). The enigma of Mayer waves: facts and models. *Cardiovasc. Res.* 70, 12–21. doi: 10.1016/j.cardiores.2005.11.008

Kalla, M., Hao, G., Tapoulal, N., Tomek, J., Liu, K., Woodward, L., et al. (2019). The cardiac sympathetic co-transmitter neuropeptide Y is pro-arrhythmic following ST-elevation myocardial infarction despite beta-blockade. *Eur Heart J.* doi: 10.1093/eurheartj/ehz852 [Epub ahead of print].

Kocsis, B. (1994). Basis for differential coupling between rhythmic discharges of sympathetic efferent nerves. *Am. J. Physiol.* 267(4 Pt 2), R1008–R1019. doi: 10.1152/ajpregu.1994.267.4.R1008

Kocsis, B., Gebber, G. L., Barman, S. M., and Kenney, M. J. (1990). Relationships between activity of sympathetic nerve pairs: phase and coherence. *Am. J. Physiol.* 259(3 Pt 2), R549–R560. doi: 10.1152/ajpregu.1990.259.3.R549

Kocsis, B., and Gyimesi-Pelczer, K. (1998). Spinal segments communicating resting sympathetic activity to postganglionic nerves of the stellate ganglion. *Am. J. Physiol.* 275, R400–R409. doi: 10.1152/ajpregu.1998.275.2.R400

Kollai, M., and Koizumi, K. (1980). Patterns of single unit activity in sympathetic postganglionic nerves. *J. Auton. Nerv. Syst.* 1, 305–312. doi: 10.1016/0165-1838(80)90025-9

Kumar, R., Wilders, R., Joyner, R. W., Jongsma, H. J., Verheijck, E. E., Golod, D. A., et al. (1996). Experimental model for an ectopic focus coupled to ventricular cells. *Circulation* 94, 833–841. doi: 10.1161/01.cir.94.4.833

Larsen, P. D., Lewis, C. D., Gebber, G. L., and Zhong, S. (2000). Partial spectral analysis of cardiac-related sympathetic nerve discharge. *J. Neurophysiol.* 84, 1168–1179. doi: 10.1152/jn.2000.84.3.1168

Lewis, D. I., and Coote, J. H. (1996). Evidence that the firing pattern of sympathetic preganglionic neurones is determined by an interaction between amines and an excitatory amino acid. *Boll. Soc. Ital. Biol. Sper.* 72, 279–294.

Lipski, J., Kanjhan, R., Kruszewska, B., and Rong, W. (1996). Properties of presympathetic neurones in the rostral ventrolateral medulla in the rat: an intracellular study "in vivo'. *J. Physiol.* 490(Pt 3), 729–744. doi: 10.1113/jphysiol.1996.sp021181

Lisman, J. E. (1997). Bursts as a unit of neural information: making unreliable synapses reliable. *Trends Neurosci.* 20, 38–43. doi: 10.1016/s0166-2236(96)10070-9

Logan, S. D., Pickering, A. E., Gibson, I. C., Nolan, M. F., and Spanswick, D. (1996). Electrotonic coupling between rat sympathetic preganglionic neurones in vitro. *J. Physiol.* 495(Pt 2), 491–502. doi: 10.1113/jphysiol.1996.sp021609

Lombardi, F., Della Bella, P., Casati, R., and Malliani, A. (1981). Effects of intracoronary administration of bradykinin on the impulse activity of afferent sympathetic unmyelinated fibers with left ventricular endings in the cat. *Circ. Res.* 48, 69–75. doi: 10.1161/01.res.48.1.69

Lombardi, F., Montano, N., Finocchiaro, M. L., Ruscone, T. G., Baselli, G., Cerutti, S., et al. (1990). Spectral analysis of sympathetic discharge in decerebrate cats. *J. Auton. Nerv. Syst.* 30(Suppl.), S97–S99. doi: 10.1016/0165-1838(90)90109-v

Lorentz, C. U., Alston, E. N., Belcik, T., Lindner, J. R., Giraud, G. D., and Habecker, B. A. (2010). Heterogeneous ventricular sympathetic innervation, altered beta-adrenergic receptor expression, and rhythm instability in mice lacking the p75 neurotrophin receptor. *Am. J. Physiol. Heart Circ. Physiol.* 298, H1652–H1660. doi: 10.1152/ajpheart.01128.2009

Macefield, V. G. (2013). Sympathetic microneurography. *Handb. Clin. Neurol.* 117, 353–364. doi: 10.1016/B978-0-444-53491-0.00028-6

Maling, H. M., and Moran, N. C. (1957). Ventricular arrhythmias induced by sympathomimetic amines in unanesthetized dogs following coronary artery occlusion. *Circ. Res.* 5, 409–413. doi: 10.1161/01.res.5.4.409

Malliani, A., Pagani, M., Lombardi, F., and Cerutti, S. (1991). Cardiovascular neural regulation explored in the frequency domain. *Circulation* 84, 482–492. doi: 10.1161/01.cir.84.2.482

Malliani, A., Schwartz, P. J., and Zanchetti, A. (1969). A sympathetic reflex elicited by experimental coronary occlusion. *Am. J. Physiol.* 217, 703–709. doi: 10.1152/ajplegacy.1969.217.3.703

Malpas, S. C. (1998). The rhythmicity of sympathetic nerve activity. *Prog. Neurobiol.* 56, 65–96. doi: 10.1016/s0301-0082(98)00030-6

Mantravadi, R., Gabris, B., Liu, T., Choi, B. R., de Groat, W. C., Ng, G. A., et al. (2007). Autonomic nerve stimulation reverses ventricular repolarization sequence in rabbit hearts. *Circ. Res.* 100, e72–e80. doi: 10.1161/01.RES.0000264101.06417.33

Marina, N., Abdala, A. P., Korsak, A., Simms, A. E., Allen, A. M., Paton, J. F., et al. (2011). Control of sympathetic vasomotor tone by catecholaminergic C1 neurones of the rostral ventrolateral medulla oblongata. *Cardiovasc. Res* 91, 703–710. doi: 10.1093/cvr/cvr128

Marina, N., Becker, D. L., and Gilbey, M. P. (2008). Immunohistochemical detection of connexin36 in sympathetic preganglionic and somatic motoneurons in the adult rat. *Auton. Neurosci* 139, 15–23. doi: 10.1016/j.autneu.2007.12.004

Marina, N., Taheri, M., and Gilbey, M. P. (2006). Generation of a physiological sympathetic motor rhythm in the rat following spinal application of 5-HT. *J. Physiol* 571(Pt 2), 441–450. doi: 10.1113/jphysiol.2005.100677

Martinez, D. G., Nicolau, J. C., Lage, R. L., Toschi-Dias, E., de Matos, L. D., Alves, M. J., et al. (2011). Effects of long-term exercise training on autonomic control in myocardial infarction patients. *Hypertension* 58, 1049–1056. doi: 10.1161/HYPERTENSIONAHA.111.176644

Matsukawa, K., Ninomiya, I., and Nishiura, N. (1993). Effects of anesthesia on cardiac and renal sympathetic nerve activities and plasma catecholamines. *Am. J. Physiol.* 265(4 Pt 2), R792–R797. doi: 10.1152/ajpregu.1993.265.4.R792

Meijborg, V. M., Conrath, C. E., Opthof, T., Belterman, C. N., de Bakker, J. M., and Coronel, R. (2014). Electrocardiographic T wave and its relation with ventricular repolarization along major anatomical axes. *Circ. Arrhythm. Electrophysiol.* 7, 524–531. doi: 10.1161/CIRCEP.113.001622

Montano, N., Barman, S. M., Gnecchi-Ruscone, T., Porta, A., Lombardi, F., and Malliani, A. (1995). [Role of low-frequency neuronal activity in the medulla in the regulation of the cardiovascular system]. *Cardiologia* 40, 41–46.

Montano, N., Cogliati, C., da Silva, V. J., Gnecchi-Ruscone, T., Massimini, M., Porta, A., et al. (2000). Effects of spinal section and of positive-feedback excitatory reflex on sympathetic and heart rate variability. *Hypertension* 36, 1029–1034. doi: 10.1161/01.hyp.36.6.1029

Montano, N., Furlan, R., Guzzetti, S., McAllen, R. M., and Julien, C. (2009). Analysis of sympathetic neural discharge in rats and humans. *Philos. Trans. A Math. Phys. Eng. Sci.* 367, 1265–1282. doi: 10.1098/rsta.2008.0285

Montano, N., Gnecchi-Ruscone, T., Porta, A., Lombardi, F., Malliani, A., and Barman, S. M. (1996). Presence of vasomotor and respiratory rhythms in the discharge of single medullary neurons involved in the regulation of cardiovascular system. *J. Auton. Nerv. Syst.* 57, 116–122. doi: 10.1016/0165-1838(95)00113-1

Montano, N., Lombardi, F., Gnecchi Ruscone, T., Contini, M., Finocchiaro, M. L., Baselli, G., et al. (1992). Spectral analysis of sympathetic discharge, R-R interval and systolic arterial pressure in decerebrate cats. *J. Auton. Nerv. Syst.* 40, 21–31. doi: 10.1016/0165-1838(92)90222-3

Moravec, M., and Moravec, J. (1989). Adrenergic neurons and short proprioceptive feedback loops involved in the integration of cardiac function in the rat. *Cell Tissue Res.* 258, 381–385. doi: 10.1007/bf00239458

Moravec, M., Moravec, J., and Forsgren, S. (1990). Catecholaminergic and peptidergic nerve components of intramural ganglia in the rat heart. An immunohistochemical study. *Cell Tissue Res.* 262, 315–327. doi: 10.1007/bf00309887

Morris, K. F., Nuding, S. C., Segers, L. S., Baekey, D. M., Shannon, R., Lindsey, B. G., et al. (2010). Respiratory and Mayer wave-related discharge patterns of raphe and pontine neurons change with vagotomy. *J. Appl. Physiol. (*1985) 109, 189–202. doi: 10.1152/japplphysiol.01324.2009

Myles, R. C., Wang, L., Kang, C., Bers, D. M., and Ripplinger, C. M. (2012). Local beta-adrenergic stimulation overcomes source-sink mismatch to generate focal arrhythmia. *Circ. Res.* 110, 1454–1464. doi: 10.1161/CIRCRESAHA.111.262345

Nabauer, M., Beuckelmann, D. J., Uberfuhr, P., and Steinbeck, G. (1996). Regional differences in current density and rate-dependent properties of the transient outward current in subepicardial and subendocardial myocytes of human left ventricle. *Circulation* 93, 168–177. doi: 10.1161/01.cir.93.1.168

Nilsson, H., Ljung, B., Sjoblom, N., and Wallin, B. G. (1985). The influence of the sympathetic impulse pattern on contractile responses of rat mesenteric arteries and veins. *Acta Physiol. Scand.* 123, 303–309. doi: 10.1111/j.1748-1716.1985.tb07592.x

Ninomiya, I., Akiyama, T., and Nishiura, N. (1990). Mechanism of cardiac-related synchronized cardiac sympathetic nerve activity in awake cats. *Am. J. Physiol.* 259(3 Pt 2), R499–R506. doi: 10.1152/ajpregu.1990.259.3.R499

Ninomiya, I., Malpas, S. C., Matsukawa, K., Shindo, T., and Akiyama, T. (1993). The amplitude of synchronized cardiac sympathetic nerve activity reflects the number of activated pre- and postganglionic fibers in anesthetized cats. *J. Auton. Nerv. Syst.* 45, 139–147. doi: 10.1016/0165-1838(93)90125-e

Ninomiya, I., Matsukawa, K., Honda, T., Nishiura, N., and Shirai, M. (1986). Cardiac sympathetic nerve activity and heart rate during coronary occlusion in awake cats. *Am. J. Physiol.* 251(3 Pt 2), H528–H537. doi: 10.1152/ajpheart.1986.251.3.H528

Ninomiya, I., Nishiura, N., Matsukawa, K., and Akiyama, T. (1989). Fundamental rhythm of cardiac sympathetic nerve activity in awake cats at rest and during body movement. *Jpn. J. Physiol.* 39, 743–753. doi: 10.2170/jjphysiol.39.743

Nishikawa, K., Terai, T., Morimoto, O., Yukioka, H., and Fujimori, M. (1994). Effects of intravenous lidocaine on cardiac sympathetic nerve activity and A-V conduction in halothane-anesthetized cats. *Acta Anaesthesiol. Scand.* 38, 115–120. doi: 10.1111/j.1399-6576.1994.tb03851.x

Nolan, M. F., Logan, S. D., and Spanswick, D. (1999). Electrophysiological properties of electrical synapses between rat sympathetic preganglionic neurones in vitro. *J. Physiol.* 519(Pt 3), 753–764. doi: 10.1111/j.1469-7793.1999.0753n.x

Opthof, T., Coronel, R., Wilms-Schopman, F. J., Plotnikov, A. N., Shlapakova, I. N., Danilo, P., et al. (2007). Dispersion of repolarization in canine ventricle and the electrocardiographic T wave: Tp-e interval does not reflect transmural dispersion. *Heart Rhythm* 4, 341–348. doi: 10.1016/j.hrthm.2006.11.022

Opthof, T., Remme, C. A., Jorge, E., Noriega, F., Wiegerinck, R. F., Tasiam, A., et al. (2017). Cardiac activation-repolarization patterns and ion channel expression mapping in intact isolated normal human hearts. *Heart Rhythm* 14, 265–272. doi: 10.1016/j.hrthm.2016.10.010

Pagani, M., Lombardi, F., Guzzetti, S., Rimoldi, O., Furlan, R., Pizzinelli, P., et al. (1986). Power spectral analysis of heart rate and arterial pressure variabilities as a marker of sympatho-vagal interaction in man and conscious dog. *Circ. Res.* 59, 178–193. doi: 10.1161/01.res.59.2.178

Panikkath, R., Reinier, K., Uy-Evanado, A., Teodorescu, C., Hattenhauer, J., Mariani, R., et al. (2011). Prolonged Tpeak-to-tend interval on the resting ECG is associated with increased risk of sudden cardiac death. *Circ. Arrhythm. Electrophysiol.* 4, 441–447. doi: 10.1161/CIRCEP.110.960658

Pickering, A. E., Spanswick, D., and Logan, S. D. (1994). 5-Hydoxytryptamine evokes depolarizations and membrane potential oscillations in rat sympathetic preganglionic neurones. *J. Physiol.* 480(Pt 1), 109–121. doi: 10.1113/jphysiol.1994.sp020345

Pierce, M. L., Deuchars, J., and Deuchars, S. A. (2010). Spontaneous rhythmogenic capabilities of sympathetic neuronal assemblies in the rat spinal cord slice. *Neuroscience* 170, 827–838. doi: 10.1016/j.neuroscience.2010.07.007

Poelzing, S., and Rosenbaum, D. S. (2004). Altered connexin43 expression produces arrhythmia substrate in heart failure. *Am. J. Physiol. Heart Circ. Physiol.* 287, H1762–H1770. doi: 10.1152/ajpheart.00346.2004

Pogwizd, S. M., and Bers, D. M. (2004). Cellular basis of triggered arrhythmias in heart failure. *Trends Cardiovasc. Med.* 14, 61–66. doi: 10.1016/j.tcm.2003.12.002

Pogwizd, S. M., Qi, M., Yuan, W., Samarel, A. M., and Bers, D. M. (1999). Upregulation of Na(+)/Ca(2+) exchanger expression and function in an arrhythmogenic rabbit model of heart failure. *Circ. Res.* 85, 1009–1019. doi: 10.1161/01.res.85.11.1009

Pogwizd, S. M., Schlotthauer, K., Li, L., Yuan, W., and Bers, D. M. (2001). Arrhythmogenesis and contractile dysfunction in heart failure: roles of sodium-calcium exchange, inward rectifier potassium current, and residual beta-adrenergic responsiveness. *Circ. Res.* 88, 1159–1167. doi: 10.1161/hh1101.091193

Priori, S. G., and Corr, P. B. (1990). Mechanisms underlying early and delayed afterdepolarizations induced by catecholamines. *Am. J. Physiol.* 258(6 Pt 2), H1796–H1805. doi: 10.1152/ajpheart.1990.258.6.H1796

Pueyo, E., Orini, M., Rodriguez, J. F., and Taggart, P. (2016). Interactive effect of beta-adrenergic stimulation and mechanical stretch on low-frequency oscillations of ventricular action potential duration in humans. *J. Mol. Cell. Cardiol.* 97, 93–105. doi: 10.1016/j.yjmcc.2016.05.003

Rajendran, P. S., Nakamura, K., Ajijola, O. A., Vaseghi, M., Armour, J. A., Ardell, J. L., et al. (2016). Myocardial infarction induces structural and functional remodelling of the intrinsic cardiac nervous system. *J. Physiol.* 594, 321–341. doi: 10.1113/JP271165

Rizas, K. D., Hamm, W., Kaab, S., Schmidt, G., and Bauer, A. (2016). Periodic repolarisation dynamics: a natural probe of the ventricular response to sympathetic activation. *Arrhythm. Electrophysiol. Rev.* 5, 31–36. doi: 10.15420/aer.2015:30:2

Rizas, K. D., McNitt, S., Hamm, W., Massberg, S., Kaab, S., Zareba, W., et al. (2017). Prediction of sudden and non-sudden cardiac death in post-infarction patients with reduced left ventricular ejection fraction by periodic repolarization dynamics: MADIT-II substudy. *Eur. Heart J.* 38, 2110–2118. doi: 10.1093/eurheartj/ehx161

Rizas, K. D., Nieminen, T., Barthel, P., Zurn, C. S., Kahonen, M., Viik, J., et al. (2014). Sympathetic activity-associated periodic repolarization dynamics predict mortality following myocardial infarction. *J. Clin. Invest.* 124, 1770–1780. doi: 10.1172/JCI70085

Ross, C. A., Armstrong, D. M., Ruggiero, D. A., Pickel, V. M., Joh, T. H., and Reis, D. J. (1981). Adrenaline neurons in the rostral ventrolateral medulla innervate thoracic spinal cord: a combined immunocytochemical and retrograde transport demonstration. *Neurosci. Lett.* 25, 257–262. doi: 10.1016/0304-3940(81)90401-8

Schmidt, G., Malik, M., Barthel, P., Schneider, R., Ulm, K., Rolnitzky, L., et al. (1999). Heart-rate turbulence after ventricular premature beats as a predictor of mortality after acute myocardial infarction. *Lancet* 353, 1390–1396. doi: 10.1016/s0140-6736(98)08428-1

Schreihofer, A. M., and Guyenet, P. G. (1997). Identification of C1 presympathetic neurons in rat rostral ventrolateral medulla by juxtacellular labeling in vivo. *J. Comp. Neurol.* 387, 524–536. doi: 10.1002/(sici)1096-9861(19971103)387:4<524::aid-cne4>3.0.co;2-4

Shannon, T. R., Pogwizd, S. M., and Bers, D. M. (2003). Elevated sarcoplasmic reticulum Ca2+ leak in intact ventricular myocytes from rabbits in heart failure. *Circ. Res.* 93, 592–594. doi: 10.1161/01.RES.0000093399.11734.B3

Shen, E., Wu, S. Y., and Dun, N. J. (1994). Spontaneous and transmitter-induced rhythmic activity in neonatal rat sympathetic preganglionic neurons in vitro. *J. Neurophysiol.* 71, 1197–1205. doi: 10.1152/jn.1994.71.3.1197

Smith, J. E., Jansen, A. S., Gilbey, M. P., and Loewy, A. D. (1998). CNS cell groups projecting to sympathetic outflow of tail artery: neural circuits involved in heat loss in the rat. *Brain Res.* 786, 153–164. doi: 10.1016/s0006-8993(97)01437-6

Sourioux, M., Bertrand, S. S., and Cazalets, J. R. (2018). Cholinergic-mediated coordination of rhythmic sympathetic and motor activities in the newborn rat spinal cord. *PLoS Biol.* 16:e2005460. doi: 10.1371/journal.pbio.2005460

Spanswick, D., and Logan, S. D. (1990). Spontaneous rhythmic activity in the intermediolateral cell nucleus of the neonate rat thoracolumbar spinal cord in vitro. *Neuroscience* 39, 395–403. doi: 10.1016/0306-4522(90)90276-a

Srinivasan, N. T., Orini, M., Providencia, R., Simon, R., Lowe, M., Segal, O. R., et al. (2019). Differences in the upslope of the precordial body surface ECG T wave reflect right to left dispersion of repolarization in the intact human heart. *Heart Rhythm* 16, 943–951. doi: 10.1016/j.hrthm.2018.12.006

Srinivasan, N. T., Orini, M., Simon, R. B., Providencia, R., Khan, F. Z., Segal, O. R., et al. (2016). Ventricular stimulus site influences dynamic dispersion of repolarization in the intact human heart. *Am. J. Physiol. Heart Circ. Physiol.* 311, H545–H554. doi: 10.1152/ajpheart.00159.2016

Su, C. K. (2001). Intraspinal amino acid neurotransmitter activities are involved in the generation of rhythmic sympathetic nerve discharge in newborn rat spinal cord. *Brain Res.* 904, 112–125. doi: 10.1016/s0006-8993(01)02495-7

Sun, M. K., Hackett, J. T., and Guyenet, P. G. (1988a). Sympathoexcitatory neurons of rostral ventrolateral medulla exhibit pacemaker properties in the presence of a glutamate-receptor antagonist. *Brain Res.* 438, 23–40. doi: 10.1016/0006-8993(88)91320-0

Sun, M. K., Young, B. S., Hackett, J. T., and Guyenet, P. G. (1988b). Reticulospinal pacemaker neurons of the rat rostral ventrolateral medulla with putative sympathoexcitatory function: an intracellular study in vitro. *Brain Res.* 442, 229–239. doi: 10.1016/0006-8993(88)91508-9

Tseng, W. T., Chen, R. F., Tsai, M. L., and Yen, C. T. (2009). Correlation of discharges of rostral ventrolateral medullary neurons with the low-frequency sympathetic rhythm in rats. *Neurosci. Lett.* 454, 22–27. doi: 10.1016/j.neulet.2009.02.057

Tsuchimochi, H., Matsukawa, K., Komine, H., and Murata, J. (2002). Direct measurement of cardiac sympathetic efferent nerve activity during dynamic exercise. *Am. J. Physiol. Heart Circ. Physiol.* 283, H1896–H1906. doi: 10.1152/ajpheart.00112.2002

Vaquero, M., Calvo, D., and Jalife, J. (2008). Cardiac fibrillation: from ion channels to rotors in the human heart. *Heart Rhythm* 5, 872–879. doi: 10.1016/j.hrthm.2008.02.034

Veldkamp, M. W., Verkerk, A. O., van Ginneken, A. C., Baartscheer, A., Schumacher, C., de Jonge, N., et al. (2001). Norepinephrine induces action potential prolongation and early afterdepolarizations in ventricular myocytes isolated from human end-stage failing hearts. *Eur. Heart J.* 22, 955–963. doi: 10.1053/euhj.2000.2499

Verrier, R. L., Klingenheben, T., Malik, M., El-Sherif, N., Exner, D. V., Hohnloser, S. H., et al. (2011). Microvolt T-wave alternans physiological basis, methods of measurement, and clinical utility-consensus guideline by International Society for Holter and Noninvasive Electrocardiology. *J. Am. Coll. Cardiol.* 58, 1309–1324. doi: 10.1016/j.jacc.2011.06.029

Watanabe, T., Rautaharju, P. M., and McDonald, T. F. (1985). Ventricular action potentials, ventricular extracellular potentials, and the ECG of guinea pig. *Circ. Res.* 57, 362–373. doi: 10.1161/01.res.57.3.362

Wong, C. X., Brown, A., Lau, D. H., Chugh, S. S., Albert, C. M., Kalman, J. M., et al. (2019). Epidemiology of sudden cardiac death: global and regional perspectives. *Heart Lung Circ.* 28, 6–14. doi: 10.1016/j.hlc.2018.08.026

Xie, Y., Sato, D., Garfinkel, A., Qu, Z., and Weiss, J. N. (2010). So little source, so much sink: requirements for afterdepolarizations to propagate in tissue. *Biophys. J.* 99, 1408–1415. doi: 10.1016/j.bpj.2010.06.042

Yan, G. X., Lankipalli, R. S., Burke, J. F., Musco, S., and Kowey, P. R. (2003). Ventricular repolarization components on the electrocardiogram: cellular basis and clinical significance. *J. Am. Coll. Cardiol.* 42, 401–409.

Yuan, B. X., Ardell, J. L., Hopkins, D. A., and Armour, J. A. (1993). Differential cardiac responses induced by nicotine sensitive canine atrial and ventricular neurones. *Cardiovasc. Res.* 27, 760–769. doi: 10.1093/cvr/27.5.760

Zhang, Y., Post, W. S., Blasco-Colmenares, E., Dalal, D., Tomaselli, G. F., and Guallar, E. (2011). Electrocardiographic QT interval and mortality: a meta-analysis. *Epidemiology* 22, 660–670. doi: 10.1097/EDE.0b013e318225768b

15

Ion Channel Trafficking: Control of Ion Channel Density as a Target for Arrhythmias?

Elise Balse [1*] *and Hannah E. Boycott* [2]

[1] Unité de Recherche sur les Maladies Cardiovasculaires, le Métabolisme et la Nutrition, Faculté de Médecine Pitié-Salpêtrière, Sorbonne Universités, UPMC Univ. Paris VI, Inserm, UMRS 1166, Université Pierre et Marie Curie, Paris, France, [2] Department of Cardiovascular Medicine, John Radcliffe Hospital, University of Oxford, Oxford, United Kingdom

Correspondence:
Elise Balse
elise.balse@upmc.fr

The shape of the cardiac action potential (AP) is determined by the contributions of numerous ion channels. Any dysfunction in the proper function or expression of these ion channels can result in a change in effective refractory period (ERP) and lead to arrhythmia. The processes underlying the correct targeting of ion channels to the plasma membrane are complex, and have not been fully characterized in cardiac myocytes. Emerging evidence highlights ion channel trafficking as a potential causative factor in certain acquired and inherited arrhythmias, and therapies which target trafficking as opposed to pore block are starting to receive attention. In this review we present the current evidence for the mechanisms which underlie precise control of cardiac ion channel trafficking and targeting.

Keywords: potassium channels, sodium channel, arrhythmias, cardiac, trafficking, accessory proteins

FUNCTIONAL EXPRESSION OF ION CHANNELS IN THE SARCOLEMMA AND CARDIAC EXCITABILITY

The function of the heart is governed by the electrical and mechanical activity of myocytes. The functional expression of several different types of ion channels in the myocyte sarcolemma determines the shape and duration of the action potential (AP), and therefore controls the effective refractory period (ERP) of the myocardium. The ERP is a protective mechanism that keeps the heart rate in check and thus prevents arrhythmias. Any prolongation or shortening of the ERP is therefore potentially arrhythmogenic. Most genetic arrhythmias are caused by mutations which alter the biophysical properties of ion channels. However, the proper functional expression of ion channels can be disrupted at several points including at the transcriptional, translational, and post-translational levels. In the last two decades, studies have emerged in which mutations carried by ion channels have been shown to be linked to trafficking defects, resulting in retention and/or degradation of the channel early in the trafficking process.

The density of active ion channels in specific membrane domains is a dynamic process resulting from the concomitant and antagonistic action of anterograde (exocytosis, recycling) and retrograde (internalization) pathways. Targeting and stabilization of these channels by anchoring partners in specialized domains of the sarcolemma also dynamically regulate the electrical activity of the cell (Balse et al., 2012; **Figure 1**).

The majority of mutations related to trafficking defects involve endoplasmic reticulum (ER) exit defects, leading to targeting of misfolded channels to degradation by the ERAD system (endoplasmic reticulum-associated degradation, lysosomal, or proteasomal). Such mutations have been identified for *HERG* (Furutani et al., 1999), *KCNQ1* (Gouas et al., 2004), and *SCN5A* (Valdivia et al., 2004) and associated with long QT and Brugada syndromes. Sorting signals carried by ion channels also are necessary for ER and trans-Golgi network exit (TGN) (Kupershmidt et al., 2002). A mutation involving an endocytotic defect of *TRPM4* has also been identified in human progressive familial heart block type I (Kruse et al., 2009). Finally, another crucial factor is the association (early or late) of ion channels with ancillary subunits, chaperones, and anchoring partners that are involved in channel function and localization.

BEYOND CHANNELOPATHIES: TRAFFICKING PROCESSES AS REGULATORS OF CARDIAC ACTION POTENTIAL

Trafficking and targeting of integral membrane proteins, including ion channels and receptors, have been explored in other cell types such as epithelial cells and neurons. Although these studies have yielded great insights, these mechanisms have not been studied extensively in cardiomyocytes. Such research may provide insight into the regulation of cardiac excitability *via* ion channel trafficking. Although trafficking defects have been reported for certain ion channel mutations, and are associated with retention in intracellular organelles, the characterization of intracellular trafficking in control and disease conditions are largely lacking in native cardiomyocytes. The fact that these cells are highly structurally and functionally specialized suggests that trafficking and targeting of cardiac ion channels may involve unique and specific pathways. Furthermore, the propagation of electrical activation within the myocardium is a complex process controlled by the spatial/differential distribution of ion channels within single cardiomyocytes that eventually establishes the anisotropic ratio. The underlying mechanisms regulating ion channel targeting to sarcolemmal subdomains, and tethering into macromolecular complexes remains a largely unanswered, yet important question.

In acquired arrhythmias such as heart failure and atrial fibrillation, ion channel dysfunction and electrical remodeling are often associated with tissue remodeling including hypertrophy/dilatation, replacement and interstitial fibrosis, and gap junction disorganization (Rucker-Martin et al., 2006). In this context, abnormal trafficking and targeting of cardiac ion channels emerge as important pathogenic factors of the electrical remodeling (Schotten et al., 2011). Importantly, increased knowledge of the pathways underlying cardiac ion channel trafficking may yield novel drug targets which lack the problems associated with conventional pore block therapies. Such therapies are frequently highly non-selective and have numerous unwanted side effects. The purpose of this mini-review is to provide an overview of the mechanisms of trafficking of ion channels in native cardiomyocytes that could potentially result in the discovery of new targets for antiarrhythmic therapies.

HYPOKALEMIA AND HERG CHANNEL REGULATION

The I_{Kr} current is encoded by the human ether-a-go-go–related gene (*HERG,* also known as *KCNH2*) in the heart (Sanguinetti et al., 1995; Trudeau et al., 1995). *HERG* mutations resulting in reduced I_{Kr} cause type 2 long QT syndrome (LQT2), which predisposes individuals to life-threatening arrhythmias. *HERG* mutations often disrupt the forward trafficking of hERG (thereby reducing sarcolemmal expression of the channel), and subsequently result in decreased I_{Kr} (Anderson et al., 2006). The hERG channel is also a notorious target for several classes of drugs that engender acquired long QT syndrome (LQTS) (Sanguinetti and Tristani-Firouzi, 2006). For instance, LQTS and Torsades de pointes are exacerbated by hypokalemia, with a moderate increase in serum $[K^+]$ capable of correcting LQTS in some patients (Compton et al., 1996). Hypokalemia is therefore considered a risk factor for LQTS and sudden cardiac death.

Guo and colleagues elegantly revealed how the plasma membrane density of hERG channels is regulated under physiological and pathophysiological (hypokalemia) conditions. They showed that lowering extracellular potassium drastically accelerated hERG internalization and degradation both in overexpression systems and native I_{Kr} in a hypokalemia rabbit model (Guo et al., 2009). Rabbits fed with low-K^+ diet showed prolonged QTc correlated to significantly prolonged APD_{90}. *In vitro*, exposure to 0 mM K^+ medium completely and reversibly eliminated I_{Kr} without significant effects on other potassium currents. The decrease in I_{Kr} accompanied reduced expression of hERG, combined with reduced surface expression of the channel. Finally, they showed that 0 mM K^+ medium induced the internalization of hERG by increasing ubiquitylation and resulted in lysosomal degradation (Guo et al., 2009). These findings provide a potential mechanism for hypokalemia-induced exacerbation of LQTS.

LIPIDIC CONTENT AND $K_V1.5$ CHANNEL REGULATION

Cardiac excitability can be regulated by cellular lipid content. Free cholesterol is a major lipid class shown to regulate membrane fluidity, curvature, and stiffness (Lundbaek et al., 1996). The function of several cardiac ion channels are regulated directly by cholesterol, which modulates channel properties (Oliver et al., 2004; Epshtein et al., 2009).

The I_{Kur} current, carried by $K_V1.5$ channels, is an important component of atrial repolarization (Fedida et al., 1993; Wang et al., 1993) and has been implicated in the pathology of atrial fibrillation (Van Wagoner et al., 1997; Brundel et al., 2001). The groups of D. Fedida and J. Martens contributed substantially to the study of the trafficking of $K_V1.5$ channel in expression systems (McEwen et al., 2007; Steele et al., 2007). Trafficking of vesicles is regulated by several Rab GTP-ases, involved at every stage of the process; regulating sorting, tethering and docking of trafficking vesicles. The early endosome (EE), associated with Rab4, mediates fast recycling while the recycling endosome, associated with Rab11, coordinates the slow recycling of proteins back to the cell membrane.

We showed that membrane cholesterol depletion *via* methyl-β-cyclodextrin (MβCD) increased the number of functional $K_V1.5$ channels in the sarcolemma of atrial myocytes, also reducing their mobility as shown by Fluorescence recovery After Photobleaching (Balse et al., 2009). Cholesterol depletion triggers exocytosis of ion channels from sub-membrane compartments. Indeed, the overexpression of a dominant negative (DN) form of Rab11 (associated with the recycling endosome), prevented the current increase upon MβCD treatment whereas overexpression of a DN form of Rab4, associated with the early endosome, did not. The recycling endosome, considered a slow route for ion channel recycling (Steele et al., 2007), is particularly sensitive to cholesterol depletion as rapid dissociation (<10 min) of the channel from the vesicle was observed (Balse et al., 2009). These results showed that channel turnover can be modified by changes in the lipid environment and that sub-membrane storage compartments can be recruited to modify the electrical properties of cardiomyocytes.

MECHANICAL CHALLENGE AND K_V1.5 CHANNEL REGULATION

Cardiomyocytes are exposed to mechanical forces when the heart contracts. These forces consist of stretch, shear and strain constraints. Shear forces in the myocardium are primarily generated by the movement of sheets of cardiomyocytes sliding relative to each other when the muscle contracts, as well as by blood flow during the cardiac cycle (LeGrice et al., 1995; Costa et al., 1999). Increased shear stress stimulates intracellular calcium transients (Morad et al., 2005), increases the beating rate of neonatal ventricular myocytes (Lorenzen-Schmidt et al., 2006), and triggers propagating APs in monolayers of ventricular myocytes (Kong et al., 2005).

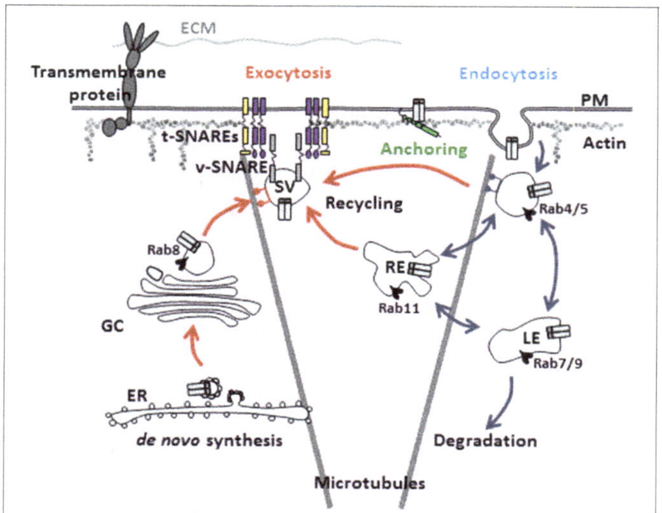

FIGURE 1 | General scheme of the various steps and regulators involved in the trafficking of ion channels. Ion channels are targeted to the plasma membrane via the anterograde and recycling pathways (red arrows). Once targeted to a specialized domain of the membrane, ion channels are stabilized by anchoring partners/associate subunits to be functional (green). Then, signals for internalization (blue arrows) lead to either degradation or recycling. PM, plasma membrane; EE, early endosome; LE, late endosome; ECM, extracellular matrix; RE, recycling endosome; GC, Golgi complex; ER, endoplasmic reticulum; SV, secretory vesicle.

We showed that in rat atrial myocytes shear stress activates a large outward current, mirrored by a decrease in AP duration (Boycott et al., 2013). The main ion channel mediating the increase in current K_V1.5, which was recruited from subcellular compartments to the sarcolemma, a phenomenon which was directly observed by TIRF microscopy. The donor compartment was again identified as the recycling endosome. K_V1.5 channel exocytosis requires integrin signaling through focal adhesion kinase (FAK) and relies on an intact microtubule system. We also found that the response was dysregulated in a model of chronic hemodynamic overload. Hypertrophied atrial myocytes had reduced K_V1.5 expression, despite an increase in basal I_{Kur}. The response of these cardiomyocytes to shear stress was reduced, and the kinetics altered. Our results suggested chronically increased mechanical stress over activates the integrin signaling pathway, resulting in an increased I_{Kur}, AP shortening and a reduction in the capability of cells to respond to shear stress (Boycott et al., 2013). Thus, pools of K_V1.5 from the slow recycling route may comprise an inducible reservoir mediating faster atrial repolarization. The shortening of the AP observed following heart failure in the atria could be partly explained by a shift in the trafficking balance toward increased exocytosis.

MODULATION OF K_V1.5 INTERNALIZATION BY ANTIARRHYTHMICS

Whereas conventional antiarrhythmic drugs generally target ion permeability by binding to the pore of the channel, increasing evidence suggests some compounds can indirectly disrupt protein trafficking. In this context, sustained efforts have been conducted to develop antiarrhythmic agents that affect channel trafficking, notably hERG channels blockers that stabilize misfolded channels and rescue hERG trafficking mutants (Wible et al., 2005).

The group of J. Martens has been at the forefront of investigations into the potential antiarrhythmic properties of drugs which acutely modulate the surface density of functional channels (Schumacher et al., 2009). The class I antiarrhythmic drug quinidine is known to inhibit I_{Kur} current through open-channel block of K_V1.5 channel. Using an immunocytochemical approach to quantify surface and internalized channels, Schumacher and colleagues showed that quinidine dose-dependently induced the internalization of K_V1.5 channel over short-time frames (10 min) in the HL-1 cell line and in dissociated neonatal mouse myocytes. The effect of quinidine was stereospecific as quinine has no effect on K_V1.5 channel surface density (despite exerting the pore-block effect of its stereoisomer) and subunit-dependent, as the K_V1.5-related channels K_V2.1 or K_V4.2 did not show internalization at the same time points and doses. In addition, quinidine-induced K_V1.5 channel internalization followed the same endocytotic pathway as constitutive endocytosis (as previously identified Choi et al., 2005), being microtubule-dependent and dynamin-mediated. Finally, whereas acute treatment allows channel recycling to the surface, chronic treatment with a clinical-compatible concentration led to channel degradation through the proteasome. This pharmacological control of $K_V1.5$ surface expression and trafficking represents a novel mechanism by which drug stimulated endocytosis of an ion channel may be utilized as an anti-arrhythmic tool.

ORGANIZATION OF ION CHANNEL MACROMOLECULAR COMPLEXES

It is noteworthy that emerging evidence challenges the assumption that ion channels function as homogeneous complexes. Rather, it seems likely that ion channels form macro-complexes with other ion channels, and that these complexes contribute to the stabilization of channels at the sarcolemma, and facilitate proper electrical conduction. The MAGUK protein SAP97 contributes to the formation of macromolecular complexes involving different ion channel families: $K_V1.5$ (Godreau et al., 2002; Abi-Char et al., 2008), $K_V4.x$ (El-Haou et al., 2009; Gillet et al., 2015), Kir2.x (Leonoudakis et al., 2001; Milstein et al., 2012; Matamoros et al., 2016), and $Na_V1.5$ (Petitprez et al., 2011; Milstein et al., 2012), SAP97 also couples ion channels to signaling pathways, allowing the regulation of $K_V4.x$ channels by CaMKII (El-Haou et al., 2009). An important recent breakthrough showed that SAP97 regulates the formation of $Na_V1.5$/Kir2.1 complexes, the two critical channels underlying I_{K1} and I_{Na}, respectively. These currents are responsible for maintenance of the resting membrane potential and rapid depolarization during the upstroke of the AP (Milstein et al., 2012). This multi-channel organization enables reciprocal modulation, contributing to maintenance of normal cardiac excitability. Interestingly, co-expression with $Na_v1.5$ seems to reduce internalization of Kir2.1, suggesting that participation in a macromolecular complex reduces anterograde trafficking of Kir2.1 (Milstein et al., 2012). Another example of multi-channel organization for $Na_V1.5$/Kir2.x, but mediated by syntrophin, has been recently reported (Matamoros et al., 2016). In addition to $Na_v1.5$, other cardiac ion channels have been shown to interact. For example, the KCNQ1/KCNE1 genes that encode I_{Ks} (Barhanin et al., 1996; Sanguinetti et al., 1996) interact with hERG, and the channels can reciprocally regulate (Ehrlich et al., 2004; Ren et al., 2010; Organ-Darling et al., 2013), with KCNQ1 also functioning as a chaperone for hERG trafficking (Biliczki et al., 2009). In the context of hypokalemia, KCNQ1/hERG co-expression slowed the internalization of mature, i.e. cell-surface expressed, hERG channels whereas KCNQ1 alone is not sensitive to hypokalemia (Guo et al., 2011). As the association between hERG and KCNQ1 only occurs at the plasma membrane, KCNQ1 likely contributes to hERG membrane stability.

MODULATION OF ION CHANNEL ANTEROGRADE TRAFFICKING BY PARTNER PROTEINS

A fascinating question relates to the nature of the molecular mechanisms which regulate ion channel targeting into distinct subdomains of the sarcolemma and their tethering in large molecular complexes. Cardiac myocytes are structurally and functionally highly polarized cells. While the transmission of the AP between myocytes occurs at the intercalated disc (ID), the AP is conducted along the myocyte at the lateral membrane (LM).

The direct targeting of hemichannels to the ID *via* the microtubule plus-end-tracking protein EB1 (Shaw et al., 2007) and the targeting of $Ca_V1.2$ to T-tubules by BIN1, a protein involved in membrane invagination and endocytotic processes (Hong et al., 2012) have been important major discoveries.

Recently, the spatial distribution of $Na_V1.5$ has received interest. Whereas $Na_V1.5$ is highly concentrated at the ID (3 to 8 fold larger current), $Na_V1.5$ channels at the LM show a lower density (Verkerk et al., 2007; Lin et al., 2011). This differential distribution of $Na_V1.5$ channels favors the anisotropic conduction of the myocardial depolarization wave (Spach, 1999). Several partners of $Na_v1.5$ have been identified such as gap junctional (i.e., connexin-43), desmosomal (plakophilin-2), actin cytoskeleton-binding (ankyrin-G), and the MAGUK protein SAP97 at the ID and syntrophin at the LM (for review see Shy et al., 2014). All these partners exert a positive regulatory effect on I_{Na} since their silencing *in vitro*, Knock Out *in vivo* or reduced expression in the Duchenne muscular dystrophy mouse model leads to reduced sodium current and localization. However, whether these proteins are involved anterograde trafficking of $Na_V1.5$ or associate with the channel once inserted in the plasma membrane to stabilize it is not clear. Recently, we have characterized a new partner of the $Na_V1.5$ channel in the myocardium, the MAGUK protein CASK. CASK is located at the LM, in association with the syntrophin/dystrophin complex. In contrast with other $Na_V1.5$ partners, CASK negatively regulates I_{Na} by impeding $Na_V1.5$ anterograde trafficking to the LM (Eichel et al., 2016). In dilated human atria, associated with AF or valve regurgitation, expression of CASK is reduced without affecting its localization. The consequence of this would likely be increased I_{Na} at the LM and could be considered detrimental for cardiac anisotropy. Keeping with the recent discovery that SAP97 is necessary for the interaction between $Na_V1.5$ and Kir2.1 (Milstein et al., 2012), MAGUK proteins could be major partners for the organization of multi-channel complexes.

CONCLUSION

Although only proven *in vitro* at present, early ER/Golgi trafficking rescue has been shown to be feasible for trafficking-defective mutant channels by temperature decrease, Hsp70 and 91 cytosolic chaperones, and pharmacological chaperones. Pharmacological chaperones include channel blockers, such as anti-histamines (Astemizole), anti-serotoninergic (Cisapride) and antiarrhythmics (e.g., E-4031 for hERG), that are difficult to manipulate as they can also block the channel and worsen the disease. However, certain pore-blocking drugs, such as fexofenadine, have been shown to rescue hERG trafficking of some mutant channels at concentrations far below the IC50 for pore-block (Rajamani et al., 2002). Furthermore, in an iPSC model of LQTS2 in which hERG was not expressed at the sarcolemma, sarcolemmal hERG expression was achieved using the proteasomal inhibitor ALLN, which allowed the re-trafficking and functional expression of the channel (Mehta et al., 2014). These studies highlight the relevance of research into pharmacological rescue of trafficking deficient mutant channels. Low molecular weight compounds such as DMSD, TMD and glycerol act as nonspecific chemical chaperones mostly likely by stabilizing proteins during folding and maturation (Kaufman and Ficker, 2003). In acquired cardiopathies, three pathways are worthy of special attention: the recycling endosome/Rab11 pathway, the endocytosis/dynamin/microtubule pathway and, the association of ion channels with specific partners for anterograde trafficking and correct targeting to specialized membrane subdomains of the myocyte. Future studies are necessary to explore the specific roles of ion channel partners on ion channel trafficking/targeting vs. membrane scaffolding to understand the relative contribution of these proteins in dictating cardiac excitability and function under normal and pathological conditions. The highly specialized architecture of the cardiomyocyte dictates that more studies in native cells are necessary to improve our understanding of the mechanisms involved, and how they impact upon the pathology of arrhythmia.

AUTHOR CONTRIBUTIONS

All authors listed have made a substantial, direct and intellectual contribution to the work, and approved it for publication.

REFERENCES

Abi-Char, J., El-Haou, S., Balse, E., Neyroud, N., Vranckx, R., Coulombe, A., et al. (2008). The anchoring protein SAP97 retains Kv1.5 channels in the plasma membrane of cardiac myocytes. *Am. J. Physiol. Heart Circ. Physiol.* 294, H1851–H1861. doi: 10.1152/ajpheart.01045.2007

Anderson, C. L., Delisle, B. P., Anson, B. D., Kilby, J. A., Will, M. L., Tester, D. J., et al. (2006). Most LQT2 mutations reduce Kv11.1 (hERG) current by a class 2 (Trafficking-Deficient) mechanism. *Circulation* 113, 365–373. doi: 10.1161/CIRCULATIONAHA.105.570200

Balse, E., El-Haou, S., Dillanian, G., Dauphin, A., Eldstrom, J., Fedida, D., et al. (2009). Cholesterol modulates the recruitment of Kv1.5 channels from Rab11-associated recycling endosome in native atrial myocytes. *Proc. Natl. Acad. Sci. U.S.A.* 106, 14681–14686. doi: 10.1073/pnas.0902809106

Balse, E., Steele, D. F., Abriel, H., Coulombe, A., Fedida, D., and Hatem, S. N. (2012). Dynamic of ion channel expression at the plasma membrane of cardiomyocytes. *Physiol. Rev.* 92, 1317–1358. doi: 10.1152/physrev.00041.2011

Barhanin, J., Lesage, F., Guillemare, E., Fink, M., Lazdunski, M., and Romey, G. (1996). K(V)LQT1 and lsK (minK) proteins associate to form the I(Ks) cardiac potassium current. *Nature* 384, 78–80. doi: 10.1038/384078a0

Biliczki, P., Girmatsion, Z., Brandes, R. P., Harenkamp, S., Pitard, B., Charpentier, F., et al. (2009). Trafficking-deficient long QT syndrome mutation KCNQ1-T587M confers severe clinical phenotype by impairment of KCNH2 membrane localization: evidence for clinically significant IKr-IKs alpha-subunit interaction. *Heart Rhythm* 6, 1792–1801. doi: 10.1016/j.hrthm.2009.08.009

Boycott, H. E., Barbier, C. S., Eichel, C. A., Costa, K. D., Martins, R. P., Louault, F., et al. (2013). Shear stress triggers insertion of voltage-gated potassium channels from intracellular compartments in atrial myocytes. *Proc. Natl. Acad. Sci. U.S.A.* 110, E3955–E3964. doi: 10.1073/pnas.1309896110

Brundel, B. J., Van Gelder, I. C., Henning, R. H., Tuinenburg, A. E., Wietses, M., Grandjean, J. G., et al. (2001). Alterations in potassium channel gene expression in atria of patients with persistent and paroxysmal atrial fibrillation: differential regulation of protein and mRNA levels for K^+ channels. *J. Am. Coll. Cardiol.* 37, 926–932. doi: 10.1016/S0735-1097(00)01195-5

Choi, W. S., Khurana, A., Mathur, R., Viswanathan, V., Steele, D. F., and Fedida, D. (2005). Kv1.5 surface expression is modulated by retrograde trafficking of newly endocytosed channels by the dynein motor. *Circ. Res.* 97, 363–371. doi: 10.1161/01.RES.0000179535.06458.f8

Compton, S. J., Lux, R. L., Ramsey, M. R., Strelich, K. R., Sanguinetti, M. C., Green, L. S., et al. (1996). Genetically defined therapy of inherited long-QT syndrome: correction of abnormal repolarization by potassium. *Circulation* 94, 1018–1022. doi: 10.1161/01.CIR.94.5.1018

Costa, K. D., Takayama, Y., McCulloch, A. D., and Covell, J. W. (1999). Laminar fiber architecture and three-dimensional systolic mechanics in canine ventricular myocardium. *Am. J. Physiol.* 276(2 Pt 2), H595–H607.

Ehrlich, J. R., Pourrier, M., Weerapura, M., Ethier, N., Marmabachi, A. M., Hébert, T. E., et al. (2004). KvLQT1 modulates the distribution and biophysical properties of HERG. A novel alpha-subunit interaction between delayed rectifier currents. *J. Biol. Chem.* 279, 1233–1241. doi: 10.1074/jbc.M309087200

Eichel, C. A., Beuriot, A., Chevalier, M. Y., Rougier, J.S., Louault, F., Dilanian, G., et al. (2016). Lateral membrane-specific MAGUK CASK down-regulates NaV1.5 channel in cardiac myocytes. *Circ. Res.* 119, 544–556. doi: 10.1161/CIRCRESAHA.116.309254

El-Haou, S., Balse, E., Neyroud, N., Dilanian, G., Gavillet, B., Abriel, H., et al. (2009). Kv4 potassium channels form a tripartite complex with the anchoring protein SAP97 and CaMKII in cardiac myocytes. *Circ. Res.* 104, 758–769. doi: 10.1161/CIRCRESAHA.108.191007

Epshtein, Y., Chopra, A. P., Rosenhouse-Dantsker, A., Kowalsky, G. B., Logothetis, D. E., and Levitan, I. (2009). Identification of a C-terminus domain critical for the sensitivity of Kir2.1 to cholesterol. *Proc. Natl. Acad. Sci. U.S.A.* 106, 8055–8060. doi: 10.1073/pnas.0809847106

Fedida, D., Wible, B., Wang, Z., Fermini, B., Faust, F., Nattel, S., et al. (1993). Identity of a novel delayed rectifier current from human heart with a Cloned K^+ channel current. *Circ. Res.* 73, 210–216. doi: 10.1161/01.RES.73.1.210

Furutani, M., Trudeau, M. C., Hagiwara, N., Seki, A., Gong, Q., Zhou, Z., et al. (1999). Novel mechanism associated with an inherited cardiac arrhythmia: defective protein trafficking by the mutant HERG (G601S) potassium channel. *Circulation* 99, 2290–2294. doi: 10.1161/01.CIR.99.17.2290

Gillet, L., Rougier, J.-S., Shy, D., Sonntag, S., Mougenot, N., Essers, M., et al. (2015). Cardiac-specific ablation of synapse-associated protein SAP97 in mice decreases potassium currents but not sodium current. *Heart Rhythm* 12, 181–192. doi: 10.1016/j.hrthm.2014.09.057

Godreau, D., Vranckx, R., Maguy, A., Rücker-Martin, C., Goyenvalle, C., Abdelshafy, S., et al. (2002). Expression, regulation and role of the MAGUK protein SAP-97 in human atrial myocardium. *Cardiovasc. Res.* 56, 433–442. doi: 10.1016/S0008-6363(02)00602-8

Gouas, L., Bellocq, C., Berthet, M., Potet, F., Demolombe, S., Forhan, A., et al. (2004). New KCNQ1 mutations leading to haploinsufficiency in a general population; defective trafficking of a KvLQT1 mutant. *Cardiovasc. Res.* 63, 60–68. doi: 10.1016/j.cardiores.2004.02.011

Guo, J., Massaeli, H., Xu, J., Jia, Z., Wigle, J. T., Mesaeli, N., et al. (2009). Extracellular K^+ concentration controls cell surface density of IKr in Rabbit Hearts and of the HERG channel in human cell lines. *J. Clin. Invest.* 119, 2745–2757. doi: 10.1172/JCI39027

Guo, J., Wang, T., Yang, T., Xu, J., Li, W., Fridman, M. D., et al. (2011). Interaction between the cardiac rapidly (IKr) and slowly (IKs) activating delayed rectifier potassium channels revealed by low K^+-induced hERG endocytic degradation. *J. Biol. Chem.* 286, 34664–34674. doi: 10.1074/jbc.M111.253351

Hong, T.T., Smyth, J. W., Chu, K. Y., Vogan, J. M., Fong, T. S., Jensen, B. C., et al. (2012). BIN1 is reduced and Cav1.2 trafficking is impaired in human failing cardiomyocytes. *Heart Rhythm* 9, 812–820. doi: 10.1016/j.hrthm.2011.11.055

Kaufman, E. S., and Ficker, E. (2003). Is restoration of intracellular trafficking clinically feasible in the long QT syndrome?: the example of HERG mutations. *J. Cardiovasc. Electrophysiol.* 14, 320–322. doi: 10.1046/j.1540-8167.2003.02363.x

Kong, C. R., Bursac, N., and Tung, L. (2005). Mechanoelectrical excitation by fluid jets in monolayers of cultured cardiac myocytes. *J. Appl. Physiol.* 98, 2328–2336; discussion: 2320. doi: 10.1152/japplphysiol.01084.2004

Kruse, M., Schulze-Bahr, E., Corfield, V., Beckmann, A., Stallmeyer, B., Kurtbay, G., et al. (2009). Impaired endocytosis of the ion channel TRPM4 is associated with human progressive familial heart block type, I. *J. Clin. Invest.* 119, 2737–2744. doi: 10.1172/JCI38292

Kupershmidt, S., Yang, T., Chanthaphaychith, S., Wang, Z., Towbin, J. A., and Roden, D. M. (2002). Defective human ether-à-go-go-related gene trafficking linked to an endoplasmic reticulum retention signal in the C terminus. *J. Biol. Chem.* 277, 27442–27448. doi: 10.1074/jbc.M112375200

LeGrice, I. J., Takayama, Y., and Covell, J. W. (1995). Transverse shear along myocardial cleavage planes provides a mechanism for normal systolic wall thickening. *Circ. Res.* 77, 182–193. doi: 10.1161/01.RES.77.1.182

Leonoudakis, D., Mailliard, W., Wingerd, K., Clegg, D., and Vandenberg, C. (2001). Inward rectifier potassium channel Kir2.2 is associated with synapse-associated protein SAP97. *J. Cell Sci.* 114(Pt 5), 987–998.

Lin, X., Liu, N., Lu, J., Zhang, J., Anumonwo, J. M., Isom, L. L., et al. (2011). Subcellular heterogeneity of sodium current properties in adult cardiac ventricular myocytes. *Heart Rhythm* 8, 1923–1930. doi: 10.1016/j.hrthm.2011.07.016

Lorenzen-Schmidt, I., Schmid-Schönbein, G. W., Giles, W. R., McCulloch, A. D., Chien, S., and Omens, J. H. (2006). Chronotropic response of cultured neonatal Rat ventricular myocytes to short-term fluid shear. *Cell Biochem. Biophys.* 46, 113–122. doi: 10.1385/CBB:46:2:113

Lundbaek, J. A., Birn, P., Girshman, J., Hansen, A. J., and Andersen, O. S. (1996). Membrane stiffness and channel function. *Biochemistry* 35, 3825–3830. doi: 10.1021/bi952250b

Matamoros, M., Pérez-Hernández, M., Guerrero-Serna, G., Amorós, I., Barana, A., Nú-ez, M., et al. (2016). Nav1.5 N-terminal domain binding to α1-syntrophin increases membrane density of human Kir2.1, Kir2.2 and Nav1.5 channels. *Cardiovasc. Res.* 110, 279–290. doi: 10.1093/cvr/cvw009

McEwen, D. P., Schumacher, S. M., Li, Q., Benson, M. D., I-iguez-Lluhí, J. A., Van Genderen, K. M., et al. (2007). Rab-GTPase-dependent endocytic recycling of Kv1.5 in atrial myocytes. *J. Biol. Chem.* 282, 29612–29620. doi: 10.1074/jbc.M704402200

Mehta, A., Sequiera, G. L., Ramachandra, C. A., Sudibyo, Y., Chung, Y., Sheng, J., et al. (2014). Re-trafficking of hERG reverses long QT syndrome 2 phenotype in human iPS-derived cardiomyocytes. *Cardiovasc. Res.* 102, 497–506. doi: 10.1093/cvr/cvu060

Milstein, M. L., Musa, H., Balbuena, D. P., Anumonwo, J. M., Auerbach, D. S., Furspan, P. B., et al. (2012). Dynamic reciprocity of sodium and potassium channel expression in a macromolecular complex controls cardiac excitability and arrhythmia. *Proc. Natl. Acad. Sci. U.S.A.* 109, E2134–E2143. doi: 10.1073/pnas.1109370109

Morad, M., Javaheri, A., Risius, T., and Belmonte, S. (2005). Multimodality of Ca2+ signaling in Rat atrial myocytes. *Ann. N. Y. Acad. Sci.* 1047, 112–121. doi: 10.1196/annals.1341.010

Oliver, D., Lien, C.-C., Soom, M., Baukrowitz, T., Jonas, P., and Fakler, B. (2004). Functional conversion between A-type and delayed rectifier K^+ channels by membrane lipids. *Science* 304, 265–270. doi: 10.1126/science.1094113

Organ-Darling, L. E., Vernon, A. N., Giovanniello, J. R., Lu, Y., Moshal, K., Roder, K., et al. (2013). Interactions between hERG and KCNQ1 α-subunits are mediated by their COOH termini and modulated by cAMP. *Am. J. Physiol. Heart Circ. Physiol.* 304, H589–H599. doi: 10.1152/ajpheart.00385.2012

Petitprez, S., Zmoos, A.-F., Ogrodnik, J., Balse, E., Raad, N., El-Haou, S., et al. (2011). SAP97 and dystrophin macromolecular complexes determine two pools of cardiac sodium channels Nav1.5 in cardiomyocytes. *Circ. Res.* 108, 294–304. doi: 10.1161/CIRCRESAHA.110.228312

Rajamani, S., Anderson, C. L., Anson, B. D., and January, C. T. (2002). Pharmacological rescue of human K^+ channel long-QT2 mutations: human ether-a-go-go-related gene rescue without block. *Circulation* 105, 2830–2835. doi: 10.1161/01.CIR.0000019513.50928.74

Ren, X. Q., Liu, G. X., Organ-Darling, L. E., Zheng, R., Roder, K., Jindal, H. K., et al. (2010). Pore mutants of HERG and KvLQT1 downregulate the reciprocal currents in stable cell lines. *Am. J. Physiol. Heart Circ. Physiol.* 299, H1525–H1534. doi: 10.1152/ajpheart.00479.2009

Rucker-Martin, C., Milliez, P., Tan, S., Decrouy, X., Recouvreur, M., Vranckx, R., et al. (2006). Chronic hemodynamic overload of the Atria is an important factor for gap junction remodeling in human and Rat hearts. *Cardiovasc. Res.* 72, 69–79. doi: 10.1016/j.cardiores.2006.06.016

Sanguinetti, M. C., Curran, M. E., Zou, A., Shen, J., Spector, P. S., Atkinson, D. L., et al. (1996). Coassembly of K(V)LQT1 and minK (IsK) proteins to form cardiac I(Ks) potassium channel. *Nature* 384, 80–83. doi: 10.1038/384080a0

Sanguinetti, M. C., Jiang, C., Curran, M. E., and Keating, M. T. (1995). A mechanistic link between an inherited and an acquired cardiac arrthytmia: HERG encodes the IKr potassium channel. *Cell* 81, 299–307. doi: 10.1016/0092-8674(95)90340-2

Sanguinetti, M. C., and Tristani-Firouzi, M. (2006). hERG potassium channels and cardiac arrhythmia. *Nature* 440, 463–469. doi: 10.1038/nature04710

Schotten, U., Verheule, S., Kirchhof, P., and Goette, A. (2011). Pathophysiological mechanisms of Atrial fibrillation: a translational appraisal. *Physiol. Rev.* 91, 265–325. doi: 10.1152/physrev.00031.2009

Schumacher, S. M., McEwen, D. P., Zhang, L., Arendt, K. L., Van Genderen, K. M., and Martens, J. R. (2009). Antiarrhythmic drug-induced internalization of the atrial-specific k^+ channel kv1.5. *Circ. Res.* 104, 1390–1398. doi: 10.1161/CIRCRESAHA.108.192773

Shaw, R. M., Fay, A. J., Puthenveedu, M. A., von Zastrow, M., Jan, Y. N., and Jan, L. Y. (2007). Microtubule plus-end-tracking proteins target gap junctions directly from the cell interior to adherens junctions. *Cell* 128, 547–560. doi: 10.1016/j.cell.2006.12.037

Shy, D., Gillet, L., and Abriel, H. (2014). Targeting the sodium channel NaV1.5 to specific membrane compartments of cardiac cells: not a simple task! *Circ. Res.* 115, 901–903. doi: 10.1161/CIRCRESAHA.114.305305

Spach, M. S. (1999). Anisotropy of cardiac tissue: a major determinant of conduction? *J. Cardiovasc. Electrophysiol.* 10, 887–90. doi: 10.1111/j.1540-8167.1999.tb00271.x

Steele, D. F., Eldstrom, J., and Fedida, D. (2007). Mechanisms of cardiac potassium channel trafficking. *J. Physiol.* 582(Pt 1), 17–26. doi: 10.1113/jphysiol.2007.130245

Trudeau, M. C., Warmke, J. W., Ganetzky, B., and Robertson, G. A. (1995). HERG, a human inward rectifier in the voltage-gated potassium channel family. *Science* 269, 92–95. doi: 10.1126/science.7604285

Valdivia, C. R., Tester, D. J., Rok, B. A., Porter, C. B., Munger, T. M., Jahangir, A., et al. (2004). A trafficking defective, brugada syndrome-causing SCN5A mutation rescued by drugs. *Cardiovasc. Res.* 62, 53–62. doi: 10.1016/j.cardiores.2004.01.022

Van Wagoner, D. R., Pond, A. L., McCarthy, P. M., Trimmer, J. S., and Nerbonne, J. M. (1997). Outward K^+ current densities and Kv1.5 expression are reduced in chronic human atrial fibrillation. *Circ. Res.* 80, 772–781. doi: 10.1161/01.RES.80.6.772

Verkerk, A. O., van Ginneken, A. C., van Veen, T. A., and Tan, H. L. (2007). Effects of heart failure on brain-type Na+ channels in Rabbit ventricular myocytes. *Europace* 9, 571–577. doi: 10.1093/europace/eum121

Wang, Z., Fermini, B., and Nattel, S. (1993). Sustained depolarization-induced outward current in human atrial myocytes. evidence for a novel delayed rectifier K^+ current similar to Kv1.5 cloned channel currents. *Circ. Res.* 73, 1061–1076. doi: 10.1161/01.RES.73.6.1061

Wible, B. A., Hawryluk, P., Ficker, E., Kuryshev, Y. A., Kirsch, G., and Brown, A. M. (2005). HERG-Lite: a novel comprehensive high-throughput screen for drug-induced hERG risk. *J. Pharmacol. Toxicol. Methods* 52, 136–145. doi: 10.1016/j.vascn.2005.03.008

16

Concomitant Evaluation of Heart Period and QT Interval Variability Spectral Markers to Typify Cardiac Control in Humans and Rats

Beatrice De Maria*[1]*, Vlasta Bari*[2]*, Andrea Sgoifo*[3,4]*, Luca Carnevali*[3,4]*, Beatrice Cairo*[5]*, Emanuele Vaini*[2]*, Aparecida Maria Catai*[6]*, Anielle Cristhine de Medeiros Takahashi*[6]*, Laura Adelaide Dalla Vecchia*[1] *and Alberto Porta*[2,5]**

[1] *IRCCS Istituti Clinici Scientifici Maugeri, Milan, Italy,* [2] *Department of Cardiothoracic, Vascular Anesthesia and Intensive Care, IRCCS Policlinico San Donato, Milan, Italy,* [3] *Stress Physiology Laboratory, Department of Chemistry, Life Sciences and Environmental Sustainability, University of Parma, Parma, Italy,* [4] *Microbiome Research Hub, University of Parma, Parma, Italy,* [5] *Department of Biomedical Sciences for Health, University of Milan, Milan, Italy,* [6] *Department of Physiotherapy, Federal University of São Carlos, São Carlos, Brazil*

***Correspondence:**
Alberto Porta
alberto.porta@unimi.it

The variability of heart period, measured as the time distance between two consecutive QRS complexes from the electrocardiogram (RR), was exploited to infer cardiac vagal control, while the variability of the duration of the electrical activity of the heart, measured as the time interval from Q-wave onset to T-wave end (QT), was proposed as an indirect index of cardiac sympathetic modulation. This study tests the utility of the concomitant evaluation of RR variability (RRV) and QT variability (QTV) markers in typifying cardiac autonomic control of humans under different experimental conditions and of rat groups featuring documented differences in resting sympatho-vagal balance. We considered: (i) 23 healthy young subjects in resting supine position (REST) undergoing head-up tilt at 45° (T45) and 90° (T90) followed by recovery to the supine position; (ii) 9 Wistar (WI) and 14 wild-type Groningen (WT) rats in unstressed conditions, where the WT animals were classified as non-aggressive (non-AGG, $n = 9$) and aggressive (AGG, $n = 5$) according to the resident intruder test. In humans, spectral analysis of RRV and QTV was performed over a single stationary sequence of 250 consecutive values. In rats, spectral analysis was iterated over 10-min recordings with a frame length of 250 beats with 80% overlap and the median of the distribution of the spectral markers was extracted. Over RRV and QTV we computed the power in the low frequency (LF, from 0.04 to 0.15 Hz in humans and from 0.2 to 0.75 Hz in rats) band (LF_{RR} and LF_{QT}) and the power in the high frequency (HF, from 0.15 to 0.5 Hz in humans and from 0.75 to 2.5 Hz in rats) band (HF_{RR} and HF_{QT}). In humans the HF_{RR} power was lower during T90 and higher during recovery compared to REST, while the LF_{QT} power was higher during T90. In rats the HF_{RR} power was lower in WT rats compared to WI rats and the LF_{QT} power was higher in AGG than in non-AGG animals. We concluded that RRV and QTV provide complementary information in describing the functioning of vagal and sympathetic limbs of the autonomic nervous system in humans and rats.

Keywords: power spectral analysis, heart rate variability, QTV, ventricular repolarization, autonomic nervous system, wild-type rat, Wistar, head-up tilt

INTRODUCTION

Heart period, measured as the time distance between two consecutive QRS complexes from the electrocardiogram (RR), exhibits spontaneous fluctuations usually referred to as RR variability (RRV). The analysis of RRV provides some markers that have been found useful to infer the state of the cardiac autonomic control (Task Force of the European Society of Cardiology and the North American Society of Pacing and Electrophysiology,, 1996). Short-term RRV markers in humans are mainly associated with vagal modulation given that the magnitude of RR changes is dramatically reduced by full vagal blockade (Pomeranz et al., 1985). This consideration holds not only in humans but also in rats (Japundzic et al., 1990; Cerutti et al., 1991; Silva et al., 2017) and this analogy strengthened the use of rats as an animal model of human autonomic cardiac control. The amplitude of the respiratory sinus arrhythmia is one of the most utilized RRV indexes to typify cardiac vagal control (Hirsch and Bishop, 1981): it is frequently estimated via spectral analysis as the power of RRV in the high frequency (HF) band in both humans and rats, even though the definition of the HF band was adapted to account for the differences between the respiratory rates in the two species, namely from 0.15 to 0.5 Hz in humans and from 0.75 to 2.5 Hz in rats (Japundzic et al., 1990; Cerutti et al., 1991; Rubini et al., 1993). In particular, in humans the HF power of RRV is known to decrease during physiological conditions characterized by sympathetic activation and vagal withdrawal, such as during graded orthostatic challenge (Montano et al., 1994; Cooke et al., 1999; Porta et al., 2011; Marchi et al., 2016) or physical exercise (Shin et al., 1995a,b; Brenner et al., 1997; Porta et al., 2018). Similarly, in rats the HF power of RRV was utilized to typify the autonomic response to several types of stressors either pharmacological, interventional, or social (Akselrod et al., 1987; Japundzic et al., 1990; Cerutti et al., 1991; Rubini et al., 1993; Stauss et al., 1997; Sgoifo et al., 1998, 1999; Jaenisch et al., 2011; Carnevali et al., 2013; Carnevali and Sgoifo, 2014; Silva et al., 2016, 2017).

More recently, in parallel with the more traditional RRV analysis, the variability of the overall duration of the electrical activity of the heart, comprising depolarization and repolarization periods, usually quantified as the time interval from Q-wave onset to T-wave end (QT) from the electrocardiogram, has been proposed and validated as a marker of cardiac sympathetic control in humans (Berger, 2009; Malik, 2009; Porta et al., 2010; Baumert et al., 2016). QT variability (QTV) markers computed in the low frequency (LF) band (i.e., from 0.04 to 0.15 Hz in humans) have been found to increase in situations where sympatho-vagal balance is shifted toward sympathetic activation and vagal withdrawal, especially when the sympathetic drive is particularly high (Lombardi et al., 1996; Porta et al., 1998a, 2010, 2011; Yeragani et al., 2000a,b; Piccirillo et al., 2001, 2006; Bar et al., 2007; Baumert et al., 2008, 2011; El-Hamad et al., 2015), with relevant clinical consequences in risk stratification (Berger et al., 1997; Atiga et al., 1998; Porta et al., 2015). Conversely, no information was provided about the possibility to use QTV in rats, mainly because of the technical difficulties in reliably assessing QT fluctuations due to the very limited signal-to-noise ratio of QTV (Laguna et al., 1990; Speranza et al., 1993; Lombardi et al., 1996; Porta et al., 1998b) and the peculiarities of cardiac repolarization in rodents (Conrath and Opthof, 2006; Fabritz et al., 2010; Speerschneider and Thomsen, 2013; Boukens et al., 2014).

The aim of the present study is to propose the concomitant evaluation of RRV and QTV to provide a more complete view on cardiac autonomic control and to test whether this strategy could be fruitfully exploited in both humans and rats. The hypothesis of the study is that the concomitant evaluation of RRV and QTV markers can describe simultaneously cardiac vagal control via the analysis of the RRV and cardiac sympathetic regulation via the analysis of the QTV in both humans and rats. In humans we evaluated two situations of sympathetic activation and vagal withdrawal of different intensities, namely head-up tilt at 45° and 90° (Montano et al., 1994), and the following recovery to supine position during which a progressive decline of sympathetic control and a gradual vagal rebound are expected. In rats, we considered two strains with documented differences in resting cardiac sympatho-vagal balance, namely the Wistar (WI) and wild-type Groningen (WT) rats (Carnevali and Sgoifo, 2014), and, within the WT population, two subgroups featuring opposite levels of aggressiveness that have been linked to different states of the cardiac autonomic control (Carnevali et al., 2013).

MATERIALS AND METHODS

Experimental Protocol on Humans

We studied 23 young healthy volunteers (11 males, age: 26.3 ± 5.6 years). A detailed medical history and examination excluded the evidence of any disease. The subjects did not take any medication and consume any caffeine or alcohol-containing beverages in the 24 h before the recording session. Each subject underwent two consecutive head-up tilt tests with different table inclination angles, namely 45° (T45) and 90° (T90). T45 and T90 sessions were carried out in a random order, lasted 10 min and were followed by 40 min of recovery (R45 and R90, respectively) starting when the tilt table was moved back to the horizontal position. The first tilt session was preceded by a 10-min recording period in supine position (REST). Subjects lay on the tilt table supported by two belts at the level of the thigh and waist, respectively, and with both feet touching the footrest of the tilt table. During the recording sessions, subjects breathed spontaneously but were not allowed to talk. The electrocardiographic activity from a modified lead II was recorded (Biosignal Conditioning Device, Marazza, Monza, Italy) throughout all the experimental sessions and sampled at 1000 Hz. Attention was paid during the positioning of the electrodes to prevent flat or biphasic T-waves. All subjects were able to complete the protocol without experiencing any sign of presyncope. The duration of the phases was never varied.

Informed consent was obtained from all subjects before taking part in the study. The study adheres to the principles of the Declaration of Helsinki for medical research involving human subjects. The Human Research and Ethical Review Board of the L. Sacco Hospital, Milan, Italy, approved the protocol.

Experimental Protocol on Rats

We studied two different strains of rats: 9 male WI rats (age: 5.5 ± 0.5 months; weight: 436 ± 34 g) and 14 male WT rats (age: 4.4 ± 0.5 months; weight: 395 ± 40 g). Initially WT rats were classified into non-aggressive (non-AGG, $n = 5$) and aggressive (AGG, $n = 9$) WT rats, according to the resident intruder test described in Carnevali et al. (2013).

After the preliminary behavioral tests in WT rats, all rats were implanted, under tiletamine hydrochloride plus zolazepam hydrochloride anesthesia (Zoletil Virbac, France, 20 mg kg^{-1}), with radiotelemetric transmitters (TA11CTA-F40, Data Sciences International, St. Paul, MN, United States) for the recording of the cardiac electrical activity. Electrocardiograms were picked up by platform receivers (RPC-1, Data Sciences Int., St. Paul, MN, United States) located under the animal's cage and acquired via ART-Gold 4.2 data acquisition system (Data Sciences International, St. Paul, MN, United States) at a sampling rate of 1000 Hz. Animals were individually housed and kept in rooms with controlled temperature (22 ± 2°C) and lighting (lights on from 7:00 P.M. to 7:00 A.M.). After a 14-day recovery period from surgery, electrocardiograms were recorded in all rats for 1 h during the dark (active) phase of the light–dark cycle (i.e., between 10:00 A.M. and 11:00 A.M.) on different days.

The experimental protocol was approved by the Veterinarian Animal Care and Use Committee of the University of Parma, Parma, Italy, and the animals were cared in accordance with the European Community Council Directives of 22 September 2010 (2010/63/UE).

Extraction of the Beat-to-Beat RRV and QTV Series

The electrocardiographic traces recorded in both healthy humans and rats were processed with a software, developed in house, automatically measuring RR and QT (Porta et al., 1998b). The peak of the QRS complex (i.e., the R-wave) was automatically located via a method based on a threshold on the first derivative of the electrocardiogram. The peak of the QRS complex was fixed via parabolic interpolation. The RR was measured as the time distance between two consecutive QRS complex peaks. The QT was approximated as the time interval between the peak of the QRS complex and the T-wave offset (RTend) (Porta et al., 2010, 2011). The end of the T-wave was automatically delineated where the absolute value of the first derivative calculated on T-wave downslope became smaller than 30% of the absolute value of the steepest slope of the T-wave. **Figure 1** shows an example of the automatic detection of the T-wave end in a healthy subject (top panel), a WI rat (middle panel), and a WT rat (bottom panel). The detections of the QRS complex were visually checked and corrected in case of identification errors and in this case the T-wave offset delineation procedure was run again starting from the new position of the QRS complex. T-wave end detections were checked to assure the quality of the T-wave delineation. Problematic T-wave morphologies such as biphasic shapes were not observed and the first return to the isoelectric line after the onset of the T-wave always denotes the offset of the repolarization period in both humans and rats. The effects

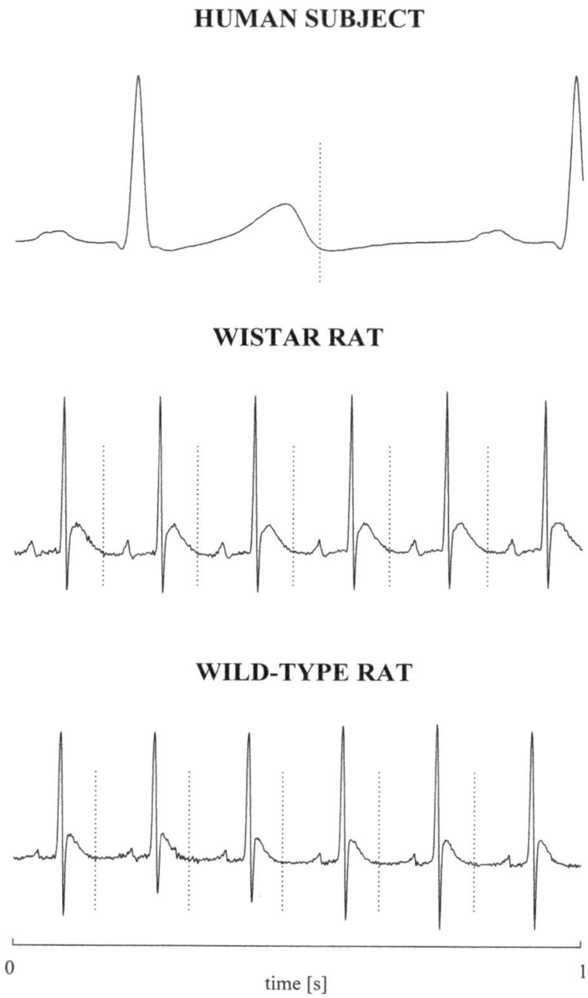

FIGURE 1 | Examples of T-wave end delineation in ECG signals of a healthy young human subject **(top)**, WI rat **(middle)**, and WT rat **(bottom)** in basal condition. T-wave end is marked with a vertical dotted line.

of isolated ectopic beats on RR and QT beat-to-beat series were corrected by means of cubic spline interpolation starting from the RR and QT measures unaffected by non-sinus cardiac beats. Corrections never exceeded the 5% of the total beats. Within each experimental session of the human protocol (i.e., REST, T45, R45, T90, and R90) segments of 250 consecutive RR and QT measures were selected. Stationarity of the selected sequences was tested according to Magagnin et al. (2011). The first stationary sequence found 3 min after the onset of posture changes was taken as the representative segment during T45 and T90 sessions and the first stationary sequence 10 min after returning to the supine position after head-up tilt was taken as the representative segment during R45 and R90 sessions. As to the animal protocol, a 10-min segment was selected in a random position within the overall recording session. The analysis was carried out over the 10-min segments divided into adjacent windows of 250 consecutive RR and QT measures with 80% overlap. The median of the distribution was chosen as the representative value of the whole series. **Figure 2** shows some examples of beat-to-beat RRV and QTV series derived from a human subject at REST (**Figures 2A,D**), from a WI rat (**Figures 2B,E**) and a WT rat (**Figures 2C,F**) in unstressed conditions.

Time and Frequency Domain RRV and QTV Analyses

In the time domain, we computed the mean of RR and QT beat-to-beat series (μ_{RR} and μ_{QT}, respectively). μ_{RR} and μ_{QT} were expressed in ms. Linear detrending procedure, subtracting from the original series the best fit linear trend, was exploited to prevent the drift of the mean and favor stationarity. After linear detrending of the series, the variances of RR and QT beat-to-beat series (σ^2_{RR} and σ^2_{QT}, respectively) were calculated and expressed in ms^2. Parametric power spectral analysis was performed. RRV and QTV series were modeled as realizations of an autoregressive process. The coefficients of the autoregressive process and the variance of the white noise corrupting the determinist part of the process were estimated via least squares method solved via the Levinson–Durbin recursion (Kay and Marple, 1981). The number of coefficients was optimized via Akaike's (1974) criterion within the range from 10 to 16. Power spectral density was decomposed into power spectral components (Baselli et al., 1997), classified as LF or HF component, according to their central frequency. The LF band range was 0.04–0.15 Hz for humans (Task Force of the European Society of Cardiology and the North American Society of Pacing and Electrophysiology,, 1996) and 0.2–0.75 Hz for rats (Carnevali et al., 2013), while the HF band range was 0.15–0.5 Hz for humans (Task Force of the European Society of Cardiology and the North American Society of Pacing and Electrophysiology,, 1996) and 0.75–2.5 Hz for rats (Carnevali et al., 2013). The sum of the absolute power of all HF components of the RR series was termed as HF_{RR} and considered to be an index of vagal modulation directed to the sinus node (Pomeranz et al., 1985), whereas the sum of the absolute power of all LF components of the QT series was labeled LF_{QT} and considered to be an index of sympathetic modulation directed to the heart (Porta et al., 2010, 2011; Baumert et al., 2011; El-Hamad et al., 2015). The power of RRV in the LF band, indicated as LF_{RR}, and the power of the QTV in the HF band, labeled as HF_{QT}, were computed as well. LF_{RR}, HF_{RR}, LF_{QT}, and HF_{QT} indexes were given in absolute units and expressed in ms^2. Spectral analysis was carried out over the linearly detrended RRV and QTV series.

Statistical Analysis

In the human protocol one-way repeated measures analysis of variance (Dunnett's test for multiple comparisons) was performed to check the significance of the differences of T45, R45, T90, and R90 versus REST. If the Kolmogorov–Smirnov normality test was not passed, Friedman one-way repeated measures analysis of variance on ranks (Dunnett's test for multiple comparisons) was carried out. In the animal protocol unpaired *t*-test was performed to assess the significance of the differences between the strains (WI versus WT) and subgroups (AGG versus non-AGG). If the Kolmogorov–Smirnov normality test was not passed, Mann–Whitney rank sum test was carried out. Statistical analysis was carried out using a commercial statistical program (Sigmaplot, Systat Software, Inc., Chicago, IL, United States, version 11.0). A $p < 0.05$ was always considered as significant.

RESULTS

Box-and-whisker plots of **Figure 3** show the results of RRV (**Figures 3A–C**) and QTV (**Figures 3D–F**) analyses performed on human data as a function of the experimental condition (i.e., REST, T45, R45, T90, and R90). Compared to REST, μ_{RR} decreased during both T45 and T90, while it was unchanged during R45 and R90 (**Figure 3A**). σ^2_{RR} was significantly higher during both R45 and R90 and was not affected by the orthostatic challenge (**Figure 3B**). HF_{RR} power significantly decreased during T90 and increased during R90 compared to REST (**Figure 3C**). μ_{QT} was significantly reduced during both T45 and T90 and did not vary during R45 and R90 (**Figure 3D**). σ^2_{QT} did not change with the experimental condition (**Figure 3E**). LF_{QT} power increased during T90 and remained stable in all the other experimental conditions (**Figure 3F**). Results relevant to time and frequency domain RRV and QTV markers derived from the experimental protocol on humans are summarized in **Table 1**. The same table reports the LF_{RR} and HF_{QT} powers as well. Both these latter markers did not vary with the experimental condition.

Box-and-whisker plots of **Figure 4** show the results of RRV (**Figures 4A–C**) and QTV (**Figures 4D–F**) analyses performe[illegible] on data derived from WI and WT rats. μ_{RR} (**Figure 4A**) ar[illegible] σ^2_{RR} (**Figure 4B**) were similar between the two strains, while [illegible] HF_{RR} power (**Figure 4C**) was higher in WI compared to [illegible] rats. μ_{QT} (**Figure 4D**) was longer in WI rats, while no [illegible] differences in σ^2_{QT} (**Figure 4E**) and LF_{QT} power (**Figure 4F**[illegible] observed. **Figure 5** has the same structure as **Figure 4** [illegible] shows the results of RRV (**Figures 5A–C**) and QTV (**Figu**[illegible] F) analyses performed on data obtained from WT [illegible] were classified as non-AGG and AGG. μ_{RR} (**Figure**[illegible] (**Figure 5B**), HF_{RR} (**Figure 5C**), and μ_{QT} (**Figure 5**[illegible] differentiate the two subgroups. On the contrary, σ^2_{QT} [illegible] and LF_{QT} (**Figure 5F**) were able to separate the [illegible] WT rats, being both σ^2_{QT} and LF_{QT} power highe[illegible] in non-AGG animals. RRV and QTV markers d[illegible] experimental protocol on rats are summarize[illegible] These tables reported LF_{RR} and HF_{QT} pow[illegible] these markers were similar in WI and WT [illegible] and they were not able to distinguish no[illegible] animals (**Table 3**).

DISCUSSION

To the best of our knowledge this is th[illegible] parameters were evaluated in rats co[illegible] RRV measures for the assessment o[illegible] and a parallel between human an[illegible] was drawn. The most important [illegible]

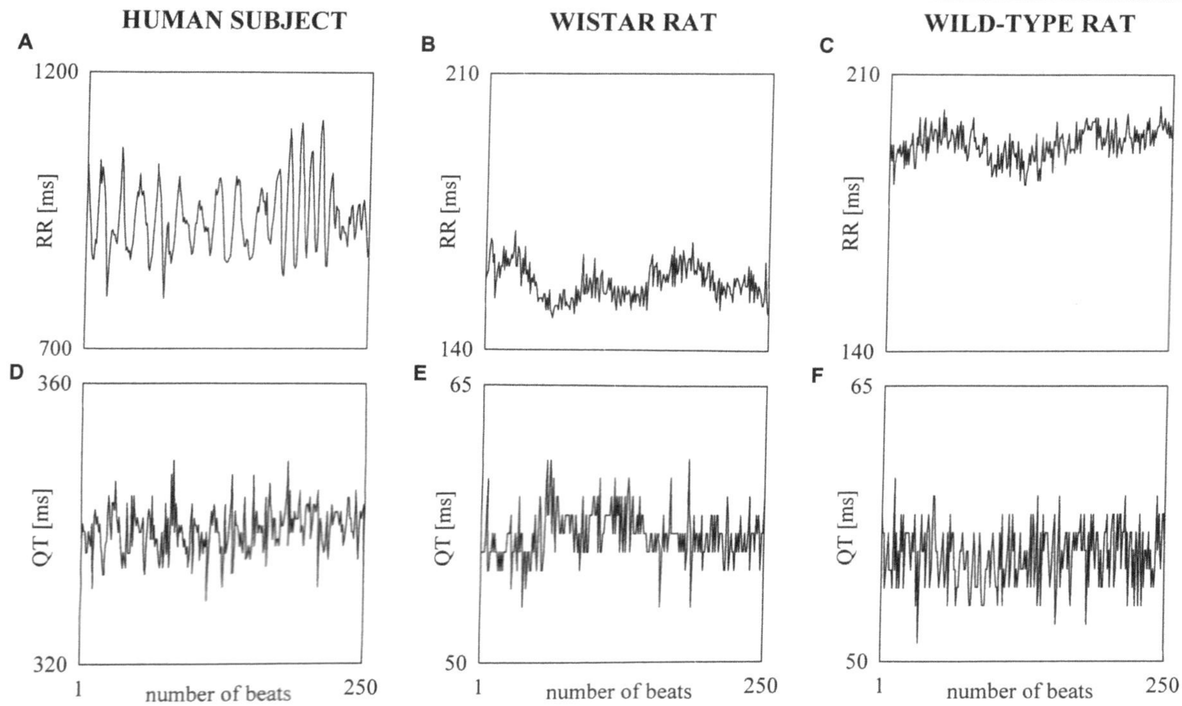

IRE 2 | The line plots show examples of beat-to-beat RRV **(A–C)** and QTV **(D–F)** series undergoing power spectral analysis recorded in a healthy young human t **(A,D)**, WI rat **(B,E)**, and WT rat **(C,F)**.

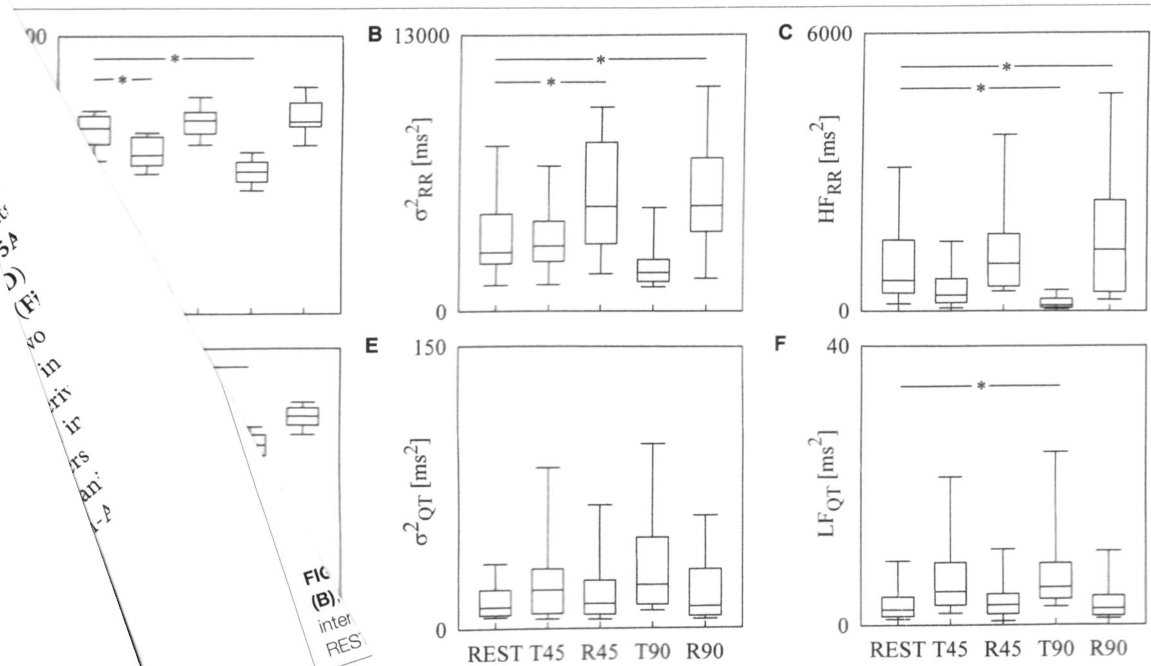

he time and frequency domain analyses of RRV and QTV in healthy young humans. The μ_{RR} **(A)**, σ^2_{RR} ction of the experimental condition (i.e., REST, T45, R45, T90, and R90). Box height represents the ent, and whiskers denote the 10th and 90th percentile. The symbol * indicates a $p < 0.05$ versus

TABLE 1 | Results of the time and frequency domain analyses of RRV and QTV in healthy young subjects.

Index	REST	T45	R45	T90	R90
μ_{RR} (ms)	937.18 (135.11)	802.56 (142.08)*	975.94 (97.25)	715.18 (96.47)*	969.17 (117.36)
σ^2_{RR} (ms^2)	2755.2 (2083.51)	3049.86 (1596.87)	4894.99 (4585.21)*	1773.36 (940.24)	4904.22 (3447.03)*
LF_{RR} (ms^2)	952.56 (1219.09)	1180.74 (1161.83)	1694.45 (1840.67)	890.56 (766.05)	1372.49 (1741.51)
HF_{RR} (ms^2)	651.6 (1095.69)	342.08 (479.25)	1016.27 (1040.69)	117.27 (182.51)*	1312.98 (1651.28)*
μ_{QT} (ms)	327.91 (33.6)	306.05 (26.65)*	336.25 (27.46)	295.09 (30.19)*	341.03 (26.73)
σ^2_{QT} (ms^2)	11.43 (12.29)	20.67 (23.11)	13.13 (16.72)	23.21 (33.49)	11.59 (23.18)
LF_{QT} (ms^2)	2.2 (3.98)	4.8 (5.71)	2.86 (2.76)	5.36 (4.78)*	2.29 (2.5)
HF_{QT} (ms^2)	4.45 (5.91)	7.43 (12.09)	3.34 (9.89)	8.62 (11.9)	4.09 (11.28)

*REST, supine position; T45, head-up tilt at 45°; R45, recovery in supine position after T45; T90, head-up tilt at 90°; R90, recovery in supine position after T90; LF, low frequency; HF, high frequency; RR, time interval between two consecutive QRS complexes; QT, time interval between the peak of the QRS complex and the T-wave offset; RRV, RR variability; QTV, QT variability; LF_{RR}, RRV power in the LF band expressed in absolute units; HF_{RR}, RRV power in the HF band expressed in absolute units; LF_{QT}, QTV power in the LF band expressed in absolute units; HF_{QT}, QTV power in the HF band expressed in absolute units. Results are presented as median with the interquartile range in round brackets. The symbol * indicates a $p < 0.05$ versus REST.*

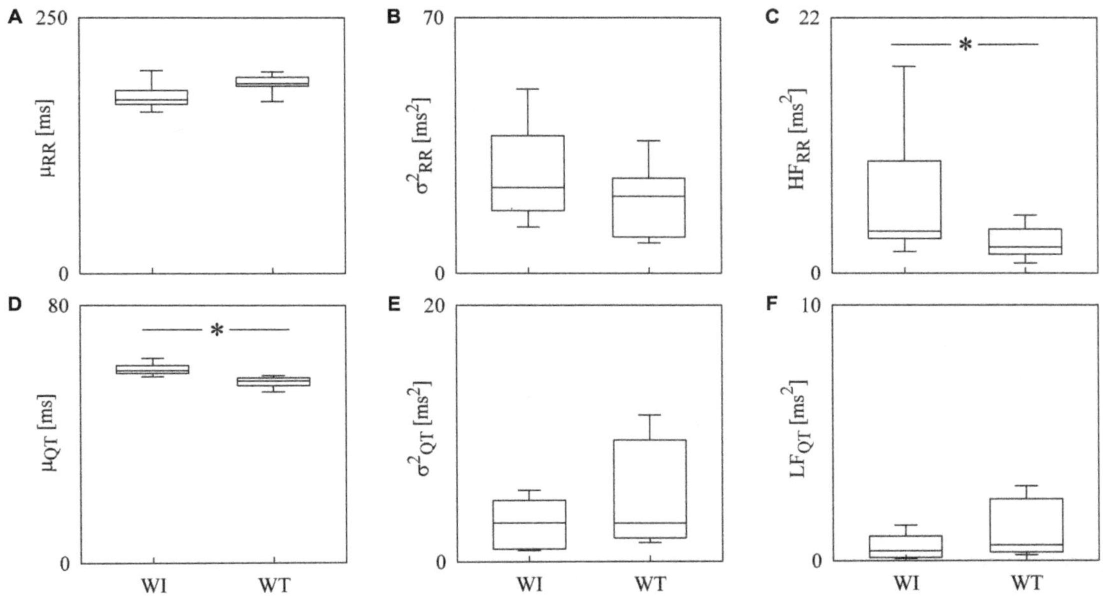

FIGURE 4 | The box-and-whisker graphs show the results of the time and frequency domain analyses of RRV and QTV in rats. The μ_{RR} **(A)**, σ^2_{RR} **(B)**, HF_{RR} **(C)**, μ_{QT} **(D)**, σ^2_{QT} **(E)**, and LF_{QT} **(F)** are given as a function of the strain (i.e., WI and WT). Box height represents the interquartile range, median is marked with a horizontal solid segment, and whiskers denote the 10th and 90th percentile. The symbol * indicates a $p < 0.05$ versus WI rats.

summarized as follows: (i) RRV is descriptive of the cardiac vagal regulation in both humans and rats; (ii) QTV is representative of cardiac sympathetic control in both humans and rats; (iii) results of RRV and QTV should be simultaneously considered to more deeply describe cardiac autonomic control in both humans and rats.

RRV and QTV Provide Complementary Information About Cardiac Autonomic Control in Humans and Rats

One of the major difficulties in exploiting RRV and spectral markers derived from RRV analysis to comprehensively characterize cardiac autonomic control is the strong link of RRV with the variation of vagal autonomic outflow, while its sensitivity to changes of the activity of the sympathetic autonomic limb is more limited. Indeed, since the initial studies on RRV (Akselrod et al., 1981; Pomeranz et al., 1985) it is well-known that the HF_{RR} power is completely abolished by full vagal blockade carried out via a high dose of atropine and that the same pharmacological challenge affects remarkably the LF_{RR} power as well. This observation suggested that the HF_{RR} power is a genuine marker of vagal modulation directed to the sinus node, while the LF_{RR} power results from the changes of the activity of both sympathetic and vagal limbs of the autonomic nervous system (Akselrod et al., 1981; Pomeranz et al., 1985). Normalization strategies attempted to limit the dependence of the LF_{RR} power on cardiac vagal control. For example, the ratio of the LF_{RR} power to σ^2_{RR} minus the RRV power in the very LF band, known as LF_{RR} power expressed

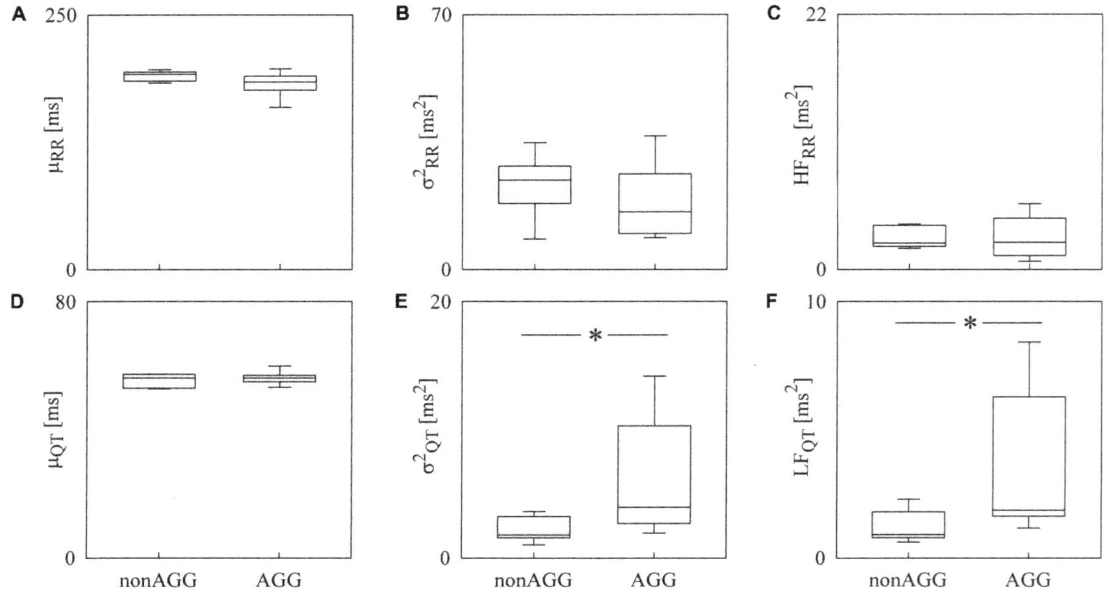

FIGURE 5 | The box-and-whisker graphs show the results of the time and frequency domain analyses of RRV and QTV in WT rats classified into non-AGG and AGG animals. The μ_{RR} **(A)**, σ^2_{RR} **(B)**, HF_{RR} **(C)**, μ_{QT} **(D)**, σ^2_{QT} **(E)**, and LF_{QT} **(F)** are given as a function of the WT subcategory (i.e., non-AGG and AGG). Box height represents the interquartile range, median is marked with a horizontal solid segment, and whiskers denote the 10th and 90th percentile. The symbol * indicates a $p < 0.05$ versus non-AGG animals.

TABLE 2 | Results of time and frequency domain analyses of RRV and QTV in WI and WT rats.

Index	WI	WT
μ_{RR} (ms)	169.99 (7.37)	185.6 (8.31)
σ^2_{RR} (ms^2)	23.76 (19.62)	21.38 (15.5)
LF_{RR} (ms^2)	1.22 (1.4)	0.58 (0.37)
HF_{RR} (ms^2)	3.69 (4.63)	2.29 (2.16)*
μ_{QT} (ms)	59.54 (2.21)	56.23 (2.32)*
σ^2_{QT} (ms^2)	2.98 (3.49)	2.95 (6.01)
LF_{QT} (ms^2)	0.38 (0.78)	0.6 (1.63)
HF_{QT} (ms^2)	1.36 (1.93)	1.68 (3.76)

*WI, Wistar rats; WT, wild-type Groningen rats; LF, low frequency; HF, high frequency; RR, time interval between two consecutive QRS complexes; QT, time interval between the peak of the QRS complex and the T-wave offset; RRV, RR variability; QTV, QT variability; LF_{RR}, RRV power in the LF band expressed in absolute units; HF_{RR}, RRV power in the HF band expressed in absolute units; LF_{QT}, QTV power in the LF band expressed in absolute units; HF_{QT}, QTV power in the HF band expressed in absolute units. Results are presented as median with the interquartile range in round brackets. The symbol * indicates a $p < 0.05$ versus WI.*

TABLE 3 | Results of time and frequency domain analyses of RRV and QTV in WT rats classified as non-AGG and AGG animals.

Index	non-AGG	AGG
μ_{RR} (ms)	191.9 (7.27)	184.22 (11.4)
σ^2_{RR} (ms^2)	24.57 (4.83)	15.86 (12.84)
LF_{RR} (ms^2)	0.66 (0.24)	0.53 (0.45)
HF_{RR} (ms^2)	2.26 (1.71)	2.32 (2.89)
μ_{QT} (ms)	56.21 (4.2)	56.25 (1.9)
σ^2_{QT} (ms^2)	1.8 (1.37)	3.98 (7.5)*
LF_{QT} (ms^2)	0.3 (0.54)	0.67 (1.96)*
HF_{QT} (ms^2)	0.92 (0.78)	1.87 (4.59)

*WT, wild-type Groningen rats; non-AGG, non-aggressive WT rats; AGG, aggressive WT rats; LF, low frequency; HF, high frequency; RR, time interval between two consecutive QRS complexes; QT, time interval between the peak of the QRS complex and the T-wave offset; RRV, RR variability; QTV, QT variability; LF_{RR}, RRV power in the LF band expressed in absolute units; HF_{RR}, RRV power in the HF band expressed in absolute units; LF_{QT}, QTV power in the LF band expressed in absolute units; HF_{QT}, QTV power in the HF band expressed in absolute units. Results are presented as median with the interquartile range in round brackets. The symbol * indicates a $p < 0.05$ versus non-AGG.*

in normalized units (Pagani et al., 1986), is one of the most frequently exploited normalized RRV indexes. The attempts of normalizing frequency domain markers of RRV to achieve a more genuine marker of sympathetic control generated some controversies (Eckberg, 1997; Pagani et al., 1997; Billman, 2013; Reyes del Paso et al., 2013). Among the most controversial issues there is the non-zero value of normalized LF_{RR} power after full vagal blockade in presence of null RR changes and the strict link between normalized LF_{RR} and normalized HF_{RR} powers given that their sum is 100 (Eckberg, 1997). The final result is that no normalization procedure solved the original problem due to the inherent contribution of vagal limb to RRV in the LF band (Akselrod et al., 1981; Pomeranz et al., 1985). More recently, some studies on QTV have suggested the possibility of monitoring cardiac sympathetic control via markers extracted from QTV (Porta et al., 1998a, 2010; Berger, 2009; Malik, 2009; El-Hamad et al., 2015; Baumert et al., 2016) and have outlined the clinical relevance of this approach in pathological populations and risk stratification (Berger et al., 1997; Atiga et al., 1998; Baumert et al., 2008, 2011; Bari et al., 2014; Porta et al., 2015).

A pragmatic route to face the issue generated by the debate on the use of RRV markers in the frequency domain was made operational in Porta et al. (2015) who proposed the simultaneous exploitation of RRV and QTV to derive a frequency domain description of the cardiac vagal control via the HF_{RR} power and of the cardiac sympathetic control via the LF_{QT} power. The strategy proposed in Porta et al. (2015) was tested in this study in humans during an experimental protocol evoking sympathetic activation and vagal withdrawal (i.e., head-up tilt) and the progressive sympathetic regulation departure and vagal control rebound during recovery after the postural challenge (Montano et al., 1994; Cooke et al., 1999; Porta et al., 2011; Marchi et al., 2016) and in rats featuring documented differences in cardiac sympatho-vagal balance at baseline (Carnevali et al., 2013; Carnevali and Sgoifo, 2014). The present study outlines the ability of the simultaneous exploitation of the HF_{RR} and LF_{QT} markers in typifying state- and trait-related modifications of the cardiac autonomic regulation in human and animal experiments. In the human protocol the significant decrease of the HF_{RR} marker during T90 and the concomitant increase of LF_{QT} power suggest, respectively, a reduced vagal and an augmented sympathetic controls as it is expected in response to the postural challenge (Montano et al., 1994; Cooke et al., 1999; Porta et al., 2011; Marchi et al., 2016). The specific ability of the HF_{RR} marker in tracking the cardiac vagal control was emphasized by the particular design of the experimental protocol in humans considering the period of recovery after the postural challenge. Indeed, the greater cardiac vagal regulation regaining after T90 was stressed by the increase of the HF_{RR} power above the levels observed at REST. The independence of the LF_{QT} power from the level of cardiac vagal control was supported by the stable values of this index during recovery compared to REST, thus stressing the complementary information that can be derived from the joint use of HF_{RR} and LF_{QT} markers. The strategy proposing the concomitant use of HF_{RR} and LF_{QT} powers excludes the utilization of the LF_{RR} power due to its mixed nature and that of the HF_{QT} power due to its non-autonomic origin. The mixed origin of the LF_{RR} power is supported by the present study as well: indeed, the constancy of the LF_{RR} power as a function of the experimental condition in the head-up tilt protocol and the inability of the LF_{RR} power to distinguish non-AGG from AGG rats is in agreement with a simultaneous increase of sympathetic modulation and a decrease of the vagal one (Porta et al., 2011). The non-autonomic origin of the HF_{QT} power results from the observation that it is likely to be the consequence of the projection of cardiac axis movements due to respiration over a single lead given that it increased when assessed over Z lead compared to X and Y ones (Porta et al., 1998b) and it is present in subjects under cardiac pacing (Lombardi et al., 1996). The non-autonomic nature of the HF_{QT} power was supported by the present study as well: indeed, it is invariable in both human and animal protocols.

The proposed strategy has the inherent limitation of disregarding the dependence of QTV on RRV due to the well-known relation linking QT to the preceding RR (Bazett, 1929). However, the selection of spectral indexes computed in different frequency bands (i.e., HF_{RR} and LF_{QT} powers) should mitigate the effects of this dependence. Our result corroborates this observation given that in humans during R90 the HF_{RR} power increased compared to REST, while the LF_{QT} marker remained stable, and in rats only the LF_{QT} power was greater in the AGG group compared to the non-AGG one while the HF_{RR} power was unvaried. However, models of the dynamical dependence of QTV on RRV should be tested (Porta et al., 1998a, 2010) in future to understand whether some normalization procedure should be applied to better represent the genuine contribution of the sympathetic drive directed to the ventricles.

RRV and QTV Can Be Fruitfully Exploited for Cardiac Autonomic Characterization in Rats

To the best of our knowledge, this is the first study in which QTV analysis was carried out on rats with the aim at assessing cardiac autonomic control and QTV markers were discussed along with those derived from RRV analysis. This approach was successfully applied with the aim at differentiating WI and WT rats and divergent subpopulations within the WT strain. WI rats are highly domesticated, docile, and placid, while WT rats exhibit a more aggressive behavior during a social conflict (Buwalda et al., 2011) than WI rats. These differences in trait aggressiveness between the two strains are mirrored by a different state of the sympatho-vagal balance in unstressed conditions, with WT rats generally showing lower indexes of cardiac vagal modulation than WI counterparts (Carnevali and Sgoifo, 2014). Our results are in agreement with Carnevali and Sgoifo (2014) given that we found a lower HF_{RR} power in WT rats than in WI rats. The expected increase of the LF_{QT} marker, suggesting a higher sympathetic control in WT rats than in WI animals, was not found even though a tendency toward an increase of the LF_{QT} power was evident. Since in presence of an active sympatho-vagal balance it is expected that a significant increase of HF_{RR} power is associated to a significant decrease of the LF_{QT} one, the decrease of HF_{RR} power in WT animals in association with an unvaried LF_{QT} index might suggest a greater complexity of the interactions between vagal and sympathetic branches of the autonomic nervous system. Complex interactions between the two branches of the autonomic nervous system are known to lead to imbalanced situations in which a vagal withdrawal is not linked to a simultaneous and proportional sympathetic activation or *vice versa* (Porta et al., 2007) or situations featuring co-activation or co-inhibition of both the autonomic nervous system limbs (Kollai and Koizumi, 1979; Paton et al., 2005). These situations might lead to non-reciprocal trends in cardiac vagal and sympathetic controls (Kollai and Koizumi, 1979). The complexity of the sympatho-vagal interactions requires a more flexible tool that does not pretend to quantify cardiac autonomic control from a unique variability series like RRV-based analysis, but considers the joint observation of RRV and QTV as a mandatory standpoint for the reliable inference of autonomic nervous system state.

The relevance of the simultaneous assessment of RRV and QTV is even more evident when the WT rats were subdivided into non-AGG and AGG animals (de Boer et al., 2003). In previous studies, AGG rats were found to be characterized by lower RRV markers in unstressed conditions compared to non-AGG rats, thus suggesting that the aggressive behavior is associated with a lower vagal control (Carnevali et al., 2013; Carnevali and Sgoifo, 2014). Such a low cardiac vagal modulation was associated with a higher arrhythmia susceptibility and a greater vulnerability to cardiac morbidity in the AGG group (Carnevali et al., 2013). Differences in resting autonomic modulation between AGG and non-AGG rats were not evident in the current study using the RRV markers given that the HF_{RR} power was similar, but they were unveiled by the QTV markers given that the LF_{QT} power was greater in AGG than in non-AGG rats. Therefore, our results suggest that the AGG rats are characterized by a higher resting sympathetic modulation that is not accompanied by a concomitant reduction of vagal modulation. This finding might be another evidence of the complexity of the cardiac control in rats where a high sympathetic drive does not imply by necessity a vagal withdrawal and further corroborates the need of an approach to the study of the cardiac autonomic control integrating different signals and not necessarily based on the concept of sympatho-vagal balance.

Time Domain RRV and QTV Parameters Versus Spectral RRV and QTV Markers

Time domain markers were commonly shown to provide the representation of the effect of a physiological challenge or an experimental maneuver on the cardiovascular system. For example, in our human protocol, the trend of the μ_{RR} suggests that the orthostatic challenge was effective because the reduction of the venous return due to posture modification provokes a tachycardic response in the attempt to prevent the arterial pressure drop (Montano et al., 1994; Cooke et al., 1999; Porta et al., 2011; Marchi et al., 2016). For example, in the same protocol the evolution of μ_{QT} suggests that the QT measures are reliable given that it is well-known that in humans μ_{QT} is shorter when μ_{RR} is reduced (Bazett, 1929). However, the limits of time domain measures in providing a complete picture appear evidently as well. For example, σ^2_{QT} was less powerful than the LF_{QT} power in describing the effect of the orthostatic challenge likely because non-autonomic effects resulting from cardiac axis movements synchronous with respiration (Porta et al., 1998b) are likely to influence more remarkably σ^2_{QT} than its portion in the LF band. For example, in non-AGG and AGG rats the μ_{RR} and μ_{QT} were similar, while the LF_{QT} power increased in the AGG group, thus stressing the non-redundant nature of time and frequency domain markers.

On the Use of Rats as an Animal Model of Human Cardiac Autonomic Control Explored via RRV and QTV Analyses

Rats are considered animals exhibiting a sympathetic dominance given that their intrinsic heart rate (i.e., the cardiac frequency under complete pharmacological autonomic blockade) is lower than the resting heart rate (Opthof, 2000). However, this observation does not imply that vagal control is absent. Indeed, the full muscarinic receptor blockade induced via a high dose of atropine dramatically reduced RRV (Japundzic et al., 1990; Cerutti et al., 1991; Silva et al., 2017), thus supporting the observation that changes of vagal activity contribute importantly to σ^2_{RR} and corroborating the use of these animals in translational studies on cardiac autonomic control. More importantly for the present study, rats respond differently to sympathetic stimulation: indeed, they show a QT prolongation, while in humans a QT shortening is observed (Conrath and Opthof, 2006; Speerschneider and Thomsen, 2013). The parallel changes of μ_{RR} and μ_{QT} reported in the present study in the human protocol and the opposite trends of μ_{RR} and μ_{QT} in WI and WT groups are in agreement with the diverse effect of an augmented sympathetic drive on μ_{RR} and μ_{QT} in humans and rats. In spite of this peculiarity, the RRV and QTV markers seem to maintain similar interpretation in both species. However, the lack of application of a stressor inducing a sympathetic activation in both WI and WT rats prevents us to deepen this issue.

Limitations of the Study and Future Developments

While our data support the association between QTV magnitude and sympathetic control, they are less informative about the shape of the relation between them. It is likely that the QTV could reflect mean sympathetic activity and its modifications about the mean when sympathetic drive is sufficiently high, while below a certain mean neural activity value QTV could be useless. We advocate pharmacological studies that could graduate the challenge in a finer manner and the contemporaneous direct recording of sympathetic activity to provide insight on the shape of this relation.

There is an open debate on the dependency of the magnitude of RRV and QTV on their means and on the need of some normalization (Sacha and Pluta, 2008; Sacha, 2013; Boyett et al., 2019; Malik et al., 2019). In the present study we tested the redundancy between QTV and μ_{QT} by calculating the normalized QT variance (QTVN), namely the ratio of the square QT standard deviation to the square μ_{QT} (Baumert et al., 2016). No difference was found either among experimental conditions in the human protocol or between groups in the animal protocol. This result might suggest a certain degree of dependency between QTV and μ_{QT}. However, the lack of significant differences is due to the enormous standard deviation of QTVN, sometimes close to two times the QTVN mean. This observation suggests some caution in using QTVN given that normalization procedure might behave differently at diverse values of μ_{QT} and the need of more deeply exploring the relation between QTV and μ_{QT}.

Since in rats the T-wave morphology is different from that in humans, due to the different shapes of the ventricular action potentials (Fabritz et al., 2010; Boukens et al., 2014), future studies should be focused on the comparison of methods based on a threshold on the first derivative (Laguna et al., 1990; Nollo et al., 1992; Porta et al., 1998b), on the tangent method taking the interception between the straight line at the steepest point of the T-wave downslope and the isoelectric line (Lepeschkin and Surawicz, 1952; Yamada et al., 1993; Porta et al., 1998b) and on template matching approach (Berger et al., 1997; Baumert et al., 2012).

CONCLUSION

In the present study, we computed frequency domain markers concurrently derived from RRV and QTV for a deeper characterization of the cardiac autonomic control. The power of RRV in the HF band and the power of QTV in the LF band were exploited to typify state- and trait-related modifications of the cardiac autonomic regulation in humans and rats. We found that the information derived from RRV and QTV spectral markers is not redundant given that trends of the HF power of RRV cannot be inferred from those of the LF power of QTV and vice versa. The complementary information was interpreted in relation to the inherent ability of RRV and QTV spectral markers to describe, respectively, cardiac vagal and sympathetic controls. Therefore, we conclude that the concomitant evaluation of RRV and QTV frequency domain markers can provide a more insightful view on cardiac autonomic function in both humans and rats than the sole exploitation of RRV indexes.

AUTHOR CONTRIBUTIONS

AP conceived and designed the study. AS, LC, AMT, and AC performed the experiments. BM analyzed the data. BM and AP drafted the manuscript and prepared the figures. BM, VB, AS, LC, BC, EV, AMT, AC, LDV, and AP interpreted the results, edited and revised the manuscript, and approved the final version of the manuscript.

REFERENCES

Akaike, H. (1974). A new look at the statistical novel identification. *IEEE Trans. Autom. Control* 19, 716–723. doi: 10.1109/tac.1974.1100705

Akselrod, S., Eliash, S., Oz, O., and Cohen, S. (1987). Hemodynamic regulation in SHR: investigation by spectral analysis. *Am. J. Physiol.* 253, H176–H183.

Akselrod, S., Gordon, D., Ubel, F. A., Shannon, D. C., Berger, A. C., and Cohen, R. J. (1981). Power spectrum analysis of heart rate fluctuation: a quantitative probe of beat-to-beat cardiovascular control. *Science* 213, 220–222. doi: 10.1126/science.6166045

Atiga, W. L., Calkins, H., Lawrence, J. H., Tomaselli, G. F., Smith, J. M., and Berger, R. D. (1998). Beat-to-beat repolarization lability identifies patients at risk for sudden cardiac death. *J. Cardiovasc. Electrophysiol.* 9:908.

Bar, K. J., Koschke, M., Boettger, M. K., Berger, S., Kabisch, A., Sauer, H., et al. (2007). Acute psychosis leads to increased QT variability in patients suffering from schizophrenia. *Schizophr. Res.* 95, 115–123. doi: 10.1016/j.schres.2007.05.034

Bari, V., Valencia, J. F., Vallverdú, M., Girardengo, G., Marchi, A., Bassani, T., et al. (2014). Multiscale complexity analysis of the cardiac control identifies asymptomatic and symptomatic patients in long QT syndrome type 1. *PLoS One* 9:e93808. doi: 10.1371/journal.pone.0093808

Baselli, G., Porta, A., Rimoldi, O., Pagani, M., and Cerutti, S. (1997). Spectral decomposition in multichannel recordings based on multi-variate parametric identification. *IEEE Trans. Biomed. Eng.* 44, 1092–1101. doi: 10.1109/10.641336

Baumert, M., Porta, A., Vos, M. A., Malik, M., Couderc, J. P., Laguna, P., et al. (2016). QT interval variability in body surface ECG: measurement, physiological basis, and clinical value: position statement and consensus guidance endorsed by the european heart rhythm association jointly with the esc working group on cardiac cellular electrophysiology. *Europace* 186, 925–944. doi: 10.1093/europace/euv405

Baumert, M., Lambert, G. W., Dawood, T., Lambert, E. A., Esler, M. D., McGrane, M., et al. (2008). QT interval variability and cardiac norepinephrine spillover in patients with depression and panic disorder. *Am. J. Physiol.* 295, H962–H968. doi: 10.1152/ajpheart.00301.2008

Baumert, M., Schlaich, M. P., Nalivaiko, E., Lambert, E., Sari, C. I., Kaye, D. M., et al. (2011). Relation between QT interval variability and cardiac sympathetic activity in hypertension. *Am. J. Physiol.* 300, H1412–H1417.

Baumert, M., Starc, V., and Porta, A. (2012). Conventional QT variability measurement vs. template matching techniques: comparison of performance using simulated and real ECG. *PLoS One* 7:e41920. doi: 10.1371/journal.pone.0041920

Bazett, H. C. (1929). An analysis of the time-relations of electrocardiograms. *Heart* 7, 353–370.

Berger, R. D. (2009). QT Interval variability: is it a measure of autonomic activity? *J. Am. Coll. Cardiol.* 54, 821–852.

Berger, R. D., Kasper, E. K., Baughman, K. L., Marban, E., Calkins, H., and Tomaselli, G. F. (1997). Beat-to-beat QT interval variability: novel evidence for repolarization lability in ischemic and nonischemic dilated cardiomyopathy. *Circulation* 96, 1557–1565. doi: 10.1161/01.cir.96.5.1557

Billman, G. E. (2013). The LF/HF ratio does not accurately measure cardiac sympatho-vagal balance. *Front. Physiol.* 4:26. doi: 10.3389/fphys.2013.00026

Boukens, B. J., Rivaud, M. R., Rentschler, S., and Coronel, R. (2014). Misinterpretation of the mouse ECG: 'musing the waves of Mus musculus'. *J. Physiol.* 592, 4613–4626. doi: 10.1113/jphysiol.2014.279380

Boyett, M., Wang, Y., and D'Souza, A. (2019). CrossTalk opposing view: heart rate variability as a measure of cardiac autonomic responsiveness is fundamentally flawed. *J. Physiol.* 597, 2599–2601. doi: 10.1113/jp277501

Malik, M., Hnatkova, K., Huikuri, H. V., Lombardi, F., Schmidt, G., and Zabel, M. (2019). CrossTalk proposal: heart rate variability is a valid measure of cardiac autonomic responsiveness. *J. Physiol.* 597, 2595–2598. doi: 10.1113/jp277500

Brenner, I. K., Thomas, S., and Shephard, R. J. (1997). Spectral analysis of heart rate variability during heat exposure and repeated exercise. *Eur. J. Appl. Physiol. Occup. Physiol.* 76, 145–156. doi: 10.1007/s004210050227

Buwalda, B., Geerdink, M., Vidal, J., and Koolhaas, J. M. (2011). Social behavior and social stress in adolescence: a focus on animal models. *Neurosci. Biobehav. Rev.* 35, 1713–1721. doi: 10.1016/j.neubiorev.2010.10.004

Carnevali, L., and Sgoifo, A. (2014). Vagal modulation of resting heart rate in rats: the role of stress, psychosocial factors, and physical exercise. *Front. Physiol.* 5:118. doi: 10.3389/fphys.2014.00118

Carnevali, L., Trombini, M., Porta, A., Montano, N., de Boer, S. F., and Sgoifo, A. (2013). Vagal withdrawal and susceptibility to cardiac arrhythmias in rats with high trait aggressiveness. *PLoS One* 87:e68316. doi: 10.1371/journal.pone.0068316

Cerutti, C., Gustin, M. P., Paultre, C. Z., Lo, M., Julien, C., Vincent, M., et al. (1991). Autonomic nervous system and cardiovascular variability in rats: a spectral analysis approach. *Am. J. Physiol.* 261, H1292–H1299.

Conrath, C. E., and Opthof, T. (2006). Ventricular repolarization: an overview of (patho)physiology, sympathetic effects and genetic aspects. *Prog. Biophys. Mol. Biol.* 92, 269–307. doi: 10.1016/j.pbiomolbio.2005.05.009

Cooke, W. H., Hoag, J. B., Crossman, A. A., Kuusela, T. A., Tahvanainen, K. U. O., and Eckberg, D. L. (1999). Human responses to upright tilt: a window on central autonomic integration. *J. Physiol.* 517, 617–628. doi: 10.1111/j.1469-7793.1999.0617t.x

de Boer, S. F., van der Vegt, B. J., and Koolhaas, J. M. (2003). Individual variation in aggression of feral rodent strains: a standard for the genetics of aggression and violence? *Behav. Genet.* 33, 485–501.

Eckberg, D. L. (1997). Sympathovagal balance: a critical appraisal. *Circulation* 96, 3224–3232. doi: 10.1161/01.cir.96.9.3224

El-Hamad, F., Lambert, E., Abbott, D., and Baumert, M. (2015). Relation between QT interval variability and muscle sympathetic nerve activity in normal subjects. *Am. J. Physiol.* 309, H1218–H1224. doi: 10.1152/ajpheart.00230.2015

Fabritz, L., Damke, D., Emmerich, M., Kaufmann, S. G., Theis, K., Blana, A., et al. (2010). Autonomic modulation and antiarrhythmic therapy in a model of long QT syndrome type 3. *Cardiovasc. Res.* 87, 60–72. doi: 10.1093/cvr/cvq029

Hirsch, J. A., and Bishop, B. (1981). Respiratory sinus arrhythmia in humans: how breathing pattern modulates heart rate. *Am. J. Physiol.* 241, H620–H629.

Jaenisch, R. B., Hentschke, V. S., Quagliotto, E., Cavinato, P. R., Schmeing, L., Xavier, L. L., et al. (2011). Respiratory muscle training improves hemodynamics, autonomic function, baroreceptor sensitivity, and respiratory mechanics in rats with heart failure. *J. Appl. Physiol.* 111, 1664–1670. doi: 10.1152/japplphysiol.01245.2010

Japundzic, N., Grichois, M. L., Zitoun, P., Laude, D., and Elghozi, J. L. (1990). Spectral analysis of blood pressure and heart rate in conscious rats: effects of autonomic blockers. *J. Auton. Nerv. Syst.* 30, 91–100. doi: 10.1016/0165-1838(90)90132-3

Kay, S. M., and Marple, S. L. (1981). Spectrum analysis: a modern perspective. *Proc. IEEE* 69, 1380–1418.

Kollai, M., and Koizumi, K. (1979). Reciprocal and non-reciprocal action of the vagal and sympathetic nerves innervating the heart. *J. Auton. Nerv. Syst.* 1, 33–52. doi: 10.1016/0165-1838(79)90004-3

Laguna, P., Thakor, N. V., Caminal, P., Jane, R., Yoon, H. R., Bayes de Luna, A., et al. (1990). New algorithm for QT interval analysis in 24-hour Holter ECG: performance and applications. *Med. Biol. Eng. Comput.* 281, 67–73. doi: 10.1007/bf02441680

Lepeschkin, E., and Surawicz, B. (1952). The measurement of the Q-T interval of the electrocardiogram. *Circulation* 6, 378–388. doi: 10.1161/01.cir.6.3.378

Lombardi, F., Sandrone, G., Porta, A., Torzillo, D., Terranova, G., Baselli, G., et al. (1996). Spectral analysis of short term R-Tapex interval variability during sinus rhythm and fixed atrial rate. *Eur. Heart J.* 17, 769–778. doi: 10.1093/oxfordjournals.eurheartj.a014945

Magagnin, V., Bassani, T., Bari, V., Turiel, M., Maestri, R., Pinna, G. D., et al. (2011). Non-stationarities significantly distort short-term spectral, symbolic and entropy heart rate variability indexes. *Physiol. Meas.* 32, 1775–1786. doi: 10.1088/0967-3334/32/11/s05

Malik, M. (2009). Beat-to-beat QT variability and cardiac autonomic regulation. *Am. J. Physiol.* 295, H923–H925.

Marchi, A., Bari, V., De Maria, B., Esler, M., Lambert, E., Baumert, M., et al. (2016). Calibrated variability of muscle sympathetic nerve activity during graded head-up tilt in humans and its link with noradrenaline data and cardiovascular rhythms. *Am J. Physiol.* 310, R1134–R1143. doi: 10.1152/ajpregu.00541.2015

Montano, N., Gnecchi-Ruscone, T., Porta, A., Lombardi, F., Pagani, M., and Malliani, A. (1994). Power spectrum analysis of heart rate variability to assess changes in sympatho-vagal balance during graded orthostatic tilt. *Circulation* 90, 1826–1831. doi: 10.1161/01.cir.90.4.1826

Nollo, G., Speranza, G., Grasso, R., Bonamini, R., Mangiardi, L., and Antolini, R. (1992). Spontaneous beat-to-beat variability of the ventricular repolarisation duration. *J. Electrocardiol.* 25, 9–17. doi: 10.1016/0022-0736(92)90124-i

Opthof, T. (2000). The normal range and determinants of the intrinsic heart rate in man. *Cardiovasc. Res.* 45, 177–184. doi: 10.1016/s0008-6363(99)00322-3

Pagani, M., Lombardi, F., Guzzetti, S., Rimoldi, O., Furlan, R., Pizzinelli, P., et al. (1986). Power spectral analysis of heart rate and arterial pressure variabilities as a marker of sympatho-vagal interaction in man and conscious dog. *Circ. Res.* 59, 178–193. doi: 10.1161/01.res.59.2.178

Pagani, M., Montano, N., Porta, A., Malliani, A., Abboud, F. M., Birkett, C., et al. (1997). Relationship between spectral components of cardiovascular variabilities and direct measures of muscle sympathetic nerve activity in humans. *Circulation* 95, 1441–1448. doi: 10.1161/01.cir.95.6.1441

Paton, J. F., Boscan, P., Pickering, A. E., and Nalivaiko, E. (2005). The yin and yang of cardiac autonomic control: vago-sympathetic interactions revisited. *Brain Res. Rev.* 49, 555–565. doi: 10.1016/j.brainresrev.2005.02.005

Piccirillo, G., Cacciafesta, M., Lionetti, M., Nocco, M., Di Giuseppe, V., Moisé, A., et al. (2001). Influence of age, the autonomic nervous system and anxiety on QT-interval variability. *Clin. Sci.* 101, 429–438. doi: 10.1042/cs1010429

Piccirillo, G., Magnanti, M., Matera, S., Di Carlo, S., De Laurentis, T., Torrini, A., et al. (2006). Age and QT variability index during free breathing, controlled breathing and tilt in patients with chronic heart failure and healthy control subjects. *Transl. Res.* 142, 72–78. doi: 10.1016/j.trsl.2006.02.001

Pomeranz, B., Macaulay, R. J. B., Caudill, M. A., Kutz, I., Adam, D., Gordon, D., et al. (1985). Assessment of autonomic function in humans by heart-rate spectral-analysis. *Am. J. Physiol.* 248, H151–H153.

Porta, A., Bari, V., Badilini, F., Tobaldini, E., Gnecchi-Ruscone, T., and Montano, N. (2011). Frequency domain assessment of the coupling strength between ventricular repolarization duration and heart period during graded head-up tilt. *J. Electrocardiol.* 44, 662–668. doi: 10.1016/j.jelectrocard.2011.08.002

Porta, A., Bari, V., De Maria, B., Cairo, B., Vaini, E., Malacarne, M., et al. (2018). Peripheral resistance baroreflex during incremental bicycle ergometer exercise: characterization and correlation with cardiac baroreflex. *Front. Physiol.* 9:688. doi: 10.3389/fphys.2018.00688

Porta, A., Baselli, G., Caiani, E., Malliani, A., Lombardi, F., and Cerutti, S. (1998a). Quantifying electrocardiogram RT-RR variability interactions. *Med. Biol. Eng. Comput.* 36, 27–34. doi: 10.1007/bf02522854

Porta, A., Baselli, G., Lombardi, F., Cerutti, S., Antolini, R., Del Greco, M., et al. (1998b). Performance assessment of standard algorithms for dynamic R-T interval measurement: comparison between R-Tapex and R-Tend approach. *Med. Biol. Eng. Comput.* 36, 35–42. doi: 10.1007/bf02522855

Porta, A., Girardengo, G., Bari, V., George, A. L. Jr., Brink, P. A., Goosen, A., et al. (2015). Autonomic control of heart rate and QT interval variability influences arrhythmic risk in long QT syndrome type I. *J. Am. Coll. Cardiol.* 65, 367–374. doi: 10.1016/j.jacc.2014.11.015

Porta, A., Tobaldini, E., Gnecchi-Ruscone, T., and Montano, N. (2010). RT variability unrelated to heart period and respiration progressively increases during graded head-up tilt. *Am. J. Physiol.* 298, H1406–H1414. doi: 10.1152/ajpheart.01206.2009

Porta, A., Tobaldini, E., Guzzetti, S., Furlan, R., Montano, N., and Gnecchi-Ruscone, T. (2007). Assessment of cardiac autonomic modulation during graded head-up tilt by symbolic analysis of heart rate variability. *Am. J. Physiol.* 293, H702–H708.

Reyes del Paso, G. A., Langewitz, W., Mulder, L. J., van Roon, A., and Duschek, S. (2013). The utility of low frequency heart rate variability as an index of sympathetic cardiac tone: a review with emphasis on a reanalysis of previous studies. *Psychophysiology* 50, 477–487. doi: 10.1111/psyp.12027

Rubini, R., Porta, A., Baselli, G., Cerutti, S., and Paro, M. (1993). Power spectrum analysis of cardiovascular variability monitored by telemetry in conscious unrestrained rats. *J. Auton. Nerv. Syst.* 45, 181–190. doi: 10.1016/0165-1838(93)90050-5

Sacha, J. (2013). Why should one normalize heart rate variability with respect to average heart rate. *Front. Physiol.* 4:306. doi: 10.3389/fphys.2013.00306

Sacha, J., and Pluta, W. (2008). Alterations of an average heart rate change heart rate variability due to mathematical reasons. *Int. J. Cardiol.* 128, 444–447. doi: 10.1016/j.ijcard.2007.06.047

Sgoifo, A., De Boer, S. F., Buwalda, B., Korte-Bouws, G., Tuma, J., Bohus, B., et al. (1998). Vulnerability to arrhythmias during social stress in rats with different sympathovagal balance. *Am. J. Physiol.* 275, H460–H466. doi: 10.1152/ajpheart.1998.275.2.H460

Sgoifo, A., Koolhaas, J., De Boer, S., Musso, E., Stilli, D., Buwalda, B., et al. (1999). Social stress, autonomic neural activation, and cardiac activity in rats. *Neurosci. Biobehav. Rev.* 237, 915–923. doi: 10.1016/s0149-7634(99)00025-1

Shin, K., Minamitani, H., Onishi, S., Yamazaki, H., and Lee, M. (1995a). The power spectral analysis of heart rate variability in athletes during dynamic exercise - Part I. *Clin. Cardiol.* 18, 583–586. doi: 10.1002/clc.4960181011

Shin, K., Minamitani, H., Onishi, S., Yamazaki, H., and Lee, M. (1995b). The power spectral analysis of heart rate variability in athletes during dynamic exercise - Part II. *Clin. Cardiol.* 18, 664–668. doi: 10.1002/clc.4960181114

Silva, L. E. V., Lataro, R. M., Castania, J. A., da Silva, C. A. A., Valencia, J. F., Murta, L. O. Jr., et al. (2016). Multiscale entropy analysis of heart rate variability in heart failure, hypertensive and sinoaortic-denervated rats: classical and refined approaches. *Am. J. Physiol.* 310, R150–R156. doi: 10.1152/ajpregu.00076.2016

Silva, L. E. V., Rezende Geraldini, V., Potratz de Oliveira, B., Aguiar Silva, C. A., Porta, A., and Fazan, R. (2017). Comparison between spectral analysis and symbolic dynamics for heart rate variability analysis in the rat. *Sci. Rep.* 7:8428. doi: 10.1038/s41598-017-08888-w

Speerschneider, T., and Thomsen, M. B. (2013). Physiology and analysis of the electrocardiographic T wave in mice. *Acta Physiol.* 209, 262–271. doi: 10.1111/apha.12172

Speranza, G., Nollo, G., Ravelli, F., and Antolini, R. (1993). Beat-to-beat measurement and analysis of the R-T interval in 24 h ECG Holter recordings. *Med. Biol. Eng. Comput.* 315, 487–494. doi: 10.1007/bf02441984

Stauss, H. M., Persson, P. B., Johnson, A. K., and Kregel, K. C. (1997). Frequency response characteristics of autonomic nervous system function in conscious rats. *Am. J. Physiol.* 273, H786–H795.

Task Force of the European Society of Cardiology and the North American Society of Pacing and Electrophysiology, (1996). Heart rate variability. Standards of measurement, physiological interpretation, and clinical use. *Eur. Heart. J.* 17, 354–381. doi: 10.1093/oxfordjournals.eurheartj.a014868

Yamada, A., Hayano, J., Horie, K., Ieda, K., Mukai, S., Yamada, M., et al. (1993). Regulation of QT interval during postural transitory changes in heart rate in normal subjects. *Am. J. Cardiol.* 71, 996–998. doi: 10.1016/0002-9149(93)90922-y

Yeragani, V. K., Pohl, R., Jampala, V. C., Balon, R., Kay, J., and Igel, G. (2000a). Effect of posture and isoproterenol on beat-to-beat heart rate and QT variability. *Neuropsychobiology* 41, 113–123. doi: 10.1159/000026642

Yeragani, V. K., Pohl, R., Jampala, V. C., Balon, R., Ramesh, C., and Srinivasan, K. (2000b). Increased QT variability in patients with panic disorder and depression. *Psychiatry Res.* 93, 225–235. doi: 10.1016/s0165-1781(00)00119-0

17

K_V4.3 Expression Modulates Na_V1.5 Sodium Current

Vincent Portero[1], *Ronald Wilders*[2], *Simona Casini*[1], *Flavien Charpentier*[3], *Arie O. Verkerk*[1,2†] *and Carol Ann Remme*[1*†]

[1] Department of Experimental Cardiology, Academic Medical Center, Amsterdam, Netherlands, [2] Department of Medical Biology, Academic Medical Center, Amsterdam, Netherlands, [3] L'Institut du Thorax, INSERM, CNRS, Université de Nantes, Nantes, France

***Correspondence:**
Carol Ann Remme
c.a.remme@amc.uva.nl

† These authors have contributed equally to this work.

In cardiomyocytes, the voltage-gated transient outward potassium current (I_{to}) is responsible for the phase-1 repolarization of the action potential (AP). Gain-of-function mutations in *KCND3*, the gene encoding the I_{to} carrying K_V4.3 channel, have been associated with Brugada syndrome (BrS). While the role of I_{to} in the pro-arrhythmic mechanism of BrS has been debated, recent studies have suggested that an increased I_{to} may directly affect cardiac conduction. However, the effects of an increased I_{to} on AP upstroke velocity or sodium current at the cellular level remain unknown. We here investigated the consequences of K_V4.3 overexpression on Na_V1.5 current and consequent sodium channel availability. We found that overexpression of K_V4.3 protein in HEK293 cells stably expressing Na_V1.5 (HEK293-Na_V1.5 cells) significantly reduced Na_V1.5 current density without affecting its kinetic properties. In addition, K_V4.3 overexpression decreased AP upstroke velocity in HEK293-Na_V1.5 cells, as measured with the alternating voltage/current clamp technique. These effects of K_V4.3 could not be explained by alterations in total Na_V1.5 protein expression. Using computer simulations employing a multicellular *in silico* model, we furthermore demonstrate that the experimentally observed increase in K_V4.3 current and concurrent decrease in Na_V1.5 current may result in a loss of conduction, underlining the potential functional relevance of our findings. This study gives the first proof of concept that K_V4.3 directly impacts on Na_V1.5 current. Future studies employing appropriate disease models should explore the potential electrophysiological implications in (patho)physiological conditions, including BrS associated with *KCND3* gain-of-function mutations.

Keywords: transient outward current, sodium current, channels, action potential, myocyte, arrhythmias, computer simulation

INTRODUCTION

The cardiac sodium current (I_{Na}), generated by the *SCN5A*-encoded voltage-gated Na^+ channel (Na_V1.5) (Gellens et al., 1992), is responsible for the initial fast upstroke of the cardiac action potential (AP). It determines excitability of myocardial cells and ensures proper conduction of the electrical impulse within the heart. Consequently, Na_V1.5 channel dysfunction may lead to conduction slowing, ventricular arrhythmias, and sudden cardiac death. In particular, *SCN5A* mutations leading to loss of sodium channel function are associated with isolated (progressive) conduction slowing or block (Schott et al., 1999), sick sinus syndrome (Benson et al., 2003), and Brugada syndrome (BrS) (Chen et al., 1998; Crotti et al., 2012; Le Scouarnec et al., 2015).

In cardiomyocytes, the voltage-gated transient outward K^+ current (I_{to}) is responsible for the phase-1 repolarization of the cardiac AP and thereby contributes to the refractory period and inotropic state of the myocardium. In human, I_{to} is generated by the $K_V4.3$ channel, which is encoded by the gene *KCND3* (Niwa and Nerbonne, 2010). Gain-of-function mutations in *KCND3*, or its regulatory subunits, have also been associated with BrS (Delpón et al., 2008; You et al., 2015; Portero et al., 2016), giving rise to an ongoing discussion on the apparent role of I_{to} in the pro-arrhythmic mechanism of BrS (Wilde et al., 2010). Previous studies have suggested that an increased I_{to} may directly affect cardiac conduction due to a current-to-load mismatch during the depolarization process (Hoogendijk et al., 2010a,b). However, the effects of a gain-of-function of I_{to} on the AP upstroke velocity at the cellular level remain unknown. The characterization of various knock-out mouse models of α-subunits generating the fast component of I_{to} (*Kcnd3, Kcnd2*) confirmed the involvement of I_{to} in phase-1 repolarization, but its impact on AP upstroke velocity or I_{Na} density were not investigated (Niwa et al., 2008; Liu et al., 2015). We recently evaluated the effects of an *in silico* I_{to} injection on AP upstroke and repolarization velocity using the dynamic clamp technique (Verkerk et al., 2016). In that study, we observed a minimal effect (≈2%) of *in-silico* I_{to} injection on upstroke velocity but only when the injected current was large and rapidly activated at very negative potentials (around −50 mV). However, while an I_{to}-like current does not appear to directly affect the fast depolarization, evidence is increasing that various ion channel proteins may interact and thus modulate each other's expression, function, or membrane trafficking (Balse and Boycott, 2017). For example, studies highlighted an interaction and co-regulation of the Kir2.1 and $Na_V1.5$ proteins with a direct effect on their electrophysiological properties and thus important for cardiac excitability (Milstein et al., 2012). Moreover, a recent study demonstrated a direct interaction between the $K_V4.3$ and hERG proteins, resulting in an increase in hERG current density upon co-expression of hERG with $K_V4.3$ (Zhao et al., 2017). Considering these novel studies and the involvement of both I_{Na} and I_{to} in BrS, we hypothesized that the level of expression of $K_V4.3$ may impact on I_{Na}.

We addressed this hypothesis by evaluating the impact of $K_V4.3$ protein overexpression on $Na_V1.5$-based current and sodium channel availability in HEK293 cells stably expressing $Na_V1.5$ (HEK293-$Na_V1.5$). We show that an overexpression of $K_V4.3$ channels leads to a reduction of $Na_V1.5$ current density and lower AP upstroke velocity, as measured with the alternating voltage/current clamp (VC/CC) technique. These effects of $K_V4.3$ overexpression could not be explained by alterations in total $Na_V1.5$ protein expression. Computer simulations furthermore indicate that the experimentally observed decreased upstroke velocity is not directly due to an increase in the $K_V4.3$-based I_{to}, but instead a consequence of the $K_V4.3$ protein itself. We also demonstrate that an increase in I_{to} as well as a decrease in I_{Na} can affect cardiac conduction and that a combination of both can lead to dramatic consequences, underlining the potential functional relevance of our findings.

MATERIALS AND METHODS

HEK293-$Na_V1.5$ Cell Culture and Transfection

To avoid artifacts due to co-transfections, we evaluated the effect of the overexpression of $K_V4.3$ protein on $Na_V1.5$ currents using a genetically modified cell line constitutively overexpressing the human $Na_V1.5$ channel (van Bemmelen et al., 2004). HEK293 cells stably expressing h$Na_V1.5$ (HEK293-$Na_V1.5$, kindly provided by Drs. Hugues Abriel and Jean-Sébastien Rougier) were cultured in DMEM (Gibco) supplemented with 10% FBS (Biowest), L-glutamine (Gibco), penicillin-streptomycin (Gibco), and Zeomycin (Invitrogen) in a 5% CO_2 incubator at 37°C. Cells were transfected at 70% confluency in 36.8 mm culture wells with 1 μg IRES-GFP or 1 μg *KCND3*-IRES-GFP cDNA using lipofectamine (Invitrogen, Carlsbad, USA). Both IRES-GFP and *KCND3*-IRES-GFP (human *KCND3* transcript reference: NM_004980.4) constructs contained the same M61 vector plasmid backbone (Addgene). Gene-transfer was monitored by means of green fluorescence from the IRES-GFP or *KCND3*-IRES-GFP bicistronic vector. Patch clamp experiments were performed on single fluorescent cells 2 days after transfection.

Ventricular Cell Preparation

Animal procedures were performed in accordance with governmental and institutional guidelines for animal use in research and were approved by the Animal Experimental Committee of the Academic Medical Center, Amsterdam, The Netherlands. Single left ventricular myocytes were isolated from 3 to 5 months old FVB/N mice by enzymatic dissociation (Remme et al., 2006). Therefore, mice were anesthetized by an intraperitoneal injection of pentobarbital prior to cervical dislocation, after which the heart was excised, cannulated, and mounted on a Langendorff perfusion set-up. The hearts were perfused for 5 min with Tyrode's solution containing (in mM): 140 NaCl, 5.4 KCl, 1.8 $CaCl_2$, 1 $MgCl_2$, 5.5 glucose, 5 HEPES; pH 7.4 (NaOH). Subsequently, the heart was perfused for 8 min with a similar solution in which the calcium concentration was lowered to 1 μM, after which the enzyme Liberase Blendzyme type 4 (Roche; 0.05 mg/ml) and trypsin (Boehringer, 1 μl/ml of 2.5% solution) were added for 10 minutes. Single myocytes were obtained by gently triturating the digested tissue in the low calcium enzyme solution supplemented with bovine serum albumin (BSA, 50 mg/ml). Myocytes were washed twice in normal calcium Tyrode's solution and quiescent, rod-shaped cross-striated cells with smooth surface were selected for measurements.

Western Blot Experiment for Total $Na_V1.5$ Quantification

Forty-eight hours after transfection (1 μg IRES-GFP or 1 μg *KCND3*-IRES-GFP plasmid), HEK293-$Na_V1.5$ cells were washed twice with PBS and lysed in PBS containing 0.1% Triton and complete mini EDTA-free protease inhibitor mixture tablet (Roche). Cell lysates were then sonicated twice for 10 s and centrifuged for 10 min at 8.000 rpm. The supernatant was quantified using the BCA kit and 40 μg of each separated cell lysate was loaded on a 4–20% gradient gel (Bio-Rad) after 5 min of denaturation at 60°C in Laemmli buffer. The RbαGFP antibody used for Western blotting was purchased from Santa Cruz Biotechnology, RbαCalnexin from Calbiochem, and RbαNa_V1.5 from Sigma-Aldrich. Goat anti-rabbit horseradish peroxidase-conjugated secondary antibodies were purchased from GE Healthcare Life Science. Chemo luminescence signal was acquired with the ImageQuant LAS 4000 instrument. Band intensities were quantified using the public domain ImageJ software (USA National Institutes of Health). Total Na_V1.5 protein expression protein was normalized to the calnexin signal.

Electrophysiology

Data Acquisition

Na_V1.5 and K_V4.3 currents and upstroke velocities (dV/dt) were measured in the whole-cell configuration of the patch-clamp technique using an Axopatch 200B amplifier (Molecular Devices Corporation, Sunnyvale, CA, USA) or a custom-made amplifier, capable of fast switching between voltage clamp (VC) and current clamp (CC) modes (Berecki et al., 2010). Voltage control, data acquisition, and analysis were accomplished using custom software. Potentials were corrected for the calculated liquid junction potentials (Barry and Lynch, 1991). Signals were low-pass filtered with a cut-off frequency of 5 kHz and digitized at 20, 4, and 40 kHz for Na_V1.5, K_V4.3, and upstroke velocities, respectively. Patch pipettes were pulled from borosilicate glass (Harvard Apparatus) and had resistances of ≈2.0 MΩ after filling with the solutions as indicated below. Series resistance was compensated by ≥80%. Cell membrane capacitance (C_m) was calculated by dividing the time constant of the decay of the capacitive transient upon 5 mV hyperpolarizing voltage step from −40 mV by the series resistance. The average C_m was not significantly different between the IRES-GFP and K_V4.3-IRES-GFP cells [IRES-GFP: 12.27 ± 0.76 pF ($n = 36$); K_V4.3-IRES-GFP: 12.00 ± 0.99 pF ($n = 37$); mean±standard error of the mean (SEM)].

K_V4.3 and Na_V1.5 Current Measurements With Conventional VC

Na_V1.5 current was measured at room temperature (21°C) with patch pipettes containing (in mM): 60 CsCl, 50 aspartic acid, 11 EGTA, 1.0 $CaCl_2$, 1.0 $MgCl_2$, 5.0 Na_2ATP, 10 HEPES, pH 7.2 (CsOH). Bath solution for Na_V1.5 current measurements contained (in mM): 20 NaCl, 130 CsCl, 2 $CaCl_2$, 1 $MgCl_2$, 5 glucose, 10 HEPES, pH 7.4 (CsOH). K_V4.3 current was measured at 37°C in Tyrode's solution with the aforementioned composition. Patch pipettes for K_V4.3 current measurements were filled with solution containing (in mM): 125 K-gluc, 20 KCl, 5 NaCl, 1 $MgCl_2$, 10 BAPTA, 5 MgATP, 10 HEPES, pH 7.2 (NMDG-OH).

Current density and gating properties were determined by means of custom voltage-clamp protocols as indicated in figure insets. Cycle lengths were 5 and 10 s for Na_V1.5 and K_V4.3 current, respectively. Both Na_V1.5 and K_V4.3 current densities were defined as the difference between peak and steady-state current, divided by C_m. To determine the activation characteristics of Na_V1.5 current, current-voltage (I-V) curves were corrected for driving force and normalized to maximum peak current. Steady-state activation and inactivation curves were fitted using the Boltzmann equation $I/I_{max} = A/\{1.0+\exp[(V_{1/2}-V)/k]\}$ to determine $V_{1/2}$ (membrane potential for the half-maximal (in)activation) and the slope factor k.

Upstroke Velocity Measurements Using Alternating VC/CC

The alternating VC/CC technique was used to measure Na_V1.5 current-driven upstrokes at physiological temperature and Na^+ concentrations, as described previously (Berecki et al., 2010). Patch pipette and bath solutions were similar to those used for K_V4.3 current measurements (see above). HEK293-Na_V1.5 cells and freshly isolated myocytes were voltage clamped at a holding potential of −85 mV, a value close to the resting membrane potential of working cardiomyocytes. Next, upstroke and repolarization were elucidated by switching for 20 ms to the CC mode of the patch clamp amplifier. Upstrokes were elicited by 1.2× threshold current pulses through the patch pipette at 0.5 Hz and the stimulus current was present during the entire 20 ms in CC mode. Maximal upstroke velocity (dV/dt_{max}) during VC/CC, offline corrected for the contribution of stimulus current (I_{stim}), served as an indicator of Na_V1.5 current availability.

Computer Simulations

Numerical Reconstruction of Na_V1.5 and K_V4.3 Currents in HEK293 Cells

Alternating VC/CC experiments in HEK293 cells expressing Na_V1.5 and K_V4.3 channels were simulated in a standard cell model with intracellular and extracellular sodium and potassium concentrations similar to those of the patch-clamp experiments. The cell model contained equations for I_{Na}, I_{to}, and I_{stim}. The I_{Na} and I_{to} equations were taken from the human ventricular cell model by Ten Tusscher and Panfilov (2006) with the I_{Na} and I_{to} densities scaled by a factor of 1.8 and 6.0, respectively, to arrive at the experimentally observed values for the maximum upstroke velocity and repolarization velocity. I_{stim} was set to 6.5 pA/pF to ensure that the maximum upstroke velocity was reached at ≈4 ms after the stimulus onset as in the experiments. For numerical integration of the differential equations we applied a simple and efficient Euler-type integration scheme (Rush and Larsen, 1978) with a 1-μs time step.

Maximum Upstroke Velocity and Repolarization Velocity in Murine Left Ventricular Myocytes

The alternating VC/CC protocol of the experiments on single left ventricular myocytes was implemented in the CellML code (Cuellar et al., 2003) of the apical version of the mouse ventricular AP model by Bondarenko et al. (2004). The amplitude of the 20 ms stimulus current was set to 10 pA/pF, which made the AP upstroke occur at ≈4 ms after the stimulus onset. The maximum upstroke velocity and repolarization velocity were determined from the time derivative of the action potential trace. The CellML code was edited and run in version 0.9.31.1409 of the Windows based Cellular Open Resource (COR) environment (Garny et al., 2003) with its standard CVODE integrator.

Action Potential Transfer in Human Left Ventricular Myocytes

AP transfer was studied in a one-dimensional strand of human left ventricular myocytes. The strand consisted of 80 longitudinally coupled cells, each described by the Ten Tusscher and Panfilov model of a single human ventricular myocyte (Ten Tusscher and Panfilov, 2006). The intercellular coupling conductance was set to 6 nS and the myoplasmic resistivity was set to 150 Ω·cm. The first cell of the strand was stimulated at a rate of 1 Hz with a 2-ms, ≈20% supra-threshold stimulus current with an amplitude of 3.2 nA. As in other studies (Shaw and Rudy, 1997; Thomas et al., 2003; Wilders, 2012), the entire cell length (of 74 μm) was used as the spatial discretization element, with elements connected by the lumped myoplasmic resistance (calculated from the myocyte dimensions and the myoplasmic resistivity of 150 Ω·cm) and gap junctional resistance. At the selected gap junctional conductance of 6 nS, this lumped resistance was almost completely determined by the gap junctional resistance (Wilders, 2012). The aforementioned Euler-type integration scheme was used for numerical integration.

Statistics

Data are expressed as mean±SEM. Mann-Whitney Rank Sum test, Student *t*-test, or Two-Way Repeated Measures ANOVA followed by pairwise comparison using the Student-Newman-Keuls test were used when appropriate. The level of statistical significance was set to $p < 0.05$.

RESULTS

Characterization of K_V4.3 Current in HEK293 Cells Stably Expressing Na_V1.5

First, we characterized the K_V4.3-driven current resulting from transfection of the *KCND3*-IRES-GFP plasmid in HEK293 cells stably expressing Na_V1.5 (HEK293-Na_V1.5). **Figure 1A** shows representative currents measured between −100 to 40 mV (with 10 mV increment) during 1-s voltage clamp steps from a holding potential of −80 mV in a HEK293-Na_V1.5 cell transfected with either IRES-GFP (top) or *KCND3*-IRES-GFP (bottom). A prepulse of 5 ms to −40 mV was applied to activate and inactivate the Na_V1.5-based sodium current present in these HEK293-Na_V1.5 cells (**Figure 1A**, inset). Similar to previous reports, cells transfected with IRES-GFP showed a small endogenous current upon depolarization (**Figure 1A**, top) (Niwa et al., 2008). In contrast, cells transfected with *KCND3*-IRES-GFP displayed a large K_V4.3 current which started to activate around −40 mV and increased in amplitude upon further depolarization due to enhanced activation and increased K^+ driving force (**Figure 1A**, bottom) (Giles and van Ginneken, 1985). **Figure 1B** shows the average I-V relationships of the K_V4.3 current, which was defined as the difference between the peak and steady-state current. Its density was defined as the current amplitude divided by the membrane capacitance (C_m), amounting to ≈450 pA/pF at 40 mV in the *KCND3*-IRES-GFP transfected HEK293-Na_V1.5 cells, and >20 times smaller in the IRES-GFP transfected cells. **Figure 1C** shows the voltage-dependency of inactivation for the K_V4.3 current in the cells transfected with *KCND3*-IRES-GFP, measured using a two-pulse protocol with a 1-s prepulse to a potential between −100 and 40 mV followed by a 500-ms test pulse to 40 mV, demonstrating that the K_V4.3 current is fully available at −70 mV and more negative potentials. The $V_{1/2}$ and k of the voltage-dependency of inactivation were −45.9 ± 2.6 and −5.6 ± 0.4 mV, respectively. **Figure 1D** shows the recovery from inactivation in *KCND3*-IRES-GFP transfected HEK293-Na_V1.5 cells analyzed with 200-ms pulses to 40 mV with variable inter-pulse intervals. The time constant of recovery from inactivation, analyzed with a mono-exponential fit (**Figure 1D**, dashed line) was 160 ± 29 ms, demonstrating that recovery from inactivation was completed with an inter-pulse interval of 1 s and longer. The K_V4.3 current biophysical properties are summarized in Table S1. These data indicate that overexpression of *KCND3*-IRES-GFP in HEK293-Na_V1.5 cells results in a large I_{to}, confirming the functional expression of K_V4.3 channels at the cell membrane.

K_V4.3 Expression Reduces Na_V1.5 Current in HEK293-Na_V1.5 Cells

Secondly, we characterized the effects of K_V4.3 overexpression on Na_V1.5-based current in HEK293-Na_V1.5 cells. **Figure 2A** shows representative Na_V1.5 current activated by 500-ms depolarizing voltage clamp steps of 5 mV increment from a holding potential of −120 mV in a IRES-GFP or *KCND3*-IRES-GFP transfected HEK293-Na_V1.5 cell. In both conditions, Na_V1.5 current started to activate around −60 mV, peaked around −30 mV, and subsequently decreased in amplitude due to the reduction in Na^+ driving force. As shown in the average I-V relationships in **Figure 2B**, Na_V1.5 current density was significantly smaller in the *KCND3*-IRES-GFP transfected cells compared to IRES-GFP transfected cells. For example, at −40 mV Na_V1.5 current density was −609 ± 62 and −447 ± 61 pA/pF ($p < 0.05$; pairwise comparison using a Student-Newman-Keuls test following two-way repeated measures ANOVA) in IRES-GFP and *KCND3*-IRES-GFP transfected HEK293-Na_V1.5 cells, respectively, indicating a decrease in Na_V1.5 current density by ≈25% due to K_V4.3 overexpression. Next, we determined whether the Na_V1.5 current density decrease was accompanied by gating property changes. Because the current decay could not be reliably fit to a 2-exponential function, the time course of inactivation was instead determined by analyzing the time required for 50% of current decay to occur ($t_{50\%}$) at −30 mV (Remme et al., 2006). $t_{50\%}$ did not differ significantly between IRES-GFP and *KCND3*-IRES-GFP transfected cells [0.88 ± 0.06 ms ($n = 15$) vs. 0.84 ± 0.03 ms ($n = 19$), respectively, $p = 0.41$; Student's *t*-test]. For determining the voltage-dependency of activation for IRES-GFP and *KCND3*-IRES-GFP transfected cells, I-V relationships, as shown in **Figure 2B**, were first corrected for the Na^+ driving force. Of note, the reversal potential of Na_V1.5 current calculated using the Nernst equation is evaluated at +17.58 mV, which is in line with the sodium current recordings represented in **Figure 2A**. Next, currents were normalized to their maximal amplitude and the curves were fitted to a Boltzmann distribution curve. **Figure 2C** shows overlapping curves of voltage-dependency of inactivation. The latter curves were constructed by normalizing currents to their maximal

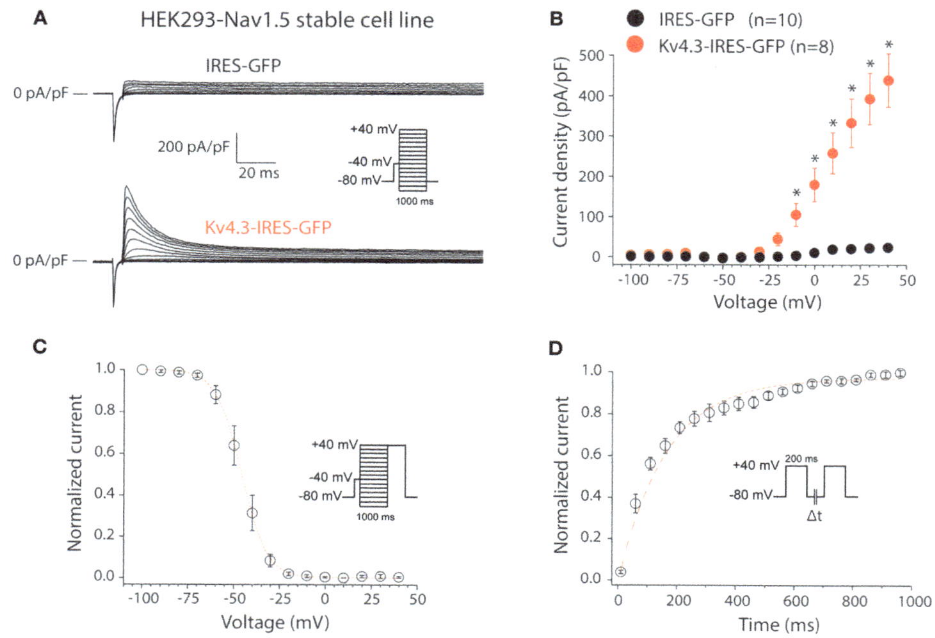

FIGURE 1 | $K_V4.3$ currents in HEK293-$Na_V1.5$ cells transfected with *KCND3*. **(A)** Typical current traces in response to voltage clamp steps to test potentials ranging from −100 to 40 mV recorded from HEK293 cells stably expressing $Na_V1.5$ (HEK293-$Na_V1.5$) and transfected with IRES-GFP (top) or *KCND3*-IRES-GFP (bottom). Inset: voltage clamp protocol used. **(B)** Current-voltage (I-V) relationships of the peak outward current in *KCND3*-IRES-GFP and IRES-GFP transfected cells. Asterisks denote $p < 0.05$. **(C)** Voltage-dependency of $K_V4.3$ inactivation in $K_V4.3$-IRES-GFP cells ($n = 8$). The dotted line is the Boltzmann fit to the average data. Inset: voltage clamp protocol used. **(D)** Average recovery from inactivation curve measured with two subsequent 200-ms pulses from −80 to +40 mV with variable inter-pulse durations (Δt) of 1–1,000-ms ($n = 4$). Inset: voltage clamp protocol used. The red dashed line is a mono-exponential fit of the average data.

current during the voltage clamp step to −20 mV. Similarly, **Figure 2D** shows overlapping curves of voltage-dependency of activation for IRES-GFP and *KCND3*-IRES-GFP transfected cells. These data demonstrate that neither the voltage-dependency of activation nor the voltage-dependency of inactivation of $Na_V1.5$ current were affected by $K_V4.3$ expression. The $Na_V1.5$ current biophysical properties are summarized in Table S1. Western blot analysis showed no differences in $Na_V1.5$ protein expression levels between HEK293-$Na_V1.5$ cells with overexpression of *KCND3*-IRES-GFP or GFP (**Figure 3**; original images provided in the Supplementary Material, Figure S1). Thus, our data demonstrate that $K_V4.3$ expression reduces $Na_V1.5$ current without affecting its gating properties or the $Na_V1.5$ expression level.

$K_V4.3$ Expression Reduces Action Potential Upstroke Velocity

Thirdly, we assessed upstroke velocities in the HEK293-$Na_V1.5$ cells, transfected with either IRES-GFP or *KCND3*-IRES-GFP plasmids. Noteworthy, HEK293 cells expressing $Na_V1.5$ display fast depolarizations upon switching from voltage clamp (VC) to current clamp (CC) due to Na^+ channel activation as previously shown (Berecki et al., 2010; Verkerk et al., 2016; Lieve et al., 2017). Thus, the alternating VC/CC technique allows for a more dynamic assessment of $Na_V1.5$ current as compared to measurements in VC configuration, in the setting of more physiological temperature and Na^+ gradients across the membrane. **Figure 4A** shows typical upstrokes (top) and their time derivatives (bottom) measured upon switching from a holding potential of −85 mV in VC to CC for 20-ms. Upstrokes were evoked at 0.5 Hz, a stimulus frequency at which $K_V4.3$ current is fully available (cf. **Figure 1D**). **Figure 4B** summarizes the maximum upstroke velocities (top) and maximum repolarization velocities (bottom). On average, the maximum upstroke velocity of *KCND3*-IRES-GFP transfected cells was 21% lower than that of IRES-GFP transfected cells (441 ± 17 vs. 556 ± 24 V/s; $p < 0.05$). Both cell types displayed a repolarization phase following the upstroke (**Figure 4A**) with a significantly larger maximum velocity (73 ± 13 vs. 22 ± 3 V/s) in *KCND3*-IRES-GFP as compared to IRES-GFP transfected cells (**Figure 4B**, bottom). In **Figure 4C**, we plotted for each cell its maximum repolarization velocity vs. its maximum upstroke velocity, further demonstrating an inverse relationship between $Na_V1.5$-induced depolarization and $K_V4.3$-induced repolarization velocities: $K_V4.3$ expression increases repolarization velocity, but reduces upstroke velocity.

Relation Between Repolarization and Depolarization in Ventricular Myocytes of Mice

The above presented data indicate that $K_V4.3$ (over)expression decreases $Na_V1.5$ current (**Figure 2B**) and upstroke velocity

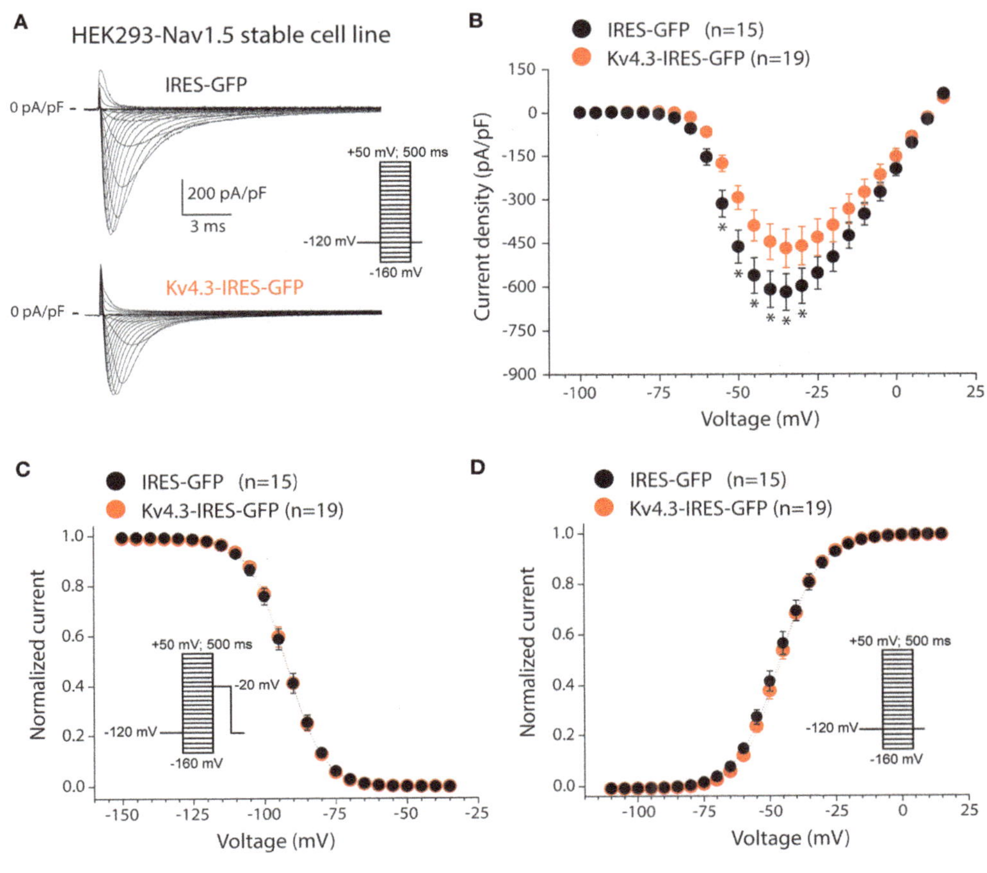

FIGURE 2 | $K_V4.3$ overexpression reduces $Na_V1.5$ currents. **(A)** Typical $Na_V1.5$ current traces in response to 500-ms depolarizing voltage steps from a holding potential of −120 mV to test potentials ranging from −160 to 50 mV in IRES-GFP (top) and *KCND3*-IRES-GFP (bottom) transfected HEK293-$Na_V1.5$ cells. Inset: voltage clamp protocol used. **(B)** Average I-V relationships of the $Na_V1.5$ peak current in IRES-GFP and *KCND3*-IRES-GFP transfected cells. Asterisks denote $p < 0.05$. **(C,D)** Average steady-state inactivation **(C)** and activation **(D)** curves. Insets: voltage clamp protocol used. Voltage-dependency of inactivation was measured using a two-pulse protocol where a 500-ms conditioning prepulse to membrane potentials between −160 and 50 mV (to induce steady-state inactivation), was followed by a 50-ms test pulse to −20 mV. Voltage-dependency of activation was measured using the same protocol described as described in **(A)**.

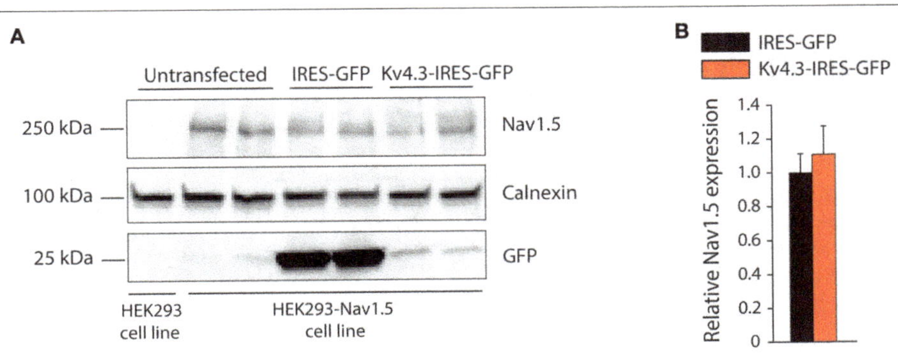

FIGURE 3 | $Na_V1.5$ total expression is not affected by $K_V4.3$ overexpression. **(A)** Representative Western blots of $Na_V1.5$, calnexin and GFP protein expression in HEK293-$Na_V1.5$ cells. Data from IRES-GFP and *KCND3*-IRES-GFP transfected cells as well as untransfected cells. Total lysate of HEK293 cells lacking the $Na_V1.5$ overexpression cassette (leftmost lane) was used as negative control for $Na_V1.5$ antibody specificity. **(B)** Average total $Na_V1.5$ expression normalized to calnexin protein expression in *KCND3*-IRES-GFP transfected HEK293-$Na_V1.5$ cells, compared to IRES-GFP transfected HEK293-$Na_V1.5$ cells ($n = 6$, 3 different blots).

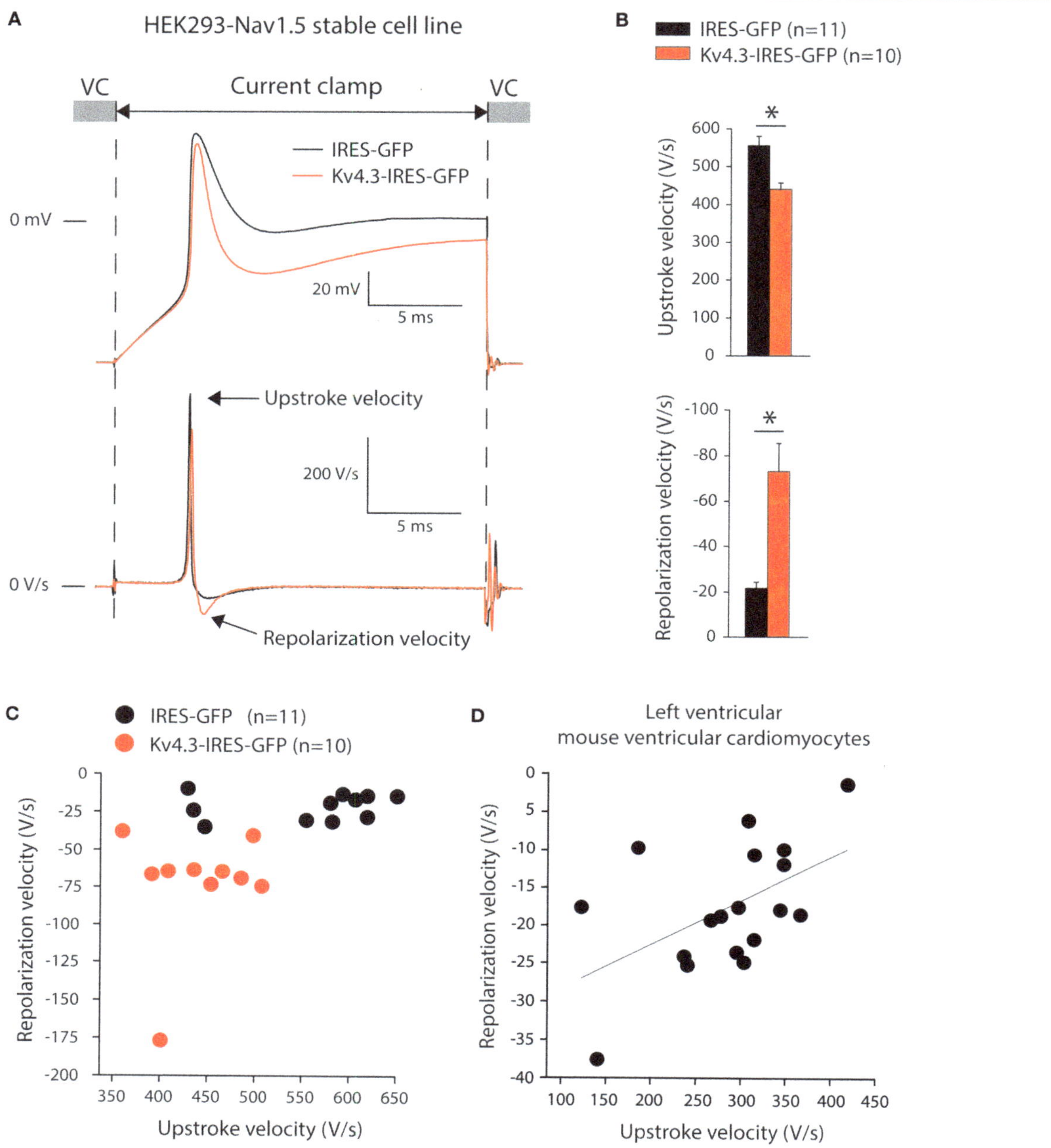

FIGURE 4 | $K_V4.3$ overexpression reduces upstroke velocities. **(A)** Typical examples of upstrokes in *KCND3*-IRES-GFP and IRES-GFP transfected HEK293-$Na_V1.5$ cells measured with the alternating voltage/current clamp (VC/CC) technique (top) and time derivatives of these upstrokes (bottom). Arrows indicate the maximum AP upstroke and repolarization velocities. **(B)** Average AP upstroke (top) and repolarization velocities (bottom). Asterisks denote $p < 0.05$. **(C)** Relationship of upstroke and repolarization velocities in HEK293-$Na_V1.5$ cells. **(D)** Relationship of AP upstroke and repolarization velocities in murine isolated left ventricular myocytes. The solid line represents the linear fit (Pearson's coefficient: $r = 0.53$).

(**Figure 4B**), resulting in an inverse relationship between the maximum velocities of depolarization and repolarization (**Figure 4C**). Next, we determined whether a relationship between repolarization and depolarization also exists in cardiomyocytes. Therefore, we re-analyzed data of alternating VC/CC measurements in murine isolated left ventricular myocytes performed for a previous study (Remme et al., 2006).

In mouse ventricular myocytes, the maximum upstroke and repolarization velocities were 285 ± 19 and −18 ± 2 V/s (n = 18), respectively. In **Figure 4D**, we plotted for each cell its maximum repolarization velocity vs. its maximum upstroke velocity, demonstrating an inverse relationship, similar to our experiments on HEK293 cells (**Figure 4C**).

Computer Simulations

To assess the functional relevance of the aforementioned findings, we first carried out computer simulations to explore whether the presence of a $K_V4.3$-based I_{to} *per se* may affect the maximum upstroke velocity of the HEK293-$Na_V1.5$ cells. To this end, we constructed a model of a HEK293 cell expressing both I_{Na} and I_{to} channels to further explore the findings of the alternating VC/CC experiment of **Figures 4A,B**. The I_{Na} and I_{to} equations were taken from the human ventricular cell model by Ten Tusscher and Panfilov (2006). The characteristics of the simulated I_{Na} and I_{to} are shown in **Figures 5A–D** (and also in Figures S2, S3). As illustrated in **Figures 5E–G**, I_{to} is effectively zero at the moment of maximum upstroke velocity, indicating that this maximum upstroke velocity is fully determined by I_{Na}. Conversely, I_{Na} is almost zero at the moment of maximum repolarization velocity. Accordingly, there is no direct contribution of I_{Na} to the maximum repolarization velocity, although it must be noted that I_{Na} may still affect repolarization velocity through its effect on AP shape. If the voltage-dependency of the I_{to} channels is shifted by −30 mV, thus letting them start to activate near −40 mV, I_{to} is still effectively zero at the moment of maximum upstroke velocity (data not shown).

Next, we established to which extent the $K_V4.3$-based I_{to} and the $Na_V1.5$-based I_{Na} *per se* modulate the maximum upstroke velocity and repolarization velocity of murine left

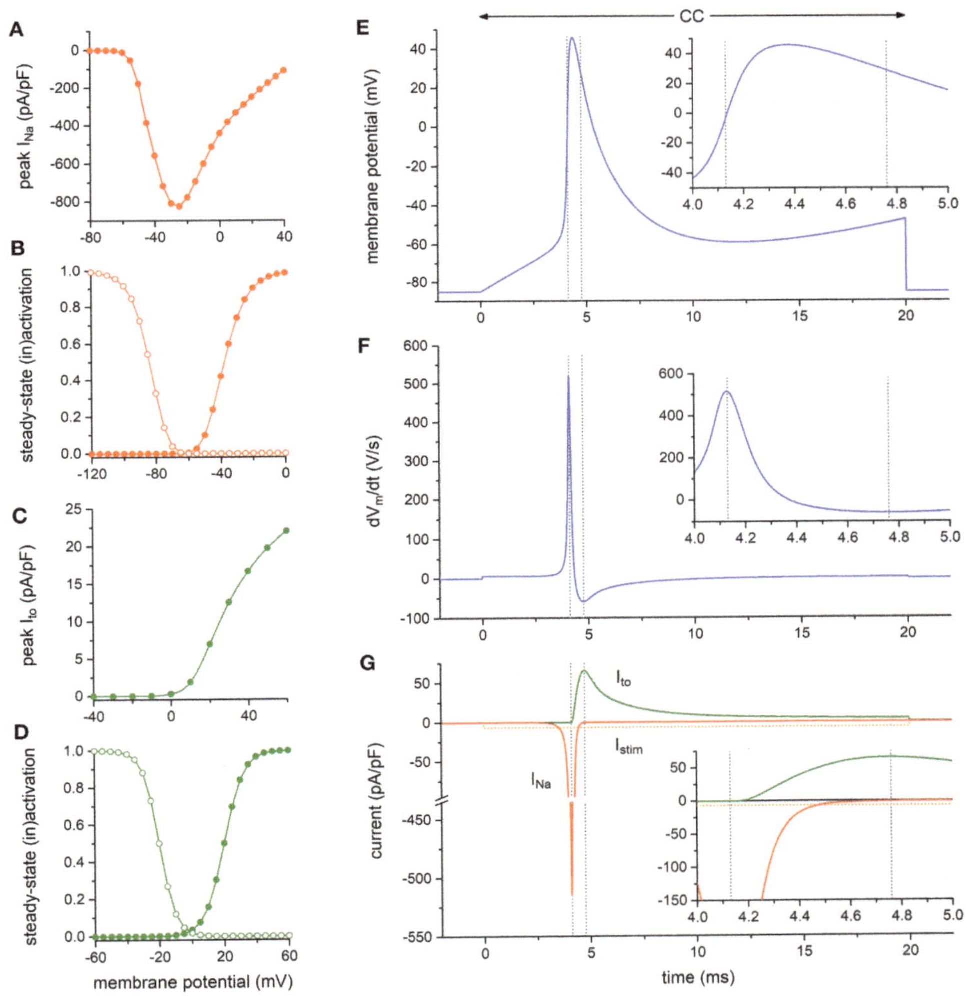

FIGURE 5 | Numerical reconstruction of $Na_V1.5$ and $K_V4.3$ currents in alternating VC/CC experiments. **(A–D)** Characteristics of the simulated $hNa_V1.5$ driven fast sodium current (I_{Na}) and $hK_V4.3$ driven transient outward current (I_{to}). **(A)** I_{Na} peak current as obtained with the voltage clamp protocol of **Figure 2**. **(B)** I_{Na} steady-state activation and inactivation curves (closed and open symbols, respectively) as obtained with the voltage clamp protocol of **Figure 2**. **(C)** I_{to} peak current as obtained with the voltage clamp protocol of **Figure 1**. **(D)** I_{to} steady-state activation and inactivation curves (closed and open symbols, respectively). **(E–G)** Reconstruction of the alternating VC/CC experiment. **(E)** Membrane potential (V_m) during the 20-ms current clamp (CC) phase. Inset: V_m on an expanded time scale. **(F)** Time derivative of the membrane potential trace of **(E)**. Inset: dV_m/dt on an expanded time scale. **(G)** Individual time courses of I_{Na}, I_{to}, and the 20-ms inward stimulus current (I_{stim}). Note the axis break. Inset: I_{Na}, I_{to}, and I_{stim} on an expanded time scale. The vertical dashed lines in **(E–G)** indicate the time of the maximum upstroke velocity (left lines) and the time of the maximum repolarization velocity (right lines). Alternating VC/CC protocol as in the patch-clamp experiments on HEK293-$Na_V1.5$ cells.

ventricular myocytes. To this end, we ran computer simulations of the alternating VC/CC experiment on mouse ventricular myocytes of **Figure 4D** using the apical version of the mouse ventricular AP model by Bondarenko et al. (2004), in which we increased or decreased the density of either I_{to} or I_{Na}. The characteristics of I_{Na} and I_{to} of the Bondarenko et al. (2004) model are shown in **Figures 6A–C** (and also in Figures S2, S3). As shown in **Figure 6D**, and as expected from **Figure 5**, the maximum upstroke velocity is independent of I_{to} conductance (G_{to}), whereas G_{to} is an important determinant of repolarization velocity. The maximum repolarization velocity increases almost linearly with G_{to} (**Figure 6D**, open squares), albeit not in a 1:1 fashion—a four times increase in G_{to} (from 40 to 160% of its control value) results in a 2.3 times increase in maximum repolarization velocity, which can be explained by accompanying changes in AP shape (and thus in channel activation and inactivation) as well as the presence of other membrane currents. As shown in **Figure 6E**, the maximum upstroke velocity is strongly dependent on I_{Na} conductance (G_{Na}), whereas repolarization velocity is only substantially affected by G_{Na} at lower values of G_{Na}. At these lower values, the AP reaches a considerably lower peak (data not shown), which in turn results in less activation of I_{to} channels as well as a lower driving force for these channels. At control or higher values

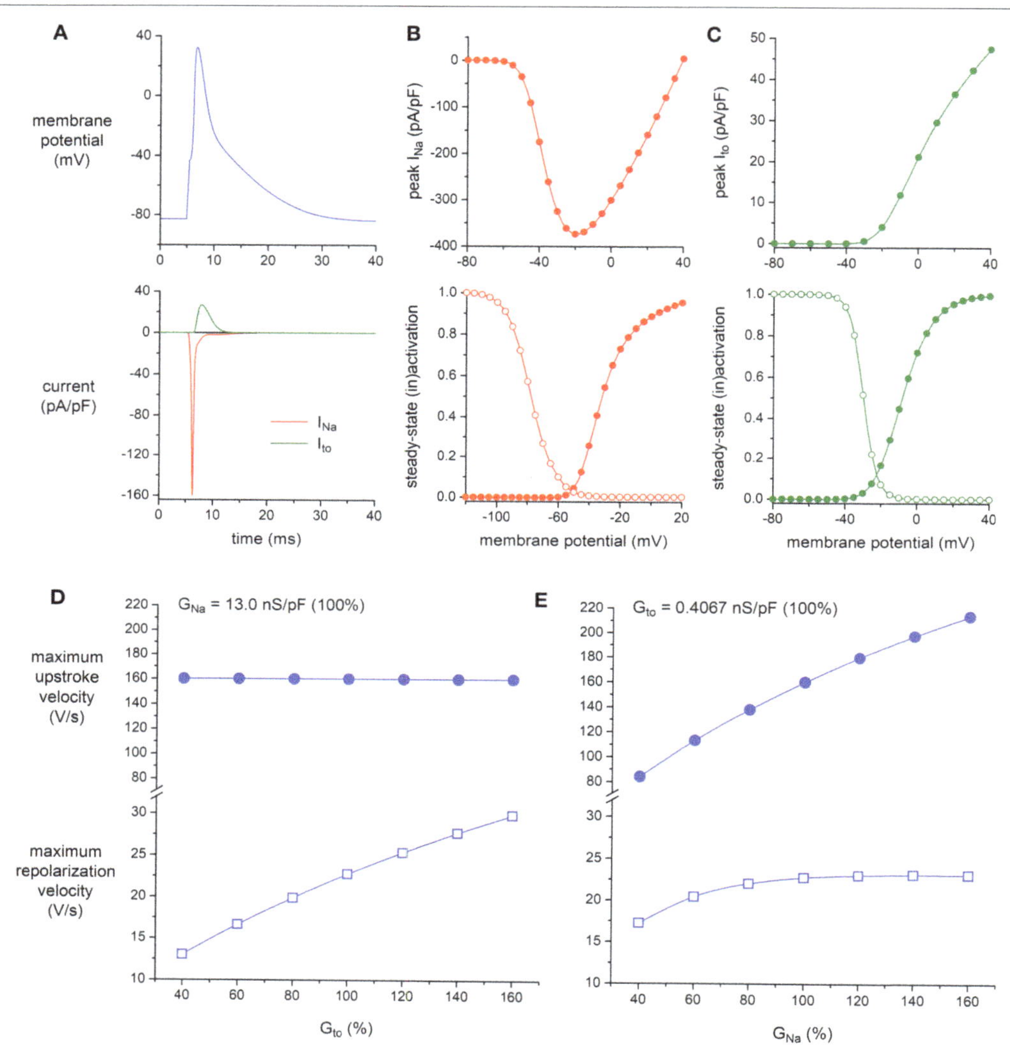

FIGURE 6 | Effect of I_{Na} and I_{to} density on maximum upstroke and repolarization velocity in simulated murine left ventricular myocytes. **(A–C)** Characteristics of the computer model of apical mouse ventricular myocytes (Bondarenko et al., 2004) used in the simulations. **(A)** Action potential (top) and associated I_{Na} and I_{to} (bottom). **(B)** I_{Na} peak current (top) and steady-state activation and inactivation curves (bottom; closed and open symbols, respectively), as obtained with the voltage clamp protocol of **Figure 2**. **(C)** I_{to} peak current (top) and steady-state activation and inactivation curves (bottom; closed and open symbols, respectively), as obtained with the voltage clamp protocol of **Figure 1**. **(D,E)** Maximum upstroke velocity and maximum repolarization velocity as obtained in a reconstruction of the alternating VC/CC experiment. **(D)** Maximum upstroke velocity (filled symbols) and maximum repolarization velocity (open symbols) as a function of I_{to} conductance (G_{to}) at a constant value of I_{Na} conductance (G_{Na}). **(E)** Maximum upstroke velocity and maximum repolarization velocity as a function of G_{Na} at a constant value of G_{to}. Alternating VC/CC protocol as in the patch-clamp experiments on murine left ventricular myocytes.

of G_{Na}, repolarization velocity is not notably dependent on G_{Na}.

Finally, we tested whether a decrease in G_{Na} can result in a loss of conduction in the presence of a concomitant increase in G_{to}. This was studied in a one-dimensional strand of poorly coupled human left ventricular myocytes, as illustrated in **Figure 7A**. Under control conditions (100% G_{Na} and 100% G_{to}), the stimulated leftmost cell of the strand was able to drive its neighboring cells (**Figure 7B**). This was also observed upon a 20% increase in G_{to} or a 50% decrease in G_{Na} (**Figures 7C,D**, respectively). The main effect of the decrease in G_{Na} was a slowing of conduction (cf. **Table 1**). However, the introduction of a concomitant 20% increase in G_{to} led to loss of conduction: an action potential was elicited in the first cell of the strand, but this cell was unable to transfer this action potential to its neighboring cells (**Figure 7E**). Thus, a simultaneous increase in I_{to} and decrease in I_{Na} in the setting of a compromised cellular coupling, as may occur on a microscopic scale in BrS patients, may result in severe conduction alteration.

DISCUSSION

In the present study, we report for the first time a direct effect of $K_V4.3$ expression on $Na_V1.5$ current and consequent sodium channel availability. We found that overexpression of $K_V4.3$ protein reduces $Na_V1.5$ current density (**Figure 2**) without affecting total $Na_V1.5$ protein expression. Moreover, $K_V4.3$ overexpression decreased the upstroke velocity, which was not due to a direct effect of the current generated by $K_V4.3$. These findings suggest that the observed effects of $K_V4.3$ on $Na_V1.5$ are due to a functional interaction between the two channel proteins rather than an electrophysiological interference. The physiological relevance of our findings was demonstrated in a multicellular *in silico* model where we found that an I_{to} increase and concomitant I_{Na} decrease is capable of impairing conduction (**Figure 7**).

Decreased AP Upstroke Velocity Secondary to $K_V4.3$ Overexpression

Using the alternating VC/CC technique, we observed in HEK293 cells stably expressing $Na_V1.5$ a decrease in upstroke velocity secondary to overexpression of $K_V4.3$. Upstroke velocity decreased to a similar extent as $Na_V1.5$ sodium current density (≈25%) in cells overexpressing $K_V4.3$ compared to cells overexpressing only GFP. Although the alternating VC/CC technique is not commonly used in cardiac electrophysiology, it allows detailed I_{Na} studies in a dynamic fashion under close-to-physiological conditions as occurring during cardiac action potentials (Berecki et al., 2010). Previously it has been used to demonstrate changes in I_{Na} during heart failure (Berecki et al., 2010), changes in intracellular Ca^{2+} concentration (Casini et al., 2009), and in the setting of *SCN5A* mutations (Remme et al., 2006; Lieve et al., 2017). Using dynamic clamp, we have recently assessed the effect of an I_{to}-like current on the upstroke velocity in HEK293 cells transiently overexpressing $Na_V1.5$ channels. That study revealed only a minor influence of I_{to}, if any, on

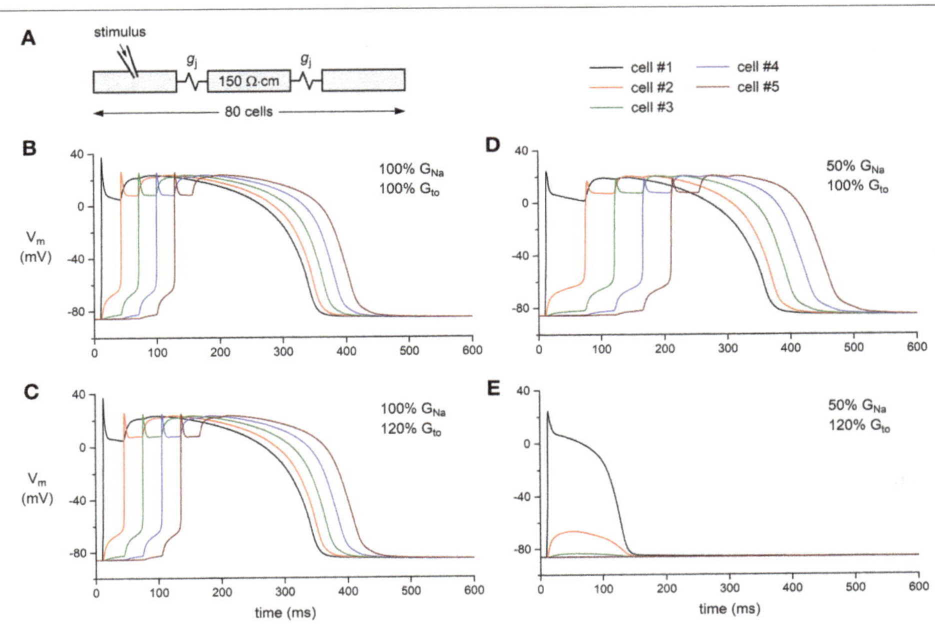

FIGURE 7 | Effect of I_{Na} and I_{to} density on action potential propagation in a simulated strand of human left ventricular myocytes. **(A)** Geometry of the strand. The intercellular coupling conductance (g_j) was set to 6 nS and the myoplasmic resistivity was set to 150 Ω·cm. **(B–E)** Action potential propagation in the strand as a function of I_{Na} conductance (G_{Na}) and I_{to} conductance (G_{to}). **(B)** Control conditions: G_{Na} and G_{to} both set to 100% of their control value. **(C)** Slight slowing of action potential propagation upon an increase in G_{to} to 120% of its control value. **(D)** Slowing of action potential propagation upon a decrease in G_{Na} to 50% of its control value. **(E)** Failure of action potential propagation upon a concomitant decrease in G_{Na} and increase in G_{to}.

TABLE 1 | Action potential parameters and propagation in a strand of human left ventricular myocytes.

Settings	APA (mV)	$(dV_m/dt)_{max}$ (V/s)	APD_{90} (ms)	CV (cm/s)
100% G_{Na}, 100% G_{to}	111.3	223.5	275.6	0.260
100% G_{Na}, 120% G_{to}	110.5	217.1	272.1	0.245
50% G_{Na}, 100% G_{to}	104.6	79.0	248.1	0.163

Data obtained from computer simulations with an intercellular coupling conductance of 6 nS. APA, action potential amplitude; $(dV_m/dt)_{max}$, maximum upstroke velocity; APD_{90}, action potential duration at 90% repolarization; CV, conduction velocity in the strand. Action potential parameters for cells in the middle of the strand.

upstroke velocity (Verkerk et al., 2016). Here, we confirmed these results using computer simulations based on the current densities recorded (**Figure 5**). The I_{to} current is not yet present at the time of the maximum upstroke velocity confirming that I_{to} does not affect the upstroke velocity in single cells. Moreover, no correlation between I_{to} density and AP upstroke velocity was observed during simulations of the electrical activity of cardiomyocytes (**Figure 6**). Thus, the observed $K_V4.3$-induced decrease in upstroke velocity is not a consequence of an increased $K_V4.3$ current.

In freshly isolated left ventricular myocytes of mice, we found an inverse relationship between the maximum upstroke velocity and repolarization velocity (**Figure 4D**). It is tempting to speculate that such a relationship is due to effects of $K_V4.3$ expression, but this observation might also be due to different currents or transcription gradient of both *Kcnd3* and *Scn5a* through the myocardial wall. Nevertheless, it indicates that depolarization and repolarization are not independent factors. Future overexpression or knock-down experiments in myocytes are needed to provide further insight into the potential relevance of our observation.

Modulation of $Na_V1.5$ Current by $K_V4.3$ Expression

We found that $K_V4.3$ overexpression resulted in a significantly decreased $Na_V1.5$ current density, while neither current kinetics nor total $Na_V1.5$ protein expression were affected. Several studies have previously reported interactions and consequent inter-relationships between sodium and potassium channels, or their associated subunits, leading to electrophysiological modifications of either current (Hu et al., 2012; Milstein et al., 2012; Matamoros et al., 2016; Utrilla et al., 2017). For instance, Kir2.1 and $Na_V1.5$ channels when co-expressed exert a synergic effect on current density due to a distinct trafficking process as compared to when these channels are expressed separately (Utrilla et al., 2017). Concerning the direct interaction of $K_V4.3$ and $Na_V1.5$, a mutation in the *SCN1B* gene encoding the cardiac sodium channel β1 subunit has been found in BrS and sudden infant death syndrome patients (Hu et al., 2012). This specific *SCN1B* mutation led to a decreased I_{Na} together with an increased I_{to}, suggesting that $Na_v1.5$ may physically interact with $K_V4.3$ via β1 to form a macromolecular complex. In neurons, both sodium and potassium channels mainly localize at the axon initial segment (AIS), a subcellular region involved in AP genesis. Ion channel recruitment to the AIS is highly dependent on the cytoskeleton and associated proteins which densely populate this region (Brachet et al., 2010; Leterrier et al., 2011; Vacher et al., 2011). A comparable structure is observed at the intercalated discs in adult cardiomyocytes, a subcellular region also characterized by a high density of sodium channels (Agullo-Pascual et al., 2014; Marsman et al., 2014; El Refaey et al., 2017). Our findings, together with existing knowledge, may suggest a potential subcellular co-localization of $K_V4.3$ and $Na_V1.5$ in cardiomyocytes and a possible explanation for the co-regulation of channel function. Further studies should aim at unraveling the molecular mechanism involved in our observation. A recent work also highlighted the synergic impact of $K_V4.3$ expression on hERG channels in HEK293 cells (Zhao et al., 2017). This study together with our findings strongly suggest that the overexpression or knock-down of $K_V4.3$ in cardiomyocytes may lead to a complex modulation of ion channels initially seen as unrelated including $Na_V1.5$, hERG, and Kir2.1 channels.

Potential (Patho)Physiological Implications

Our computer simulations show that a concomitant increase in I_{to} and decrease in I_{Na} are capable of significantly affecting cardiac conduction. Our current observations may thus be particularly relevant in the phenotypical explanation of BrS patients presenting with mutations in the *KCND3* gene or in genes encoding $K_V4.3$ associated subunits leading to gain-of-function through an increased protein stability or membrane trafficking of $K_V4.3$ channels. In this context, an increased I_{to} current could be associated with a simultaneous decrease in I_{Na} and consequent conduction slowing (Kucera et al., 2017). Such an effect is likely even more prominent within the subepicardium, a region with relatively low I_{Na} and high I_{to}. This may be of particular relevance in the right ventricular subepicardium and right ventricular outflow tract, where fractionated signals indicative of slowed conduction are often observed in BrS patients (Nademanee et al., 2011). Importantly, concomitant cardiac structural abnormalities, for example age-dependent development of fibrosis (Coronel et al., 2005), may further compromise conduction and hence unmask the impact of increased I_{to} (Hoogendijk et al., 2010a). Moreover, one may speculate that the known gender differences in I_{to} magnitude may also contribute to the male preponderance for BrS via an indirect effect on I_{Na} (Di Diego et al., 2002).

Limitations

While we clearly demonstrated that $K_V4.3$ is capable of decreasing $Na_V1.5$ current density, extrapolation to physiological cardiomyocyte conditions must be done with some caution. The upstroke velocities measured in our experiments are in the same range of values as recorded in cardiomyocytes (Berecki et al., 2010; Veerman et al., 2017). However, *KCND3* overexpression resulted in $K_V4.3$ currents larger than the I_{to} previously reported in various animal species and human ventricular cardiomyocytes (Niwa and Nerbonne, 2010).

Consequently, the $K_V4.3$-induced ≈25% reduction of $Na_V1.5$ current density and upstroke velocity reported in this study is likely smaller in animal species and human. Moreover, our experiments in HEK293 cells were performed without β subunits of either $Na_V1.5$ or $K_V4.3$. We therefore cannot exclude a supplementary complexity of $Na_V1.5$ macromolecular complexes in cardiomyocytes. Nevertheless, our myocyte data at least demonstrate that depolarization is not independent of repolarization.

CONCLUSION

Overall, this study gives the first proof of concept that the $K_V4.3$ protein directly impacts on $Na_V1.5$ current. Future studies employing appropriate disease models should explore the potential electrophysiological implications in (patho)physiological conditions, including BrS associated with gain-of-function mutations in *KCND3*.

AUTHOR CONTRIBUTIONS

Experimental design: VP, RW, FC, AV, and CR; Data acquisition: VP, RW, and AV; Analysis and interpretation of data: VP, RW, SC, AV, and CR; Drafting manuscript: VP, RW, AV, and CR; Editing manuscript, and approval: VP, RW, SC, FC, AV, and CR; Funding: CR.

ACKNOWLEDGMENTS

We thank Drs. Hugues Abriel and Jean-Sebastien Rougier (Institute of Biochemistry and Molecular Medicine, Bern, Switzerland) for kindly providing the HEK293-$Na_V1.5$ cell line, Dr. Ruben Coronel (Academic Medical Center, Amsterdam, The Netherlands) for inspiring discussions, and Jan G. Zegers and Dr. Antoni C.G van Ginneken (Academic Medical Center, Amsterdam, The Netherlands) for developing and providing technical assistance with the soft- and hardware.

REFERENCES

Agullo-Pascual, E., Lin, X., Leo-Macias, A., Zhang, M., Liang, F.-X., Li, Z., et al. (2014). Super-resolution imaging reveals that loss of the C-terminus of connexin43 limits microtubule plus-end capture and $Na_V1.5$ localization at the intercalated disc. *Cardiovasc. Res.* 104, 371–381. doi: 10.1093/cvr/cvu195

Balse, E., and Boycott, H. E. (2017). Ion channel trafficking: control of ion channel density as a target for arrhythmias? *Front. Physiol.* 8:808. doi: 10.3389/fphys.2017.00808

Barry, P. H., and Lynch, J. W. (1991). Liquid junction potentials and small cell effects in patch-clamp analysis. *J. Membr. Biol.* 121, 101–117. doi: 10.1007/BF01870526

Benson, D. W., Wang, D. W., Dyment, M., Knilans, T. K., Fish, F. A., Strieper, M. J., et al. (2003). Congenital sick sinus syndrome caused by recessive mutations in the cardiac sodium channel gene (*SCN5A*). *J. Clin. Invest.* 112, 1019–1028. doi: 10.1172/JCI18062

Berecki, G., Wilders, R., de Jonge, B., van Ginneken, A. C. G., and Verkerk, A. O. (2010). Re-evaluation of the action potential upstroke velocity as a measure of the Na^+ current in cardiac myocytes at physiological conditions. *PLoS ONE* 5:e15772. doi: 10.1371/journal.pone.0015772

Bondarenko, V. E., Szigeti, G. P., Bett, G. C. L., Kim, S.-J., and Rasmusson, R. L. (2004). Computer model of action potential of mouse ventricular myocytes. *Am. J. Physiol. Heart Circ. Physiol.* 287, H1378–H1403. doi: 10.1152/ajpheart.00185.2003

Brachet, A., Leterrier, C., Irondelle, M., Fache, M.-P., Racine, V., Sibarita, J.-B., et al. (2010). Ankyrin G restricts ion channel diffusion at the axonal initial segment before the establishment of the diffusion barrier. *J. Cell. Biol.* 191, 383–395. doi: 10.1083/jcb.201003042

Casini, S., Verkerk, A. O., van Borren, M. M. G. J., van Ginneken, A. C. G., Veldkamp, M. W., de Bakker, J. M. T., et al. (2009). Intracellular calcium modulation of voltage-gated sodium channels in ventricular myocytes. *Cardiovasc. Res.* 81, 72–81. doi: 10.1093/cvr/cvn274

Chen, Q., Kirsch, G. E., Zhang, D., Brugada, R., Brugada, J., Brugada, P., et al. (1998). Genetic basis and molecular mechanism for idiopathic ventricular fibrillation. *Nature* 392, 293–296. doi: 10.1038/32675

Coronel, R., Casini, S., Koopmann, T. T., Wilms-Schopman, F. J. G., Verkerk, A. O., de Groot, J. R., et al. (2005). Right ventricular fibrosis and conduction delay in a patient with clinical signs of Brugada syndrome: a combined electrophysiological, genetic, histopathologic, and computational study. *Circulation* 112, 2769–2777. doi: 10.1161/CIRCULATIONAHA.105.532614

Crotti, L., Marcou, C. A., Tester, D. J., Castelletti, S., Giudicessi, J. R., Torchio, M., et al. (2012). Spectrum and prevalence of mutations involving BrS1- through BrS12-susceptibility genes in a cohort of unrelated patients referred for Brugada syndrome genetic testing: implications for genetic testing. *J. Am. Coll. Cardiol.* 60, 1410–1418. doi: 10.1016/j.jacc.2012.04.037

Cuellar, A. A., Lloyd, C. M., Nielsen, P. F., Bullivant, D. P., Nickerson, D. P., and Hunter, P. J. (2003). An overview of CellML 1.1, a biological model description language. *Simulation* 79, 740–747. doi: 10.1177/0037549703040939

Delpón, E., Cordeiro, J. M., Núñez, L., Thomsen, P. E. B., Guerchicoff, A., Pollevick, G. D., et al. (2008). Functional effects of *KCNE3* mutation and its role in the development of Brugada syndrome. *Circ. Arrhythm. Electrophysiol.* 1, 209–218. doi: 10.1161/CIRCEP.107.748103

Di Diego, J. M., Cordeiro, J. M., Goodrow, R. J., Fish, J. M., Zygmunt, A. C., Pérez, G. J., et al. (2002). Ionic and cellular basis for the predominance of the Brugada syndrome phenotype in males. *Circulation* 106, 2004–2011. doi: 10.1161/01.CIR.0000032002.22105.7A

El Refaey, M. M., and Mohler, P. J. (2017). Ankyrins and spectrins in cardiovascular biology and disease. *Front. Physiol.* 8:852. doi: 10.3389/fphys.2017.00852

Garny, A., Kohl, P., and Noble, D. (2003). Cellular open resource (COR): a public CellML based environment for modelling biological function. *Int. J. Bifurcat. Chaos* 13, 3579–3590. doi: 10.1142/S021812740300882X

Gellens, M. E., George, A. L., Chen, L. Q., Chahine, M., Horn, R., Barchi, R. L., et al. (1992). Primary structure and functional expression of the human cardiac tetrodotoxin-insensitive voltage-dependent sodium channel. *Proc. Natl. Acad. Sci. U.S.A.* 89, 554–558. doi: 10.1073/pnas.89.2.554

Giles, W. R., and van Ginneken, A. C. G. (1985). A transient outward current in isolated cells from the crista terminalis of rabbit heart. *J. Physiol.* 368, 243–264. doi: 10.1113/jphysiol.1985.sp015856

Hoogendijk, M. G., Opthof, T., Postema, P. G., Wilde, A. A. M., de Bakker, J. M. T., and Coronel, R. (2010a). The Brugada ECG pattern: a marker of channelopathy, structural heart disease, or neither? Toward a unifying mechanism of the Brugada syndrome. *Circ. Arrhythm. Electrophysiol.* 3, 283–290. doi: 10.1161/CIRCEP.110.937029

Hoogendijk, M. G., Potse, M., Linnenbank, A. C., Verkerk, A. O., den Ruijter, H. M., van Amersfoorth, S. C. M., et al. (2010b). Mechanism of right precordial ST-segment elevation in structural heart disease: excitation failure by current-to-load mismatch. *Heart Rhythm* 7, 238–248. doi: 10.1016/j.hrthm.2009.10.007

Hu, D., Barajas-Martínez, H., Medeiros-Domingo, A., Crotti, L., Veltmann, C., Schimpf, R., et al. (2012). A novel rare variant in *SCN1Bb* linked to Brugada syndrome and SIDS by combined modulation of $Na_V1.5$ and $K_V4.3$ channel currents. *Heart Rhythm* 9, 760–769. doi: 10.1016/j.hrthm.2011.12.006

Kucera, J. P., Rohr, S., and Kleber, A. G. (2017). Microstructure, cell-to-cell coupling, and ion currents as determinants of electrical propagation and arrhythmogenesis. *Circ. Arrhythm. Electrophysiol.* 10:e004665. doi: 10.1161/CIRCEP.117.004665

Le Scouarnec, S., Karakachoff, M., Gourraud, J.-B., Lindenbaum, P., Bonnaud, S., Portero, V., et al. (2015). Testing the burden of rare variation in arrhythmia-susceptibility genes provides new insights into molecular diagnosis for Brugada syndrome. *Hum. Mol. Genet.* 24, 2757–2763. doi: 10.1093/hmg/ddv036

Leterrier, C., Vacher, H., Fache, M.-P., d'Ortoli, S. A., Castets, F., Autillo-Touati, A., et al. (2011). End-binding proteins EB3 and EB1 link microtubules to ankyrin G in the axon initial segment. *Proc. Natl. Acad. Sci. U.S.A.* 108, 8826–8831. doi: 10.1073/pnas.1018671108

Lieve, K. V., Verkerk, A. O., Podliesna, S., van der Werf, C., Tanck, M. W., Hofman, N., et al. (2017). Gain-of-function mutation in *SCN5A* causes ventricular arrhythmias and early onset atrial fibrillation. *Int. J. Cardiol.* 236, 187–193. doi: 10.1016/j.ijcard.2017.01.113

Liu, J., Kim, K.-H., Morales, M. J., Heximer, S. P., Hui, C.-C., and Backx, P. H. (2015). Kv4.3-encoded fast transient outward current is presented in Kv4.2 knockout mouse cardiomyocytes. *PLoS ONE* 10:e0133274. doi: 10.1371/journal.pone.0133274

Marsman, R. F. J., Bezzina, C. R., Freiberg, F., Verkerk, A. O., Adriaens, M. E., Podliesna, S., et al. (2014). Coxsackie and adenovirus receptor is a modifier of cardiac conduction and arrhythmia vulnerability in the setting of myocardial ischemia. *J. Am. Coll. Cardiol.* 63, 549–559. doi: 10.1016/j.jacc.2013.10.062

Matamoros, M., Pérez-Hernández, M., Guerrero-Serna, G., Amorós, I., Barana, A., Núñez, M., et al. (2016). Nav1.5 N-terminal domain binding to α1-syntrophin increases membrane density of human Kir2.1, Kir2.2 and Nav1.5 channels. *Cardiovasc. Res.* 110, 279–290. doi: 10.1093/cvr/cvw009

Milstein, M. L., Musa, H., Balbuena, D. P., Anumonwo, J. M. B., Auerbach, D. S., Furspan, P. B., et al. (2012). Dynamic reciprocity of sodium and potassium channel expression in a macromolecular complex controls cardiac excitability and arrhythmia. *Proc. Natl. Acad. Sci. U.S.A.* 109, E2134–E2143. doi: 10.1073/pnas.1109370109

Nademanee, K., Veerakul, G., Chandanamattha, P., Chaothawee, L., Ariyachaipanich, A., Jirasirirojanakorn, K., et al. (2011). Prevention of ventricular fibrillation episodes in Brugada syndrome by catheter ablation over the anterior right ventricular outflow tract epicardium. *Circulation* 123, 1270–1279. doi: 10.1161/CIRCULATIONAHA.110.972612

Niwa, N., and Nerbonne, J. M. (2010). Molecular determinants of cardiac transient outward potassium current (I_{to}) expression and regulation. *J. Mol. Cell. Cardiol.* 48, 12–25. doi: 10.1016/j.yjmcc.2009.07.013

Niwa, N., Wang, W., Sha, Q., Marionneau, C., and Nerbonne, J. M. (2008). Kv4.3 is not required for the generation of functional $I_{to,f}$ channels in adult mouse ventricles. *J. Mol. Cell. Cardiol.* 44, 95–104. doi: 10.1016/j.yjmcc.2007.10.007

Portero, V., Le Scouarnec, S., Es-Salah-Lamoureux, Z., Burel, S., Gourraud, J.-B., Bonnaud, S., et al. (2016). Dysfunction of the voltage-gated K^+ channel β2 subunit in a familial case of Brugada syndrome. *J. Am. Heart. Assoc.* 5:e003122. doi: 10.1161/JAHA.115.003122

Remme, C. A., Verkerk, A. O., Nuyens, D., van Ginneken, A. C. G., van Brunschot, S., Belterman, C. N. W., et al. (2006). Overlap syndrome of cardiac sodium channel disease in mice carrying the equivalent mutation of human SCN5A-1795insD. *Circulation* 114, 2584–2594. doi: 10.1161/CIRCULATIONAHA.106.653949

Rush, S., and Larsen, H. (1978). A practical algorithm for solving dynamic membrane equations. *IEEE Trans. Biomed. Eng.* 25, 389–392. doi: 10.1109/TBME.1978.326270

Schott, J. J., Alshinawi, C., Kyndt, F., Probst, V., Hoorntje, T. M., Hulsbeek, M., et al. (1999). Cardiac conduction defects associate with mutations in SCN5A. *Nat. Genet.* 23, 20–21. doi: 10.1038/12618

Shaw, R. M., and Rudy, Y. (1997). Ionic mechanisms of propagation in cardiac tissue: roles of the sodium and L-type calcium currents during reduced excitability and decreased gap junction coupling. *Circ. Res.* 81, 727–741. doi: 10.1161/01.RES.81.5.727

Ten Tusscher, K. H. W. J., and Panfilov, A. V. (2006). Cell model for efficient simulation of wave propagation in human ventricular tissue under normal and pathological conditions. *Phys. Med. Biol.* 51, 6141–6156. doi: 10.1088/0031-9155/51/23/014

Thomas, S. P., Kucera, J. P., Bircher-Lehmann, L., Rudy, Y., Saffitz, J. E., and Kléber, A. G. (2003). Impulse propagation in synthetic strands of neonatal cardiac myocytes with genetically reduced levels of connexin43. *Circ. Res.* 92, 1209–1216. doi: 10.1161/01.RES.0000074916.41221.EA

Utrilla, R. G., Nieto-Marín, P., Alfayate, S., Tinaquero, D., Matamoros, M., Pérez-Hernández, M., et al. (2017). Kir2.1-Nav1.5 channel complexes are differently regulated than Kir2.1 and Nav1.5 channels alone. *Front. Physiol.* 8:903. doi: 10.3389/fphys.2017.00903

Vacher, H., Yang, J.-W., Cerda, O., Autillo-Touati, A., Dargent, B., and Trimmer, J. S. (2011). Cdk-mediated phosphorylation of the Kvβ2 auxiliary subunit regulates Kv1 channel axonal targeting. *J. Cell. Biol.* 192, 813–824. doi: 10.1083/jcb.201007113

van Bemmelen, M. X., van, Rougier, J.-S., Gavillet, B., Apothéloz, F., Daidié, D., Tateyama, M., et al. (2004). Cardiac voltage-gated sodium channel Na_V1.5 is regulated by Nedd4-2 mediated ubiquitination. *Circ. Res.* 95, 284–291. doi: 10.1161/01.RES.0000136816.05109.89

Veerman, C. C., Podliesna, S., Tadros, R., Lodder, E. M., Mengarelli, I., de Jonge, B., et al. (2017). The Brugada syndrome susceptibility gene *HEY2* modulates cardiac transmural ion channel patterning and electrical heterogeneity. *Circ. Res.* 121, 537–548. doi: 10.1161/CIRCRESAHA.117.310959

Verkerk, A. O., Veerman, C. C., Zegers, J. G., and Wilders, R. (2016). Effects of the transient outward potassium current on action potential upstroke velocities tested using the dynamic clamp technique. *Comput. Cardiol.* 43, 257–260. doi: 10.22489/CinC.2016.076-143

Wilde, A. A. M., Postema, P. G., Di Diego, J. M., Viskin, S., Morita, H., Fish, J. M., et al. (2010). The pathophysiological mechanism underlying Brugada syndrome: depolarization versus repolarization. *J. Mol. Cell. Cardiol.* 49, 543–553. doi: 10.1016/j.yjmcc.2010.07.012

Wilders, R. (2012). Arrhythmogenic right ventricular cardiomyopathy: considerations from *in silico* experiments. *Front. Physiol.* 3:168. doi: 10.3389/fphys.2012.00168

You, T., Mao, W., Cai, B., Li, F., and Xu, H. (2015). Two novel Brugada syndrome-associated mutations increase K_V4.3 membrane expression and function. *Int. J. Mol. Med.* 36, 309–315. doi: 10.3892/ijmm.2015.2223

Zhao, X.-J., Zhu, C., Tian, L.-Y., Fu, Y.-C., Zhang, Y., Chen, X., et al. (2017). Kv4.3 modulates the distribution of hERG. *Sci. Rep.* 7:17757. doi: 10.1038/s41598-017-17837-6

18

Voltage-Gated Sodium Channel β1/β1B Subunits Regulate Cardiac Physiology and Pathophysiology

*Nnamdi Edokobi and Lori L. Isom**

Department of Pharmacology, University of Michigan Medical School, Ann Arbor, MI, United States

***Correspondence:**
Lori L. Isom
lisom@umich.edu

Cardiac myocyte contraction is initiated by a set of intricately orchestrated electrical impulses, collectively known as action potentials (APs). Voltage-gated sodium channels (Na_Vs) are responsible for the upstroke and propagation of APs in excitable cells, including cardiomyocytes. Na_Vs consist of a single, pore-forming α subunit and two different β subunits. The β subunits are multifunctional cell adhesion molecules and channel modulators that have cell type and subcellular domain specific functional effects. Variants in *SCN1B*, the gene encoding the Na_V-β1 and -β1B subunits, are linked to atrial and ventricular arrhythmias, e.g., Brugada syndrome, as well as to the early infantile epileptic encephalopathy Dravet syndrome, all of which put patients at risk for sudden death. Evidence over the past two decades has demonstrated that Na_V-β1/β1B subunits play critical roles in cardiac myocyte physiology, in which they regulate tetrodotoxin-resistant and -sensitive sodium currents, potassium currents, and calcium handling, and that Na_V-β1/β1B subunit dysfunction generates substrates for arrhythmias. This review will highlight the role of Na_V-β1/β1B subunits in cardiac physiology and pathophysiology.

Keywords: sodium channel, B subunit, arrhythmia, epilepsy, cell adhesion, electrophysiology

INTRODUCTION

The heart contracts to pump blood throughout the body. It consists of specialized cells called cardiac myocytes (CMs), and contraction of CMs is initiated by electrical impulses called action potentials (APs) (Nerbonne and Kass, 2005). Cardiac APs are generated and propagated through the coordinated signaling of ion channels. Upon membrane depolarization, voltage-gated sodium channels (Na_Vs) activate and inactivate rapidly to allow sodium influx (Hille and Catterall, 2012). This is responsible for the rising phase and propagation of the AP in mammalian CMs (Nerbonne and Kass, 2005). Na_Vs are heterotrimeric transmembrane proteins consisting of one pore-forming α and two β subunits (Catterall, 2000). Na_V-β subunits are expressed in mammalian heart (Isom et al., 1992; Makita et al., 1994) and their functional loss can result in electrical abnormalities that predispose patients to arrhythmias. Variants in the gene *SCN1B,* encoding the splice variants Na_V-β1 and Na_V-β1B, are implicated in a variety of inherited pathologies including epileptic encephalopathy (O'Malley and Isom, 2015), Brugada syndrome (BrS) (Watanabe et al., 2008; Hu et al., 2012), long-QT syndrome (LQTS) (Riuró et al., 2014), atrial arrhythmias (Watanabe et al., 2009), and sudden infant death syndrome (SIDS) (Hu et al., 2012) (**Figure 1**, **Table 1**). Remarkably, regardless of disease etiology, patients with *SCN1B* mutations have an increased risk of sudden death. Classically, the Na_V-β subunits were characterized as modulators of the Na_V ion-conducting pore. However, from research over the past two decades, we know that Na_V-β subunits are dynamic,

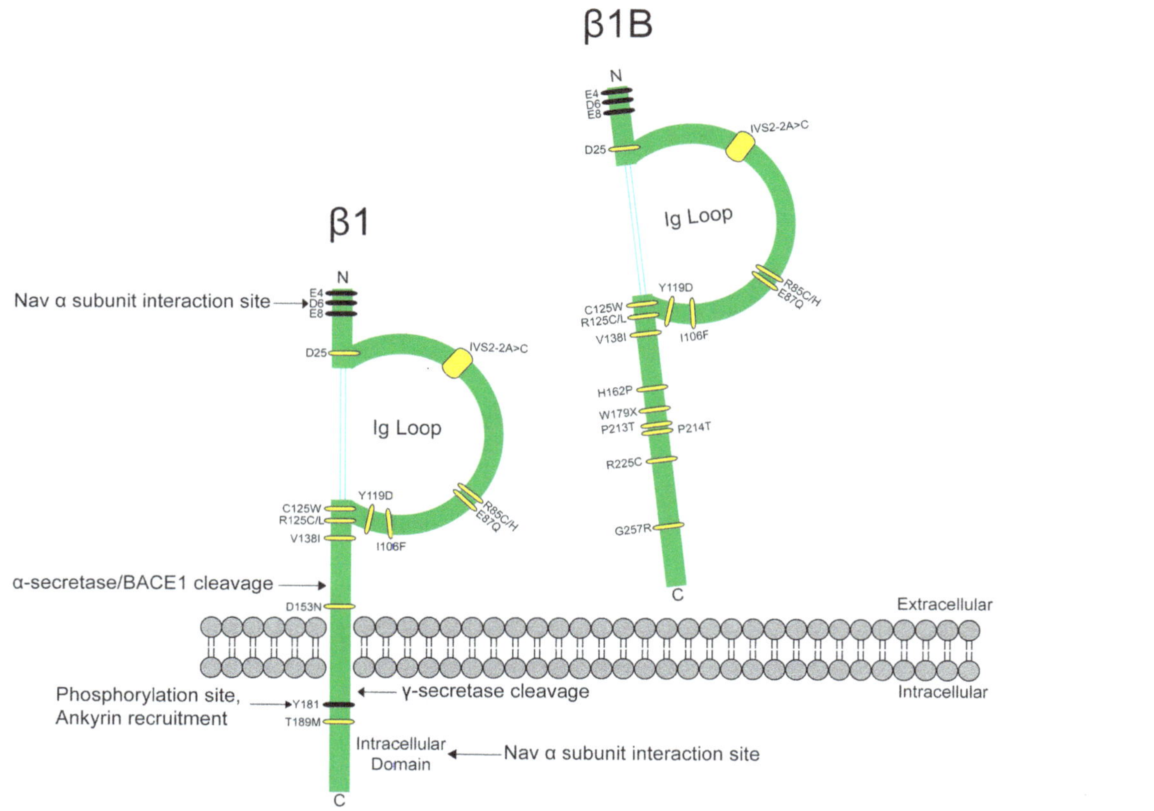

FIGURE 1 | *SCN1B* variants are linked to epilepsy syndromes and cardiac conduction diseases. *SCN1B* encodes Na_V-β1 (**left**) and its secreted splice variant Na_V-β1B (**right**). Sites for β1-α interaction, ankyrin binding, phosphorylation, and proteolytic cleavage are indicated. Ig: immunoglobulin. Human disease variants in β1 or β1B are indicated in yellow and are described in **Table 1**. Adapted from O'Malley and Isom (2015).

multifunctional proteins that play important roles in cardiac physiology (O'Malley and Isom, 2015). Here, we will focus our review on the current understanding of Na_V-β1/β1B function in CMs and discuss disease implications.

NA$_V$S ARE DIFFERENTIALLY EXPRESSED IN CARDIAC MYOCYTES

To understand Na_V-β subunit physiology in heart, one must first consider the associated Na_V-α subunits. Na_V1.5 is the predominantly expressed Na_V-α in CMs and the primary contributor to recorded sodium current (I_{Na}) density (Rogart et al., 1989; Gellens et al., 1992; Catterall, 2000; Maier et al., 2002). Na_V1.5 is a "tetrodotoxin resistant (TTX-R)" channel (Catterall et al., 2005), in contrast to "TTX-sensitive (TTX-S)" channels, e.g., Na_Vs normally found in brain, for which TTX has nanomolar affinity (Catterall et al., 2005). TTX has micromolar affinity for Na_V1.5 due to the presence of a cysteine residue in the selectivity filter in a position that is otherwise filled by an aromatic amino acid in TTX-S channels (Satin et al., 1992). TTX-S channels, Na_V1.1, Na_V1.3, and Na_V1.6, are expressed in heart as well as in brain (Malhotra et al., 2001; Lopez-Santiago et al., 2007). They are preferentially localized in the transverse tubules (T-tubules) (Malhotra et al., 2001, 2002; Lopez-Santiago et al., 2007) where they are postulated to function in excitation-contraction coupling (Maier et al., 2002) (**Figure 2**).

CMs associate at the intercalated disk (ID), where adherens junctions, gap junctions, and desmosomes participate in intercellular communication (Vermij et al., 2017) (**Figure 3A**). Na_V1.5 channels cluster at cell–cell junction sites at the ID, where they co-localize with the cardiac gap junction (GJ) protein, connexin-43 (Cx43) (Maier et al., 2002, 2004) (**Figure 3B**). Na_V1.5 clustering may contribute to rapid AP conduction from cell-to-cell, similar to the node-to-node saltatory conducting function of TTX-S Na_Vs in myelinated nerves (Freeman et al., 2016). Na_V1.5 channels are also expressed at the CM lateral membrane (**Figure 2**), where they have differing biophysical properties and binding partners from those at the ID (Lin et al., 2011; Petitprez et al., 2011; Shy et al., 2013), suggesting two distinct Na_V1.5 pools.

CARDIAC NA$_V$S FORM MULTI-PROTEIN COMPLEXES

Na_V-α subunits interact with multi-protein complexes that are subcellular domain specific in heart. These interactions,

TABLE 1 | *SCN1B* variants linked to human disease.

Disease	β1	β1B
Atrial fibrillation	R85H (Watanabe et al., 2009), D153N (Watanabe et al., 2009)	R85H (Watanabe et al., 2009), D153N (Watanabe et al., 2009)
Brugada syndrome	E87Q (Watanabe et al., 2008)	E87Q (Watanabe et al., 2008), H162P (Holst et al., 2012), W179X, R214Q (Holst et al., 2012; Hu et al., 2012)
Dravet syndrome	I106F (Ogiwara et al., 2012), Y119D (Ramadan et al., 2017), C121W (Wallace et al., 1998), R125C (Patino et al., 2009)	I106F (Ogiwara et al., 2012), Y119D (Ramadan et al., 2017),C121W (Wallace et al., 1998), R125C (Patino et al., 2009)
Generalized Epilepsy with Febrile Seizures Plus (GEFS+)	D25N (Orrico et al., 2009), R85H (Scheffer et al., 2006), R85C (Scheffer et al., 2006), R125L (Fendri-Kriaa et al., 2011), five amino acid deletions (IVS2-2A>C) (Audenaert et al., 2003)	D25N (Orrico et al., 2009), R85H (Scheffer et al., 2006), R85C (Scheffer et al., 2006), R125L (Fendri-Kriaa et al., 2011), five amino acid deletions (IVS2-2A>C) (Audenaert et al., 2003)
Idiopathic epilepsy		G257R (Patino et al., 2011)
Sudden Infant Death Syndrome (SIDS)		R214Q (Hu et al., 2012), R225C (Neubauer et al., in press)
Sudden Unexpected Nocturnal Death Syndrome (SUNDS)	V138I (Liu et al., 2014), T189M (Liu et al., 2014)	V138I (Liu et al., 2014)
Long QT Syndrome (LQTS)		P213T (Riuró et al., 2014)

which involve Na_V-β1, as discussed throughout this review, are essential for proper cardiac electrical signaling (**Figure 3C**, **Table 2**). Ankyrin-G, a cytoskeletal adaptor protein, is necessary for normal expression of $Na_V1.5$ and coupling of the channel to the actin cytoskeleton (Mohler et al., 2004). A human *SCN5A* BrS variant eliminates $Na_V1.5$-ankyrin-G interactions (Mohler et al., 2004). This mutation, located in the $Na_V1.5$ DII–III loop, prevents channel cell surface expression in ventricular CMs and alters channel properties. In agreement with this result, rat CMs with reduced expression of ankyrin-G have reduced levels of $Na_V1.5$ expression and I_{Na}. Abnormal $Na_V1.5$ localization can be rescued in ankyrin-G deficient CMs through exogenous over-expression of ankyrin-G (Lowe et al., 2008). Ankyrin-G recruits βIV spectrin, which forms important scaffolding structures and plays a role in the maintenance and integrity of the plasma membrane and cytoskeleton (Yang et al., 2007). βIV spectrin associates with and targets a subpopulation of Ca^{2+}/calmodulin-dependent protein kinase II (CaMKIIδ) to the ID to phosphorylate a critical serine residue in the $Na_V1.5$ I–II linker (Hund et al., 2010; Makara et al., 2014). Mouse CMs expressing a mutant form of βIV spectrin show a positive shift in I_{Na} steady-state inactivation, elimination of late I_{Na}, shortened APD, and decreased QT intervals (Hund et al., 2010), confirming that formation of the $Na_V1.5$-ankyrin-G signaling complex is critical for maintaining normal cardiac excitability.

Cytoskeletal integrity is a pre-requisite for normal electrical coupling. During cardiac development, GJ proteins and $Na_V1.5$ appear at the ID after formation of adherens junctions (Vreeker et al., 2014). The perinexus, a newly identified region of the ID, is defined as the area surrounding the plaque of functional GJs (Rhett et al., 2013) (**Figure 3B**). Here, free connexons appear at the periphery of the GJ, after which they bind to zonula occludens1 (ZO-1). GJs form when ZO-1 free connexons from one cell associate with ZO-1 free connexons of a neighboring cell (Rhett et al., 2011). Disruption of Cx43/ZO-1 interactions increases GJ size (Hunter, 2005), and in a ZO-1 null model, GJ plaques are larger (Palatinus et al., 2010). Cx43 also interacts with $Na_V1.5$ in the perinexus (Rhett et al., 2012). The presence of $Na_V1.5$ at the perinexus may suggest that, in addition to GJ proteins, Na_Vs may participate in coupling across the extracellular space, with increasing evidence supporting that both Cx43 and $Na_V1.5$ are necessary for cell-to-cell transmission of APs (Gutstein et al., 2001; Lin et al., 2011; Jansen et al., 2012).

$Na_V1.5$ contributes to at least two distinct multiprotein complexes in ventricular CMs, one at the lateral membrane containing dystrophin and syntrophin (**Figure 2**), and the other at the ID involving the membrane-associated guanylate kinase (MAGUK) protein adapter protein, synapse-associated protein 97 (SAP97), and ankyrin-G (Petitprez et al., 2011) (**Figure 3C**). In heterologous cells, surface expression of $Na_V1.5$ is regulated by its interaction with SAP97 via a PDZ-domain (post-synaptic density protein-PSD95, disc large tumor suppressor-Dlg1, zonula occludens1-ZO1). Either the truncation of the fourth domain of $Na_V1.5$ (Shy et al., 2014) or depletion of SAP97 (Matsumoto et al., 2012) results in reduced channel cell surface expression, with a subsequent decrease of I_{Na}.

$Na_V1.5$ also interacts with fibroblast growth factor homologous factor 1B (FHF1B) (Liu et al., 2003), calmodulin (Kim et al., 2004; Young and Caldwell, 2005), Nedd4-like-ubiqutin-protein ligases (Van Bemmelen et al., 2004; Rougier et al., 2005), and is phosphorylated by Fyn (Ahern et al., 2005), a src family tyrosine kinase, all of which are involved in the regulation of channel subcellular localization and activity (**Figure 3C**). Taken together, these results accentuate the idea that cardiac Na_Vs associate with protein complexes that are specific to subcellular domains, and these interactions are critical to cardiac physiology. Undoubtedly, changes in one component of a given complex results in significant consequences to overall cardiac excitability and synchrony.

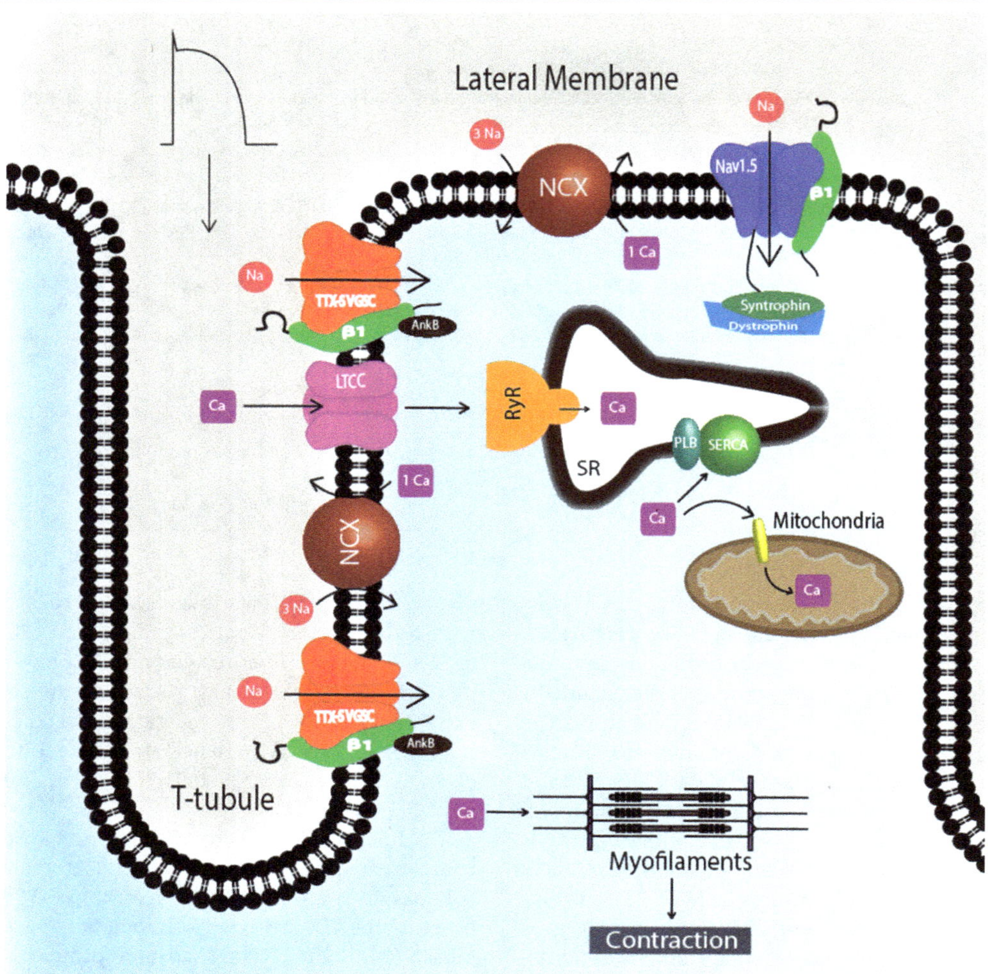

FIGURE 2 | TTX-S Na_Vs are localized to T-tubules. TTX-S Na_Vs, including $Na_V1.1$, $Na_V1.3$, and $Na_V1.6$, are located at the T-tubules of CMs where they are thought to participate in the regulation of excitation-contraction coupling. Non-phosphorylated Na_V-β1 subunits are co-localized with TTX-S Na_V-α subunits at the T-tubules where they play roles in calcium signaling and homeostasis. $Na_V1.5$ is localized at the lateral membrane as well as the ID (**Figure 3**). At the lateral membrane, $Na_V1.5$ is complexed with syntrophin and dystrophin. Abbreviations: L-type calcium channel (LTCC), phospholamban (PLB), ryanodine receptor (RyR), sarcoplasmic reticulum Ca^{2+}-ATPase (SERCA), sodium-calcium exchanger (NCX), transverse tubules (T-tubule).

NA$_V$-β SUBUNITS MODULATE CARDIAC EXCITABILITY

In mammalian genomes, five Na_V-β subunits are encoded by four genes, *SCN1B-SCN4B* (O'Malley and Isom, 2015). Na_V-β1-β4 are transmembrane proteins with type 1 topology consisting of an extracellular N-terminus containing an immunoglobulin (Ig) domain, a transmembrane segment, and an intracellular C-terminus (Brackenbury and Isom, 2011) (**Figure 1**). Na_V-β1B, a splice variant of *SCN1B*, contains the Na_V-β1 N-terminal and Ig domains, but lacks a transmembrane domain (Kazen-Gillespie et al., 2000), resulting in a secreted protein (Patino et al., 2011) (**Figure 1**). Na_V-β subunits can interact both covalently and non-covalently with Na_V-α subunits: Na_V-β1 and -β3 interact non-covalently with Na_V-α via their N- and C-termini (McCormick et al., 1998; Meadows et al., 2001), while Na_V-β2 and -β4 interact covalently with Na_V-α via a single N-terminal cysteine located in the extracellular Ig loop (Chen et al., 2012; Gilchrist et al., 2013).

Canonically, Na_V-βs are known as modulators of Na_V electrophysiological properties and cell surface expression (Brackenbury and Isom, 2011). Heterologous expression systems and mouse models have shown that Na_V-βs modulate Na_V – αs in cell type specific manners, thus the Na_V α/β subunit composition of a given cell confers unique biophysical properties that can be finely tuned (Calhoun and Isom, 2014). Not surprisingly, Na_V-β1 modulation of $Na_V1.5$ varies depending on the system studied. In *Xenopus* oocytes, the amplitude of $Na_V1.5$ expressed I_{Na} increases with increasing amounts of β1 mRNA (Qu et al., 1995). Antisense-mediated post-transcriptional silencing of *Scn1b* in H9C2, a CM line, alters TTX-S and TTX-R

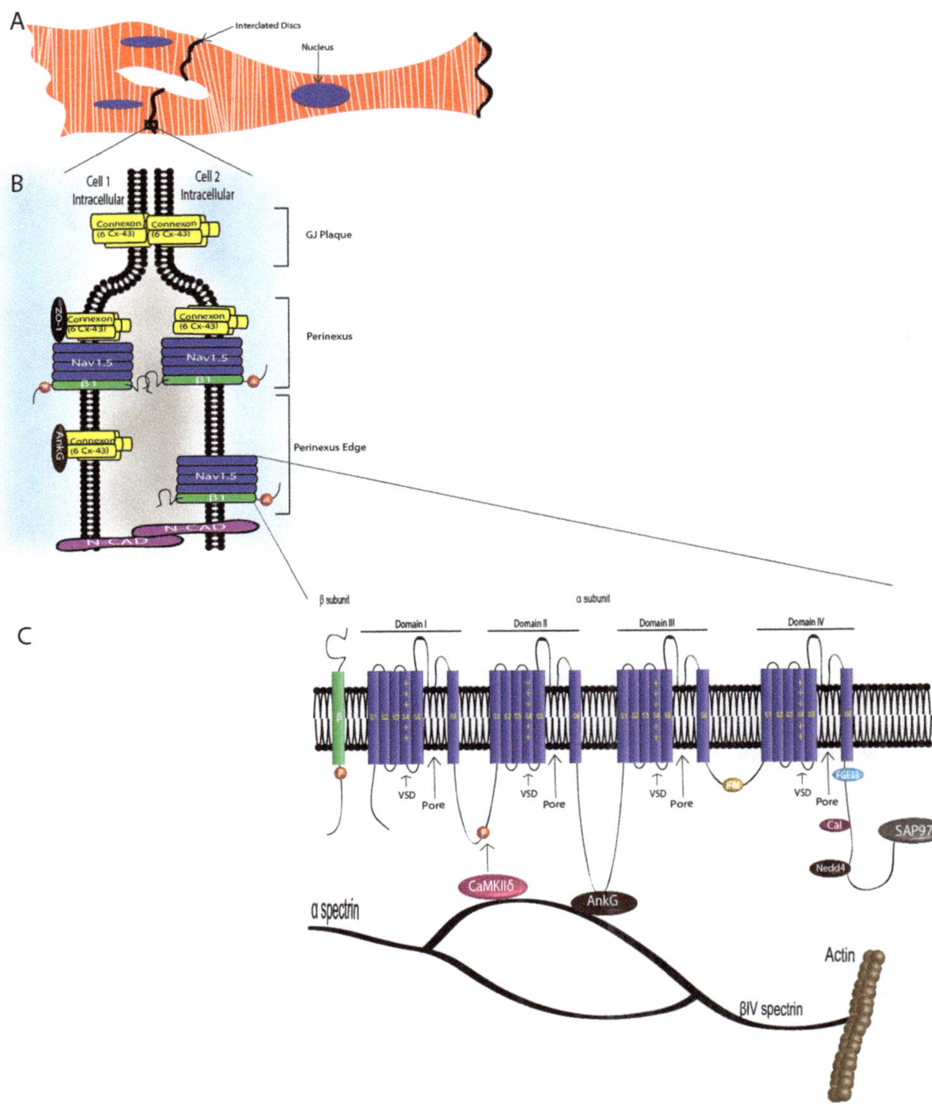

FIGURE 3 | VGSC complexes at the cardiac intercalated disk. CMs associate at the ID, where $Na_V1.5$, Nav-β1 subunits, adherens junctions, gap junctions, and desmosomes define intercellular communication. **(A)** Associated CMs. **(B)** Proposed model of the GJ plaque, perinexus, and perinexus edge. Nav-β1 subunits at the ID are tyrosine phosphorylated, possibly through Fyn kinase activation, and may function in cell–cell adhesion in the perinexus and perinexus edge. **(C)** At the ID, Nav1.5 associates with a multi-protein complex (also see **Table 2**). The S4 segment of each Na_V-α subunit homologous domain forms the voltage sensing domain (VSD) and segments 5 and 6 in each domain create the ion-conducting pore. Three hydrophobic amino acids, IFM, form the inactivation gate. Abbreviations: Ankyrin-G (AnkG), Calmodulin (Cal), Ca^{2+}/calmodulin-dependent protein kinase II (CaMKIIδ), Fibroblast growth factor homologous factor 1B (FHF1B), N-Cadherin (N-Cad), Nedd4-like-ubiqutin-protein ligases (Nedd4), Synapse-associated protein 97 (SAP97).

Na_V-α mRNA and protein expression, resulting in decreased I_{Na} (Baroni et al., 2014). In contrast, *Scn1b* null mouse CMs have increased expression of *Scn3a* and *Scn5a*, along with increased TTX-S and TTX-R I_{Na} (Lopez-Santiago et al., 2007). In heterologous cells, Na_V-β1 expression results in slight changes in $Na_V1.5$ I_{Na}, but significant effects on voltage-dependence and channel kinetics. In Tsa201 cells transfected with $Na_V1.5$, co-expression of Na_V-β1 positively shifts the voltage-dependence of inactivation (Malhotra et al., 2001). Co-expression of Na_V-β1 with $Na_V1.5$ in *Xenopus* oocytes causes a depolarizing shift in steady-state inactivation compared with WT alone (Zhu et al., 2017), suggesting that β1 may allow the α subunit voltage-sensing domains to recover more rapidly to the resting state. Thus, Na_V-β1 may initiate fine-tuned acute and chronic feedback mechanisms that differentially control expression and function of Na_V-αs in the heart.

Na_V-β1B is expressed in fetal brain and in heart at all developmental time points. When expressed alone or in the

TABLE 2 | $Na_V1.5$ ID interacting proteins.

Interacting protein	Effects on $Na_V1.5$	Reference(s)
Ankyrin-G (AnkG)	Proper expression at plasma membrane and coupling to actin cytoskeleton	Mohler et al., 2004
Calmodulin (Cal)	Regulates biophysical properties	Tan et al., 2002; Kim et al., 2004; Young and Caldwell, 2005; Gabelli et al., 2014
Ca^{2+}/calmodulin-dependent protein kinase II (CaMKIIδ)	Phosphorylation and modulates excitability	Hund et al., 2010; Makara et al., 2014
Fibroblast growth factor homologous factor 1B (FHF1B)	Modulate channel gating	Liu et al., 2003
Nedd4-like-ubiqutin-protein ligases (Nedd4)	Ubiquitination and regulated internalization. Possible mechanism in modulation of channel density at the plasma membrane	Van Bemmelen et al., 2004; Rougier et al., 2005
Synapse-associated protein 97 (SAP97)	Stability and anchoring to the cell membrane	Petitprez et al., 2011; Matsumoto et al., 2012

presence of TTX-S Na_V-αs in a heterologous expression system, Na_V-β1B is secreted (Patino et al., 2011). Secreted Na_V-β1B functions as a CAM ligand to promote signal transduction in cultured neurons (Patino et al., 2011). In contrast, Na_V-β1B is retained at the cell surface when co-expressed with $Na_V1.5$ (Patino et al., 2011) and Na_V-β1B co-expression increases I_{Na} density compared to $Na_V1.5$ alone (Watanabe et al., 2008). The disease variant, β1B-G257R (**Figure 1**, **Table 1**), causes Na_V-β1B to be retained inside the cell, resulting in a functional null phenotype (Patino et al., 2011). The variant, β1B-W179X (**Figure 1**, **Table 1**), fails to increase $Na_V1.5$ I_{Na} density, suggesting that it may also be a functional null mutation (Watanabe et al., 2008). A number of Na_V-β1B variants have now been linked to cardiac arrhythmias (**Figure 1**, **Table 1**), thus this subunit is critical to cardiac physiology.

While the Na_V-αs are known to form and function as monomers, recent evidence suggests that they can also form dimers, and that dimerization is mediated through an interaction site within the first intracellular loop (Clatot et al., 2017). Na_V-α dimers display coupled gating properties, which are mediated through the action of 14-3-3 proteins (Clatot et al., 2017). The 14-3-3 family of proteins is important for the regulation of cardiac I_{Na}, and disrupted 14-3-3 expression may exert pro-arrhythmic effects on cardiac electrical properties (Allouis et al., 2006; Sreedhar et al., 2016). The functional importance of cardiac Na_V-α dimerization may be to target and enhance the density of channels at specific subcellular domains. $Na_V1.5$-R1432G, a surface localization defective *SCN5A* mutant, displays a dominant negative effect on WT $Na_V1.5$, but only in the presence of Na_V-β1 (Mercier et al., 2012). Thus, Na_V-β1 may normally mediate physical interactions between $Na_V1.5$ dimers, however further research must be performed.

NA_V-βS DO MORE THAN MODULATE I_{NA}

Na_V-β subunits are multifunctional (O'Malley and Isom, 2015). In addition to modulating channel gating and cell surface expression/localization, Na_V-βs are Ig superfamily cell adhesion molecules (CAMs) that facilitate cell–cell communication and initiate intracellular signaling cascades. Na_V-β1 and -β2 participate in *trans*-homophilic cell adhesion, resulting in the recruitment of ankyrin-G to the plasma membrane at sites of cell–cell contact (Malhotra et al., 2000). Importantly, this occurs both in the presence and absence of Na_V-α, at least *in vitro*. Na_V-β1 and -β2 also participate in cell–matrix adhesion, binding tenascin-R and tenascin- C to modulate cell migration (Srinivasan et al., 1998; Xiao et al., 1999). The Na_V-β3 amino acid sequence is most similar to Na_V-β1 compared to the other Na_V-β subunits (Morgan et al., 2000). While Na_V-β3 does not function as a CAM when expressed in *Drosophila* S2 cells, as shown for Na_V-β1 and -β2 (Chen et al., 2012), it does so in mammalian cells where *trans* homophilic adhesion was shown to require an intact Cys2–Cys24 disulfide bond (Yereddi et al., 2013).

Na_V-β function, localization, and expression are regulated by multiple post-translational modifications including phosphorylation, glycosylation, and proteolytic cleavage (Calhoun and Isom, 2014). All Na_V-βs have highly glycosylated N-terminal domains, containing 3 to 4 N-linked glycosylation sites each (Isom et al., 1992; McCormick et al., 1998; Johnson et al., 2004), and these modifications contribute to cell surface expression and channel modulation (Johnson et al., 2004). Lastly, Na_V-βs are targets for sequential proteolytic cleavage by α-secretase/BACE1 and γ-secretase, resulting in the release of N-terminal and C-terminal domains (Wong et al., 2005). These cleavage products may have important physiological effects on transcriptional regulation of Na_V-α subunit genes. For example, γ-secretase cleavage of Na_V-β2 in neurons *in vitro* leads to translocation of the intracellular domain to the nucleus, where it increases *SCN1A* mRNA expression and $Na_V1.1$ protein (Kim et al., 2007).

Of the five Na_V-β subunits, Na_V-β1 has been the most studied in terms of its CAM function. In the heart, Na_V-β1 ID localization suggests a role in cardiac cell–cell contact. *Scn1b* and *Scn5a* have overlapping temporal and spatial expression profiles during heart development (Domínguez et al., 2005). In ventricular CMs, Na_V-β1 is co-localized at the ID (Kaufmann et al., 2010) with $Na_v1.5$ (Maier et al., 2004), as well as at the T-tubules with TTX-S channels (Malhotra et al., 2001; Lopez-Santiago et al., 2007). Recent evidence suggests that Na_V-β1-mediated cell–cell adhesion may occur at the perinexal membrane, and this putative interaction can be acutely inhibited by βadp1, a novel peptide mimetic of the Na_V-β1 CAM domain (Veeraraghavan et al., 2016). Dose-dependent administration of βadp1 decreased cellular adhesion in Na_V-β1-overexpressing fibroblasts. 75% of βadp1-treated hearts exhibited spontaneous ventricular tachycardias, revealing preferential slowing of transverse conduction. These data support a role for *trans* Na_V-β1-mediated cell–cell adhesion at the perinexal membrane and suggest a role for adhesion in conduction (**Figure 3B**). Because a large proportion of *SCN1B* disease variants affect the Ig domain (**Figure 1**), it is likely that disruption of Na_V-β1-mediated cell–cell adhesion contributes to disease mechanisms and, if so, that restoring adhesion may be a future therapeutic target.

The Na_V-β1 intracellular domain can be phosphorylated at tyrosine (Y) residue 181 (Malhotra et al., 2002, 2004; McEwen et al., 2004), possibly through activation of Fyn kinase (Brackenbury et al., 2008; Nelson et al., 2014) (**Figure 1**). β1Y181E, a phosphomimetic, participates in cell adhesion but does not interact with ankyrin or modulate I_{Na}, suggesting that Y181 is an important regulatory point for cytoskeletal association and channel modulation (Malhotra et al., 2002). In CMs, tyrosine-phosphorylated Na_V-β1 and non-phosphorylated Na_V-β1 are differentially localized to subcellular domains where they interact with specific cytoskeletal and signaling proteins (Malhotra et al., 2004). At the T-tubules, non-phosphorylated Na_V-β1 interacts with TTX-S Na_Vs and ankyrin-B (**Figure 2**) (Malhotra et al., 2004). In contrast, tyrosine-phosphorylated Na_V-β1 is localized to the ID where it interacts with $Na_v1.5$ and N-cadherin (**Figures 3B,C**) (Malhotra et al., 2004). We do not yet know whether phosphorylation targets Na_V-β1 to specialized subcellular regions or whether Na_V-β1 is differentially phosphorylated upon arrival. Phosphorylation may be a signaling mechanism by which cells regulate the density and localization of Na_V-β1, and by association Na_v-αs, to specific subcellular domains. In summary, Na_V-β1 subunits serve as critical links between the extracellular and intracellular signaling environments of cells through ion channel modulation as well as cell–cell adhesion.

NA$_V$-β1 MODULATES POTASSIUM CHANNELS

Na_V-β1 can interact with and modulate voltage-gated potassium channels (K_vs) in addition to Na_Vs. K_v-α subunits assemble as tetramers that normally associate with modulatory Kv-β subunits (Snyders, 1999). The $K_v4.x$ subfamily of channels express rapidly activating, inactivating, and recovering cardiac transient outward currents (I_{to}) (Snyders, 1999). Co-expression of Na_V-β1 with $K_v4.3$ results in a ~four-fold increase in I_{to} density (Deschênes and Tomaselli, 2002). Additionally, Na_V-β1 alters the voltage-dependence and kinetics of channel gating compared to $K_v4.3$ expressed alone (Deschênes and Tomaselli, 2002). Importantly, Na_V-β1 associates with $K_v4.2$ and enhances its surface expression (Marionneau et al., 2012). Whole-cell voltage-clamp recordings obtained from cells expressing $K_v4.2$ with Na_V-β1 resulted in higher I_{to} densities compared to $K_v4.2$ alone (Marionneau et al., 2012). Na_V-β1 can also interact with and modulate K_v1 ($K_v1.1$, $K_v1.2$, $K_v1.3$, or $K_v1.6$) and K_v7 ($K_v7.2$) channels (Nguyen et al., 2012). Lastly, Na_V-β1B can also associate with $K_v4.3$, resulting in increased I_{to} (Hu et al., 2012). Thus, K_v currents can be modulated by Na_V-β subunits, at least in heterologous expression systems. Transfection of neonatal rat ventricular myocytes with siRNA targeting Na_V-β1 significantly reduced the expression of $K_v4.x$ protein and reduced both I_{Na} and I_{to} (Deschênes et al., 2008), suggesting that Na_V-β1 can modulate K_v currents in the heart *in vivo*.

The inward rectifier current I_{K1}, expressed by Kir2.1, is critical for setting the resting membrane potential and modulating the late-phase of repolarization and AP duration in CMs (Nerbonne and Kass, 2005). Similar to $Na_v1.5$, Kir2.x channels contain a C-terminal PDZ-binding domain which mediates interaction with SAP97 and syntrophin (Matamoros et al., 2016). It is thought that Kir2.x channels associate in microdomains that include caveolin 3, $Na_v1.5$, SAP97, and syntrophin (Vaidyanathan et al., 2013). $Na_v1.5$ interacts with α1-syntrophin via an internal N-terminal PDZ-like binding domain in addition to the C-terminal PDZ-binding domains (Matamoros et al., 2016). Importantly, $Na_v1.5$-β1 co-expression increases Kir2.1 and Kir2.2, but not Kir2.3, currents, again suggesting that these channels are functionally linked and that Na_v-β1 is critical to the formation of multi-ion channel complexes.

IN VIVO ROLES OF *SCN1B*

Animal models have been instrumental in understanding the role of *Scn1b* in cardiac excitability. *Scn1b* deletion in mice results in severe seizures, ventricular arrhythmias, and sudden death prior to weaning (Chen, 2004). *Scn1b* null ventricular CMs exhibit prolonged AP repolarization, increased *Scn5a*/$Na_v1.5$ gene and protein expression, increased *Scn3a* expression, increased transient and persistent I_{Na} density, and prolonged QT and RR intervals (Lopez-Santiago et al., 2007). In agreement with an adhesive role for β1, cytoskeletal disruption in CMs also results in increased persistent I_{Na} (Undrovinas et al., 1995). Consistent with this, ventricular CMs isolated from cardiac-specific *Scn1b* null mice have increased I_{Na} density, increased susceptibility to polymorphic ventricular arrhythmias, and altered intracellular calcium handling that is TTX-S (Lin et al., 2015). These data indicate that loss of *Scn1b* expression is arrhythmogenic, mediated by altered ion channel gene and protein expression, I_{Na}, I_K, and calcium handling. Cardiac specific *Scn1b* deletion increases the duration of calcium signaling, resulting in delayed afterdepolarizations (Lin et al., 2015). It will be interesting to determine if expression of disease-associated *SCN1B* variants leads to dysfunctional ryanodine receptor signaling, which can also result in altered levels of intracellular calcium and the generation of arrhythmias (Bers, 2008; Fearnley et al., 2011; Glasscock, 2014).

The cardiac AP relies on the orchestration of multiple ion channels in concert. Na_V-β1 is an important modulator of Na_V-α as well as some K_V- and Kir-α subunits. Na_V and K channels may be functionally linked through Na_V-β1/β1B, and if so, defects in this mechanism may contribute to cardiac disease. It will be critical to determine the physiological effects of Na_V-β1 interaction with other K channels, calcium channels, or other calcium-handling proteins at the T-tubules. It is intriguing to consider that Na_V-β1 may serve as a central communication hub between sodium, potassium, and calcium channel families to coordinate depolarization, repolarization, and calcium signaling in CMs.

SCN1B AND HUMAN DISEASE

SCN1B variants are implicated in a variety of inherited pathologies, including epileptic encephalopathy and cardiac arrhythmias (O'Malley and Isom, 2015) (**Figure 1**, **Table 1**). The epileptic encephalopathy Dravet syndrome is linked to heterozygous variants in *SCN1A* leading to haploinsufficiency in most patients, however, a subset of patients has *SCN1B* homozygous loss-of-function variants (Patino et al., 2009). The leading cause of mortality in Dravet syndrome is Sudden Unexpected Death in Epilepsy (SUDEP) (Nobili et al., 2011; Kalume, 2013; Devinsky et al., 2016). *SCN1B* variants are also linked to inherited cardiac arrhythmia syndromes that increase the risk of sudden death, including BrS (Hu et al., 2012), LQTS (Riuró et al., 2014), atrial arrhythmias (Watanabe et al., 2009), and SIDS (Hu et al., 2012). Diagnostic overlap between epilepsy and cardiac conduction disease can confound causative links between the two phenotypes (Ravindran et al., 2016). Cardiac conduction abnormalities can be poorly recognized in patients with epilepsy and vice versa (Zaidi et al., 2000). A retrospective electrocardiography study revealed that abnormal ventricular conduction was more common in SUDEP cases than in epileptic controls (Chyou et al., 2016). We propose that variants in *SCN1B*, including those linked to epilepsy, predispose patients to compromised cardiac electrical abnormalities. Thus, cardiovascular evaluation may be helpful in treating epileptic encephalopathy patients.

SUMMARY

Na_V-β1 and -β1B are multifunctional molecules that associate with Na_v and K channels, cytoskeletal proteins, CAMs, and extracellular matrix molecules in the heart and brain. In addition, Na_V-β1/β1B modulate multiple ionic currents, channel expression levels, and channel subcellular localization. Thus, it is not surprising that variants in *SCN1B* are linked to devastating cardiac and neurological diseases with a high risk of sudden death. In the field of cardiac physiology, important questions remain regarding specific cardiac Na_V-β1 binding partners, potential effects of Na_V-β1 on calcium-handling, the potential role of Na_V-β1 in Na_v1.5 dimerization, and the mechanism of phosphorylation events that affect Na_V-β1 targeting to and association with subcellular domain specific signaling complexes at the ID, lateral membrane, and T-tubules. Understanding the functions of Na_V-β1 within these protein complexes will help to elucidate underlying mechanisms of cardiac arrhythmias and associated sudden death, as well as lead to the discovery of novel biomarkers and therapeutic targets for human disease.

AUTHOR CONTRIBUTIONS

All authors listed have made a substantial, direct and intellectual contribution to the work, and approved it for publication.

REFERENCES

Ahern, C. A., Zhang, J. F., Wookalis, M. J., and Horn, R. (2005). Modulation of the cardiac sodium channel Nav1.5 by Fyn, a Src family tyrosine kinase. *Circ. Res.* 96, 991–998. doi: 10.1161/01.RES.0000166324.00524.dd

Allouis, M., Le Bouffant, F., Wilders, R., Péroz, D., Schott, J. J., Noireaud, J., et al. (2006). 14-3-3 Is a regulator of the cardiac voltage-gated sodium channel Nav1.5. *Circ. Res.* 98, 1538–1546. doi: 10.1161/01.RES.0000229244.97497.2c

Audenaert, D., Claes, L., Ceulemans, B., Löfgren, a, Van Broeckhoven, C., and De Jonghe, P. (2003). A deletion in SCN1B is associated with febrile seizures and early-onset absence epilepsy. *Neurology* 61, 854–856. doi: 10.1212/01.WNL.0000080362.55784.1C

Baroni, D., Picco, C., Barbieri, R., and Moran, O. (2014). Antisense-mediated post-transcriptional silencing of SCN1B gene modulates sodium channel functional expression. *Biol. Cell* 106, 13–29. doi: 10.1111/boc.201300040

Bers, D. M. (2008). Calcium cycling and signaling in cardiac myocytes. *Annu. Rev. Physiol.* 70, 23–49. doi: 10.1146/annurev.physiol.70.113006.100455

Brackenbury, W. J., Davis, T. H., Chen, C., Slat, E., Detrow, M. J., Dickendesher, T. L., et al. (2008). Voltage-gated Na+ channel beta1 subunit-mediated neurite outgrowth requires Fyn kinase and contributes to postnatal CNS development *in vivo*. *J. Neurosci.* 28, 3246–3256. doi: 10.1523/JNEUROSCI.5446-07.2008

Brackenbury, W. J., and Isom, L. L. (2011). Na+ channel β1 subunits: overachievers of the ion channel family. *Front. Pharmacol.* 2:53. doi: 10.3389/fphar.2011.00053

Calhoun, J. D., and Isom, L. L. (2014). The role of non-pore-forming β subunits in physiology and pathophysiology of voltage-gated sodium channels. in voltage gated sodium channels. *Handb. Exp. Pharmacol.* 221, 51–89. doi: 10.1007/978-3-642-41588-3_4

Catterall, W. A. (2000). From ionic currents to molecular mechanisms: the structure and function of voltage-gated sodium channels. *Neuron* 26, 13–25. doi: 10.1016/S0896-6273(00)81133-2

Catterall, W., Goldin, A. L., and Waxman, S. G. (2005). International Union of Pharmacology. XLVII. Nomenclature and structure-function relationships of voltage-gated sodium channels. *Pharmacol. Rev.* 57, 397–409. doi: 10.1124/pr.57.4.4

Chen, C. (2004). Mice lacking sodium channel 1 subunits display defects in neuronal excitability, sodium channel expression, and nodal architecture. *J. Neurosci.* 24, 4030–4042. doi: 10.1523/JNEUROSCI.4139-03.2004

Chen, C., Calhoun, J. D., Zhang, Y., Lopez-Santiago, L., Zhou, N., Davis, T. H., et al. (2012). Identification of the cysteine residue responsible for disulfide linkage of Na+channel α and β2 subunits. *J. Biol. Chem.* 287, 39061–39069. doi: 10.1074/jbc.M112.397646

Chyou, J. Y., Friedman, D., Cerrone, M., Slater, W., Guo, Y., Taupin, D., et al. (2016). Electrocardiographic features of sudden unexpected death in epilepsy. *Epilepsia* 57, e135–e139. doi: 10.1111/epi.13411

Clatot, J., Hoshi, M., Wan, X., Liu, H., Jain, A., Shinlapawittayatorn, K., et al. (2017). Voltage-gated sodium channels assemble and gate as dimers. *Nat. Commun.* 8:2077. doi: 10.1038/s41467-017-02262-0

Deschênes, I., Armoundas, A., a, Jones, S. P., and Tomaselli, G. F. (2008). Post-transcriptional gene silencing of KChIP2 and Navbeta1 in neonatal rat cardiac myocytes reveals a functional association between Na and Ito currents. *J. Mol. Cell. Cardiol.* 45, 336–346. doi: 10.1016/j.yjmcc.2008.05.001

Deschênes, I., and Tomaselli, G. F. (2002). Modulation of Kv4.3 current by accessory subunits. *FEBS Lett.* 528, 183–188. doi: 10.1016/S0014-5793(02)03296-9

Devinsky, O., Hesdorffer, D. C., Thurman, D. J., Lhatoo, S., and Richerson, G. (2016). Sudden unexpected death in epilepsy: epidemiology, mechanisms, and prevention. *Lancet Neurol.* 15, 1075–1088. doi: 10.1016/S1474-4422(16)30158-2

Domínguez, J. N., Navarro, F., Franco, D., Thompson, R. P., and Aránega, A. E. (2005). Temporal and spatial expression pattern of beta1 sodium channel subunit during heart development. *Cardiovasc. Res.* 65, 842–850. doi: 10.1016/j.cardiores.2004.11.028

Fearnley, C. J., Llewelyn Roderick, H., and Bootman, M. D. (2011). Calcium signaling in cardiac myocytes. *Cold Spring Harb. Perspect. Biol.* 3:a004242. doi: 10.1101/cshperspect.a004242

Fendri-Kriaa, N., Kammoun, F., Salem, I. H., Kifagi, C., Mkaouar-Rebai, E., Hsairi, I., et al. (2011). New mutation c.374C>T and a putative disease-associated haplotype within SCN1B gene in Tunisian families with febrile seizures. *Eur. J. Neurol.* 18, 695–702. doi: 10.1111/j.1468-1331.2010.03216.x

Freeman, S. A., Desmazières, A., Fricker, D., Lubetzki, C., and Sol-Foulon, N. (2016). Mechanisms of sodium channel clustering and its influence on axonal impulse conduction. *Cell. Mol. Life Sci.* 73, 723–735. doi: 10.1007/s00018-015-2081-1

Gabelli, S. B., Boto, A., Kuhns, V. H., Bianchet, M. A., Farinelli, F., Aripirala, S., et al. (2014). Regulation of the NaV1.5 cytoplasmic domain by calmodulin. *Nat. Commun.* 5:5126. doi: 10.1038/ncomms6126

Gellens, M. E., George, A. L., Chen, L. Q., Chahine, M., Horn, R., Barchi, R. L., et al. (1992). Primary structure and functional expression of the human cardiac tetrodotoxin-insensitive voltage-dependent sodium channel. *Proc. Natl. Acad. Sci. U.S.A.* 89, 554–558. doi: 10.1073/pnas.89.2.554

Gilchrist, J., Das, S., Van Petegem, F., and Bosmans, F. (2013). Crystallographic insights into sodium-channel modulation by the β4 subunit. *Proc. Natl. Acad. Sci.U.S.A.* 110, E5016–E5024. doi: 10.1073/pnas.1314557110

Glasscock, E. (2014). Genomic biomarkers of SUDEP in brain and heart. *Epilepsy Behav.* 38, 172–179. doi: 10.1016/j.yebeh.2013.09.019

Gutstein, D. E., Morley, G. E., Tamaddon, H., Vaidya, D., Schneider, M. D., Chen, J., et al. (2001). Conduction slowing and sudden Arrhythmic death in mice with cardiac-restricted inactivation of connexin43. *Circ. Res.* 88, 333–339. doi: 10.1161/01.RES.88.3.333

Hille, B., and Catterall, W. A. (2012). "Chapter 4 – Electrical excitability and ion channels," in *Basic Neurochemistry, 8th edn, Principles of Molecular, Cellular, and Medical Neurobiology*, eds S. T. Brady, G. J. Siegel, R. W. Albers, and D. L. Price (Amsterdam; Boston, MA; Heidelberg; London; New York, NY; Oxford; Paris; San Diego, CA; San Francisco, CA; Singapore; Sydney; Tokyo: Elsevier; Academic Press), 63–80.

Holst, A. G., Saber, S., Houshmand, M., Zaklyazminskaya, E. V., Wang, Y., Jensen, H. K., et al. (2012). Sodium current and potassium transient outward current genes in Brugada syndrome: screening and bioinformatics. *Can. J. Cardiol.* 28, 196–200. doi: 10.1016/j.cjca.2011.11.011

Hu, D., Barajas-Martínez, H., Medeiros-Domingo, A., Crotti, L., Veltmann, C., Schimpf, R., et al. (2012). A novel rare variant in SCN1Bb linked to Brugada syndrome and SIDS by combined modulation of Nav1.5 and Kv4.3 channel currents. *Heart Rhythm* 9, 760–769. doi: 10.1016/j.hrthm.2011.12.006

Hund, T. J., Koval, O. M., Li, J., Wright, P. J., Qian, L., Snyder, J. S., et al. (2010). A β IV -spectrin / CaMKII signaling complex is essential for membrane excitability in mice. *J. Clin. Invest.* 120, 3508–3519. doi: 10.1172/JCI43621

Hunter, A. W. (2005). Zonula occludens-1 alters connexin43 gap junction size and organization by influencing channel accretion. *Mol. Biol. Cell* 16, 5686–5698. doi: 10.1091/mbc.E05-08-0737

Isom, L. L., De Jongh, K. S., Patton, D. E., Reber, B. F., Offord, J., Charbonneau, H., et al. (1992). Primary structure and functional expression of the beta 1 subunit of the rat brain sodium channel. *Science* 256, 839–842. doi: 10.1126/science.1375395

Jansen, J. A., Noorman, M., Musa, H., Stein, M., De Jong, S., Van Der Nagel, R., et al. (2012). Reduced heterogeneous expression of Cx43 results in decreased Nav1.5 expression and reduced sodium current that accounts for arrhythmia vulnerability in conditional Cx43 knockout mice. *Heart. Rhythm* 9, 600–607. doi: 10.1016/j.hrthm.2011.11.025

Johnson, D., Montpetit, M. L., Stocker, P. J., and Bennett, E. S. (2004). The sialic acid component of the beta1 subunit modulates voltage-gated sodium channel function. *J. Biol. Chem.* 279, 44303–44310. doi: 10.1074/jbc.M408900200

Kalume, F. (2013). Sudden unexpected death in Dravet syndrome: respiratory and other physiological dysfunctions. *Respir Physiol Neurobiol.* 189, 324–328. doi: 10.1016/j.resp.2013.06.026

Kaufmann, S. G., Westenbroek, R. E., Zechner, C., Maass, A. H., Bischoff, S., Muck, J., et al. (2010). Functional protein expression of multiple sodium channel alpha- and beta-subunit isoforms in neonatal cardiomyocytes. *J. Mol. Cell. Cardiol.* 48, 261–269. doi: 10.1016/j.yjmcc.2009.04.017

Kazen-Gillespie, K., a, Ragsdale, D. S., D'Andrea, M. R., Mattei, L. N., Rogers, K. E., and Isom, L. L. (2000). Cloning, localization, and functional expression of sodium channel beta1A subunits. *J. Biol. Chem.* 275, 1079–1088. doi: 10.1074/jbc.275.2.1079

Kim, D. Y., Carey, B. W., Wang, H., Ingano, L. A. M., Binshtok, A. M., Wertz, M. H., et al. (2007). BACE1 regulates voltage-gated sodium channels and neuronal activity. *Nat. Cell Biol.* 9, 755–764. doi: 10.1038/ncb1602

Kim, J., Ghosh, S., Liu, H., Tateyama, M., Kass, R. S., and Pitt, G. S. (2004). Calmodulin mediates Ca^{2+} sensitivity of sodium channels. *J. Biol. Chem.* 279, 45004–45012. doi: 10.1074/jbc.M407286200

Lin, X., Liu, N., Lu, J., Zhang, J., Anumonwo, J. M. B., Isom, L. L., et al. (2011). Subcellular heterogeneity of sodium current properties in adult cardiac ventricular myocytes. *Heart. Rhythm* 8, 1923–1930. doi: 10.1016/j.hrthm.2011.07.016

Lin, X., O'Malley, H., Chen, C., Auerbach, D., Foster, M., Shekhar, A., et al. (2015). *Scn1b* deletion leads to increased tetrodotoxin-sensitive sodium current, altered intracellular calcium homeostasis and arrhythmias in murine hearts. *J. Physiol.* 593, 1389–1407. doi: 10.1113/jphysiol.2014.277699

Liu, C., Dib-Hajj, S. D., Renganathan, M., Cummins, T. R., and Waxman, S. G. (2003). Modulation of the cardiac sodium channel Nav1.5 by fibroblast growth factor homologous factor 1B. *J. Biol. Chem.* 278, 1029–1036. doi: 10.1074/jbc.M207074200

Liu, C., Tester, D. J., Hou, Y., Wang, W., Lv, G., Ackerman, M. J., et al. (2014). Is sudden unexplained nocturnal death syndrome in Southern China a cardiac sodium channel dysfunction disorder? *Forensic Sci. Int.* 236, 38–45. doi: 10.1016/j.forsciint.2013.12.033

Lopez-Santiago, L. F., Meadows, L. S., Ernst, S. J., Chen, C., Malhotra, J. D., McEwen, D. P., et al. (2007). Sodium channel Scn1b null mice exhibit prolonged QT and RR intervals. *J. Mol. Cell. Cardiol.* 43, 636–647. doi: 10.1016/j.yjmcc.2007.07.062

Lowe, J. S., Palygin, O., Bhasin, N., Hund, T. J., Boyden, P. A., Shibata, E., et al. (2008). Voltage-gated Nav channel targeting in the heart requires an ankyrin-G-dependent cellular pathway. *J. Cell Biol.* 180, 173–186. doi: 10.1083/jcb.200710107

Maier, S. K. G., Westenbroek, R. E., McCormick, K. A., Curtis, R., Scheuer, T., and Catterall, W. A. (2004). Distinct subcellular localization of different sodium channel α and β subunits in single ventricular myocytes from mouse heart. *Circulation* 109, 1421–1427. doi: 10.1161/01.CIR.0000121421.61896.24

Maier, S. K. G., Westenbroek, R. E., Schenkman, K. A., Feigl, E. O., Scheuer, T., and Catterall, W. A. (2002). An unexpected role for brain-type sodium channels in coupling of cell surface depolarization to contraction in the heart. *Proc. Natl. Acad. Sci. U.S.A.* 99, 4073–4078. doi: 10.1073/pnas.261705699

Makara, M. A., Curran, J., Little, S. C., Musa, H., Polina, I., Smith, S. A., et al. (2014). Ankyrin-G coordinates intercalated disc signaling platform to regulate cardiac excitability *in vivo*. *Circ. Res.* 115, 929–938. doi: 10.1161/CIRCRESAHA.115.305154

Makita, N., Bennett, P. B., and George, A. L. (1994). Voltage-gated Na+ channel beta 1 subunit mRNA expressed in adult human skeletal muscle, heart, and brain is encoded by a single gene. *J. Biol. Chem.* 269, 7571–7578.

Malhotra, J. D., Chen, C., Rivolta, I., Abriel, H., Malhotra, R., Mattei, L. N., et al. (2001). Characterization of sodium channel alpha- and beta-subunits in rat and mouse cardiac myocytes. *Circulation* 103, 1303–1310. doi: 10.1161/01.CIR.103.9.1303

Malhotra, J. D., Kazen-Gillespie, K., Hortsch, M., and Isom, L. L. (2000). Sodium channel β subunits mediate homophilic cell adhesion and recruit ankyrin to points of cell-cell contact. *J. Biol. Chem.* 275, 11383–11388. doi: 10.1074/jbc.275.15.11383

Malhotra, J. D., Koopmann, M. C., Kazen-Gillespie, K. A., Fettman, N., Hortsch, M., and Isom, L. L. (2002). Structural requirements for interaction of sodium channel beta 1 subunits with ankyrin. *J. Biol. Chem.* 277, 26681–26688. doi: 10.1074/jbc.M202354200

Malhotra, J. D., Thyagarajan, V., Chen, C., and Isom, L. L. (2004). Tyrosine-phosphorylated and nonphosphorylated sodium channel β1 subunits are differentially localized in cardiac myocytes. *J. Biol. Chem.* 279, 40748–40754. doi: 10.1074/jbc.M407243200

Marionneau, C., Carrasquillo, Y., Norris, A. J., Townsend, R. R., Isom, L. L., Link, A. J., et al. (2012). The sodium channel accessory subunit Navβ1 regulates neuronal excitability through modulation of repolarizing voltage-gated K^+ channels. *J. Neurosci.* 32, 5716–5727. doi: 10.1523/JNEUROSCI.6450-11.2012

Matamoros, M., Perez-Hernández, M., Guerrero-Serna, G., Amorós, I., Barana, A., Núñez, M., et al. (2016). Nav1.5 N-terminal domain binding to α1-syntrophin increases membrane density of human Kir2.1, Kir2.2 and Nav1.5 channels. *Cardiovasc. Res.* 110, 279–290. doi: 10.1093/cvr/cvw009

Matsumoto, M., Fujikawa, A., Suzuki, R., Shimizu, H., Kuboyama, K., Hiyama, T. Y., et al. (2012). SAP97 promotes the stability of Nax channels at the plasma membrane. *FEBS Lett.* 586, 3805–3812. doi: 10.1016/j.febslet.2012.09.018

McCormick, K. A., Isom, L. L., Ragsdale, D., Smith, D., Scheuer, T., and Catterall, W. A. (1998). Molecular determinants of Na+ channel function in the extracellular domain of the beta1 subunit. *J. Biol. Chem.* 273, 3954–3962. doi: 10.1074/jbc.273.7.3954

McEwen, D. P., Meadows, L. S., Chen, C., Thyagarajan, V., and Isom, L. L. (2004). Sodium channel β1 subunit-mediated modulation of Nav1.2 currents and Cell surface density is dependent on interactions with contactin and ankyrin. *J. Biol. Chem.* 279, 16044–16049. doi: 10.1074/jbc.M400856200

Meadows, L., Malhotra, J. D., Stetzer, a, Isom, L. L., and Ragsdale, D. S. (2001). The intracellular segment of the sodium channel beta 1 subunit is required for its efficient association with the channel alpha subunit. *J. Neurochem.* 76, 1871–1878. doi: 10.1046/j.1471-4159.2001.00192.x

Mercier, A., Clément, R., Harnois, T., Bourmeyster, N., Faivre, J. F., Findlay, I., et al. (2012). The β1-Subunit of Nav1.5 Cardiac Sodium Channel Is Required for a Dominant Negative Effect through α-α Interaction. *PLoS ONE* 7:e48690. doi: 10.1371/journal.pone.0048690

Mohler, P. J., Rivolta, I., Napolitano, C., LeMaillet, G., Lambert, S., Priori, S. G., et al. (2004). Nav1.5 E1053K mutation causing Brugada syndrome blocks binding to ankyrin-G and expression of Nav1.5 on the surface of cardiomyocytes. *Proc. Natl. Acad. Sci.U.S.A.* 101, 17533–17538. doi: 10.1073/pnas.0403711101

Morgan, K., Stevens, E. B., Shah, B., Cox, P. J., Dixon, A. K., Lee, K., et al. (2000). Beta 3: an additional auxiliary subunit of the voltage-sensitive sodium channel that modulates channel gating with distinct kinetics. *Proc. Natl. Acad. Sci. U.S.A.* 97, 2308–2313. doi: 10.1073/pnas.030362197

Nelson, M., Millican-Slater, R., Forrest, L. C., and Brackenbury, W. J. (2014). The sodium channel β1 subunit mediates outgrowth of neurite-like processes on breast cancer cells and promotes tumour growth and metastasis. *Int. J. Cancer* 135, 2338–2351. doi: 10.1002/ijc.28890

Nerbonne, J. M., and Kass, R. S. (2005). Molecular physiology of cardiac repolarization. *Physiol. Rev.* 85, 1205–1253. doi: 10.1152/physrev.00002.2005

Neubauer, J., Rougier, J.-S., Abriel, H., and Haas, C. (in press). Functional implications of a rare variant in the sodium channel β1B subunit (SCN1B) in a five-month old male sudden infant death syndrome (SIDS) case. *Heart. Case Rep.* doi: 10.1016/j.hrcr.2018.01.010

Nguyen, H. M., Miyazaki, H., Hoshi, N., Smith, B. J., Nukina, N., Goldin, A. L., et al. (2012). Modulation of voltage-gated K+ channels by the sodium channel β1 subunit. *Proc. Natl. Acad. Sci. U.S.A.* 109, 18577–18582. doi: 10.1073/pnas.1209142109

Nobili, L., Proserpio, P., Rubboli, G. B., Montano, N. C., Didato, G., D., and Tassinari, C. (2011). Sudden unexpected death in epilepsy (SUDEP) and sleep. *Sleep Med. Rev.* 15, 237–246. doi: 10.1016/j.smrv.2010.07.006

O'Malley, H. A., and Isom, L. L. (2015). Sodium channel β subunits: emerging targets in channelopathies. *Annu. Rev. Physiol.* 77, 481–504. doi: 10.1146/annurev-physiol-021014-071846

Ogiwara, I., Nakayama, T., Yamagata, T., Ohtani, H., Mazaki, E., Tsuchiya, S., et al. (2012). A homozygous mutation of voltage-gated sodium channel beta(I) gene SCN1B in a patient with Dravet syndrome. *Epilepsia* 53, e200–e203. doi: 10.1111/epi.12040

Orrico, A., Galli, L., Grosso, S., Buoni, S., Pianigiani, R., Balestri, P., et al. (2009). Mutational analysis of the SCN1A, SCN1B and GABRG2 genes in 150 Italian patients with idiopathic childhood epilepsies. *Clin. Genet.* 75, 579–581. doi: 10.1111/j.1399-0004.2009.01155.x

Palatinus, J. A., O'Quinn, M. P., Barker, R. J., Harris, B. S., Jourdan, J., and Gourdie, R. G. (2010). ZO-1 determines adherens and gap junction localization at intercalated disks. *Am. J. Physiol. Heart. Circ. Physiol.* 300, H583–H594. doi: 10.1152/ajpheart.00999.2010

Patino, G. A., Brackenbury, W. J., Bao, Y., Lopez-Santiago, L. F., O'Malley, H. A., Chen, C., et al. (2011). Voltage-gated Na+ channel beta1B: a secreted cell adhesion molecule involved in human epilepsy. *J. Neurosci.* 31, 14577–14591. doi: 10.1523/JNEUROSCI.0361-11.2011

Patino, G. A., Claes, L. R. F., Lopez-Santiago, L. F., Slat, E. A., Dondeti, R. S. R., Chen, C., et al. (2009). A functional null mutation of SCN1B in a patient with Dravet Syndrome. *J. Neurosci.* 29, 10764–10778. doi: 10.1523/JNEUROSCI.2475-09.2009

Petitprez, S., Zmoos, A. F., Ogrodnik, J., Balse, E., Raad, N., El-Haou, S., et al. (2011). SAP97 and dystrophin macromolecular complexes determine two pools of cardiac sodium channels Nav1.5 in cardiomyocytes. *Circ. Res.* 108, 294–304. doi: 10.1161/CIRCRESAHA.110.228312

Qu, Y., Isom, L. L., Westenbroek, R. E., Rogers, J. C., Tanada, T. N., McCormick, K. A., et al. (1995). Modulation of cardiac Na+ channel expression in Xenopus oocytes by beta 1 subunits. *J. Biol. Chem.* 270, 25696–25701. doi: 10.1074/jbc.270.43.25696

Ramadan, W., Patel, N., Anazi, S., Kentab, A. Y., Bashiri, F. A., Hamad, M. H., et al. (2017). Confirming the recessive inheritance of SCN1B mutations in developmental epileptic encephalopathy. *Clin. Genet.* 92, 327–331. doi: 10.1111/cge.12999

Ravindran, K., Powell, K. L., Todaro, M., and O'Brien, T. J. (2016). The pathophysiology of cardiac dysfunction in epilepsy. *Epilepsy Res.* 127, 19–29. doi: 10.1016/j.eplepsyres.2016.08.007

Rhett, J. M., Jourdan, J., and Gourdie, R. G. (2011). Connexin 43 connexon to gap junction transition is regulated by zonula occludens-1. *Mol. Biol. Cell* 22, 1516–1528. doi: 10.1091/mbc.E10-06-0548

Rhett, J. M., Ongstad, E. L., Jourdan, J., and Gourdie, R. G. (2012). Cx43 associates with Nav1.5 in the cardiomyocyte perinexus. *J. Membr. Biol.* 245, 411–422. doi: 10.1007/s00232-012-9465-z

Rhett, J. M., Veeraraghavan, R., Poelzing, S., and Gourdie, R. G. (2013). The perinexus: Sign-post on the path to a new model of cardiac conduction? *Trends Cardiovasc. Med.* 23, 222–228. doi: 10.1016/j.tcm.2012.12.005

Riuró, H., Campuzano, O., Arbelo, E., Iglesias, A., Batlle, M., Pérez-Villa, F., et al. (2014). A missense mutation in the sodium channel β1b subunit reveals SCN1B as a susceptibility gene underlying long QT syndrome. *Heart Rhythm* 11, 1202–1209. doi: 10.1016/j.hrthm.2014.03.044

Rogart, R. B., Cribbs, L. L., Muglia, L. K., Kephart, D. D., and Kaiser, M. W. (1989). molecular cloning of a putative tetrodotoxin-resistant rat heart Na+ channel isoform. *Proc. Natl. Acad. Sci. U.S.A.* 86, 8170–8174. doi: 10.1073/pnas.86.20.8170

Rougier, J.-S., van Bemmelen, M. X., Bruce, M. C., Jespersen, T., Gavillet, B., Apothéloz, F., et al. (2005). Molecular determinants of voltage-gated sodium channel regulation by the Nedd4/Nedd4-like proteins. *Am. J. Physiol. Cell Physiol.* 288, C692–C701. doi: 10.1152/ajpcell.00460.2004

Satin, J., Kyle, J. W., Chen, M., Bell, P., Cribbs, L. L., Fozzard, H. A., et al. (1992). A mutant of TTX-resistant cardiac sodium channels with TTX-sensitive properties. *Science* 256, 1202–1205. doi: 10.1126/science.256.5060.1202

Scheffer, I. E., Harkin, L. A., Grinton, B. E., Dibbens, L. M., Turner, S. J., Zielinski, M. A., et al. (2006). Temporal lobe epilepsy and GEFS+ phenotypes associated with SCN1B mutations. *Brain* 130, 100–109. doi: 10.1093/brain/awl272

Shy, D., Gillet, L., and Abriel, H. (2013). Cardiac sodium channel NaV1.5 distribution in myocytes via interacting proteins: the multiple pool model. *Biochim. Biophys. Acta* 1833, 886–894. doi: 10.1016/j.bbamcr.2012.10.026

Shy, D., Gillet, L., Ogrodnik, J., Albesa, M., Verkerk, A. O., Wolswinkel, R., et al. (2014). PDZ domain-binding motif regulates cardiomyocyte compartment-specific navl.5 channel expression and function. *Circulation* 130, 147–160. doi: 10.1161/CIRCULATIONAHA.113.007852

Snyders, D. J. (1999). Structure and function of cardiac potassium channels. *Cardiovasc. Res.* 42, 377–390. doi: 10.1016/S0008-6363(99)00071-1

Sreedhar, R., Arumugam, S., Thandavarayan, R. A., Giridharan, V. V., Karuppagounder, V., Pitchaimani, V., et al. (2016). Depletion of cardiac 14-3-3η protein adversely influences pathologic cardiac remodeling during myocardial infarction after coronary artery ligation in mice. *Int. J. Cardiol.* 202, 146–153. doi: 10.1016/j.ijcard.2015.08.142

Srinivasan, J., Schachner, M., and Catterall, W., a. (1998). Interaction of voltage-gated sodium channels with the extracellular matrix molecules tenascin-C and tenascin-R. *Proc. Natl. Acad. Sci. U.S.A.* 95, 15753–15757. doi: 10.1073/pnas.95.26.15753

Tan, H. L., Kupershmidt, S., Zhang, R., Stepanovic, S., Roden, D. M., Wilde, A. A. M., et al., (2002). A calcium sensor in the sodium channel modulates cardiac excitability. *Nature* 415, 442–447. doi: 10.1038/415442a

Undrovinas, A. I., Shander, G. S., and Makielski, J. C. (1995). Cytoskeleton modulates gating of voltage-dependent sodium channel in heart. *Am. J. Physiol.* 269, H203–H214. doi: 10.1152/ajpheart.1995.269.1.H203

Vaidyanathan, R., Vega, A. L., Song, C., Zhou, Q., Tan, B., Berger, S., et al. (2013). The interaction of caveolin 3 protein with the potassium inward rectifier channel Kir2.1: physiology and pathology related to long QT syndrome 9 (LQT9). *J. Biol. Chem.* 288, 17472–17480. doi: 10.1074/jbc.M112.435370

Van Bemmelen, M. X., Rougier, J. S., Gavillet, B., Apothéloz, F., Daidié, D., Tateyama, M., et al. (2004). Cardiac voltage-gated sodium channel Nav1.5 is regulated by Nedd4-2 mediated ubiquitination. *Circ. Res.* 95, 284–291. doi: 10.1161/01.RES.0000136816.05109.89

Veeraraghavan, R., Hoeker, G. S., Poelzing, S., and Gourdie, R. G. (2016). Abstract 13129: Acute Inhibition of Sodium Channel Beta Subunit (β1) -mediated Adhesion is Highly Proarrhythmic. *Circulation* 134, A13129 LP-A13129.

Vermij, S. H., Abriel, H., and van Veen, T. A. B. (2017). Refining the molecular organization of the cardiac intercalated disc. *Cardiovasc. Res.* 113, 259–275. doi: 10.1093/cvr/cvw259

Vreeker, A., van Stuijvenberg, L., Hund, T. J., Mohler, P. J., Nikkels, P. G. J., and van Veen, T. A. B. (2014). Assembly of the cardiac intercalated disk during pre- and postnatal development of the human heart. *PLoS ONE* 9:e94722. doi: 10.1371/journal.pone.0094722

Wallace, R. H., Wang, D. W., Singh, R., Scheffer, I. E., George, A. L., Phillips, H. et al. (1998). Febrile seizures and generalized epilepsy associated with a mutation in the Na+-channel betal subunit gene SCN1B. *Nat. Genet.* 19, 366–370. doi: 10.1038/1252

Watanabe, H., Darbar, D., Kaiser, D. W., Jiramongkolchai, K., Chopra, S., Donahue, B. S., et al. (2009). Mutations in sodium channel β1- and β2-subunits associated with atrial fibrillation. *Circ. Arrhythm. Electrophysiol.* 2, 268–275. doi: 10.1161/CIRCEP.108.779181

Watanabe, H., Koopmann, T. T., Scouarnec, S., Le, Y. T., Ingram, C. R., Schott, J., et al. (2008). Sodium channel β1 subunit mutations associated with Brugada syndrome and cardiac conduction disease in humans. *Structure* 118, 268–275. doi: 10.1172/JCI33891

Wong, H. K., Sakurai, T., Oyama, F., Kaneko, K., Wada, K., Miyazaki, H., et al. (2005). β subunits of voltage-gated sodium channels are novel substrates of β-site amyloid precursor protein-cleaving enzyme (BACE1) and γ-secretase. *J. Biol. Chem.* 280, 23009–23017. doi: 10.1074/jbc.M414648200

Xiao, Z. C., Ragsdale, D. S., Malhotra, J. D., Mattei, L. N., Braun, P. E., Schachner, M., et al. (1999). Tenascin-R is a functional modulator of sodium channel β subunits. *J. Biol. Chem.* 274, 26511–26517. doi: 10.1074/jbc.274.37.26511

Yang, Y., Ogawa, Y., Hedstrom, K. L., and Rasband, M. N. (2007). βIV spectrin is recruited to axon initial segments and nodes of Ranvier by ankyrinG. *J. Cell Biol.* 176, 509–519. doi: 10.1083/jcb.200610128

Yereddi, N. R., Cusdin, F. S., Namadurai, S., Packman, L. C., Monie, T. P., Slavny, P., et al. (2013). The immunoglobulin domain of the sodium channel β3 subunit contains a surface-localized disulfide bond that is required for homophilic binding. *FASEB J.* 27, 568–580. doi: 10.1096/fj.12-209445

Young, K. A., and Caldwell, J. H. (2005). Modulation of skeletal and cardiac voltage-gated sodium channels by calmodulin. *J. Physiol.* 565, 349–370. doi: 10.1113/jphysiol.2004.081422

Zaidi, A., Clough, P., Cooper, P., Scheepers, B., and Fitzpatrick, A. P. (2000). Misdiagnosis of epilepsy: many seizure-like attacks have a cardiovascular cause. *J. Am. Coll. Cardiol.* 36, 181–184. doi: 10.1016/S0735-1097(00)00700-2

Zhu, W., Voelker, T. L., Varga, Z., Schubert, A. R., Nerbonne, J. M., and Silva, J. R. (2017). Mechanisms of noncovalent β subunit regulation of Na $_V$ channel gating. *J. Gen. Physiol.* 149, 813–831. doi: 10.1085/jgp.201711802

19

Cx43 Isoform GJA1-20k Promotes Microtubule Dependent Mitochondrial Transport

Ying Fu [1†], *Shan-Shan Zhang* [1†], *Shaohua Xiao* [1†], *Wassim A. Basheer* [1], *Rachel Baum* [1], *Irina Epifantseva* [1], *TingTing Hong* [1,2] and *Robin M. Shaw* [1,2*]

[1] Cedars-Sinai Medical Center, Cedars-Sinai Heart Institute, Los Angeles, CA, United States, [2] Department of Medicine, University of California, Los Angeles, Los Angeles, CA, United States

***Correspondence:**
Robin M. Shaw
robin.shaw@cshs.org

† These authors have contributed equally to this work.

Connexin 43 (Cx43, encoded by *GJA1*) is a cell-cell communication gap junction protein expressed in all organ systems. It was recently found that *GJA1* mRNA undergoes alternative translation to generate N-terminal truncated isoforms, of which GJA1-20k is the most abundant. Here we report a surprising finding that, unlike full length GJA1-43k, GJA1-20k has a strong tropism for mitochondria. Exploring function, we found that GJA1-20k appears to be an organelle chaperone and that overexpression of GJA1-20k is sufficient to rescue mitochondrial localization to the cell periphery upon exposure to hydrogen peroxide, which effectively limits the network fragmentation that occurs with oxidative stress. By high-resolution fluorescent imaging and electron microscopy, we determined that GJA1-20k is enriched at the interface between mitochondria and microtubules, appearing to load organelles for transport. Mutagenesis experiments revealed that although the microtubule-binding domain (MTBD) in GJA1-20k is not necessary for protein localization to mitochondria, the MTBD is essential for GJA1-20k to facilitate mitochondrial transport and maintain mitochondrial localization at the periphery. These results reveal an unexpected role for the alternatively translated isoform of the Cx43 gap junction protein, GJA1-20k, which is to facilitate microtubule-based mitochondrial transport and to maintain mitochondrial network integrity during cellular stress.

Keywords: gap junction protein, Cx43, alternative translation, mitochondria, microtubule, oxidative stress

INTRODUCTION

Connexin 43 (Cx43) is the most widely expressed of the 21 human connexins, occurring in all organ systems and is best recognized as a cell-cell communication protein (Beyer et al., 1987). Alternations of Cx43 expression and function are associated with numerous diseases including cardiac arrhythmias (Luke and Saffitz, 1991; Smith et al., 1991; Beardslee et al., 1998), cancer (Solan et al., 2012), ischemic injury (Beardslee et al., 2000), connective tissue disease (Paznekas et al., 2003), and heart failure (Akar et al., 2007; Basheer and Shaw, 2016). The mechanistic relationship between a cell-cell coupling protein and most non-arrhythmic diseases is not well understood.

Human Cx43 is encoded by the *GJA1* gene in which the entire coding sequence is within the second exon (Fishman et al., 1991). Thus, *GJA1* cannot produce different protein isoforms via alternative splicing. It was recently found that ribosomal translation initiating at internal AUG start codons within the mRNA coding sequence, commonly known as alternative translation, generates multiple endogenous carboxyl-terminal (C-terminal) segments of Cx43 protein. These products of alternative translation are N-terminal truncations of the full length Cx43 protein. Alternative translation of *GJA1* occurs widely in cell lines (Smyth and Shaw, 2013; Salat-Canela et al., 2014), primary cells (Salat-Canela et al., 2014; Ul-Hussain et al., 2014), and human heart (Smyth and Shaw, 2013). Mammalian target of rapamycin (mTOR) and MAP kinase-interacting serine/threonine-protein kinases 1/2 (Mnkl/2) signaling pathways (Smyth and Shaw, 2013; Salat-Canela et al., 2014) have been found to regulate alternative translation and inhibition of either mTOR or Mnkl/2 increases expression of the truncated isoforms (Smyth and Shaw, 2013; Salat-Canela et al., 2014). Pathway dependence implies alternative translation of *GJA1* can be turned on or off, depending on metabolic condition. Hypoxic stress is another condition that induces endogenous expression of the smaller isoforms (Ul-Hussain et al., 2014).

The role of the smaller alternatively translated isoforms of GJA1 is largely unknown. Of the isoforms, GJA1-20k is commonly the most highly expressed (Smyth and Shaw, 2013; Salat-Canela et al., 2014; Ul-Hussain et al., 2014). We have previously reported that GJA1-20k occurs in endoplasmic reticulum and aids full length Cx43 trafficking to cell-cell borders (Smyth and Shaw, 2013; Basheer et al., 2017), indicating that GJA1-20k can act as a chaperone in forward trafficking.

In this study, we report the surprising finding that in additional to full length Cx43 trafficking, GJA1-20k also targets to mitochondria. Furthermore, upon H_2O_2-induced stress, GJA1-20k but not full-length Cx43 is sufficient to preserve localization of mitochondria at the cell periphery. Using electron microscopy, we identified GJA1-20k at the mitochondria and the interface between microtubules and mitochondria, appearing to load mitochondria for transport. Mutagenesis experiments reveal that the previously identified tubulin-binding domain in GJA1-20k (Saidi Brikci-Nigassa et al., 2012) is not required for its mitochondrial localization but is essential for rescue of mitochondrial network integrity upon H_2O_2 treatment. In addition, under control conditions, GJA1-20k promotes microtubule-based mitochondrial transport, which is lost when the tubulin-interacting residues are removed. Taken together, these findings introduce the alternatively translated GJA1-20k isoform of the traditional Cx43 gap junction protein as a regulator of microtubule-based mitochondrial transport, which protects the organelle network during stress.

MATERIALS AND METHODS

Molecular Biology

Human *GJA1* cDNAs (Open Biosystems) encoding full-length Cx43 and small isoforms were first cloned into pDONR/221 to generate Gateway entry clones (Thermo Fisher Scientific) as previously described. Destination vectors (pDEST) encoding C-terminal GFP-, mCherry-, and HA-tagged proteins were subsequently made for mammalian cell expression. All constructs are driven by the cytomegalovirus (CMV) promoter, and contain internal methionine start sites mutagenized to leucine to ensure single isoform expression. Mutagenesis was carried out with the Quick Change Lightning Mutagenesis Kit (Agilent) according to manufacturer's instructions. Mutagenesis primers used to remove all six tubulin-interacting residues (Saidi Brikci-Nigassa et al., 2012) in GJA1-20k-del6 are: 5′ AAG GGC GTT AAG GAT AAG GGA AAG AGC GAC CCT AGT GGT GCG CTG AGC 3′, and 5′ GCT CAG CGC ACC ACT AGG GTC GCT CTT TCC CTT ATC CTT AAC GCC CTT 3′. The mito-BFP plasmid was a gift from Dr. Gia Voeltz (Addgene plasmid # 49151).

Cell Lines and Primary Cell Isolation

HeLa, HaCaT, and HEK293T cell lines (ATCC) were maintained at 37°C in a humidified atmosphere of 5% CO_2 in fully supplemented media containing DMEM with 10% fetal bovine serum (FBS), nonessential amino acids, sodium pyruvate (Thermo Fisher Scientific), and Mycozap-CL (Lonza). Primary cardiac fibroblasts were isolated from neonatal mouse hearts as described (Zhang et al., 2014). Fibroblasts adhering to the dish during the pre-plating step were enriched for 1 week in DMEM:F12 supplemented with 3.5% FBS and 1x Mycozap-PR (Lonza). Primary glial cells were isolated from neonatal mouse brains as previously described (He et al., 2007; Habas et al., 2013).

Biochemistry

Co-immunoprecipitation was carried out using HeLa cells expressing HA-tagged GJA1-20k. Cytoskeletal-protein interactions were stabilized by the addition of phalloidin (25 μM, Sigma-Aldrich) during cell lysis in 0.5% NP40 buffer (in mM, 150 KCl, 20 HEPES, 2 $MgCl_2$, 2 K_2HPO_4, 1 DTT, 1 NaF, 0.1 Na_3VO_4, 0.5% NP40, pH7.4 with halt protease inhibitor). Cells were rotated for 30 min and spun down at 10,000 × g for 20 min at 4°C to remove insoluble debris. Following protein normalization, cell lysates were precleared using Dynabeads protein G (Thermo Fisher Scientific) for 30 min with rotation at 4°C. Beads were discarded, and 2 mg of precleared lysate was used for each reaction. Immunoprecipitation was undertaken using 5 μg of either mouse anti-HA (4C12, Abcam), or mouse anti-GST (B-14, Santa-Cruz Biotechnology) as negative isotype control at 4°C for 4 h with rotation. Dynabeads protein G (20 μl) was added to each reaction, and the tubes were rotated for an additional 45 min at room temperature. Protein complexes were washed 3 times with lysis buffer using a Dynamag-2 magnet. Proteins were then eluted with 30 μl 2X NuPAGE sample buffer containing 100 mM DTT, incubated at 37° for 20 min, and subjected to SDS-PAGE electrophoresis and Western blotting. Membranes were imaged using the ChemiDoc MP detection system (Bio-Rad). The experiments were repeated three times.

Mitochondrial Fractionation

Mitochondria fractionation of HeLa cells transfected with HA-tagged GJA1-43k or GJA1-20k, was performed as previously described (Singh et al., 2012). Cells were manually homogenized

Abbreviations: mRNA, messenger RNA; C-terminal, carboxyl-terminal; ER, endoplasmic reticulum; PDI, protein disulfide-isomerase; TMRM, indicator tetramethylrhodamine methyl ester; Tom20, translocase of outer membrane 20; TEM, transmission electron microscopy; NMR, nuclear magnetic resonance; MTBD, microtubule-binding domain; H_2O_2, hydrogen peroxide; Noc, nocodazole; DMSO, dimethyl sulfoxide.

in isolation buffer A with BSA (mM): 230 mannitol, 70 sucrose, 10 HEPES, 2 EDTA pH 7.2 with KOH, and 1 mg/mL fatty acid free BSA using a Potter Elvehjem homogenizer (Sigma-Aldrich). Homogenates were centrifuged at 1,300 × g for 3 min at 4°C. The resulting supernatants were collected and centrifuged at 10,000 × g for 10 min at 4°C. The supernatant fraction (F0) was saved for Western blotting. Pellets containing crude mitochondria were overlaid on 30% (v/v) Percoll (Sigma-Aldrich) in buffer B (mM): 250 sucrose, 10 HEPES-Na, 1 EDTA-Na_2, pH 7.4. Samples were centrifuged (Optima MAX-XP, Beckman Coulter) in a fixed angle rotor at 50,000 × g at 4°C for 45 min. After ultracentrifugation, three fractions were collected and labeled as F1, F2, and F3 from cell samples. Fractions were pelleted at 12,000 × g for 5 min at 4°C for Western blotting. Three independent experiments were conducted and the representative blots were shown.

Confocal Fixed and Live-Cell Imaging

Images were acquired using a Nikon Eclipse T*i* imaging system with a ×100/1.49 Apo TIRF or a x20/0.75 Plan Apo objective, a spinning disk confocal unit (Yokogowa CSU-X1) with 486, 561, and 647-nm diode-pumped solid state lasers, and an ORCA-Flash 4.0 Hamamatsu camera (C11440), controlled by NIS Elements software. Live cell imaging was carried out in transiently transfected HeLa cells as previously described (Zhang et al., 2014). Glass-bottomed dishes were coated with human fibronectin (10 µg/ml, Corning) and 0.1% gelatin (Sigma-Aldrich). Cells were grown on these dishes at 37°C in a humidified atmosphere of 5% CO_2 in fully supplemented media. Cells were cotransfected with fluorescently tagged GJA1 isoforms and mito-BFP using Lipofectamine 2000 according to manufacture's instructions (Thermo Fisher Scientific). At 16–24 h post transfection, cells were immersed in imaging solution containing HBSS supplemented with 10% FBS, and 1x Mycozap-CL. Images were acquired at 37°C using our Nikon Eclipse T*i* imaging system described above. Active mitochondria were labeled by loading cells for 30 min with imaging solution containing 2.5 µM TMRM (Thermo Fisher Scientific). Pearson's coefficient was calculated using the ImageJ JACoP plugin (Bolte and Cordelières, 2006). Three independent experiments were conducted and 5-10 cells were imaged from each experiment.

H_2O_2 Treatment and Mitochondrial Analysis

HeLa cells were plated on coated glass-bottom dishes and transfected with the following plasmids: GST-GFP, GJA1-43k-GFP, and GJA1-20k-GFP. At 24 h post transfection, samples were treated with 300 µM H_2O_2 (Sigma-Aldrich) or PBS in fully supplemented medium for 4 h. Cells were fixed in 4% PFA (Electron Microscopy Services) in PBS for 20 min at RT. Immunolabeling: rabbit anti-Tom20 (1:100, Santa Cruz Biotechnology) and chicken anti-GFP (1:500, Abcam). Alexa Fluors (Thermo Fisher Scientific) were used for secondary antibody detection for 1 h at RT. ProLong Gold Antifade containing DAPI was used to mount samples. Using ImageJ (NIH), the peripheral/central fluorescence ratio was determined by dividing peripheral Tom20 signal by that of the perinuclear and Golgi regions. First, each image is background-subtracted using a rolling ball radius of 50 pixels. Thresholding for the inner region of interest (ROI) encompassing the nucleus was set based on 1/6 of the maximal Tom20 intensity of the entire cell. Signal from the nuclear ROI was removed from the cell. The middle ROI (perinuclear/Golgi) boundary was set by expanding the inner ROI by 4 micrometers. Finally, signal density from the remaining outer ROI (periphery) is divided by the sum of that of the inner and middle ROIs to obtain the ratio (Figure S10). Percentages of cells with connected mitochondria were determined by scoring blinded datasets of immunolabeled Tom20 signal from at least 4 experimental replicates.

Electron Microscopy

HeLa cells were transfected with GST-GFP or GJA1-20k-GFP plasmids as described above. Cells were fixed in 2% glutaraldehyde in PBS at RT for 10 min, scraped, and pelleted by centrifugation at 4,200 × g followed by 16,000 × g. Pellets were fixed for 2 additional hours, and then post fixed with 1% osmium tetroxide followed by incubation with 3% uranyl acetate. Samples were dehydrated in ethanol, treated with propylene oxide, embedded in Spurr resin (Electron Microscopy Services), and sectioned using an ultramicrotome (UCT, Leica). Sections were then mounted on EM grids and stained with uranyl acetate and lead citrate. Images were acquired using the JEM1200-EX, JEOL microscope equipped with a digital camera (BioScan 600W, Gatan). For immunogold labeling, cells were fixed in 4% formaldehyde and 0.1% glutaraldehyde in PBS at RT for 10 min, scraped, and pelleted as described above. Cells were fixed overnight at 4°C in 4% formaldehyde and 0.1% glutaraldehyde in PBS and thereafter mixed with 1.5% low melting temperature agarose. Small pieces of agarose with embedded cells were incubated overnight in 1.85 M sucrose/20% PVP-10/50 mM Hepes pH 7.4. Each piece was mounted on an aluminum pin and snap frozen in liquid nitrogen. Ultra-thin sections were prepared using a cryo-ultramicrotome (UC6, Leica) with an F6 cryo-attachment and a Diatome cryoimmuno (35°) diamond knife. The sections were incubated with rabbit anti-GFP primary antibody (1:200; Abcam) at 4°C overnight. The sections were then incubated with secondary antibody conjugated with 10 nm gold particles (1:20; Ted Pella) and imaged as described above. Electron microscopy work was done by the Electron Imaging Center at California NanoSystems Institute, University of California Los Angeles.

Tracking of Mitochondrial Movement

Live cell imaging was performed 24 h post transfection of GST-GFP, GJA1-20k-GFP, or GJA1-20k-del6-GFP together with mito-BFP. Fresh imaging solution, containing either 25 µM nocodazole (to disrupt microtubules) or 0.08% DMSO, was added to cells for 45 min prior to image acquisition. Mito-BFP signal was tracked every 5 s for 5 min. To determine mitochondrial velocity and displacement, the MTrackJ plugin (Meijering et al., 2012) for ImageJ (NIH) was used to track individual mitochondrion moving toward the cell tip within a 60 × 60 μm^2 ROI. Four separate experiments were performed.

Statistical Analysis

All quantitative data were expressed as mean ± SEM and analyzed using Prism 6 software (GraphPad). For comparison between two groups, unpaired two-tail Student's *t*-test was performed. For comparison among three and more groups, one-way ANOVA followed by either Tukey's or Bonferroni's post-hoc test was performed. For comparison between groups with or without H_2O_2 treatment, two-way ANOVA followed by Tukey's post-hoc test was performed. A *P* value of less than 0.05 was deemed statistically significant. For tracking data, histograms of mean velocities of each condition were used for nonlinear Gaussian fitting. Single Gaussian fitting generated the following coefficients of determination (R^2) to assess the goodness of fit: 0.93 (GST control), 0.95 (GST treated with nocodazole), 0.78 (GJA1-20k), and 0.85 (GJA1-20k-del6). Based on these values, data for GJA1-20k and GJA1-20k-del6 were fitted with the sum of two Gaussian distributions to yield R^2-values of 0.91 and 0.97, respectively.

RESULTS

GJA1-20k Is Localized Outside of the ER

In addition to the full-length Cx43 protein, endogenous GJA1-20k (see cartoon in Figure S1A) is highly expressed in primary cardiomyocytes and astrocytes, as well as many cell lines including cancer models (Smyth and Shaw, 2013; Salat-Canela et al., 2014; Ul-Hussain et al., 2014). We previously reported that GJA1-20k primarily localizes to the cytoplasm in reticular structures that correspond to ER/Golgi suggesting a role for GJA1-20k in the Cx43 vesicular transport pathway (Smyth and Shaw, 2013). In detailed confocal imaging of immunofluorescence of HeLa cells labeled with exogenous GJA1-20k-GFP, we also found GJA1-20k positive signal throughout the cell (Figure S1B, arrows). As seen in Figure S1C, there is localization of GJA1-20k-GFP (green) with the ER marker protein disulfide-isomerase (PDI, red) (Pearson's coefficient: $r = 0.722$). However, the more intense clusters do not appear to share ER localization. The larger GJA1-20k clusters either overlap with ER (arrowhead) or exist in shapes independent of ER (arrow). These results prompted us to determine the identity of the structures associated with GJA1-20k.

GJA1-20k Delineates the Mitochondrial Network

It is recognized that the ER is closely associated with mitochondrial network, participating in dynamic mitochondrial regulation (Friedman et al., 2011). Additionally, accumulating evidence has supported that full length Cx43 is associated with mitochondria (Boengler et al., 2005; Srisakuldee et al., 2014; Gadicherla et al., 2017). Therefore, we decided to examine the association of GJA1-20k with mitochondria. As seen in **Figure 1A**, while full-length Cx43 (upper panel) (GJA1-43k, with internal start sites mutated to produce only the full-length protein) only partially localizes with the mitochondrial marker mito-BFP (arrows), GJA1-20k strongly co-localizes with mito-BFP (middle panel) as well as with actively respiring mitochondria marked by the membrane potential indicator tetramethylrhodamine methyl ester (TMRM) (bottom panel). GJA1-20k localization is indistinguishable from that of the two mitochondrial markers and appears to function as a mitochondrial marker itself. To address the concern that a GFP tag may interfere with cellular localization of GJA1 isoforms, we took advantage of the previously characterized cervical carcinoma cell line, C33A, that expresses endogenous GJA1-20k (Salat-Canela et al., 2014). Using anti- C-terminal and N-terminal antibodies for Cx43, we can distinguish localization patterns between GJA1-43k (anti- N and C terminal Cx43 antibody positive) and smaller GJA1 isoforms (anti-C terminal Cx43 antibody positive only). As seem in Figure S2, it is primarily the anti C-terminal antibody which outlines mitochondria, indicating that alternatively translated GJA1-20k are preferentially localized to mitochondria, consistent with observation of exogenously expressed GFP-tagged protein. Furthermore, as seen in the same figure, localization of endogenous protein to mitochondria occurs in the peripheral cortex of the cell rather than in more central locations. The imaging data in Figure S2 confirm that even endogenous alternatively translated GJA1-20k preferentially localizes to mitochondria.

We then performed biochemical fractionation to confirm mitochondrial enrichment of GJA1-20k in transfected cells. As seen in **Figure 1B**, translocase of outer membrane 20 (Tom20) marks mitochondrial fraction and is substantially enriched in fractions F2 and F3. This is concurrent with a corresponding decrease in plasma membrane markers including Na^+/K^+-ATPase and N-cadherin. In addition to full length GJA1-43k, GJA1-20k protein is highly enriched in mitochondrial fractions F2 and F3, which supports the mitochondrial localization of GJA1-20k observed in immunofluorescence experiments (**Figure 1A**). These data indicate that in HeLa cells transfected GJA1-20k has a strong tropism to mitochondria and delineates the entire mitochondrial network.

Since both imaging and biochemical data support enrichment of GJA1-20k in mitochondria, we next sought to confirm that these findings are not restricted to HeLa cells. We obtained human keratinocytes (HaCaT), HEK293 cells, isolated primary neonatal mouse glial cells and cardiac fibroblasts. As seen in **Figure 1C**, mitochondrial expression of exogenous GJA1-20k is detected in all three types of cells. We have yet to identify cells in which GJA1-20k does not strongly localize to the mitochondrial network.

GJA1-20k Localizes to the Interface of Mitochondria and Microtubules

We have previously reported that GJA1-20k can organize the cytoskeleton trafficking pathways of Cx43 (Smyth and Shaw, 2013; Basheer et al., 2017), which occurs along microtubules (Giepmans et al., 2001; Lauf et al., 2002; Shaw et al., 2007). Microtubule-dependent transport has also been reported for organelles such as mitochondria (Chan, 2006; Wang and Schwarz, 2009; Tanaka et al., 2011). We are interested in the possibility of interaction between GJA1-20k and the

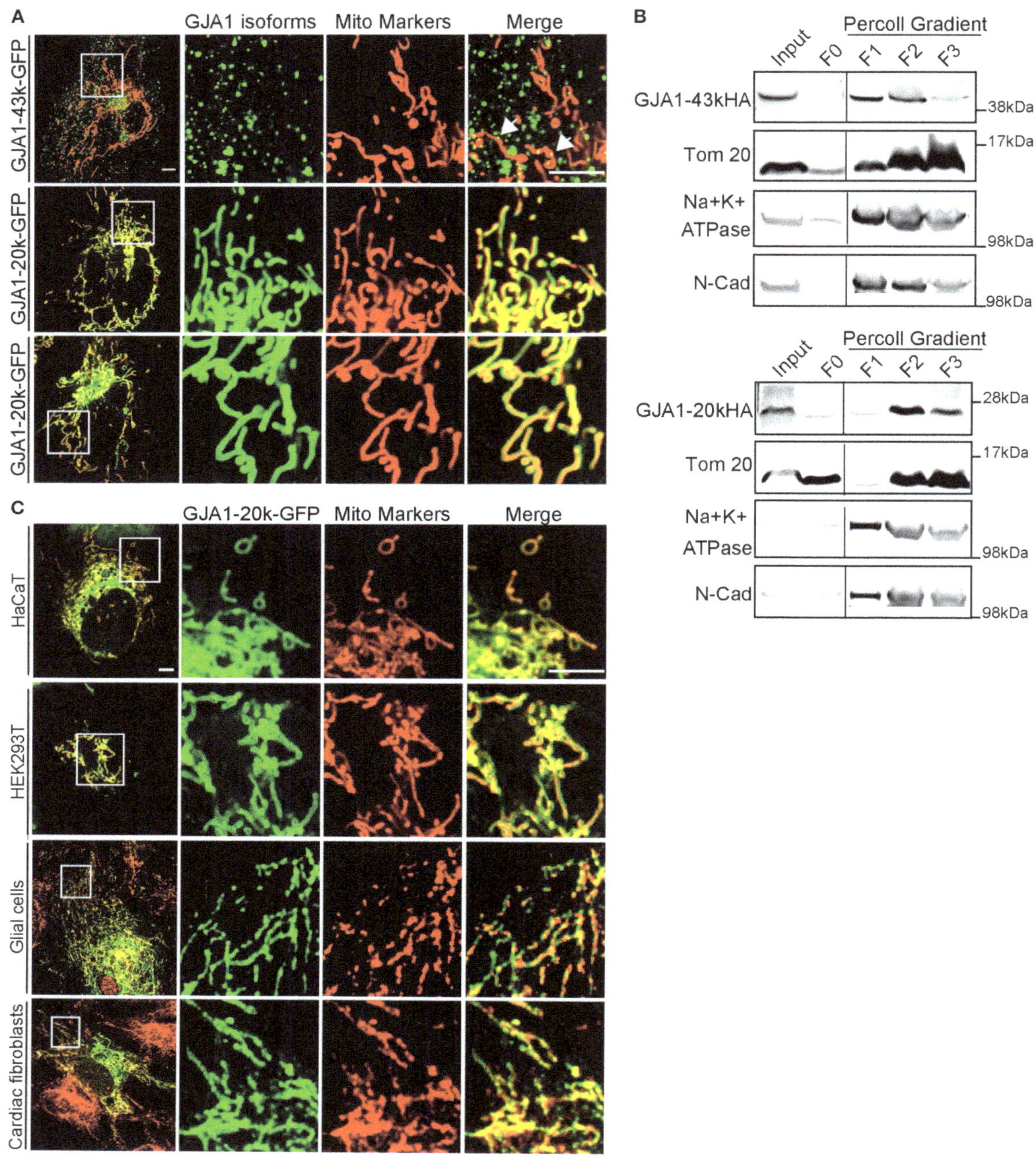

FIGURE 1 | GJA1-20k delineates the mitochondrial network. **(A)** Imaging of live HeLa cells expressing GFP-tagged GJA1-43k or GJA1-20k (green) and mitochondrial markers (red). GJA1-43k associates with mitochondria as small puncta (arrows). GJA1-20k colocalizes with mito-BFP (middle panel) and TMRM (bottom panel). Scale bar = 5 μm. **(B)** Relative enrichment of HA-tagged isoforms in total cell lysate (input), the cytosol supernatant (F0), and membrane fractions of crude mitochondrial pellet (F1–F3). Mitochondria (Tom20). Plasma membrane (Na^+K^+ATPase, N-cadherin). Full blots were in Figures S7, S8. **(C)** Live cell imaging of HaCat and HEK293T cells cotransfected with mito-BFP and GJA1-20k-GFP. Immunofluorescence of GFP and Tom20 in primary glial cells and cardiac fibroblasts transfected with GJA1-20k-GFP. Scale bar = 5 μm.

microtubule network in respect to mitochondrial transport. As seen in **Figure 2A**, we found positive co-immunoprecipitation between HA-tagged GJA1-20k and alpha-tubulin, indicating interaction between GJA1-20k and the microtubule highway. Next, using live-cell imaging, we identified that movements of mitochondria containing GJA1-20k signal, when recorded over 45 s, follow trajectories defined by microtubules (**Figures 2B,C** and Supplemental Video 1), indicating that microtubules might function as guides for GJA1-20k associated mitochondrial movement.

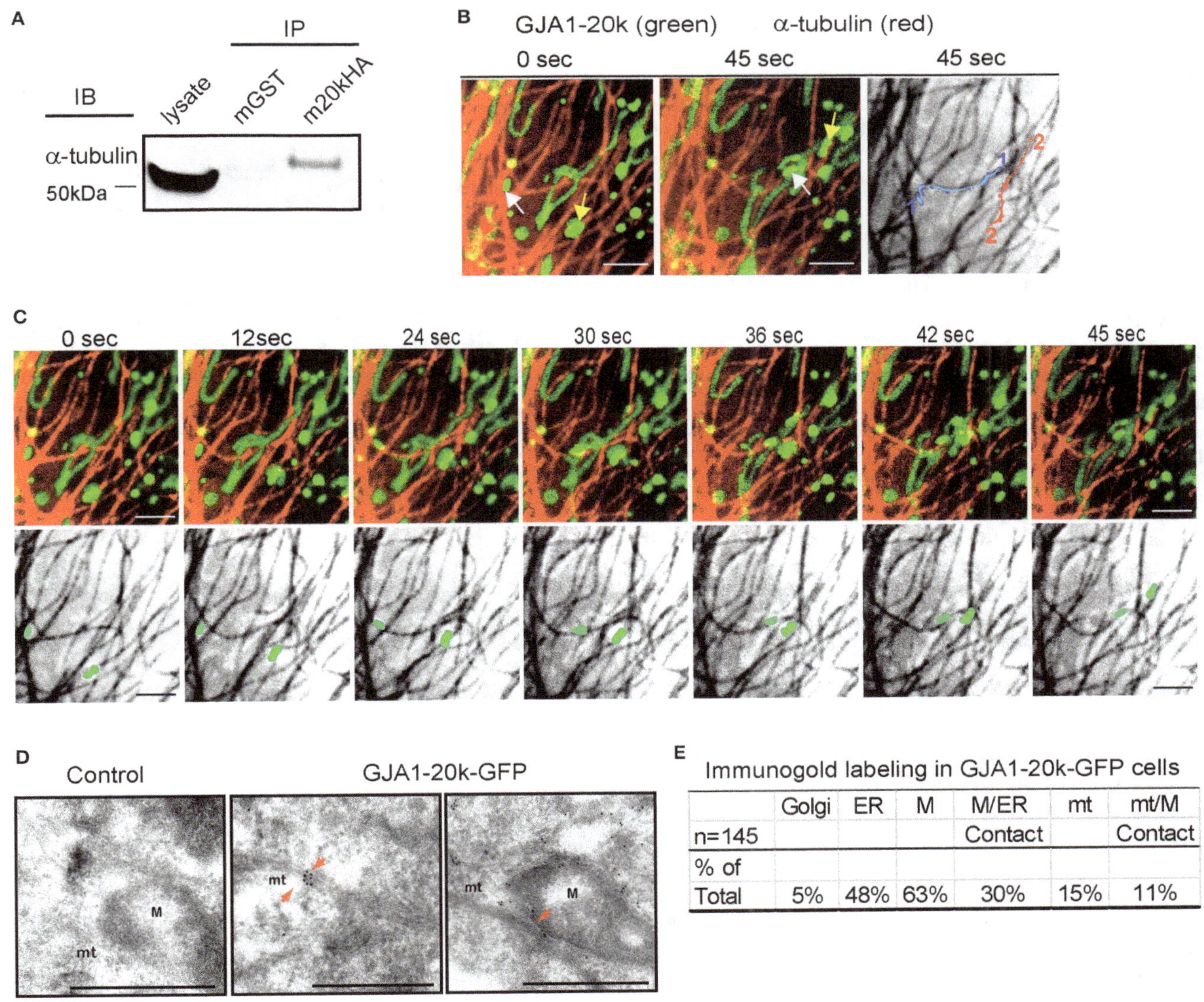

n=145	Golgi	ER	M	M/ER Contact	mt	mt/M Contact
% of Total	5%	48%	63%	30%	15%	11%

FIGURE 2 | GJA1-20k binds α-tubulin, targeting to the microtubule/mitochondria interface. **(A)** Coimmunoprecipitation between GJA1-20k-HA (IP) and α-tubulin (IB). Antibodies used for IP were labeled as mGST (mouse GST antibody) and m20kHA (mouse HA antibody). Full blot is in Figure S9. **(B)** Live-cell confocal of GJA1-20k-mCherry and α-tubulin-GFP in HeLa cells. Individual GJA1-20k tracks (45 s). **(C)** Time-lapse of merged and tubulin images with moving mitochondria. **(D)** TEM images of GJA1-20k-GFP (immunogold labeled for GFP) occurring along a microtubule bundle, a mitochondrion, and the interface between these structures (arrows) in HeLa cells. Non-transfected negative control (left panel). Microtubules (mt). Mitochondria (M). Scale bar = 500 nm. **(E)** The percent of total images (145) with positive immunogold labeling of each respective organelle is listed in the table. A total of 145 images with gold particles are analyzed.

If GJA1-20k facilitates mitochondrial interaction with microtubules, then its localization is expected to be enriched at points of interaction. The confocal live cell imaging clearly demonstrates that mitochondria follow microtubule tracks. However, live cell confocal imaging cannot provide sufficient detail on spatial localization of GJA1-20k GFP due to the resolution of confocal imaging, especially when projecting signals of the three-dimensional organelle to two-dimensional images. Therefore, we used transmission electron microscopy (TEM) together with immunogold labeling of exogenous GJA1-20k to explore in high resolution the spatial relationship among GJA1-20k, mitochondria, and microtubules. Consistent with the confocal imaging results, mitochondria in GJA1-20k-expressing cells are closely associated with microtubules, stretching along them (**Figure 2D**, and Figure S3). Moreover, immunogold labeling further confirmed that GJA1-20k targets to mitochondria. More than 60% of total immunogold positive images contain gold particle-labeled GJA1-20k in mitochondria (**Figure 2E**), which is further enriched at mitochondrial membrane. Not surprisingly, cellular organelles such as ER and Golgi were also identified by immunogold labeling in GJA1-20k transfected cells. Although only 15% (22) of all 145 images contain gold particle-labeled GJA1-20k at microtubules, the majority (16/22, 73%) of them are associated with mitochondria at the microtubule interface, which is within 0.1 micron of microtubules (**Figures 2D,E**). It appears that GJA1-20k helps to load the mitochondrion along the microtubule for transport. Together, the data in **Figure 2** provide biochemical, live-cell imaging, and TEM evidence in support of a role for GJA1-20k in microtubule-based mitochondrial transport.

GJA1-20k Mediates Microtubule-Based Mitochondrial Transport

GJA1-20k, beginning with amino acid 213, contains a portion of the fourth transmembrane domain of Cx43, and the entire cytoplasmic C-terminal tail (Figure S1A). Like its full-length counterpart, this 170 amino acid isoform includes the microtubule-binding domain (MTBD), which occurs at amino acids 234–259 of Cx43 (Giepmans et al., 2001; Saidi Brikci-Nigassa et al., 2012) (Figure S3). Six residues (^{239}RV^{240} and ^{247}YHAT^{250}) in MTBD have been found critical for microtubule/Cx43 interaction (Saidi Brikci-Nigassa et al., 2012).

Based on the association between GJA1-20k with mitochondria (**Figures 1**, **2**) and microtubules (**Figure 2**), we tested whether GJA1-20k mediates microtubule-based mitochondrial transport. We generated a mutant lacking the six residues essential for microtubule interaction (GJA1-20k-del6) (**Figure 3A**; Figure S11). GJA1-20k and mutated GJA1-20k-del6 were overexpressed in HeLa cells. Interestingly, as seen in **Figure 3B,** GJA1-20k-del6 retains a mitochondrial localization which is indistinguishable from wildtype GJA1-20k, suggesting that the MTBD is not necessary for GJA1-20k localization to mitochondria.

We next examined how the mutation of MTBD affects dynamics of mitochondrial transport in transfected cells. Mitochondrial movements were assessed by tracking individual mitochondrion over a 5-min period. Representative tracks are presented in **Figure 3C**, with original movies in Supplemental Videos S2–S5. Mitochondria were tracked in the presence of GJA1-20k, GJA1-20k-del6, or the microtubule disruptor nocodazole (noc). Quantitative analysis (**Figures 3D,E**) revealed that nocodazole significantly reduces average mitochondrial transport speed and net displacement relative to DMSO treated control cells. In contrast, GJA1-20k increases average mitochondrial speed, while average mitochondrial speed and displacement in GJA1-20k-del6 transfected cells were not significantly different from control. Frequency distribution analyses of individual average mitochondrial speeds (per 5 min windows) were fit with single Gaussian curves (single Gaussian unless R^2 fit was less than 0.9 and then double Gaussian curves were used to fit the data, **Figure 3F**). The original histograms on which the curve fits are based have been removed for clarity in **Figure 3F**. The interested reader is referred to Figure S4 for the original data. The primary peaks of GST (black), GJA1-20k (blue), and GJA1-20k-del6 (red) curves were similar at an average speed of

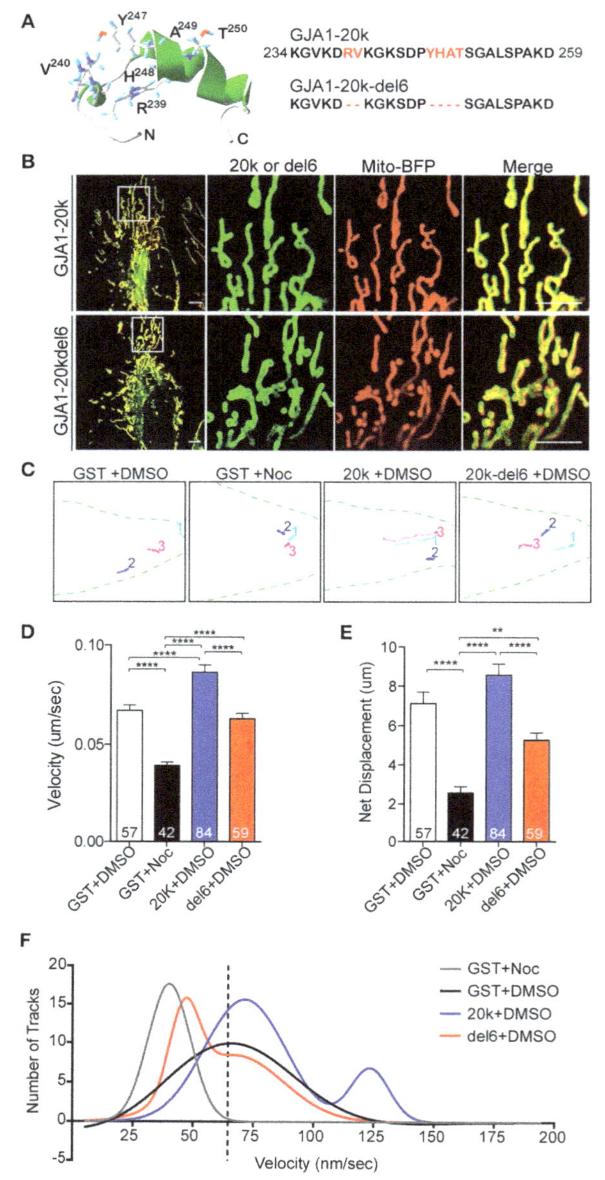

FIGURE 3 | Key microtubule-interacting residues mediate trafficking. **(A)** Swiss PDB Viewer rendering of the MTBD. Six residues (red) were removed in GJA1-20k-del6. **(B)** Live-cell images of GJA1-20k vs. GJA1-20k-del6 (green). Mito-BFP (red). Scale bar = 5 μm. Noc = nocodazole. **(C)** Live-cell mitochondrial tracks (mito-BFP) in each group. **(D–E)** Tracked speed and displacement, respectively. Data are mean ± SEM (n = 4 experimental repeats, 10–30 tracked mitochondria from 5 to 10 cells from each repeat were included. N in each column is number of mitochondria tracked), $^{**}p < 0.01$, $^{****}p < 0.0001$, one-way ANOVA, Tukey's *post hoc* test. **(F)** Nonlinear Gaussian fitting of track velocity frequency and distribution. The R^2 coefficient of Gaussian fitting are: 0.93 (GST, single Gaussian fitting), 0.95 (GST+Noc, single Gaussian fitting), 0.91 (20 k, double Gaussian fitting), 0.97 (del6, double Gaussian fitting).

~65 nm/s. Nocodazole shifted the GST curve to the left (gray), indicating a loss of fast mitochondrial movement on microtubules, whereas a secondary curve to the right (movement at higher speeds) occurred only with GJA1-20k cells (blue) and the area under the curve indicates about 24% population of mitochondria are traveling at the higher speed. These data indicate that in cells with exogenous GJA1-20k containing an intact MTBD, a subpopulation of mitochondria travels at twice the median speed, which is consistent with kinesin-based transport (Wang and Schwarz, 2009; Tanaka et al., 2011). In contrast, the secondary peak of GJA1-20k-del6 cells is shifted to the left (lower speeds, red), closer to the nocodazole peak, indicating loss of mitochondrial transport on microtubules. This is further supported by reduced tubulin interaction with GJA1-20k-del6 (Figure S11). Thus, we conclude that exogenous GJA1-20k increases the instances of mitochondria utilizing microtubule-based transport. The rapid outward-directed movement supports the role of GJA1-20k in increasing microtubule-based transport of mitochondria to the cell periphery.

GJA1-20k Preserves Mitochondrial Distribution during Stress

Since our results indicate that GJA1-20k mediates mitochondrial movement along microtubules (**Figures 2**, **3**), we next asked whether GJA1-20k can safeguard a distributed mitochondrial network during cellular stress. Mitochondrial morphology in fixed cells, as determined by Tom20 immunofluorescence, was observed in HeLa cells subjected to PBS or 300 μM H_2O_2 for 4 h. Confocal imaging of cells expressing GFP-tagged GST, GJA1-43k, or GJA1-20k revealed a distributed mitochondrial network in all groups treated with PBS (**Figure 4A**, left panels and Figure S5). Upon H_2O_2 treatment however, mitochondria became centralized and fragmented in cells expressing GST and GJA1-43k, indicating a damaged mitochondrial network. Interestingly, the majority of GJA1-20k transfected cells retained well distributed network and elongated mitochondrial morphology (**Figure 4A**, right panels). We quantified mitochondrial localization as a ratio of peripheral to central distribution and observed that GJA1-20k significantly rescued mitochondrial peripheralization during H_2O_2 stress (**Figure 4B**). We then quantified elongated mitochondria and found that GJA1-20k rescued mitochondrial morphology as well, when cells were treated with H_2O_2 (**Figure 4C**). These data indicate that introduction of GJA1-20k maintains peripheral mitochondria, limiting organelle network collapse when subjected to metabolic stress. It is possible that GJA1-20k could confer a protective and pro-survival effect through its regulation of mitochondrial distribution and morphology.

In **Figure 3** we introduced the GJA1-20k-del6 mutant which lacks the key residues in the MTBD of GJA1-20k, and observed persistent mitochondrial localization of GJA1-20k-del6 but impaired microtubule transport (**Figures 3B,F**). We tested whether GJA1-20k-del6 could rescue mitochondrial localization and morphology when cells are subjected to H_2O_2 stress. The results, in **Figures 4A,D,E** are negative. Apparently without the microtubule binding capacity, GJA1-20k-del6 loses the capability of GJA1-20k to rescue mitochondrial network integrity during stress, indicating the importance of microtubule based transport for mitochondrial response to oxidative stress.

DISCUSSION

The present study identified that GJA1-20k, produced via alternative translation from the same mRNA encoding gap junction protein Cx43, preferentially localizes to mitochondria and mitochondria/microtubule interfaces. We find that GJA1-20k facilitates microtubule-dependent trafficking of mitochondria to cell periphery, thereby preserving distributed mitochondrial network and preventing mitochondrial fragmentation induced by oxidative stress (depicted in the cartoon in **Figure 5**). This work reveals a novel function of GJA1-20k in regulating mitochondrial distribution in response to cellular stress.

Alternative Translation of Cx43 and Its Functional Significance

It is commonly accepted that, in eukaryotic cells, mature mRNA molecules encode and correspond to single protein products. In recent years, accumulating evidence has suggested that alternative translation start sites are highly conserved in the mammalian genome and that proteome diversity produced via alternative translation may be more important than previously thought (Kochetov, 2008; Bazykin and Kochetov, 2011; de Klerk and 't Hoen, 2015). Cx43 is the first mammalian ion channel identified to undergo alternative translation (Smyth and Shaw, 2013; Salat-Canela et al., 2014; Ul-Hussain et al., 2014). Up to six alternatively translated Cx43 isoforms are produced from *GJA1* mRNA in the heart (Smyth and Shaw, 2013), all of which are N-terminal truncated and contain either the entire or distal portion of the C-terminal tail. The loss of one or more transmembrane domains of full length Cx43 gives rise to different protein solubility which can result in different cellular distribution, biophysical properties and their functions. In addition to its role as a chaperone to facilitate full-length GJA1-43k protein trafficking to the cell-cell border (Smyth and Shaw, 2013; Basheer et al., 2017), we now report that by interacting with microtubules GJA1-20k also aids trafficking and distribution of mitochondrial organelles (**Figures 2**, **3**), resulting in cellular protection from stress (**Figure 4**). With the microtubule binding domain located at proximal C-terminus, it is likely that the N-terminal partial fourth transmembrane domain of GJA1-20k can interact with mitochondrial membrane lipids and/or other mitochondrial adaptor proteins to mediate microtubule dependent interaction and transport of mitochondria.

Alternative translation is a highly regulated process. In this study, we took advantage of HeLa cell lines with little endogenous expression of Cx43 which provides a clear background to study function of alternatively translated smaller isoforms. However, it is known that cellular stress may act as a trigger for alternative translation to generate isoforms that increase survival. For instance, the protein level of GJA1-20k in mouse primary astrocytes nearly doubled following exposure to intermittent hypoxia for 120 min (Ul-Hussain et al., 2014). Similarly, signaling

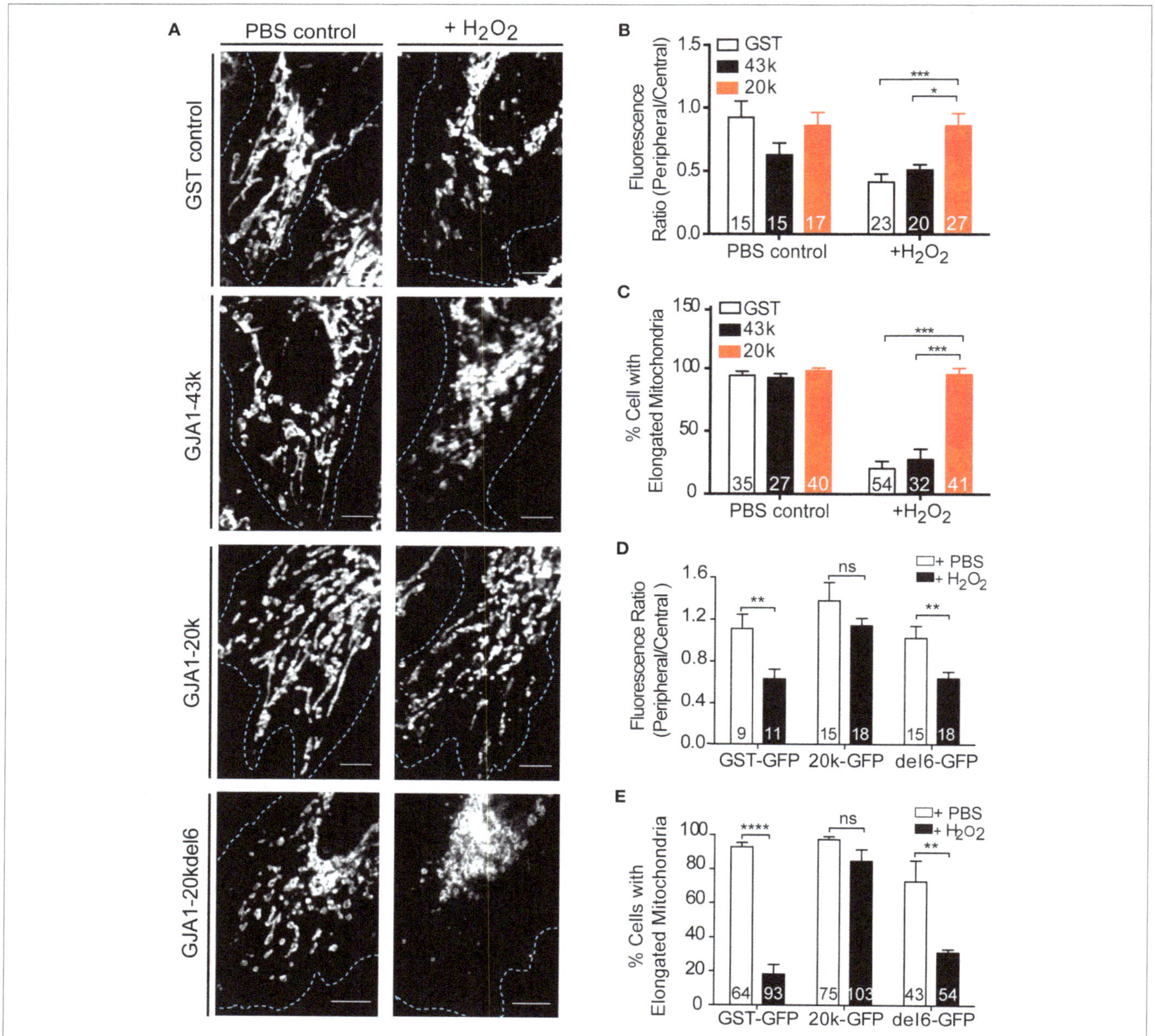

FIGURE 4 | GJA1-20k limits mitochondrial fragmentation upon oxidative stress. **(A)** Mitochondria morphology and distribution (Tom20) in HeLa cells expressing GFP-tagged GST, GJA1-43k, or GJA1-20k, or GJA1-20kdel6 treated with PBS or 300 μM H_2O_2. Cell borders (blue). Scale bar = 5 μm. See also Figure S6. **(B)** Periphery versus cell center Tom20 fluorescence intensity and **(C)** percentage of cells containing elongated mitochondria comparing GFP-tagged GST, GJA1-43k and GJA1-20k. **(D)** Peripheral vs. central mitochondria (Tom20) (See Figure S10) and **(E)** percentage of cells with elongated mitochondria comparing GFP-tagged GST, 20k, 20k-del6 in PBS or H_2O_2. All data are mean ± SEM (n = 4 repeats), $^*p < 0.05$, $^{**}p < 0.01$, $^{***}p < 0.001$, $^{****}p < 0.0001$, two-way ANOVA, Tukey's *post-hoc*-test.

pathways involved in survival, such as mTOR and Mnk1/2 have been linked to upregulation of GJA1-20k by between 2- and 50-fold (Smyth and Shaw, 2013; Salat-Canela et al., 2014). Therefore, our study, though in a heterologous expression system, provides a glimpse of functional impact of GJA1-20k. Given the dynamic regulation of alternative translation, understanding the function of smaller isoforms of Cx43 provides a rare opportunity to identify novel protein targets required for cell survival.

Microtubule-Based Mitochondrial Transport and Distribution

Mitochondria form an extensively regulated and highly dynamic organelle network that is responsible for energy production, calcium homeostasis, cell signaling, cell growth and survival (Frederick and Shaw, 2007). Highly regulated intracellular movement of mitochondria and their appropriate distribution are crucial for the function and integrity of the overall network

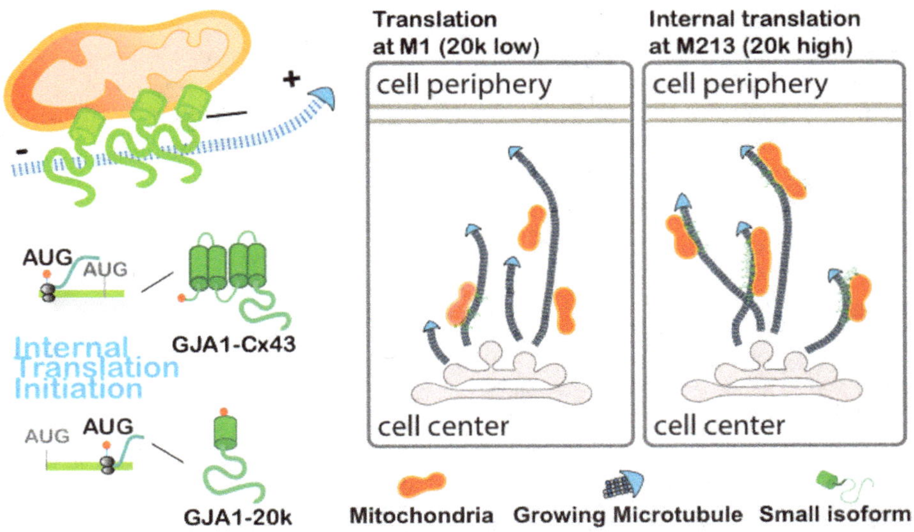

FIGURE 5 | Graphical illustration demonstrates that GJA1-20k localizes to mitochondria and facilitates microtubule-dependent mitochondrial transport to cell periphery and limits mitochondrial fragmentation upon oxidative stress.

(Chan, 2006). Spatial mobility is one of the primary means by which the mitochondria can alter their function to adapt to environmental changes and cellular stresses.

In multicellular eukaryotes, mitochondria move along microtubule tracks by attaching to motors such as kinesin for anterograde transport and dynein for retrograde transport (Hollenbeck and Saxton, 2005; Russo et al., 2009). Impaired mitochondrial movement and the resulting aberrant distribution are detrimental for the cell function, which is particularly manifest in highly polarized cells (Frederick and Shaw, 2007; Saotome et al., 2008). Here we find that, even in HeLa cells, pharmaceutical disruption of microtubules dramatically reduces mitochondrial transport (**Figure 3**), confirming the role of microtubules in mitochondrial movement. The alternatively translated small isoform of Cx43, GJA1-20k, when expressed exogenously, facilitates mitochondrial trafficking along microtubules. Our finding demonstrates that GJA1-20k not only regulates microtubule dependent vesicular protein cargo trafficking (Smyth and Shaw, 2013; Basheer et al., 2017), but also microtubule dependent organelle transport (**Figures 3**, **4**). A mutant of GJA1-20k (GJA1-20k-del6) which lacks ability to bind microtubules still reaches mitochondrial membrane, suggesting microtubule transport is not needed for mitochondrial affinity and possibly GJA1-20k-del6 may localize to mitochondria at earlier stages of mitogenesis. However GJA1-20k-del6 fails to rescue mitochondrial mobility and to maintain mitochondrial network distribution in presence of H_2O_2 (**Figure 4**). Through its interaction with microtubules, GJA1-20k may act as an adaptor protein to facilitate loading of mitochondria onto microtubule trafficking highways for movement and distribution within the cell. In future studies, it will be important to address whether GJA1-20k also interacts with known microtubule-based motor/adaptor transport complex proteins (Chan, 2006; Wang and Schwarz, 2009; Tanaka et al., 2011) which regulate mitochondrial trafficking velocity and directionality.

Of note and in additional to spatial mobility, mitochondria engage in repeating cycles of fusion and fission to intermix membrane lipids and matrix contents to ensure organelle network health and function (Ong et al., 2010, 2013; Huang et al., 2013). Maintenance of an intact network of elongated mitochondria protects against mitophagy and cell death through evasion of autophagosome engulfment (Gomes et al., 2011; Rambold et al., 2011). To buffer against damage and dysfunction, impaired mitochondria undergo fission and are distributed throughout the remaining healthy network (Nakada et al., 2001; Ono et al., 2001). In all cells, there exists a dynamic equilibrium between mitochondrial fission and fusion. Both fission and fusion are carried out by a distinct group of proteins, including Drp1, FIS1, OPA1, and mitofusin 1/2. It is possible that, through interaction with one or more of these proteins, GJA1-20k tips the balance between fission and fusion in favor of elongated morphology of mitochondria.

CONCLUSIONS

We have identified that GJA1-20k enriches at mitochondria and facilitates microtubule-based mitochondrial transport which preserves organelle network integrity upon oxidative stress. GJA1-20k, a protein that was only recently recognized to exist by alternative translation (Smyth and Shaw, 2013; Salat-Canela et al., 2014; Ul-Hussain et al., 2014), provides a means by which otherwise traditional Cx43 gap junction protein can have a highly diverse repertoire of non-canonical roles. It is possible that the GJA1-20k peptide could be developed into a therapeutic to prevent mitochondrial fragmentation in situations of cellular stress.

AUTHOR CONTRIBUTIONS

YF, S-SZ, and SX contribute equally to the experimental design, acquisition, interpretation of data and drafting the manuscript. WB, RB, and IE contribute to experimental design, data acquisition and drafting the manuscript. TH and RS contributed to all aspects of this work. All authors agree to be accountable for accuracy and integrity of the work.

ACKNOWLEDGMENTS

We thank L.Y. Jan and M. Petkovic for critical review of the manuscript and helpful discussions; S. Ryazantsev at the Electron Imaging Center at California NanoSystems Institute of UCLA for his expertise in electron microscopy; as well as T. Hitzeman, R. Naami and E. Naami for technical assistance. All constructs generated in this study are available at the Addgene plasmid repository.

REFERENCES

Akar, F. G., Nass, R. D., Hahn, S., Cingolani, E., Shah, M., Hesketh, G. G., et al. (2007). Dynamic changes in conduction velocity and gap junction properties during development of pacing-induced heart failure. *Am. J. Physiol. Heart Circ. Physiol.* 293, H1223–H1230. doi: 10.1152/ajpheart.00079.2007

Basheer, W. A., Xiao, S., Epifantseva, I., Fu, Y., Kleber, A. G., Hong, T., et al. (2017). GJA1-20k arranges actin to guide Cx43 delivery to cardiac intercalated discs. *Circ. Res.* 121, 1069–1080. doi: 10.1161/CIRCRESAHA.117.311955

Basheer, W., and Shaw, R. (2016). The "tail" of Connexin43: an unexpected journey from alternative translation to trafficking. *Biochim. Biophys. Acta* 1863, 1848–1856. doi: 10.1016/j.bbamcr.2015.10.015

Bazykin, G. A., and Kochetov, A. V. (2011). Alternative translation start sites are conserved in eukaryotic genomes. *Nucleic Acids Res.* 39, 567–577. doi: 10.1093/nar/gkq806

Beardslee, M. A., Laing, J. G., Beyer, E. C., and Saffitz, J. E. (1998). Rapid turnover of connexin43 in the adult rat heart. *Circ. Res.* 83, 629–635. doi: 10.1161/01.RES.83.6.629

Beardslee, M. A., Lerner, D. L., Tadros, P. N., Laing, J. G., Beyer, E. C., Yamada, K. A., et al. (2000). Dephosphorylation and intracellular redistribution of ventricular connexin43 during electrical uncoupling induced by ischemia. *Circ. Res.* 87, 656–662. doi: 10.1161/01.RES.87.8.656

Beyer, E. C., Paul, D. L., and Goodenough, D. A. (1987). Connexin43: a protein from rat heart homologous to a gap junction protein from liver. *J. Cell Biol.* 105, 2621–2629. doi: 10.1083/jcb.105.6.2621

Boengler, K., Dodoni, G., Rodriguez-Sinovas, A., Cabestrero, A., Ruiz-Meana, M., Gres, P., et al. (2005). Connexin 43 in cardiomyocyte mitochondria and its increase by ischemic preconditioning. *Cardiovasc. Res.* 67, 234–244. doi: 10.1016/j.cardiores.2005.04.014

Bolte, S., and Cordelières, F. P. (2006). A guided tour into subcellular colocalization analysis in light microscopy. *J. Microsc.* 224, 213–232. doi: 10.1111/j.1365-2818.2006.01706.x

Chan, D. C. (2006). Mitochondria: dynamic organelles in disease, aging, and development. *Cell* 125, 1241–1252. doi: 10.1016/j.cell.2006.06.010

de Klerk, E., and 't Hoen, P.A. (2015). Alternative mRNA transcription, processing, and translation: insights from RNA sequencing. *Trends Genet.* 31, 128–139. doi: 10.1016/j.tig.2015.01.001

Fishman, G. I., Eddy, R. L., Shows, T. B., Rosenthal, L., and Leinwand, L. A. (1991). The human connexin gene family of gap junction proteins: distinct chromosomal locations but similar structures. *Genomics* 10, 250–256. doi: 10.1016/0888-7543(91)90507-B

Frederick, R. L., and Shaw, J. M. (2007). Moving mitochondria: establishing distribution of an essential organelle. *Traffic* 8, 1668–1675. doi: 10.1111/j.1600-0854.2007.00644.x

Friedman, J. R., Lackner, L. L., West, M., Dibenedetto, J. R., Nunnari, J., and Voeltz, G. K. (2011). ER tubules mark sites of mitochondrial division. *Science* 334, 358–362. doi: 10.1126/science.1207385

Gadicherla, A. K., Wang, N., Bulic, M., Agullo-Pascual, E., Lissoni, A., De Smet, M., et al. (2017). Mitochondrial Cx43 hemichannels contribute to mitochondrial calcium entry and cell death in the heart. *Basic Res. Cardiol.* 112:27. doi: 10.1007/s00395-017-0618-1

Giepmans, B. N., Verlaan, I., Hengeveld, T., Janssen, H., Calafat, J., Falk, M. M., et al. (2001). Gap junction protein connexin-43 interacts directly with microtubules. *Curr. Biol.* 11, 1364–1368. doi: 10.1016/S0960-9822(01)00424-9

Gomes, L. C., Di Benedetto, G., and Scorrano, L. (2011). During autophagy mitochondria elongate, are spared from degradation and sustain cell viability. *Nat. Cell Biol.* 13, 589–598. doi: 10.1038/ncb2220

Habas, A., Hahn, J., Wang, X., and Margeta, M. (2013). Neuronal activity regulates astrocytic Nrf2 signaling. *Proc. Natl. Acad. Sci. U.S.A.* 110, 18291–18296. doi: 10.1073/pnas.1208764110

He, Y., Dupree, J., Wang, J., Sandoval, J., Li, J., Liu, H., et al. (2007). The transcription factor Yin Yang 1 is essential for oligodendrocyte progenitor differentiation. *Neuron* 55, 217–230. doi: 10.1016/j.neuron.2007.06.029

Hollenbeck, P. J., and Saxton, W. M. (2005). The axonal transport of mitochondria. *J. Cell Sci.* 118, 5411–5419. doi: 10.1242/jcs.02745

Huang, X., Sun, L., Ji, S., Zhao, T., Zhang, W., Xu, J., et al. (2013). Kissing and nanotunneling mediate intermitochondrial communication in the heart. *Proc. Natl. Acad. Sci. U.S.A.* 110, 2846–2851. doi: 10.1073/pnas.1300741110

Kochetov, A. V. (2008). Alternative translation start sites and hidden coding potential of eukaryotic mRNAs. *Bioessays* 30, 683–691. doi: 10.1002/bies.20771

Lauf, U., Giepmans, B. N., Lopez, P., Braconnot, S., Chen, S. C., and Falk, M. M. (2002). Dynamic trafficking and delivery of connexons to the plasma membrane and accretion to gap junctions in living cells. *Proc. Natl. Acad. Sci. U.S.A.* 99, 10446–10451. doi: 10.1073/pnas.162055899

Luke, R. A., and Saffitz, J. E. (1991). Remodeling of ventricular conduction pathways in healed canine infarct border zones. *J. Clin. Invest.* 87, 1594–1602. doi: 10.1172/JCI115173

Meijering, E., Dzyubachyk, O., and Smal, I. (2012). Methods for cell and particle tracking. *Meth. Enzymol.* 504, 183–200. doi: 10.1016/B978-0-12-391857-4.00009-4

Nakada, K., Inoue, K., Ono, T., Isobe, K., Ogura, A., Goto, Y. I., et al. (2001). Inter-mitochondrial complementation: mitochondria-specific system preventing mice from expression of disease phenotypes by mutant mtDNA. *Nat. Med.* 7, 934–940. doi: 10.1038/90976

Ong, S. B., Hall, A. R., and Hausenloy, D. J. (2013). Mitochondrial dynamics in cardiovascular health and disease. *Antioxid. Redox Signal.* 19, 400–414. doi: 10.1089/ars.2012.4777

Ong, S. B., Subrayan, S., Lim, S. Y., Yellon, D. M., Davidson, S. M., and Hausenloy, D. J. (2010). Inhibiting mitochondrial fission protects the heart against ischemia/reperfusion injury. *Circulation* 121, 2012–2022. doi: 10.1161/CIRCULATIONAHA.109.906610

Ono, T., Isobe, K., Nakada, K., and Hayashi, J. I. (2001). Human cells are protected from mitochondrial dysfunction by complementation of DNA products in fused mitochondria. *Nat. Genet.* 28, 272–275. doi: 10.1038/90116

Paznekas, W. A., Boyadjiev, S. A., Shapiro, R. E., Daniels, O., Wollnik, B., Keegan, C. E., et al. (2003). Connexin 43 (GJA1) mutations cause the pleiotropic phenotype of oculodentodigital dysplasia. *Am. J. Hum. Genet.* 72, 408–418. doi: 10.1086/346090

Rambold, A. S., Kostelecky, B., and Lippincott-Schwartz, J. (2011). Together we are stronger: fusion protects mitochondria from autophagosomal degradation. *Autophagy* 7, 1568–1569. doi: 10.4161/auto.7.12.17992

Russo, G. J., Louie, K., Wellington, A., Macleod, G. T., Hu, F., Panchumarthi, S., et al. (2009). Drosophila Miro is required for both anterograde and retrograde axonal mitochondrial transport. *J. Neurosci.* 29, 5443–5455. doi: 10.1523/JNEUROSCI.5417-08.2009

Saidi Brikci-Nigassa, A., Clement, M. J., Ha-Duong, T., Adjadj, E., Ziani, L., Pastre, D., et al. (2012). Phosphorylation controls the interaction of the connexin43 C-terminal domain with tubulin and microtubules. *Biochemistry* 51, 4331–4342. doi: 10.1021/bi201806j

Salat-Canela, C., Sesé, M., Peula, C., Ramón, Y., Cajal, S., and Aasen, T. (2014). Internal translation of the connexin 43 transcript. *Cell Commun. Signal.* 12:31. doi: 10.1186/1478-811X-12-31

Saotome, M., Safiulina, D., Szabadkai, G., Das, S., Fransson, A., Aspenstrom, P., et al. (2008). Bidirectional Ca^{2+}-dependent control of mitochondrial dynamics by the Miro GTPase. *Proc. Natl. Acad. Sci. U.S.A.* 105, 20728–20733. doi: 10.1073/pnas.0808953105

Shaw, R. M., Fay, A. J., Puthenveedu, M. A., Von Zastrow, M., Jan, Y. N., and Jan, L. Y. (2007). Microtubule plus-end-tracking proteins target gap junctions directly from the cell interior to adherens junctions. *Cell* 128, 547–560. doi: 10.1016/j.cell.2006.12.037

Singh, A., Yadav, V., and Prasad, R. (2012). Comparative lipidomics in clinical isolates of Candida albicans reveal crosstalk between mitochondria, cell wall integrity and azole resistance. *PLoS ONE* 7:e39812. doi: 10.1371/journal.pone.0039812

Smith, J. H., Green, C. R., Peters, N. S., Rothery, S., and Severs, N. J. (1991). Altered patterns of gap junction distribution in ischemic heart disease. An immunohistochemical study of human myocardium using laser scanning confocal microscopy. *Am. J. Pathol.* 139, 801–821.

Smyth, J. W., and Shaw, R. M. (2013). Autoregulation of connexin43 gap junction formation by internally translated isoforms. *Cell Rep.* 5, 611–618. doi: 10.1016/j.celrep.2013.10.009

Solan, J. L., Hingorani, S. R., and Lampe, P. D. (2012). Changes in connexin43 expression and localization during pancreatic cancer progression. *J. Membr. Biol.* 245, 255–262. doi: 10.1007/s00232-012-9446-2

Srisakuldee, W., Makazan, Z., Nickel, B. E., Zhang, F., Thliveris, J. A., Pasumarthi, K. B., et al. (2014). The FGF-2-triggered protection of cardiac subsarcolemmal mitochondria from calcium overload is mitochondrial connexin 43-dependent. *Cardiovasc. Res.* 103, 72–80. doi: 10.1093/cvr/cvu066

Tanaka, K., Sugiura, Y., Ichishita, R., Mihara, K., and Oka, T. (2011). KLP6: a newly identified kinesin that regulates the morphology and transport of mitochondria in neuronal cells. *J. Cell Sci.* 124, 2457–2465. doi: 10.1242/jcs.086470

Ul-Hussain, M., Olk, S., Schoenebeck, B., Wasielewski, B., Meier, C., Prochnow, N., et al. (2014). Internal Ribosomal Entry Site (IRES) activity generates endogenous carboxyl-terminal domains of Cx43 and is responsive to hypoxic conditions. *J. Biol. Chem.* 289, 20979–20990. doi: 10.1074/jbc.M113.540187

Wang, X., and Schwarz, T. L. (2009). The mechanism of $Ca2^{+}$ -dependent regulation of kinesin-mediated mitochondrial motility. *Cell* 136, 163–174. doi: 10.1016/j.cell.2008.11.046

Zhang, S. S., Hong, S., Kléber, A. G., Lee, L. P., and Shaw, R. M. (2014). A micropatterning approach for imaging dynamic Cx43 trafficking to cell-cell borders. *FEBS Lett.* 588, 1439–1445. doi: 10.1016/j.febslet.2014.01.002

20

A Systemic Mapping Approach for Right and Left Parahisian Ventricular Arrhythmias Ablation

Ling-cong Kong[†], Tian Shuang[†], Zheng Li, Zhi-guo Zou, Wen-long Jiang, Jun Pu and Xin-hua Wang**

Department of Cardiology, Ren Ji Hospital, Shanghai Jiao Tong University School of Medicine, Shanghai, China

***Correspondence:**
Xin-hua Wang
ttwwxh@126.com
Jun Pu
pujun310@hotmail.com

[†]These authors have contributed equally to this work

Background: Catheter ablation for parahisian ventricular arrhythmias (PHVA) is technically challenging and associated with increased risks of atrioventricular block (AVB). We developed a systemic mapping approach to improve the efficacy and safety of PHVA ablation.

Methods: Forty-three patients (29 males; average age 65.8 ± 10.5 years) with PHVAs were enrolled. A systemic mapping approach comprising differential electrocardiogram, sequential mapping, and ablation beneath/above the septal leaflet of the tricuspid valve (SLTV) and at the neighboring/contralateral regions (the aortic root and sub-aortic valve region) was applied for PHVA. The effectiveness and safety of this approach was evaluated at 1 year's follow-up.

Results: Sequential ablation beneath the SLTV (B-SLTV) succeeded in 24 (66.7 %) of 36 with right PHVA and ablation above the SLTV succeeded in 6 of the remaining 12 with failed B-SLTV ablation. Target-His bundle (HB) distance > 4.5 mm significantly predicted successful right PHVA ablation (OR 1.703; 95% CI 1.084–2.676, $P = 0.02$). "Seeming" right PHVA by electrocardiogram in 4 and apparent left PHVA in 3 was successfully ablated at the sub-aortic parahisian region. At 1 year's follow-up, 27 (75%) of 36 patients with right PHVA and 6 (85.7%) of 7 patients with left PHVA were free of PHVA recurrence off anti-arrhythmic drugs. The total success rate was 76.7% by using the systemic mapping approach for PHVA. One patient with A-SLTV ablation underwent pacemaker implantation due to complete AVB.

Conclusions: The systemic mapping approach was effective and safe for treating PHVA. The target-HB distance was a significant predictor for right PHVA ablation.

Keywords: parahisian ventricular arrhythmias, systemic mapping approach, radiofrequency ablation, atrioventricular block, the septal leaflet of the tricuspid valve

HIGHLIGHTS

- The systemic mapping approach comprising differential ECG, mapping and ablation beneath/above the SLTV and the neighboring/contralateral regions was effective and safe for treating right and left parahisian VAs.
- B-SLTV ablation succeeded in two thirds of patients with right parahisian VAs.
- Target-HB distance > 4.5 mm could predict successful ablation of right parahisian VAs.

BACKGROUND

Most idiopathic ventricular arrhythmias (VAs) [pre-mature ventricular contraction (PVC) and ventricular tachycardia (VT)] originate from the right ventricular outflow tract (RVOT), and can be eliminated by radiofrequency (RF) catheter ablation effectively (1, 2). Parahisian VA (PHVA), defined as the earliest activation exhibiting His potential or <1 cm away from the His bundle (HB) of the right or left ventricular side (3), are less commonly seen, with the prevalence of 3–9% in all idiopathic VAs (4, 5). Catheter ablation for PHVA is technically challenging because the septal leaflet of the tricuspid valve (SLTV) hampers catheter tip-tissue contacts by the "above SLTV (A-SLTV)" approach. In contrast to RVOT-VAs, PHVAs ablation is associated with compromised effectiveness and higher risks of conduction system injury (5–8).

A novel technical improvement is to curve the catheter tip reversely and place it beneath the SLTV (B-SLTV) to acquire good proximity to the basal interventricular septum (9, 10). The B-SLTV approach might be superior to the A-SLTV approach in terms of effectiveness and safety, and was recommended for PHVAs ablation in recent studies (10, 11); Nevertheless, catheter ablation might fail even by the B-SLTV approach in a considerable proportion of patients (11). In this scenario sequential mapping at the A-SLTV region, the neighboring left parahisian area or the aortic root might help to improve the outcomes (12). These findings reminded us to propose a systemic mapping approach for PHVAs ablation. This study was carried out to evaluate the effectiveness and safety of this approach in a consecutive cohort of patients with right and left PHVAs.

METHOD

Study Population

Forty-three patients (29 males; average age 65.8 ± 10.5 years) with PHVAs were enrolled to undergo catheter ablation from January 2017 to September 2020. PHVAs were diagnosed according to surface electrocardiograms (ECGs) (3–5), which typically manifested QRS discordance in inferior leads (lead II/III/aVF), "QS"/"Qr"/"qR"pattern in lead V1, and precordial transition earlier than lead V3/V4 (**Figure 1A**). Inclusion criteria were symptomatic monomorphic VAs; daily PVC burden >10% or total PVC exceeding 10,000 per day or concomitant with VT of identical morphology; refractory or intolerance to at least one antiarrhythmic drug (AAD), including beta-blockers, Class Ic and Class III AADs. Exclusion criteria were ischemic heart disease; primary cardiomyopathy; prior cardiac surgery; congenital heart disease. All patients provided written informed consent for the ablation.

Abbreviations: PHVA, parahisian ventricular arrhythmias; PVC, premature ventricular contraction; VA, ventricular arrhythmia; VT, ventricular tachycardia; RF, radiofrequency; HB, the His bundle; RVOT, the right ventricular outflow tract; AVB, atrioventricular block; SLTV, the septal leaflet of the tricuspid valve; AAD, antiarrhythmic drug.

The Protocol of Systemic Mapping Approach for PHVAs

The protocol of systemic mapping approach was shown in **Figure 1B**. Briefly, it could be described as three steps. Step 1: Pre-judgement of left or right PHVAs according to the QRS morphology in lead V1 and precordial transitional zone (13). The "R"/"qR(s)" pattern in V1 and precordial transitional zone ≤ V1 indicated a left PHVA. The "QS"/"rS" pattern in V1 and precordial transitional zone ≥ V2 indicated a right PHVA. Step 2: Initial ablation based on the results of parahisian mapping. For right PHVA, the B-SLTV approach was performed in all patients. For left PHVA, ablation was performed above or below the aortic valve based on the mapping results. Step 3: Subsequent mapping and ablation if the initial ablation failed, including A-SLTV ablation and anatomical ablation at the contralateral parahisian region and the adjacent structures.

Electrophysiological Mapping

The procedures were performed in fasting state and under local analgesia. A decapolar catheter was positioned within coronary sinus (CS) *via* left femoral vein or left subclavian vein. A 3.5 mm saline-irrigated catheter with or without contact-force sensing (Thermocool Navistar or SmartTouch Thermocool Navistar, Biosense Webster, CA, USA) was used for geometry reconstruction, mapping and ablation. If spontaneous VAs was insufficient for mapping, intravenous infusion of isopreterenol (2–5 μg/min) was used to provoke the clinical VAs. The result of activation mapping was displayed on the geometry in color-coded manner. The site with the highest amplitude of His potential was tagged as the "HB." Pace mapping was applied with the output just higher than the diastolic capture threshold. A matched pace mapping was defined as the morphology of paced QRS identical to that of the clinical VAs in at least 11 of 12 leads.

EP Mapping at the Preferential Regions

For right PHVAs, the B-SLTV region was preferentially mapped. To access to the subvalvular area, the ablation catheter was introduced to the right ventricle *via* a Swartz sheath (SR0 type, St. Jude Medical, MN, USA), then curved reversely and clockwise rotated the catheter and pulled it back toward the tricuspid annulus, to form catheter inversion configuration (**Figures 2A–C**). The position of the catheter tip was judged by fluoroscopy and confirmed by intracardiac echocardiography (ICE) imaging (CARTO Sound, Biosense Webster, CA, USA) (**Figures 2D,H**). For left PHVAs, the mapping catheter was advanced in the left ventricle *via* trans-aortic retrograde approach to map the left parahisian region and the septal region of mitral annulus (**Figure 3**).

The earliest activation site was tagged on the geometry and served as the initial ablation target if it was >4 mm away from the HB, and if the HB-Right bundle branch (RBB) capture threshold by pacing at the earliest activation site was higher than that at the HB site (14). However, in case of the earliest activation <4 mm away from the HB, or if HB-RBB was captured with lower threshold at this site than the HB, attempt of ablation could be tried under close monitoring of junctional rhythm/AV conduction (**Figure 4**).

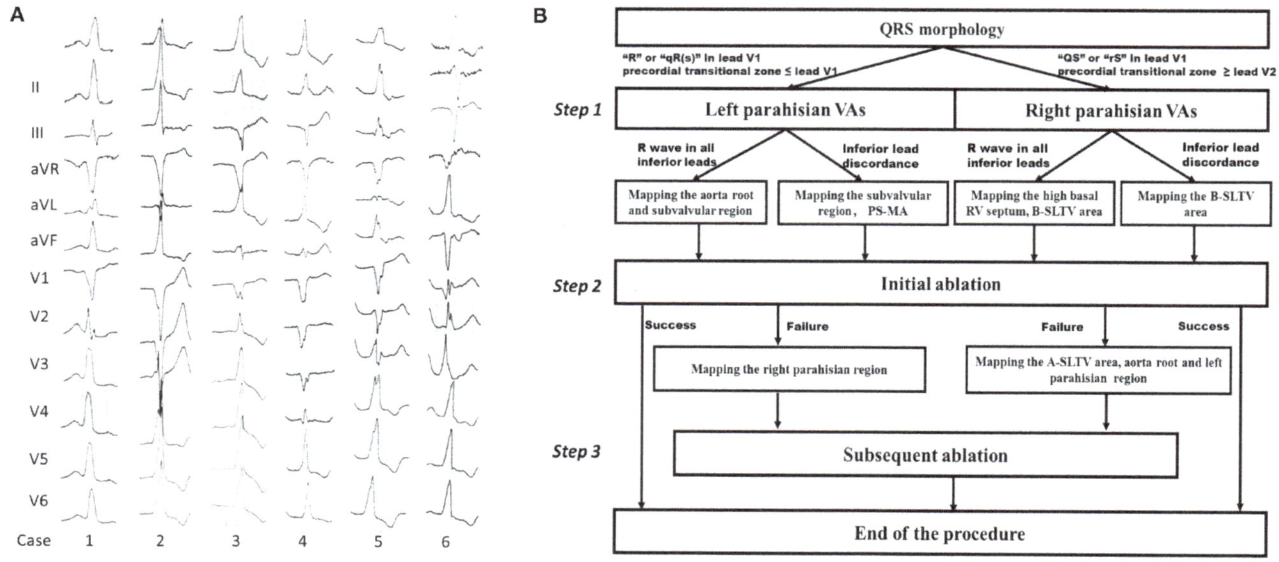

FIGURE 1 | Examples of PHVA electrocardiograms and the flow chart of the systemic mapping approach. **(A)** Typical twelve-lead electrocardiographic manifestation of parahisian VAs. Right parahisian VAs were diagnosed in Case 1–5, and left parahisian VA in Case 6. Note there were positive "R" waves/or QRS discordance in inferior leads, a "QS" wave in lead V1, precordial transition in lead V2–V4 for right parahisian VAs, and a "qR" wave in lead V1 and precordial transition in lead V1–V2 for left parahisian VA. **(B)** The flow chart of the systemic mapping approach for right and left parahisian VA.

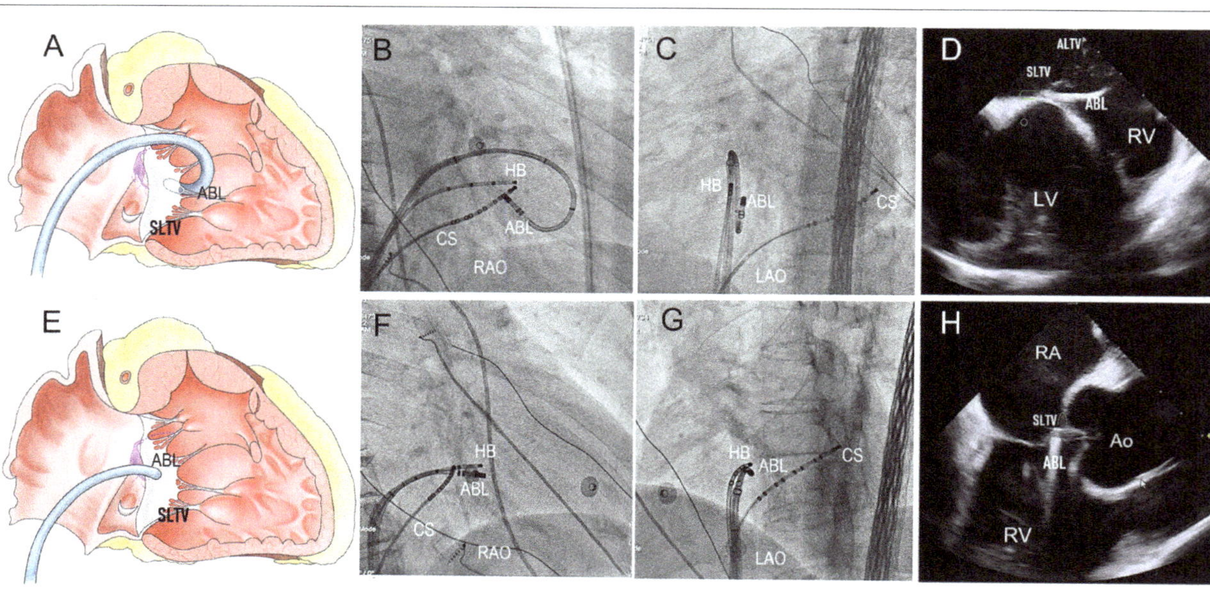

FIGURE 2 | The Catheter placement in the B-SLTV and A-SLTV approach. **(A)** The schematic diagram illustrating the catheter tip was reversely curved beneath the SLTV (RAO view). **(B,C)** The fluoroscopic images showing the catheter was reversely curved beneath the SLTV through a long sheath (RAO and LAO view). **(D,H)** The ultrasonic images confirmed the catheter placement beneath the SLTV. **(E)** The schematic diagram showing the catheter tip was directly placed above the SLTV (RAO view). **(F,G)** The fluoroscopic images showing the catheter tip was placed directly above the SLTV (RAO and LAO view). HB, the His bundle; CS, coronary sinus; ABL, the ablation catheter; SLTV, the septal leaflet of the tricuspid valve; ALTV, the anterior leaflet of the tricuspid valve; RA, the right atrium; RV, the right ventricle; LV, left ventricle; RAO, right anterior oblique; LAO, left anterior oblique.

Subsequent EP Mapping at Other Regions

If the attempt of B-SLTV ablation failed or was withdrawn due to safety concerns, the A-SLTV region (**Figures 2E–G**), contralateral parahisian regions and the neighboring structures (i.e., the coronary cusps at the aortic root) were mapped to search for an earlier activation site than the initial one, or the adjacent

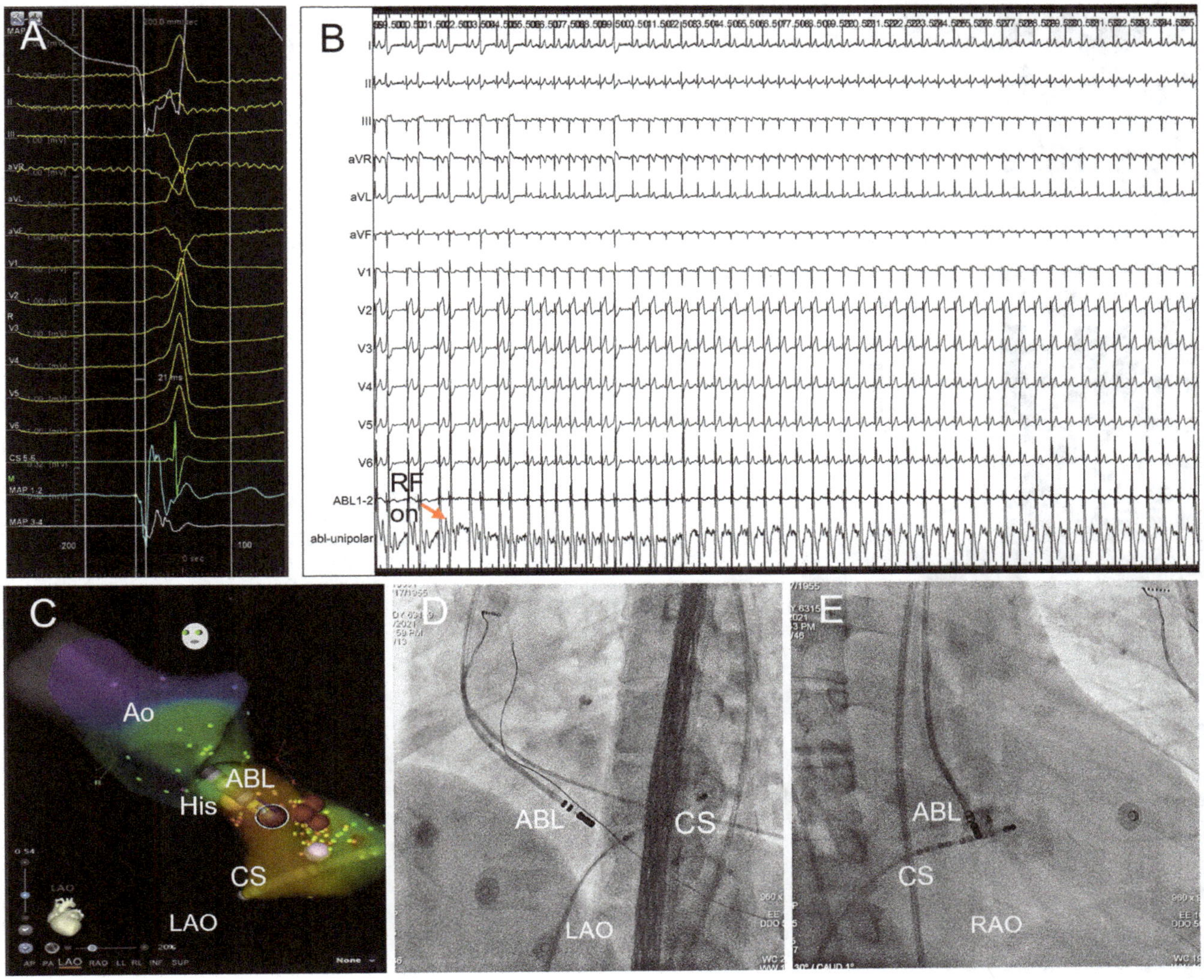

FIGURE 3 | Trans-aortic retrograde ablation of left PHVA. **(A)** Tracings were unipolar MAP1, twelve-lead surface ECG, CS_{5-6}, bipolar MAP_{1-2}, MAP_{3-4}. The local bipolar electrogram at the ablation target preceded the QRS onset by 21 ms with a sharp "QS" unipolar electrogram. **(B)** RF ablation 30W, 60s at the sub-aortic ablation target successfully eliminated the left PHVA without causing PR prolongation or AVB. **(C)** Activation mapping of the left PHVA region and the aortic root. The catheter tip was positioned at the ablation target ≈3 mm below the HB in the left ventricle. Ablation attempt (30W, 10 s) was not effective at other sites slightly away from the ablation target. Red dots represented ablation lesions. **(D,E)** The catheter placement at the left parahisian region on LAO and RAO fluoroscopic projection. Ao, the aorta; HB, the His bundle; CS, coronary sinus; ABL, the ablation catheter; RAO, right anterior oblique; LAO, left anterior oblique.

site that was just opposite to the initial lesion. They were served as a better target for subsequent ablation, or as a suitable target for anatomical ablation.

RF Ablation Settings

Once the initial ablation target was determined, irrigated RF ablation was applied for lesion creation. Typically, RF energy delivery commenced at 20W (saline-irrigation speed 17 ml/min, contact force 8–20 g if applicable), and was gradually titrated to 35–45 W (saline-irrigation speed 20–25 ml/min, contact force 8–20 g if applicable) if no sign of AV conduction injury was observed (5–10). If the clinical VAs were suppressed within 15 s, RF energy delivery was prolonged for 90–120 s, otherwise RF ablation was suspended, and re-mapping was performed. RF ablation was terminated immediately in case of PR prolongation or rapid junctional rhythm, which foreboded impending AV block (AVB).

Procedural success was deemed if no clinical VAs recurred at the end of 30 min's observation period with the challenge of intravenous isoproterenol infusion (2–5 μg/min).

Post-ablation Management and Follow-Up

Patients were discharged the next day after the procedure and were regularly followed up at the outpatient clinic for 1 year. All AADs were withdrawn if no symptomatic VAs were detected. Surface ECG and 24 h Holter monitoring were

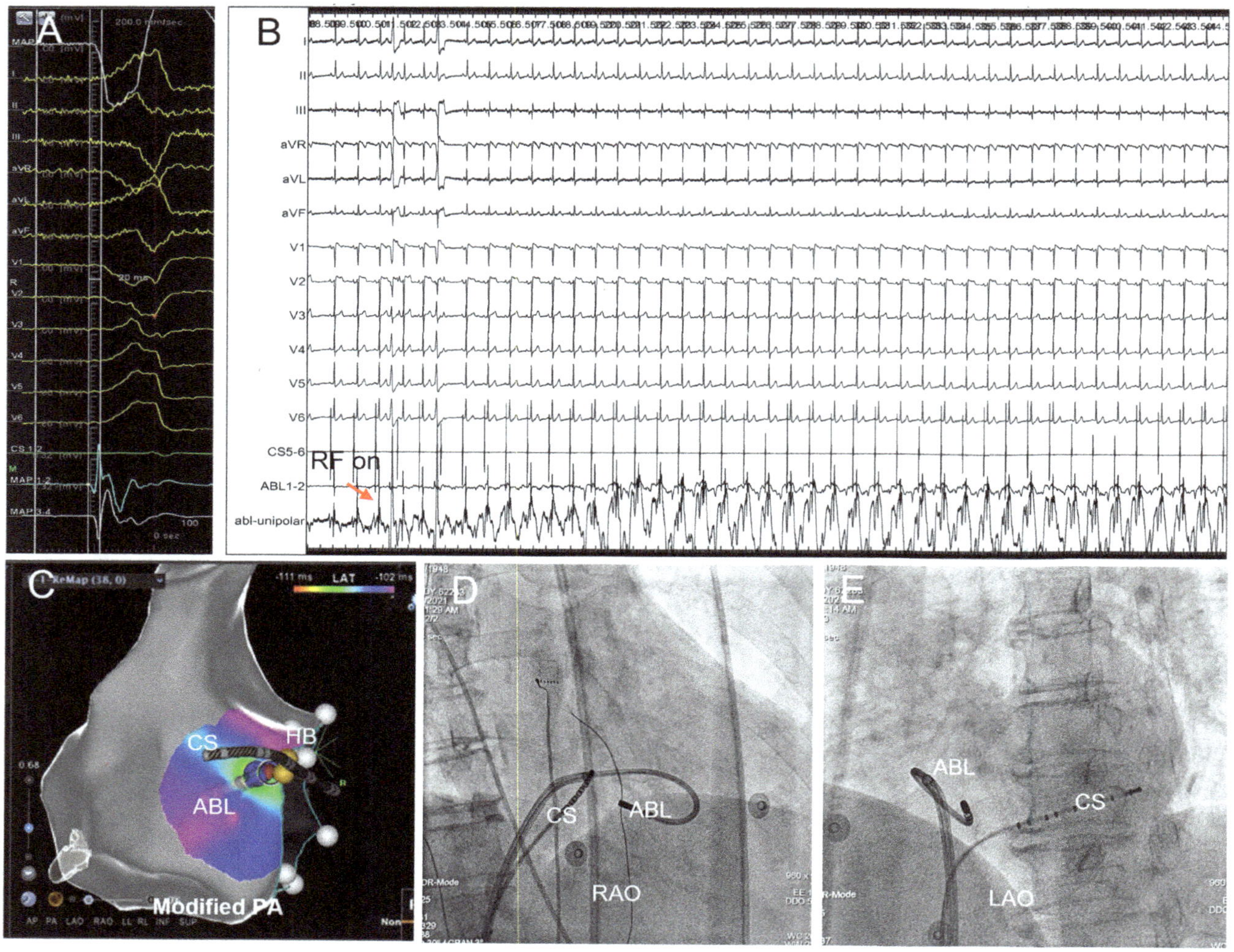

FIGURE 4 | Successful B-SLTV ablation of right PHVA with the ablation target extremely close to the HB. **(A)** Tracings were unipolar MAP_1, twelve-lead surface ECG, CS_{1-2}, bipolar MAP_{1-2}, MAP_{3-4}. The local bipolar electrogram at the ablation target preceded the QRS onset by 20 ms with a sharp "QS" unipolar electrogram. **(B)** Saline-irrigated RF energy delivery 35W, 90s at this site successfully abolished the PVC, without junctional rhythm or AV conduction impairment. **(C)** The catheter tip was positioned beneath the SLTV ≈ 2 mm away from the HB. The blue dot represented the ablation lesion. **(D,E)** The B-SLTV placement of the ablation catheter was displayed on RAO and LAO projection. HB, the His bundle; CS, coronary sinus; ABL, the ablation catheter. PA, postero-anterior; RAO, right anterior oblique; LAO, left anterior oblique.

performed at 3, 6, and 12 months after the procedure, and were performed whenever the patient experienced symptoms suggesting a VA recurrence.

Clinical success was defined as absence of clinical PHVAs on surface ECGs and reduction of clinical VAs burden by more than 90% on 24 h Holter monitoring compared with the recording prior to the procedure at the end of 1 year's follow-up off AADs.

Statistical Analysis

Continuous variables with normal distribution were expressed as mean ± standard deviation (SD) or as median and range otherwise. They were compared by Student's t-test if the variance was equal, or by Mann–Whitney U-test otherwise. Category variables were expressed as counts and percentage (%), and were compared with χ^2 or Fisher's exact test. Multivariate binary logistic regression analysis was applied to detect the independent predictors for successful right PHVA ablation, which were described as odds ratio (OR) and 95% confidence interval (CI). A receiver operating characteristic (ROC) analysis was applied to determine the cut-off value for predicting successful right PHVA ablation. A two-tailed $P < 0.05$ was considered statistically significant. Statistical analysis was performed by IBM SPSS Statistics 19.0 for Windows (IBM Corporation, Somers, NY, USA).

RESULTS

The baseline demographic parameters in all patients and in those with right / left PHVAs were listed in **Table 1**, respectively.

TABLE 1 | Patients' baseline characteristics.

Parameters	Total	Right parahisian VA	Left parahisian VA
Cases (*N*)	43	36	7
Age (years)	65.8 ± 10.5	65.7 ± 11.2	66.4 ± 5.1
Male, *n* (%)	29 (67.4)	23 (63.9)	6 (85.7)
24-h PVC count	17,603 ± 7,072	16,878 ± 7,028	21,331 ± 6,528
History of PVC (months)	5.0 (4.0, 8.0)	5.0 (4.0, 7.8)	6.0 (3.0, 24.0)
Comorbidities			
Hypertension, *n* (%)	18 (41.8)	15 (41.6)	3(42.9)
Diabetes mellitus, *n* (%)	5 (11.6)	4 (11.1)	1(14.3)
Mild coronary atherosclerosis, *n* (%)	2 (4.7)	2 (5.6)	0
LVEF 40–50%	3 (7.0)	2 (5.6)	1 (14.3)
Presenting arrhythmia			
Isolated PVC, *n* (%)	42 (97.7)	35 (97.2)	7 (100)
PVC/NSVT, *n* (%)	1(2.3)	1 (2.8)	0
AAD use			
Beta-Blocker, *n* (%)	20 (46.5)	17 (47.2)	3 (42.9)
Class Ic drug, *n* (%)	19 (44.2)	15 (41.7)	4 (57.1)
Sotalol, *n* (%)	10 (23.3)	8 (22.2)	2 (28.6)
Amiodarone, *n* (%)	6 (14.0)	6 (16.7)	0 (0)

PVC, premature ventricular complex; NSVT, non-sustained ventricular tachycardia; LVEF, left ventricular ejection fraction; AAD, antiarrhythmic drug.

There were 18 patients with hypertension, 5 with type 2 diabetes mellitus, 2 with mild coronary artery atherosclerosis detected by computed tomographic angiography, and 3 with left ventricular ejection fraction 40–50%. Forty-two patients presented with isolated PVCs and 1 with concomitant non-sustained VT. An average of 1.3 ± 0.5 AADs were used per patient. The clinical VA was primarily diagnosed as left PHVA in 3 patients and as right PHVA in the remaining 40 patients based on the ECG. PHVA was successfully ablated from the left side in 4 of 40 patients with ECG-diagnosed right PHVA, and was re-grouped as left PHVA. Totally there were 36 with right PHVA and 7 with left-sided VA.

Right PHVA Ablation

RF ablation by the B-SLTV approach succeeded in 24 (66.7%) of 36 patients with right PHVA, and failed in the remaining 12 patients (**Figure 5**). The electrocardiographic and procedural data were compared between successful and unsuccessful B-SLTV ablation in **Table 2**. There was significant greater target -HB distance and lower prevalence of junctional beats in patients with successful B-SLTV ablation than in those without. ECG morphologies, the local ventricular activation preceding QRS onset (V-QRS), proportion of small HB potential at the target, average RF power, RF duration, number of RF delivery and fluoroscopy time were comparable between successful and unsuccessful B-SLTV ablation.

Among the electrocardiographic and procedural parameters, target-HB distance was the only factor that could predict successful B-SLTV ablation for right PHVA (OR 1.703; 95% CI 1.084–2.676, $P = 0.02$). ROC analysis showed target-HB distance cutoff value was 4.5 mm (sensitivity 66.7% and specificity 83.3%; Area under the curve = 0.773, 95% CI 0.614–0.931, $P = 0.01$). There was no significant difference in RF power and duration between cases with target-HB distance > 4.5 mm and those with target-HB distance ≤ 4.5 mm (35.0 ± 2.3 vs. 36.0 ± 3.4 W, $P = 0.34$; 155.5 ± 38.1 vs. 146.3 ± 34.2 s, $P = 0.76$, respectively).

Subsequent ablation in 12 patients with unsuccessful B-SLTV ablation was listed in detail in **Supplementary Table 1**. A-SLTV ablation successfully abolished the clinical VA in 6 of them. Totally procedural success was achieved in 30 (83.3%) of 36 patients with right PHVA. The remaining 6 patients experienced ablation failure even after thorough mapping and ablation at the neighboring structures (RVOT and three coronary cusps at the aortic root) and the left- parahisian region.

Left PHVA Ablation

Sub-aortic valve ablation was successful in all seven patients with left PHVA. In each of 4 patients with failed right parahisian ablation, the V-QRS time at the left-sided target was greater than that at the right-sided target (27 vs. 24, 31 vs. 29, 16 vs. 14, 33 vs. 31 ms, respectively). Compared with right PHVA, left PHVA exhibited higher proportion of precordial transition ≤lead V2 and lower proportion of QS shape in lead V1 on ECG recordings (**Table 2**). The procedural parameters were comparable except that the target-HB distance was greater in left sided group than that in right-sided group.

Complications

Mechanical injury caused right bundle branch block in 6 patients during catheter manipulation in the RV, which recovered in all of them within 24 h post-ablation. Transient high degree AVB occurred during A-SLTV ablation 4 mm below the HB in 1 patient, and resolved completely after immediate ablation suspension. However, this patient underwent pacemaker implantation due to complete AV block one-month post-ablation.

Follow-Up Results at 1 Year

At the end of 12 months' follow-up, clinical success was achieved in 27 (75%) of 36 patients with right PHVA and in 6 (85.7%) of 7 patients with left PHVA. In this PHVA cohort, totally the clinical success was achieved in 33 (76.7%) of 43 patients off AADs by using this systemic mapping approach.

DISCUSSION

Major Findings

In this retrospective study we firstly proposed and evaluated a novel systemic mapping approach for PHVA ablation, which was a combination of ablation at the B-SLTV/A-SLTV region, the neighboring structures and the contralateral parahisian regions. Secondly the target-HB distance was the only predictor for right PHVA ablation among all the procedural parameters and

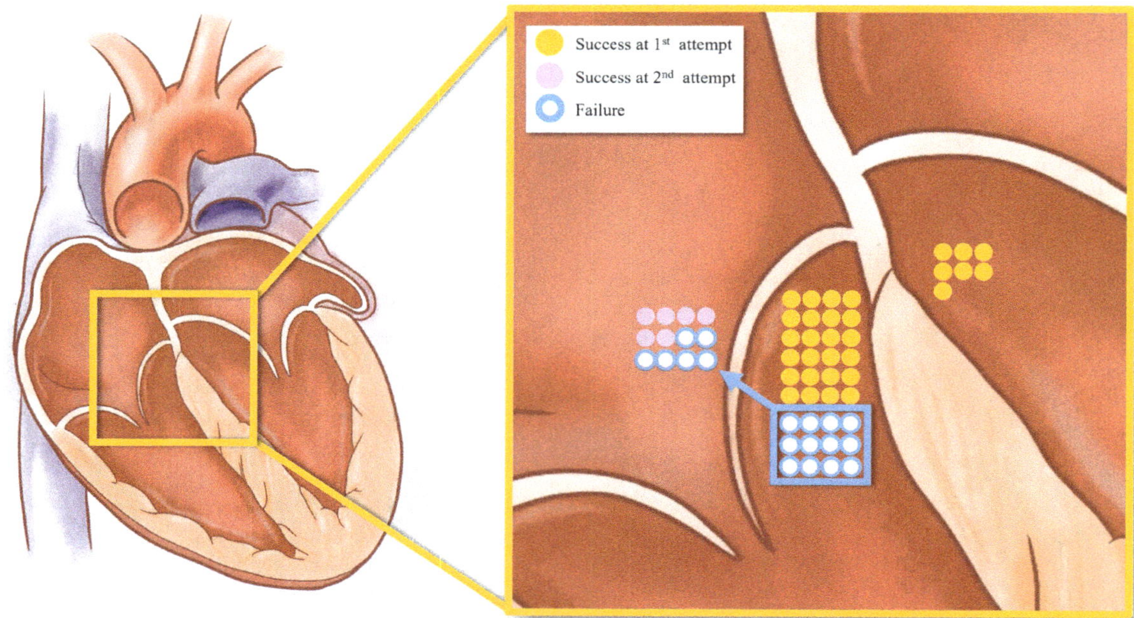

FIGURE 5 | The schematic diagram showing the acute procedural results of right and left PHVA ablation. The yellow dots represented successful cases by the B-SLTV approach and those by trans-aortic retrograde ablation. The purple dots represented success cases by the adjunctive A-SLTV approach. White dots represented cases with ablation failure.

TABLE 2 | Comparison of right and left parahisian VA ablation.

	Right parahisian VA ablation (n = 36)			**Left parahisian VA ablation (n = 7)**
	Total	**Successful B-SLTV (n = 24)**	**Unsuccessful B-SLTV (n = 12)**	
ECG morphology				
QS pattern in lead V1, n (%)	33 (91.7)$^{\$}$	23 (95.8)	10 (83.3)	2 (28.6)$^{\$}$
Precordial transition ≤ lead V2, n (%)	14 (38.9)$^{\#}$	8 (33.3)	6 (50.0)	6 (85.7)$^{\#}$
Inferior lead negative/discordance, n (%)	27 (75.0)	18 (75.0)	9 (75.0)	7 (100.0)
Procedural parameters				
V-QRS, ms	24.8 ± 7.4	25.1 ± 7.1	24.1 ± 8.4	24.1 ± 5.7
Target-HB distance, mm	5.1 ± 2.3‡	5.8 ± 2.3*	3.7 ± 1.7*	7.4 ± 1.8‡
Small HBP at the target, n (%)	11(30.6)	5 (20.8)	6 (50)	2 (28.6)
Junctional beats, n (%)	10 (27.8)	2 (8.3)*	8 (66.7)*	2 (28.6)
RF power (W)	35.5 ± 3.0	35.1 ± 1.9	36.3 ± 4.3	36.9 ± 3.1
Number of RF delivery	3.6 ± 1.3	3.3 ± 1.2	4.0 ± 1.3	4.0 ± 1.2
RF duration (s)	150.6 ± 35.9	149.2 ± 37.2	153.4 ± 34.5	165.7 ± 41.5
Fluoroscopy time (s)	519.5 ± 352.7	441.6 ± 270.1	675.5 ± 451.1	346.1 ± 108.3

$^{\$}P = 0.001$; $^{\#}P = 0.04$; $^{\ddagger}P = 0.02$ for comparison between right PHRA and left PHRA.
$^{*}P < 0.05$ for comparison between successful B-SLTV and unsuccessful B-SLTV group.
RF, radiofrequency; HBP, the His bundle potential.

this value exceeding 4.5 mm predicted successful ablation. This informative result might provide us a useful tool to estimate the effectiveness in advance and avoid excessive risks of AVB during the procedure.

Challenges and Obstacles for PHVAs Ablation

In one anatomical study it was found that the HB ran superficially without a layer of myocardial coat (the "naked" HB) in one fifth of the subjects (15). In another study it was found that the distal compact atrioventricular node (AVN) and the proximal HB had no surrounding myocardial layer (16). In this scenario RF ablation in close proximity to the AVN-HB was associated with increased risk of AVB. This severe complication became a major challenge for PHVA ablation. The major anatomical obstacle that was faced during right PHVA ablation was the SLTV. The "shield effect" of the SLTV prevented direct energy delivery to the basal myocardium. Furthermore, the movement of the SLTV might cause displacement of catheter tip, leading to insufficient lesion creation.

Technical Innovations in PHVA Ablation

In the early days, the conventional A-SLTV approach was initially used for right PHVA ablation in several small-volume studies (6–8), with modest effectiveness and safety results. Later on, the application of cryo-energy failed to demonstrate better efficacy and safety in right PHVA ablation, compared with RF energy (17). In that study, cryoablation succeeded in only 4 of 10 patients with PHVA with the cost of pacemaker implantation in 1 patient complicated with three-degree AVB. The potential advantages of cryo- over RF energy comprised reversible cryo-mapping with a temperature of −30°C, reduced risk of damage to the surrounding tissue and better catheter stability. However, the size of ice ball was bigger than that of the catheter tip during cryoablation at a temperature of −70°C, which might reduce the distance threshold to avoid AVB. Furthermore, the A-SLTV rather than the B-SLTV approach was applied in that study. The latter might be more useful to improve the effectiveness as well as safety for PHVA ablation, which would be discussed below.

In recently years, the novel B-SLTV ablation (also known as "catheter inversion" technique, "reversed C-curve technique," etc.) began to be applied for PHVA ablation, with a high success rate of 88% reported in a latest cohort study of 28 cases (11). The advantages of the B-SLTV approach over the conventional A-SLTV approach lay in two aspects: one was better catheter tip-tissue contact and more efficient energy delivery; the other was less risk of AVB, which was demonstrated in an animal study. It that study, the B-SLTV ablation carried less risk of AVB in experimental dogs compared with the A-SLTV ablation (18).

Judgement of B-SLTV placement of the catheter tip was vital for the B-SLTV approach. Although the fluoroscopic catheter inversion configuration indicated correct placement, it was doubtful that the catheter tip was at the right place in some cases. At this time the B-SLTV positioning could be judged by the fluoroscopic sign of catheter "fixation" while pulling it back, and could be further confirmed by ICE imaging (shown in **Figures 2D,H**). Even if the catheter tip was placed at the B-SLTV area, a contact-force sensing catheter was preferable and sometimes clockwise rotation of the catheter was needed to ensure appropriate catheter tip-tissue contact.

Rationale for a Systemic Mapping Approach for Right PHVA Ablation

Despite the important advantages, the B-SLTV approach was not the end of story in the course of right PHVA ablation. It might not be able to abolish left parahisian foci, intramural foci, or foci extremely close to the AVN-HB. In our cohort, the procedural success could only be achieved in 66.7% of the patients by the B-SLTV approach. The "seemingly" right PHRA turned out to be left PHVA in a small proportion of the patients. Similar to RVOT VA ablation, VA with a left-sided origin might breakout from a right-sided exit through a preferential conduction pathway (19, 20), exhibiting the ECG of a right-sided VA. In our study the earliest local activation time at the left side preceding the one at the right side supported the existence of preferential conduction. Apparently, the B-SLTV approach was not effective for left PHVAs and left parahisian ablation was necessitated. Furthermore, to abolish intramural foci, RF ablation in the contralateral region might be necessary, rather than repeated B-SLTV ablation. Moreover, to ablate the ectopic focus extremely close to the AVN-HB, the B-SLTV approach was not always effective or safe and the A-SLTV approach/anatomical ablation at the neighboring structures might be effective (11, 12). The adjunctive A-SLTV approach succeeded in 6 of 12 cases who experienced B-SLTV ablation failure in our study. Among 6 cases with adjunctive A-SLTV ablation success, the target-HB distance was only 2 mm in 2 cases. This result indicated that different catheter tip orientation and trivial adjustment of the target site might help to improve the ablation results on certain occasions, though the risk of AVB should be carefully balanced.

Predictors for Successful PHVA Ablation

There were no electrocardiographic predictors (such as QRS shape in lead V1 and the inferior leads, precordial transition, etc.) identified for successful PHVA ablation. However, among all the procedural parameters, we found only the target-HB distance > 4.5 mm could predict successful right PHVA ablation. We believed this finding might serve as a useful tool to estimate the effectiveness ahead of ablation and avoid excessive risks of AVB if the target-HB distance was markedly shorter than 4.5 mm.

Study Limitations

Several major limitations existed in our study. Firstly, this study was a retrospective, single-arm cohort study and included limited patients. The effectiveness and safety of the systemic mapping approach should be tested in a prospective, controlled, and large-scale clinical trials. However, given the fairly low prevalence of PHVA, all the published literature were mainly case reports or small case series reports, lacking randomized controlled studies. Secondly, it was possible that PHVA abolished at left side after failed at right side originated from an intramural focus rather than a true left side focus. However, as was the case in RVOT VA, the existence of preferential conduction might increase the difficulties in identifying left or right out-flow tract VAs. The earliest local activation time at the left-sided target preceding the one at the right-sided target supported the existence of preferential conduction in our study. There might be no gold standard for defining right, intramural and left foci, and the response to ablation might be a practical one. Successful ablation at the contralateral parahisian region or the adjacent structures justified the application of s systemic mapping approach in complex PHVA ablation.

CONCLUSIONS

The systemic mapping approach was effective and safe for treating right and left PHVAs. The ablation target-HB distance was a significant predictor for right PHVA ablation.

AUTHOR CONTRIBUTIONS

XW conceptualized the systemic mapping approach for PHVA ablation. LK, XW, and TS drafted the manuscript. LK drew the figures and illustrations. ZL were involved in clinical data collection. ZZ and WJ were involved in data processing. JP revised the manuscript. All authors have read and approved the final manuscript.

REFERENCES

Miller JM, Pezeshkian NG, Yadav AV. Catheter mapping and ablation of right ventricular outflow tract ventricular tachycardia. *J Cardiovasc Electrophysiol.* (2006) 17:800–2. doi: 10.1111/j.1540-8167.2006.0 0519.x

Dixit S, Gerstenfeld EP, Callans DJ, Marchlinski FE. Electrocardiographic patterns of superior right ventricular outflow tract tachycardias: distinguishing septal and free-wall sites of origin. *J Cardiovasc Electrophysiol.* (2003) 14:1–7. doi: 10.1046/j.1540-8167.2003.0 2404.x

Enriquez A, Tapias C, Rodriguez D, Liang J, Marchlinski F, Saenz L, et al. How to map and ablate parahisian ventricular arrhythmias. *Heart Rhythm.* (2018) 15:1268–74. doi: 10.1016/j.hrthm.2018.02.028

Ban J, Chen Y, Park H, Kim D, Lee D, Park Y, et al. Idiopathic ventricular arrhythmia originating from the para-hisian area: prevalence, electrocardiographic and electrophysiological characteristics. *J Arrhythm.* (2014) 30:48–54. doi: 10.1016/j.joa.2013.04.007

Enriquez A, Pathak RK, Santangeli P, Liang JJ, Al Rawahi M, Hayashi T, et al. Inferior lead discordance in ventricular arrhythmias: A specific marker for certain arrhythmia locations. *J Cardiovasc Electrophysiol.* (2017) 28:1179– 1186. doi: 10.1111/jce.13287

Yamauchi Y, Aonuma K, Takahashi A, Sekiguchi Y, Hachiya H, Yokoyama Y, et al. Electrocardiographic characteristics of repetitive monomorphic right ventricular tachycardia originating near the His-bundle. *J Cardiovasc Electrophysiol.* (2005) 16:1041–8. doi: 10.1111/j.1540-8167.2005.4 0787.x

Komatsu Y, Taniguchi H, Miyazaki S, Kusa S, Takayama K, Kakita K, et al. Two distinct electrocardiographic forms of idiopathic ventricular arrhythmia originating in the vicinity of the His bundle. *Europace.* (2012) 14:1778–85. doi: 10.1093/europace/eus160

Komatsu Y, Otomo K, Taniguchi H, Kakita K, Takayama K, Fujiwara H, et al. Catheter ablation of ventricular arrhythmias arising from the right ventricular septum close to the His bundle: features of the local electrogram at the optimal ablation site. *J Cardiovasc Electrophysiol.* (2011) 22:878–85. doi: 10.1111/j.1540-8167.2011.02014.x

Zeljko HM, Yue A. Catheter inversion technique for ablation of parahisian accessory pathway. *Europace.* (2015) 17:1707. doi: 10.1093/europace/e uv254

Clemens M, Peichl P, Kautzner J. Catheter ablation of idiopathic ventricular ectopy in the vicinity of the His bundle under the septal leaflet of the tricuspid valve. *Europace.* (2015) 17:1370. doi: 10.1093/europace/ euv084

Sun J, Zhang PP, Wang QS, Xu QF, Wang ZQ, Yu Y, et al. Catheter ablation of ventricular arrhythmias originating from the para-Hisian region with reversed C-curve technique. *J Cardiovasc Electrophysiol.* (2019) 30:2377–2386. doi: 10.1111/jce.14170

Yamada T, McElderry HT, Doppalapudi H, Kay GN. Catheter ablation of ventricular arrhythmias originating in the vicinity of the His bundle: significance of mapping the aortic sinus cusp. *Heart Rhythm.* (2008) 5:37–42. doi: 10.1016/j.hrthm.2007.08.032

Zhang SQ, Zheng C, Li YC, Ji KT, Yin RP, Lin JF, et al. Common and distinctive electrocardiographic characteristics and effective catheter ablation of idiopathic ventricular arrhythmias originating from different areas of ventricular septum adjacent to atrioventricular annulus. *J Cardiovasc Electrophysiol.* (2018) 29:1104–12. doi: 10.1111/jce.13638

Luo S, Zhan X, Ouyang F, Xue Y, Fang X, Liao H, et al. Catheter ablation of right-sided para-Hisian ventricular arrhythmias using a simple pacing strategy. *Heart Rhythm.* (2019) 16:380–7. doi: 10.1016/j.hrthm.2018. 09.015

Kawashima T, Sasaki H. A macroscopic anatomical investigation of atrioventricular bundle locational variation relative to the membranous part of the ventricular septum in elderly human hearts. *Surg Radiol Anat.* (2005) 27:206–13. doi: 10.1007/s00276-004-0302-7

Mulpuru SK, Cha YM, Asirvatham SJ. Synchronous ventricular pacing with direct capture of the atrioventricular conduction system: functional anatomy, terminology, and challenges. *Heart Rhythm.* (2016) 13:2237–46. doi: 10.1016/j.hrthm.2016.08.005

Miyamoto K, Kapa S, Mulpuru SK, Deshmukh AJ, Asirvatham SJ, Munger TM, et al. Safety and efficacy of cryoablation in patients with ventricular arrhythmias originating from the para-Hisian region. *JACC Clin Electrophysiol.* (2018) 4:366–73. doi: 10.1016/j.jacep.2017.12.013

1. Kato R, Matsumoto K, Goktekin O, Matsuo H, Watanabe H, Takahama

M. Parahisian radiofrequency catheter ablation in dogs: comparison of the above-valve and below-valve approaches. *J Interv Card Electrophysiol.* (2000) 4:359–68. doi: 10.1023/A:1009814803581

Yamada T, Murakami Y, Yoshida N, Okada T, Shimizu T, Toyama J, et al. Preferential conduction across the ventricular outflow septum in ventricular arrhythmias originating from the aortic sinus cusp. *J Am Coll Cardiol.* (2007) 50:884–91. doi: 10.1016/j.jacc.2007.05.021

Yamada T, Platonov M, McElderry HT, Kay GN. Left ventricular outflow tract tachycardia with preferential conduction and multiple exits. Circ Arrhythm Electrophysiol. (2008) 1:140–2. doi: 10.1161/CIRCEP.108.7 *CircArrhythm Electrophysiol.* (2008) 1:140–2. doi: 10.1161/CIRCEP.108.7 78563

21

Predictors and Long-Term Outcome of Ablation of Discrete Pre-Potentials in Patients with Idiopathic Ventricular Arrhythmias Originating from the Aortic Sinuses of Valsalva

Hui-Qiang Wei[1,2], *Xiao-Gang Guo*[2], *Gong-Bu Zhou*[3], *Qi Sun*[2], *Jian-Du Yang*[2], *Hai-Yang Xie*[2], *Jackson Liang*[4], *Shu Zhang*[2], *Shulin Wu*[1] *and Jian Ma*[2*]

[1] *Department of Cardiology, Guangdong Cardiovascular Institute, Guangdong Provincial People's Hospital, Guangdong Academy of Medical Sciences, Guangzhou, China,* [2] *State Key Laboratory of Cardiovascular Disease, Arrhythmia Center, National Center for Cardiovascular Diseases, Fuwai Hospital, Chinese Academy of Medical Sciences and Peking Union Medical College, Beijing, China,* [3] *Department of Cardiology, Peking University Third Hospital, Beijing, China,* [4] *Division of Cardiovascular Medicine, Electrophysiology Service, University of Michigan Health System, Ann Arbor, MI, United States*

***Correspondence:**
Jian Ma
majian_fuwai@126.com

Background: The predictability and long-term outcome of the discrete pre-potential (DPP) of idiopathic ventricular arrhythmias (VAs) arising from the aortic sinuses of Valsalva (ASV) have not been fully identified.

Methods: Of 687 consecutive patients undergoing ablation of outflow tract VAs, there were 105 (15.3%) patients with VAs originating from the ASV region who were included. Detailed mapping was performed within the ASV in all patients. Electrocardiographic, electrophysiological parameters, and long-term success rate were compared between patients with and without the DPPs.

Results: A DPP was recorded in 67 of 105 (63.8%) patients, including 38 left sinus of Valsalva (LSV)-VAs (38/105, 36.2%) and 29 right sinus of Valsalva (RSV)-VAs (29/105, 27.6%). The patients with DPPs had wider QRS duration (152 $\pm$ 17 vs. 145 $\pm$ 14 ms, $p < 0.001$). The average of earliest activation time was significantly earlier in patients with DPPs (-38.6 ± 8.5 vs. -27.7 ± 5.7 ms, $p < 0.001$). Mean time from the first lesion to elimination of VAs was shorter in patients with DPPs (2.3 $\pm$ 2.1 s vs. 4.9 $\pm$ 1.0 s, $p < 0.001$). A stepwise logistic multivariable analysis identified only younger age as a significant predictor of DPP (age $\leq$ 35.5 years predicted DPP with 92.9% positive predictive value). During a follow-up duration of 42.5 $\pm$ 22.3 months, 63 (94.0%) patients with DPPs and 30 (78.9%) patients without DPPs remained free of recurrent VAs ($p = 0.027$).

Conclusion: Discrete pre-potentials were observed in 63.8% of patients with VAs arising from the ASV. Ablation in patients with DPPs was associated with higher long-term success. DPPs were seen more commonly in younger (age $\leq$ 35.5 years) patients.

Keywords: ventricular arrhythmia, catheter ablation, sinus of Valsalva, discrete pre-potential, outcome

INTRODUCTION

The right or left ventricular outflow tracts (RVOTs or LVOTs) are the most common sites of origin for idiopathic ventricular tachycardia (VT) or premature ventricular contractions (PVCs). Radiofrequency (RF) catheter ablation has been considered as a safe and effective method to treat outflow tract ventricular arrhythmias (VAs), and arrhythmias from these sites are being increasingly recognized (1–3). Several studies have reported that a discrete pre-potential (DPP) can sometimes be recorded at the successful ablation sites within the aortic sinuses of Valsalva (ASV), and the presence of the DPPs has been considered to be useful in guiding ablation within the ASV (4–6). However, there remains a paucity of comparative data on the prevalence and predictability of identifying DPPs during mapping and ablation of idiopathic VAs arising from the ASV. Consequently, the aim of this study was to identify the electrocardiographic and electrophysiological predictors of DPPs of idiopathic VAs arising from the ASV.

METHODS

The data that support the findings of this study are available from the corresponding author upon reasonable request.

Study Population

A total of 687 patients underwent ablation of ventricular outflow tract VAs between January 2012 and December 2018 at our center (**Figure 1**). Patients who underwent repeat ablation or ablation failed were excluded in this study (the anatomic location of their VA origin could not be determined). All patients had cardiac imaging with transthoracic echocardiography to confirm the absence of structural heart disease. All patients provided written informed consent before the catheter ablation. This study was approved by the institutional review board of Fuwai Hospital.

ECG Analysis

Detailed analysis of clinical VT or PVCs was performed offline using an electrophysiological data acquisition system (LabSystem PRO, Bard Electrophysiology, Lowell, MA, USA). The following measurements were assessed during the clinical VT or PVCs using the measurement tool: (1) R- and S-wave amplitudes in leads I, II, III, and V_1 to V_3; (2) Q-wave amplitude in leads aVL, aVR, and the Q-wave ratio in lead aVL/aVR; (3) QRS duration; and (4) the precordial transitional zone (TZ); In addition, the precordial TZ was analyzed during the sinus rhythm. The TZ index was calculated as follows: TZ index = TZ score of the clinical VAs minus the TZ score of sinus rhythm (7). In cases with a QS pattern in lead I, we defined the R-amplitude as being 0 mV. The T-P segment was considered the isoelectric baseline for the measurement of R- and S-wave amplitude. All measurements were independently performed by two cardiac electrophysiologists.

Electrophysiological Study

After the withdrawal of all antiarrhythmic drugs for at least five half-lives, all patients underwent electrophysiological evaluation. An electrophysiological study was performed with the patient in the fasting, non-sedated state. Catheters were inserted into the heart under fluoroscopy *via* the femoral vessels. If clinical VAs did not appear simultaneously, programmed stimulation or intravenous isoproterenol was performed to provoke the clinical arrhythmias. Bipolar signals were filtered at 30–500 Hz, and unipolar signals were filtered at 0.05–500 Hz. Intravenous heparin was administered to maintain an activated clotting time of 250 s.

Mapping and Catheter Ablation

Three-dimensional electroanatomic mapping was applied in all patients using the CARTO mapping system (Biosense Webster, Inc., Diamond Bar, CA). Mapping and ablation were performed using a NaviStar ThermoCool catheter (Biosense Webster, Diamond Bar, California) *via* the femoral vessels. Point-by-point mapping was performed to create anatomic maps, and activation mapping was always used to identify the earliest activation site during the PVCs or VT as previously described (8). Pace mapping was also performed in some cases. An ideal target for ablation was selected based on the earliest activation time during the PVCs or VT. DPP was defined as sharp high-frequency potentials occurring after or during the local ventricular electrogram in sinus rhythm or preceding the local ventricular electrogram during PVCs that sometimes displayed double or multiple components.

When mapping and ablation were attempted in ASV, selective angiography through the irrigated catheter tip or aortic arteriography using a pigtail catheter was performed to locate the position of the ASVs. Detailed mapping in the ASV was achieved using the ablation catheter. RF energy was delivered using an initial power of 25 W with an irrigation rate of 17 mL/min. During RF delivery, if a decreased frequency or elimination of VAs occurred within the initial 15 s, the application was maintained and titrated for 60–90 s. If the earliest activation time of VAs was $<$20 ms, then additional mapping was performed below the valve, coronary venous system or retried in RVOT. After successful ablation, intravenous administration of isoproterenol and programmed ventricular stimulation were performed to reinduce clinical VAs. Acute procedural success was defined as elimination and non-inducibility of the clinical PVCs or VT with isoproterenol infusion and programmed stimulation after at least a 30-min waiting period after the last ablation lesion.

Follow-Up

Continuous telemetric monitoring was performed for 24 h in all patients postablation. Long-term success was defined as no recurrence of the clinical VAs during a Holter monitoring. After hospital discharge, patients were seen in outpatient clinic every 3 months for the 1st year postablation, and every 6 months thereafter. All patients underwent 24-h Holter monitoring and transthoracic echocardiography during follow-up. If the patients had any rhythm-related symptoms, a 12-lead ECG or 24-h 12-lead Holter monitoring was performed to document the cause of the symptoms.

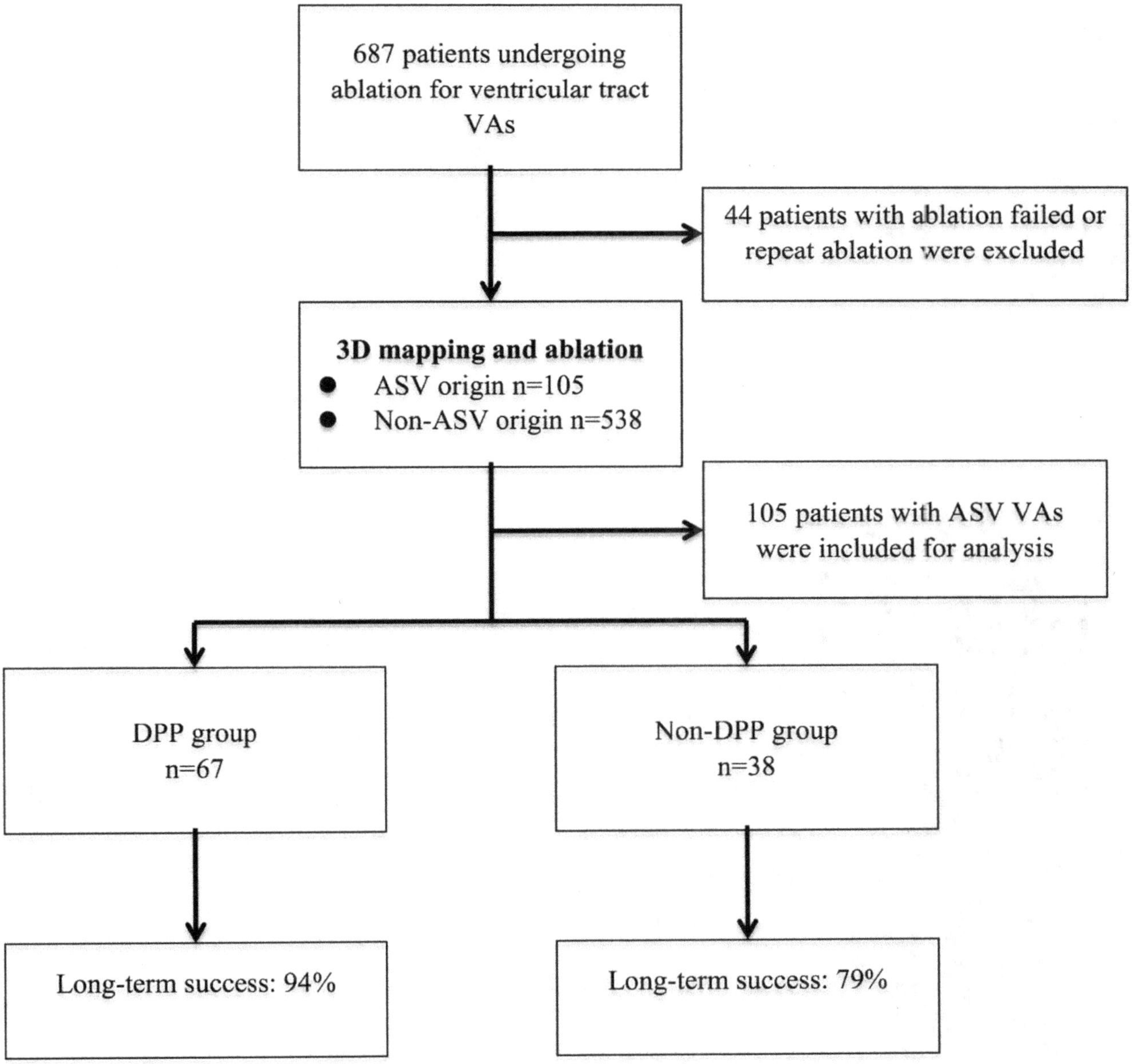

FIGURE 1 | The flow diagram of the study and long-term success rate. 3D, 3-dimensional; ASV, aortic sinus of Valsalva; DPP, discrete pre-potential; VA, ventricular arrhythmia.

Statistical Analysis

All continuous variables are expressed as mean ± SD. The categorical variables are presented as numbers and percentages. Categorical variables were compared using chi-squared analysis. Continuous variables were compared using the Student's *t*-test or Mann–Whitney *U*-test, depending on data distribution. Significant clinical characteristics and ECG parameters predicting predictors of DPPs were tested by univariately, and multivariable logistic regression models were constructed using a backward procedure with $p > 0.1$ as the default criterion for eliminating all variables. Independent variables were tested for collinearity, but no collinearity was present. Receiver operating characteristic (ROC) curves corresponding to the selected logistic regression models were constructed, and the area under the curve (AUC) was calculated to access the diagnostic value of the variables. The optimal cutoff equaled the maximum of Youden's index J, calculated from the ROC data as the cutoff with the greatest sum of sensitivity and specificity (J = sensitivity + specificity−1). A two-tailed value of $p < 0.05$ was considered statistically significant. All statistical

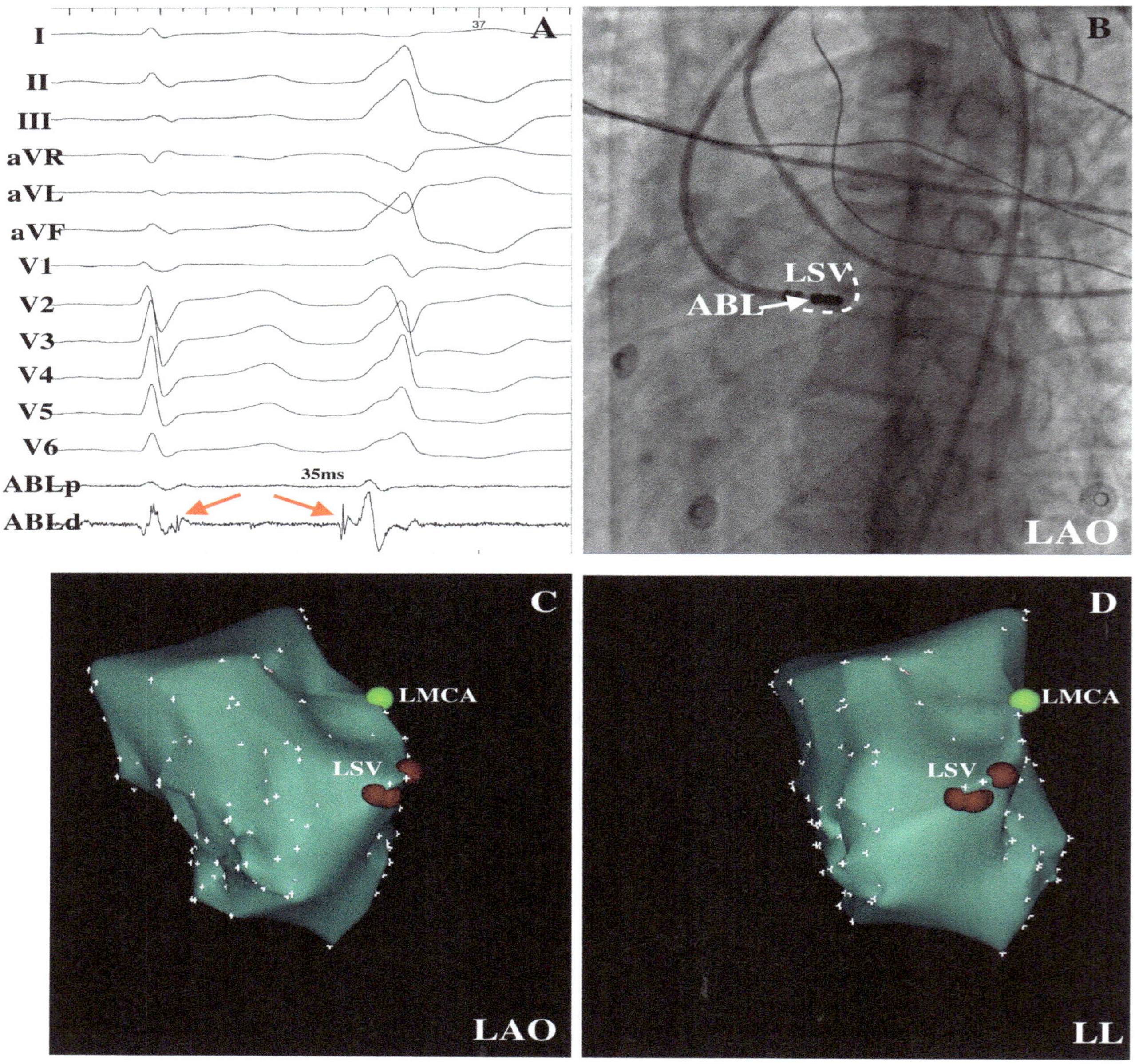

FIGURE 2 | PVCs were successfully ablated within the LSV. **(A)** Delayed potential (red arrow) was observed during the sinus rhythm, and a DPP on the LSV preceded the QRS by 35 ms at the successful ablation site was recorded. **(B)** LAO radiographic view revealed the mapping catheter within the LSV. LAO **(C)** and LL **(D)** electroanatomical maps demonstrated the successful ablation points within the LSV. LSV, left sinus of Valsalva; DPP, discrete pre-potential; LAO, left anterior oblique; LL, left lateral; ABL, ablation catheter; LMCA, left main coronary artery.

analyses were performed using SPSS 19.0 (SPSS, Inc., Chicago, IL, USA).

RESULTS

Baseline Characteristics

The successful ablation site was located within the ASV region in 105 (15.3%) of the 687 patients: 64 (61.0%) from the left sinus of Valsalva (LSV) and 41 (39.0%) from the right sinus of Valsalva (RSV). Of the 105 patients whose successful target site was from the ASV, a DPP was recorded in 67 of 105 (63.8%) patients, including 38 LSV-VAs (38/64, 59.4%) (**Figure 2**) and 29 RSV-VAs (29/41, 70.7%) (**Figure 3**). Baseline clinical and demographic data are presented in **Table 1**. Patients in whom DPPs were identified were younger in age than those without DPPs (37.6 ± 17.3 years vs. 52.2 ± 12.8 years, $p < 0.001$), and patients with DPPs were more likely to be male gender (62.7%) whereas those without DPPs were more likely to be female gender (57.9%) ($p = 0.042$)

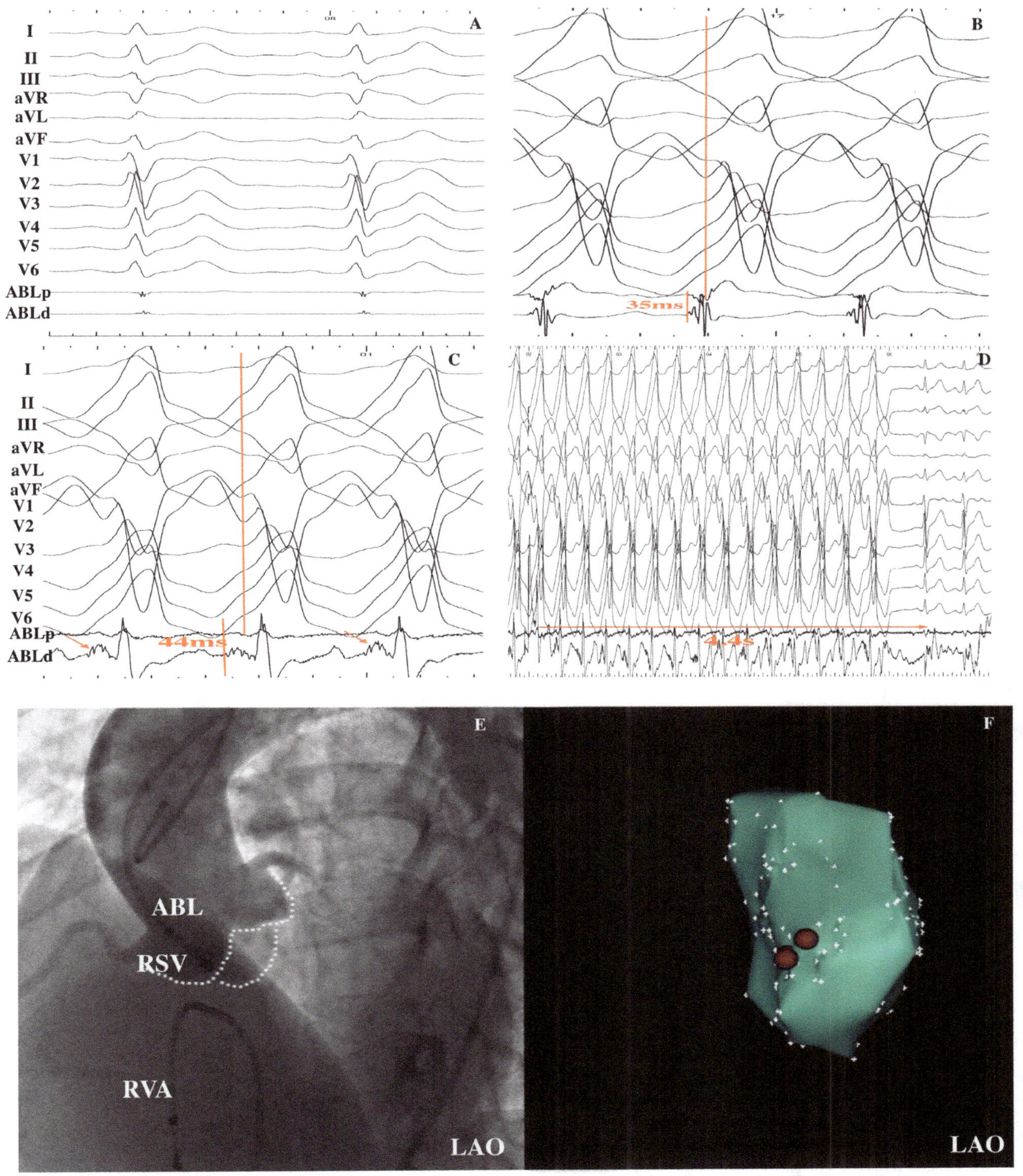

FIGURE 3 | VT was successfully ablated within the RSV in a 15-year-old male patient. **(A)** Baseline 12-lead ECG was shown; **(B)** An early ventricular activation preceded by QRS by 35 ms during the VT was recorded at the RVOT, but ablation was ineffective. **(C)** Fragmented potential (red arrow) was found at the RSV, and the interval from the potential to QRS onset was 44 ms. **(D)** After RF energy delivery, VT was terminated after 4.4 s. **(E)** LAO fluoroscopic view of the mapping catheter at the successful ablation site as demonstrated by aortic artery angiography. **(F)** Electroanatomical CARTO map of the VT in the LAO view. Red points indicate ablation points. RSV, right sinus of Valsalva; RF, radiofrequency ablation; VT, ventricular tachycardia; LAO, left anterior oblique; ABL, ablation catheter; RVA, right ventricular apex.

TABLE 1 | Baseline clinical characteristics in patients with and without DPP.

	DPP+ ($n = 67$)	DPP− ($n = 38$)	p-value
Age (years)	37.6 ± 17.3	52.2 ± 12.8	<0.001
Male	42 (62.7%)	16 (42.1%)	0.042
LVEF (%)	60.4 ± 7.5	61.3 ± 6.8	0.828
PVC burden on 24-h Holter monitoring	30,754 ± 14,740	28,466 ± 13,575	0.456
Clinical arrhythmias			0.01
Frequent PVCs	53 (79.1%)	37 (97.4%)	
Non-sustained or sustained VT	14 (20.9%)	1 (2.6%)	
Number of failed AADs	0.9 ± 0.8	1.2 ± 0.7	0.098
Structural heart disease	0	0	-

Values are described as mean ± SD or n.
DPP, discrete pre-potential; LVEF, left ventricular ejection fraction; PVC, premature ventricular contraction; VT, ventricular tachycardia; AAD, antiarrhythmic drug.

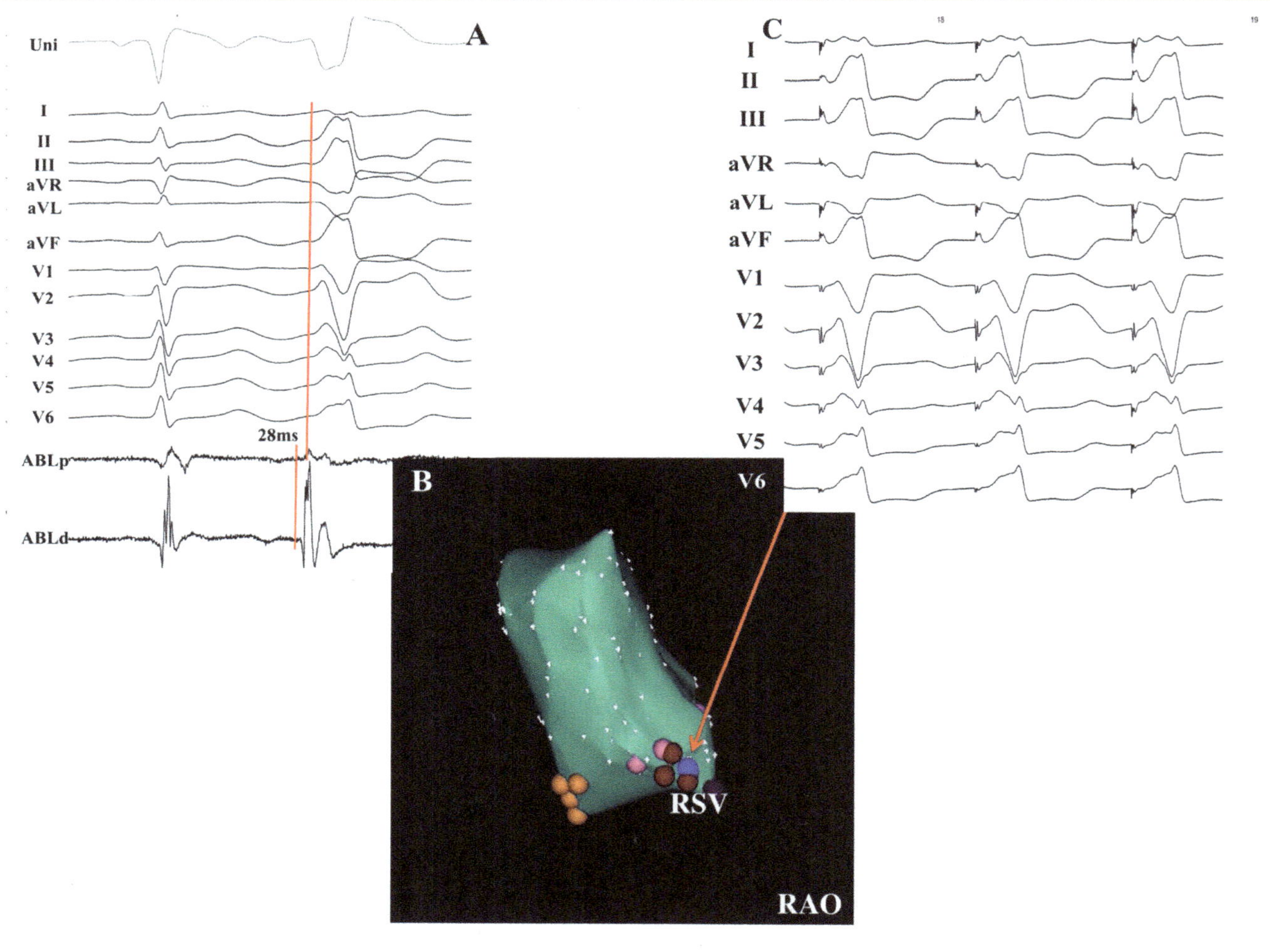

FIGURE 4 | Successful ablation of PVCs without DPPs in a 63-year-old female patient. **(A)** The earliest activation recorded at the RSV preceded the QRS complex onset by 28 ms without DPPs. **(B)** Electroanatomical CARTO map of the PVCs in the RAO view. Red points indicate the ablation points. Blue point indicates the pacing site. Orange points indicate the non-coronary sinus of Valsalva. **(C)** Pacing mapping was excellent when pacing was delivered at the ablation site. RSV, right sinus of Valsalva; DPP, discrete pre-potential; RAO, right anterior oblique.

(**Figure 4**). In addition, patients with DPPs were more likely to have non-sustained or sustained VT rather than single PVC (20.9 vs. 2.6%, $p = 0.01$).

ECG Characteristics

The VA ECG characteristics are summarized in **Table 2**. Patients with DPPs had wider QRS (152 ± 17 vs. 145 ±14 ms, $p < 0.001$).

TABLE 2 | ECG parameters during the VAs between patients with and without DPP.

	DPP+ ($n = 67$)	DPP− ($n = 38$)	p-value
QRS duration (ms)	152 ± 17	145 ± 14	0.019
R-wave amplitude in lead I (mV)	0.20 ± 0.25	0.15 ± 0.15	0.248
R-wave amplitude in lead II (mV)	1.82 ± 0.47	1.63 ± 0.37	0.105
R-wave amplitude in lead III (mV)	1.77 ± 0.61	1.63 ± 0.37	0.194
R-wave amplitude in lead aVF (mV)	1.79 ± 0.54	1.62 ± 0.31	0.117
R-wave ratio in lead II/III	1.10 ± 0.37	1.02 ± 0.17	0.260
Q-wave amplitude in lead aVL (mV)	0.86 ± 0.40	0.80 ± 0.29	0.361
Q-wave amplitude in lead aVR (mV)	0.94 ± 0.26	0.81 ± 0.16	<0.001
Q-wave ratio in lead aVL/aVR	0.96 ± 0.46	1.02 ± 0.39	0.496
R-wave amplitude in lead V_1 (mV)	0.45 ± 0.32	0.39 ± 0.27	0.285
S-wave amplitude in lead V_1 (mV)	1.03 ± 0.55	0.57 ± 0.40	<0.001
R-wave amplitude in lead V_2 (mV)	0.91 ± 0.48	0.97 ± 0.51	0.478
S-wave amplitude in lead V_2 (mV)	1.47 ± 0.91	0.90 ± 0.58	<0.001
R-wave amplitude in lead V_3 (mV)	1.41 ± 0.65	1.65 ± 0.74	0.056
Precordial TZ index	−0.53	−1.22	0.005

Values are displayed as mean ± SD.
DPP, discrete pre-potential; TZ, transitional zone.

TABLE 3 | Electrophysiological characteristics during the VAs between patients with and without DPP.

	DPP+ ($n = 67$)	DPP− ($n = 38$)	p-value
Mean activation time (ms)	−38.6 ± 8.5	−27.7 ± 5.7	<0.001
Mean time from the first RF lesion to the elimination of VAs (s)	2.3 ± 2.1	4.9 ± 1.0	<0.001
Total Number of RF application	2.1 ± 1.0	2.7 ± 0.9	<0.001
Initial mapping of right side	33 (49.3%)	12 (31.6%)	0.101

Values are demonstrated as mean ± SD or n.
DPP, discrete pre-potential; RF, radiofrequency; VA, ventricular arrhythmia.

Q-wave amplitude in lead aVR was greater in patients with DPPs (0.94 ± 0.25 vs. 0.81 ± 0.16 mV, $p < 0.001$). S-wave amplitude in leads V_1 and V_2 was greater in patients with DPPs (1.03 ± 0.55 vs. 0.57 ± 0.40 mV, $p < 0.001$; 1.47 ± 0.91 vs. 0.90 ± 0.58 mV, $p < 0.001$, respectively). The TZ index was larger in patients with DPPs compared with those without DPPs (−0.53 vs. −1.22, $p = 0.005$).

Electrophysiological Characteristics

Detailed mapping of the ASVs was performed in all patients. The average of the earliest activation time was significantly earlier in patients with DPPs than in those without DPPs (−38.6 ± 8.5 vs. −27.7 ± 5.7 ms, $p < 0.001$). RVOT mapping was initially performed in 33 (49.3%) patients with DPPs and 12 (31.6%) patients without DPPs ($p = 0.101$). The mean time from the first RF lesion to the elimination of VAs was shorter in patients with DPPs than in those without DPPs (2.3 ± 2.1 vs. 4.9 ± 1.0 s, $p <$ 0.001). The total number of RF applications in patients with DPPs was significantly less than in those without DPPs (2.1 ± 1.0 vs. 2.7 ± 0.9, $p < 0.001$) (**Table 3**).

Predictors of DPP

A stepwise logistic multivariable analysis identified only the age as a significant predictor of a DPP (OR 1.61; 95% confidence interval 1.03–2.74; $p < 0.001$). On the basis of ROC curve analysis, an age of ≤ 35.5 years produced an AUC of 0.731 with a sensitivity of 44.3% and specificity of 93.3%, with a 92.9% of positive predictive value and a 46.7% of negative predictive value (**Figure 5**).

Complications and Follow-Up

There were three peripheral vascular complications including two patients with pseudoaneurysm and one with arteriovenous fistula. There were no other major complications, including no coronary arterial damage or aortic valve injury in any patients. Over a total follow-up duration of 42.5 ± 22.3 months, 63 (94.0%) patients with DPPs and 30 (78.9%) patients without DPPs remained free of recurrent VAs in the absence of antiarrhythmic drugs. There was a significant difference in recurrent rate between patients with and without DPPs (6.0 vs. 21.1%, $p =$ 0.027). Of these patients, Seven of 12 patients received repeat ablation. Successful ablation was achieved in the same location in two patients with DPPs. However, in the other five patients without DPPs, the distribution of ablation sites was as follows: RVOT in three patients, aorto-mitral continuity (AMC) in one patient, and below RSV-LSV commissure in one patient. Repeat ablation was successful in these five patients.

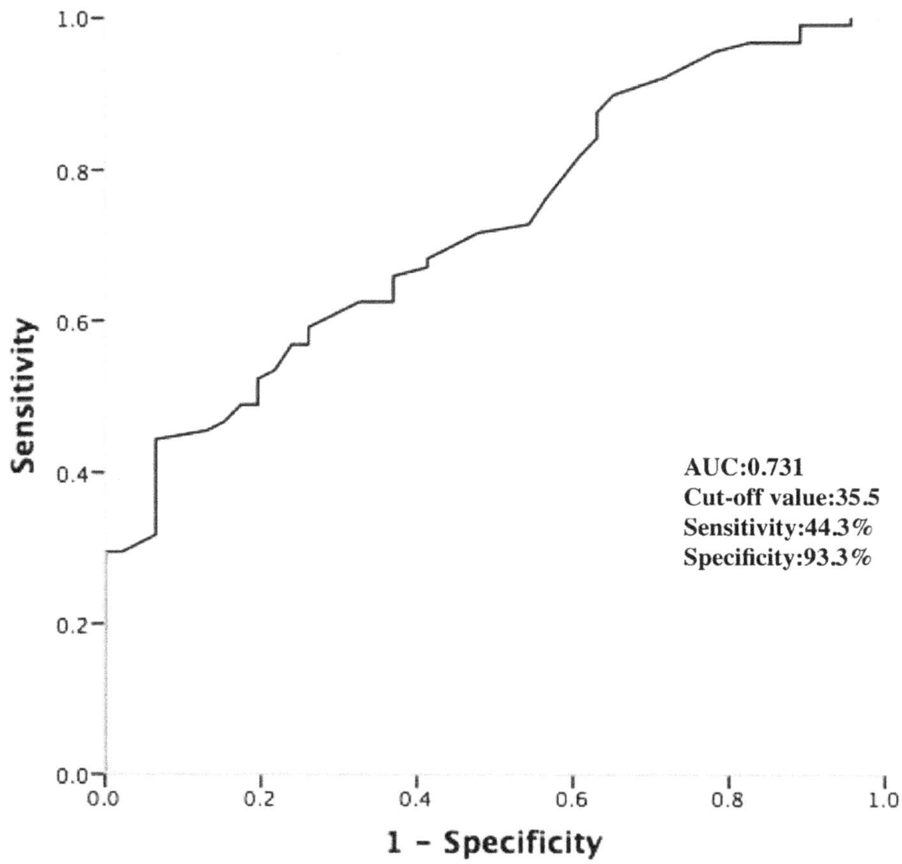

FIGURE 5 | ROC curve analyzing the age to predict the DPPs. DPP, discrete pre-potential; AUC, area under curve.

DISCUSSION

Major Findings

To the best of our knowledge, this is the first study to investigate the predictors of DPPs of VAs originating from the ASV. In this study, we found that (1) a DPP can be recorded in 63.8% of the patients whose successful ablation site locates in the LSV or RSV; (2) RF ablation in patients with DPPs was associated with a higher long-term success rate compared with those without DPPs; (3) the age is the only independent predictor of DPPs; and (4) the age $\leq$ 35.5 years can predict the presence of DPPs with a 92.9% of positive predictive value.

Presence of DPP

Previous studies have reported that extensions of the left ventricular myocardium frequently exist within the ASV (9–11). The fibrosis and fatty tissue among these muscular sleeves may create a possible VA substrate (11). The presence of DPPs of VAs originating from the ASV has been described in previous studies and considered to be useful in guiding ablation within the ASV (4–6). There has been a wide range in prevalence of DPPs during ASV and outflow tract VA ablation, ranging from 10% of all outflow tract VA ablations, 26% of all ASV ablations, and up to 100% of patients with ASV in a study by Ouyang et al. (4–6). In this study, DPPs were recorded in 67 (63.8%) of 105 patients in whom ablation from the ASV was successful in eliminating the VA. Non-sustained or sustained VT was commonly seen in the patients with DPPs, which is consistent with Ouyang's study. We surmise that the DPPs may be responsible for triggering the VA, similar to that observed from superior vena cava and pulmonary vein in patients with atrial fibrillation (12, 13). The low incidence of DPPs reported in previous studies may be due to decreased recognition of the low-amplitude DPP in some patients. The scale of the electrogram recorded in the ablation catheter should be magnified during the mapping within the ASV. In addition, small sample sizes may account for the low prevalence of the DPP.

ECG Characteristics

Few studies have described the ECG characteristics of DPPs of VAs originating from the ASV. Hachiya et al. (4) reported nine of 35 patients with DPPs and no specific ECG findings were found. In this study, using quantitative ECG analysis, several unique ECG characteristics were found in patients with DPPs. The patients with DPPs were associated with wider QRS. Q-wave amplitude in lead aVR was greater in patients with DPPs. S-wave amplitude in leads V_1 and V_2 were greater in patients with DPPs. In addition, the TZ index was larger in patients with DPPs compared with those without DPPs. The extra-ventricular myocardium extensions may be responsible for these unique ECG characteristics. These myocardial extensions were asymmetrical, with sleeves routinely found along anterior portions of the RSV and LSV (14), which might produce a vector from anterior to posterior. This activation manner results in the terminal S-wave in leads V_1 and V_2.

Predictors of DPP

The DPPs have been considered to be an indicator of successful ablation site within the ASV (4, 6). As Ouyang reported, two ventricular activation components were always recorded at the successful site in patients with VT originating from the ASV (6). In Ouyang's study, the mean age of the patients was 36.6 years. In this study, we found that the age was the independent predictor of DPPs. An age of $\leq$ 35.5 years produced an AUC of 0.731 with a sensitivity of 44.3% and specificity of 93.3%, with a high-positive predictive value, which was consistent with Ouyang's study. Younger patients were more likely to have a DPP, which might be explained by the fact that degenerative fibrosis of the myocardial extensions may occur over time with advancing age (15).

Long-Term Clinical Outcome

Several investigators have demonstrated the favorable outcome in small series of patients with DPPs of VAs originating from the ASV (4–6). In this study, during a follow-up period of 42.5 $\pm$ 22.3 months, 94% of patients with DPPs remained free of recurrent VAs. However, a higher recurrent rate was observed in patients without DPPs. This may further prove that the DPPs represent the myocardial origin of VAs, and the presence of DPPs may help to identify successful ablation sites and improve long-term success. In some cases without DPPs, although successful ablation was initially achieved in ASC, the true arrhythmia origin may not be located in ASC due to the complexity of LVOT anatomy. The larger part of the RSV and the commissure between RSV and LSV are related to the interventricular septum which forms part of the subaortic valvular region and the RVOT septal wall. Similarly, the LSV is in close relationship with the LV summit, the interventricular vein, and the AMC (16). In our study, five patients without DPPs received repeat procedures. The final ablation sites were RVOT in three patients, AMC in one patient, and below RSV-LSV commissure in one patient. Therefore, careful mapping of all the neighbor structures around the ASC may be needed in some patients without DPPs undergoing the first procedure to reduce the recurrent rate.

Study Limitations

This was a retrospective single-center study with a limited sample size. First, pace mapping was not routinely performed in all patients. Second, VAs from RSV-LSV junction were also defined as RSV or LSV-VAs and were not analyzed separately in this study. Furthermore, no non-sinus Valsalva cases were included because only four cases were found in our study, and the value of statistical analysis in such a small case series might be questioned. Third, although successful ablation was achieved within ASV in all cases, the real arrhythmia origin still could not be 100% sure. Final successful ablation in the ASV could not necessarily mean that the VAs originated from this spot. Furthermore, intracardiac echocardiography was not available in all patients due to the cost.

CONCLUSION

Discrete pre-potentials were observed in 63.8% of the patients in whom VAs were successfully eliminated with ablation from the ASV region. Ablation in patients with DPPs was associated with higher long-term success. Younger age independently predicted the DPPs. A cutoff of 35.5 years of age indicated the presence of the DPPs with a 92.9% of positive predictive value.

AUTHOR CONTRIBUTIONS

All authors listed have made a substantial, direct, and intellectual contribution to the work and approved it for publication.

REFERENCES

Calkins H, Kalbfleisch SJ, el-Atassi R, Langberg JJ, Morady F. Relation between efficacy of radiofrequency catheter ablation and site of origin of idiopathic ventricular tachycardia. *Am J Cardiol.* (1993) 71:827– 33. doi: 10.1016/0002-9149(93)90832-W

Morady F, Kadish AH, DiCarlo L, Kou WH, Winston S, deBuitlier M, et al. Long-term results of catheter ablation of idiopathic right ventricular tachycardia. *Circulation.* (1990) 82:2093–9. doi: 10.1161/01.CIR.82. 6.2093

Tsai CF, Chen SA, Tai CT, Chiang CE, Lee SH, Wen ZC, et al. Idiopathic monomorphic ventricular tachycardia: Clinical outcome, electrophysiologic characteristics and long-term results of catheter ablation. *Int J Cardiol.* (1997) 62:143–50. doi: 10.1016/S0167-5273(97)00198-8

Hachiya H, Yamauchi Y, Iesaka Y, Yagishita A, Sasaki T, Higuchi K, et al. Discrete prepotential as an indicator of successful ablation in patients with coronary cusp ventricular arrhythmia. *Circ Arrhythm Electrophysiol.* (2013) 6:898–904. doi: 10.1161/CIRCEP.113.000157

Srivathsan KS, Bunch TJ, Asirvatham SJ, Edwards WD, Friedman PA, Munger TM, et al. Mechanisms and utility of discrete great arterial potentials in the ablation of outflow tract ventricular arrhythmias. *Circ Arrhythm Electrophysiol.* (2008) 1:30–8. doi: 10.1161/CIRCEP.107.750315

Ouyang F, Fotuhi P, Ho SY, Hebe J, Volkmer M, Goya M, et al. Repetitive monomorphic ventricular tachycardia originating from the aortic sinus cusp: Electrocardiographic characterization for guiding catheter ablation. *J Am Coll Cardiol.* (2002) 39:500–8 doi: 10.1016/S0735-1097(01)01767-3

Yoshida N, Inden Y, Uchikawa T, Kamiya H, Kitamura K, Shimano M, et al. Novel transitional zone index allows more accurate differentiation between idiopathic right ventricular outflow tract and aortic sinus cusp ventricular arrhythmias. *Heart Rhythm.* (2011) 8:349–56. doi: 10.1016/j.hrthm.2010.11.023

Wei HQ, Guo XG, Liu X, Zhou GB, Sun Q, Yang JD, et al. Safety and efficacy of catheter ablation of ventricular arrhythmias with para-hisian origin via a systematic direct approach from the aortic sinus cusp. *Heart Rhythm.* (2018) 15:1626–33. doi: 10.1016/j.hrthm.2018.05.021

Ho SY. Structure and anatomy of the aortic root. *Eur J Echocardiogr.* (2009) 10:i3–10. doi: 10.1093/ejechocard/jen243

Gami AS, Noheria A, Lachman N, Edwards WD, Friedman PA, Talreja D, et al. Anatomical correlates relevant to ablation above the semilunar valves for the cardiac electrophysiologist: A study of 603 hearts. *J Interv Card Electrophysiol.* (2011) 30:5–15. doi: 10.1007/s10840-010-9523-3

Hasdemir C, Aktas S, Govsa F, Aktas EO, Kocak A, Bozkaya YT, et al. Demonstration of ventricular myocardial extensions into the pulmonary artery and aorta beyond the ventriculo-arterial junction. *Pacing Clin Electrophysiol.* (2007) 30:534–9. doi: 10.1111/j.1540-8159.2007.00704.x

Haissaguerre M, Jais P, Shah DC, Takahashi A, Hocini M, Quiniou G, et al. Spontaneous initiation of atrial fibrillation by ectopic beats originating in the pulmonary veins. *N Engl J Med.* (1998) 339:659– 66. doi: 10.1056/NEJM199809033391003

Lin WS, Tai CT, Hsieh MH, Tsai CF, Lin YK, Tsao HM, et al. Catheter ablation of paroxysmal atrial fibrillation initiated by non-pulmonary vein ectopy. *Circulation.* (2003) 107:3176–83. doi: 10.1161/01.CIR.0000074206.52056.2D

Tabatabaei N, Asirvatham SJ. Supravalvular arrhythmia: Identifying and ablating the substrate. *Circ Arrhythm Electrophysiol.* (2009) 2:316–26. doi: 10.1161/CIRCEP.108.847962

Sahasakul Y, Edwards WD, Naessens JM, Tajik AJ. Age-related changes in aortic and mitral valve thickness: Implications for two-dimensional echocardiography based on an autopsy study of 200 normal human hearts. *Am J Cardiol.* (1988) 62:424–30. doi: 10.1016/0002-9149(88)90971-X

Di Biase L, Romero J, Zado ES, Diaz JC, Gianni C, Hranitzki PM, et al. Variant of ventricular outflow tract ventricular arrhythmias requiring ablation from multiple sites: Intramural origin. *Heart Rhythm.* (2019) 16:724– 32. doi: 10.1016/j.hrthm.2018.11.028

22

Late Gadolinium Enhancement Cardiovascular Magnetic Resonance Assessment of Substrate for Ventricular Tachycardia with Hemodynamic Compromise

John Whitaker[1], Radhouene Neji[1,2], Steven Kim[3], Adam Connolly[1], Thierry Aubriot[3], Justo Juliá Calvo[4], Rashed Karim[1], Caroline H. Roney[1], Brendan Murfin[5], Carla Richardson[5], Stephen Morgan[5], Tevfik F. Ismail[1,5], James Harrison[1], Judith de Vos[6], Maurice C. G. Aalders[6], Steven E. Williams[1,7†], Rahul Mukherjee[1], Louisa O'Neill[1], Henry Chubb[1], Cory Tschabrunn[8], Elad Anter[9], Luigi Camporota[5], Steven Niederer[1], Sébastien Roujol[1], Martin J. Bishop[1], Matthew Wright[5], John Silberbauer[4], Reza Razavi[1] and Mark O'Neill[1]*

[1] School of Biomedical Engineering and Imaging Sciences, King's College, London, United Kingdom, [2] Siemens Healthcare, Frimley, United Kingdom, [3] Abbott Medical, St Paul, MN, United States, [4] Brighton and Sussex University Hospitals NHS Trust, Brighton, United Kingdom, [5] Guy's and St Thomas' NHS Foundation Trust, London, United Kingdom, [6] Department of Biomedical Engineering and Physics, Amsterdam UMC, University of Amsterdam, Amsterdam, Netherlands, [7] Centre for Cardiovascular Science, University of Edinburgh, Edinburgh, United Kingdom, [8] Division of Cardiovascular Medicine, University of Pennsylvania, Philadelphia, PA, United States, [9] Cleveland Clinic, Cleveland, OH, United States

***Correspondence:**
John Whitaker
john.whitaker@kcl.ac.uk*

Background: The majority of data regarding tissue substrate for post myocardial infarction (MI) VT has been collected during hemodynamically tolerated VT, which may be distinct from the substrate responsible for VT with hemodynamic compromise (VT-HC). This study aimed to characterize tissue at diastolic locations of VT-HC in a porcine model.

Methods: Late Gadolinium Enhancement (LGE) cardiovascular magnetic resonance (CMR) imaging was performed in eight pigs with healed antero-septal infarcts. Seven pigs underwent electrophysiology study with venous arterial-extra corporeal membrane oxygenation (VA-ECMO) support. Tissue thickness, scar and heterogeneous tissue (HT) transmurality were calculated at the location of the diastolic electrograms of mapped VT-HC.

Results: Diastolic locations had median scar transmurality of 33.1% and a median HT transmurality 7.6%. Diastolic activation was found within areas of non-transmural scar in 80.1% of cases. Tissue activated during the diastolic component of VT circuits was thinner than healthy tissue (median thickness: 5.5 mm vs. 8.2 mm healthy tissue, $p < 0.0001$) and closer to HT (median distance diastolic tissue: 2.8 mm vs. 11.4 mm healthy tissue, $p < 0.0001$). Non-scarred regions with diastolic activation were closer to steep gradients in thickness than non-scarred locations with normal EGMs (diastolic locations distance = 1.19 mm vs. 9.67 mm for non-diastolic locations, $p < 0.0001$). Sites activated late in diastole were closest to steep gradients in tissue thickness.

Conclusions: Non-transmural scar, mildly decreased tissue thickness, and steep gradients in tissue thickness represent the structural characteristics of the diastolic component of reentrant circuits in VT-HC in this porcine model and could form the basis for imaging criteria to define ablation targets in future trials.

Keywords: ventricular tachycardia, late gadolinium enhancement, cardiovascular magnetic resonance, mechanical circulatory support, venous-arterial extra corporeal membrane oxygenation (VA-ECMO)

INTRODUCTION

Viable myocytes within and on the border of dense scar display abnormal electrophysiological characteristics that promote reentrant arrhythmias (1–3). In most clinical VT ablation procedures, electrophysiological criteria alone are normally used to identify arrhythmogenic tissue (4–6). Even with a combination of ablation of clinical VT identified through activation and entrainment mapping and pace-mapping as well as substrate-based ablation (7), medium term outcomes remain modest with up to 50% of patients experiencing a recurrence of VT within a year of ablation (8).

When imaged *ex-vivo* at the near-cellular level, late-gadolinium enhanced (LGE) cardiovascular magnetic resonance (CMR) accurately identifies peri-infarct heterogeneous tissue (HT) as regions of intermediate signal intensity (ISI) (9). This tissue represents the critical substrate responsible for post-MI reentrant VT (10). These observations have been extended to *in-vivo* imaging where it has been reported that regions of ISI may also display abnormal electrophysiological properties (11, 12) described as the peri-infarct borderzone (BZ). This suggests that *in-vivo* LGE-CMR may offer a low-risk option for generating a 3D assessment of substrate that may have utility in guiding substrate-based VT ablation.

Pre-procedural cross-sectional imaging has been proposed as a non-invasive approach that may facilitate more comprehensive arrhythmogenic substrate identification and ablation (13). Effective substrate identification, either using electrophysiological or structural criteria, may be of particular importance in the context of the growing population of patients presenting with VT with hemodynamic compromise (VT-HC) (14, 15), in which only a substrate-guided approach is usually possible (6).

We hypothesized that under idealized experimental conditions the quality of LGE-CMR could be optimized in order provide accurate anatomic information about the tissue substrate for VT-HC. We aimed to characterize the tissue substrate responsible for VT-HC using high-resolution *in-vivo* 3D LGE-CMR and acquiring high-density activation mapping under hemodynamic support to identify the location of diastolic electrograms during post-MI VT-HC in a chronic porcine infarct model.

MATERIALS AND METHODS

Animal studies complied with French law and were performed at the Institut de Chirurgie Guidée par l'image (IHU), Strasbourg, France. The experimental protocol was approved by the local and national institutional animal care and ethics committee. Eight domestic pigs underwent a 180 minute balloon occlusion of the mid left anterior descending (LAD) artery to create experimental ischemia-reperfusion myocardial infarction (MI) as previously described (16). Seven weeks following MI each pig underwent late-gadolinium enhanced (LGE) cardiovascular magnetic resonance (CMR) imaging. One week later each pig underwent electrophysiology study with prophylactic hemodynamic support during which VT was induced and assessed using high-density activation mapping.

CARDIOVASCULAR MAGNETIC RESONANCE IMAGING DATA ACQUISITION

All imaging was performed on 1.5T scanner (MAGNETOM Aera, Siemens Healthineers, Erlangen, Germany) with an 18-channel body matrix coil and a 32-channel spine coil.

Clinical Standard 2D Late Gadolinium Enhanced Cardiovascular Magnetic Resonance Imaging

Ten min after 0.1 mmol/kg gadobutrol (Gadovist, Bayer Plc, Reading, UK) bolus, 2D LGE-CMR imaging was acquired. Inversion-time (TI) scout was acquired in a single mid ventricular short axis slice [free breathing, balanced steady state free precession (bSSFP); linear k-space reordering; echo time/repetition time/flip angle (TE/TR/α): 1.11 ms/2.6 ms/30°; slice thickness: 8 mm; in plane resolution: 1.8 x 1.8 mm^2; field of view (FOV): 340 x 276 mm^2]. Clinical standard 2D LGE-CMR imaging was acquired using an inversion recovery (IR) sequence with phase-sensitive IR (PSIR) reconstruction (bSSFP; linear k-space reordering; TE/TR/α: 1.21 ms/3 ms/45°; slice thickness: 6 mm; in plane resolution: 1.4 x 1.4 mm^2; FOV: 360 x 281 mm^2). Fifteen min after Gd bolus, 0.0011 mmol/kg/min Gd infusion was commenced. TI-scout was repeated at regular intervals following Gd bolus and during infusion.

3D Late Gadolinium Enhanced Cardiovascular Magnetic Resonance Imaging

Isotropic navigator-gated ECG-triggered 3D IR sequence was acquired in the mid-diastolic phase as identified from cine imaging (fat saturation prepared; bSSFP; coronal orientation; linear k-space reordering; TE/TR/α: 1.58ms/3.6ms/90°; gating window = 7 mm; parallel imaging using GRAPPA with acceleration factor 2; resolution 1.2 x 1.2 x 1.2 mm^3; FOV: 400 x 257 x 96 mm^3; 2 R-R interval ECG triggering) with full ventricular coverage. Subjective and objective parameters of image quality were compared between 2D and 3D LGE CMR imaging (further details in **Supplementary Figure 1**).

CARDIOVASCULAR MAGNETIC RESONANCE IMAGING DATA ANALYSIS

Image Segmentation

Each 3D LGE-CMR scan was manually segmented by a single observer within Seg3D2 [University of Utah, Utah, USA, https://www.sci.utah.edu/cibc-software/seg3d.html]. Based on previously reported analysis of LGE-CMR imaging from patients undergoing VT ablation (17), the segmented myocardium was thresholded for scar signal intensity (SI_{scar}) at 60% and intermediate SI ($SI_{intermediate}$) at 40% of the highest SI within the segmentation.

Tissue Thickness and Scar Transmurality Assessment

Field lines between the endocardial and epicardial surfaces were derived by solving the Laplace equation as previously described (18). Briefly, the endocardial and epicardial surfaces were tagged. To calculate the distance from endocardial to epicardial surface, the Laplace equation ($\nabla^2 u = 0$) was solved with Dirichlet boundary conditions assigned at the endocardial ($u = 0$) and epicardial ($u = 1$) surfaces. Wall thickness was evaluated as the total length of the continuous path from the endocardium to the epicardium when moving orthogonally between adjacent iso-potential surfaces. Tissue thickness gradients were assessed using a radial basis function to identify the gradient in tissue thickness (further details in **Supplementary Materials**). Transmurality of scar and HT was defined as the proportion of nodes along the path between endocardium and epicardium corresponding to each tissue type. The distance of each endocardial node to the nearest neighboring node assigned as heterogeneous tissue (HT) was automatically calculated.

Segmentations were processed to generate a surface mesh containing endocardial and epicardial surfaces, scar and aorta in the Digital Image Fusion (DIF) format for import into the Precision Electroanatomic Mapping System (EAMS, Abbott, St Paul, MN, USA) within which they were registered with the EAMS geometry, as described below.

Electrophysiology Study and Hemodynamic Support

Electrophysiology procedures were conducted 8 weeks after MI under general anesthetic (further details in **Supplementary Materials**) using the Precision electro-anatomic mapping system (EAMS, Abbott, Chicago, IL).

Prior to the EP study pigs were established on venous-arterial extra-corporeal membrane oxygenation (VA-ECMO) via the left femoral artery and vein and hemodynamic support was prophylactically instituted using a Maquet Cardiohelp machine (Maquet Getinge group, Rastatt, Germany, see **Supplementary Figure 1**). Venous and arterial access was established for the EP study and hemodynamic monitoring/drug administration. Hemodynamic compromise (HC) was defined as a rhythm associated with a mean arterial pressure (MAP) below 50 mmHg or a pulse pressure lower than 20 mmHg. During rhythms not associated with HC, VA-ECMO circuit flow was reduced to 0.5 L/min. During rhythms associated with HC, VA-ECMO flow ranged between 0.5 and 1 L to 4 L depending on hemodynamic status to maintain a MAP of 65–70 mmHg. Further details are provided in the **Supplementary Materials.**

A sensor-enabled Abbott FlexAbility™ ablation catheter was advanced to the aorta via the right femoral artery and used to acquire aortic root and coronary ostia geometry prior to gaining retrograde left ventricular (LV) access across the aortic valve. A multipolar mapping catheter [HD Grid™ or LiveWire™ duo-deca (Abbott, Chicago, IL)] was advanced through an Agilis sheath via the aorta to acquire LV endocardial geometry.

LV endocardial activation maps were acquired while pacing from the RV apex at 500 ms and then 300 ms.

An attempt was made to induce ventricular tachycardia (VT) using an adapted Wellen's VT stimulation protocol (19) with up to four extra-stimuli from right and then left ventricular sites. In the event that no VT was induced, the non-selective beta agonist isoproterenol was commenced as an infusion at an initial rate of 2 μg/min and up titrated to a maximum rate of infusion of 20 μg/min during which programmed electrical stimulation was repeated.

Activation maps were acquired using the Automap function within Precision™ using the initial deflection seen on any lead of the surface ECG leads as the timing reference with strict settings applied (EAMS, Abbott, St Paul, MN, USA) (Score = 85; speed limit = 10 mm/s; distance 1 mm; enhanced noise rejection: off). Each individual bipolar and unipolar EGM from the mapped VTs and maps during pacing were subsequently reviewed offline and the activation time reassigned when necessary. Following spontaneous or pace-termination, VT induction and mapping was subsequently repeated. Final activation maps were reviewed by at least two experienced electrophysiologists.

The extent of conduction block (identified as regions with tightly spaced isochrones in which > 15 ms separated adjacent activation points; in which activation on either side of tightly spaced isochrones from wave fronts moving in different directions, and in which double potentials identified in proximity to the boundary between adjacent waves of conduction) during RV pacing and during each mapped VT was estimated using the surface distance function within the EAMS.

Co-registration of Imaging and Electrophysiological Data

After the EP study, using the re-map function within the EAMS, a surface mesh generated from the LGE-CMR scan was imported into the EAMS in the digital image fusion (DIF) format. The EAMS LV geometry was registered to the DIF model with an initial landmark-based registration with the aorta, coronary ostia and LV apex as initial fiducial landmarks, followed by surface registration using the proprietary surface registration function within the EAMS. EAMS points manually identified as having healthy EGMs during RVP_{500} and those demonstrating diastolic activation during VT were exported from the EAMS. The location of these points from the EAMS mesh were automatically mapped to nodes on the CMR derived mesh within a 1 mm radius, to allow a node-wise assessment of the structural characteristics of tissue demonstrating diastolic activation during VT and healthy tissue could be made.

Episcopic Auto-Fluorescence Cryomicrotome Imaging

Following euthanasia, each heart was processed and then imaged using episcopic auto-fluorescence cryomicrotome imaging as previously described (20) (see **Supplementary Figure 2**).

Statistical Analysis

Normality of distribution of variables was assessed using the Shapiro-Wilks test. Normally distributed continuous variables are expressed as mean ± SD, otherwise variables are reported as medians with interquartile ranges. Normally distributed data were compared using a two tailed, paired sample *t*-test.

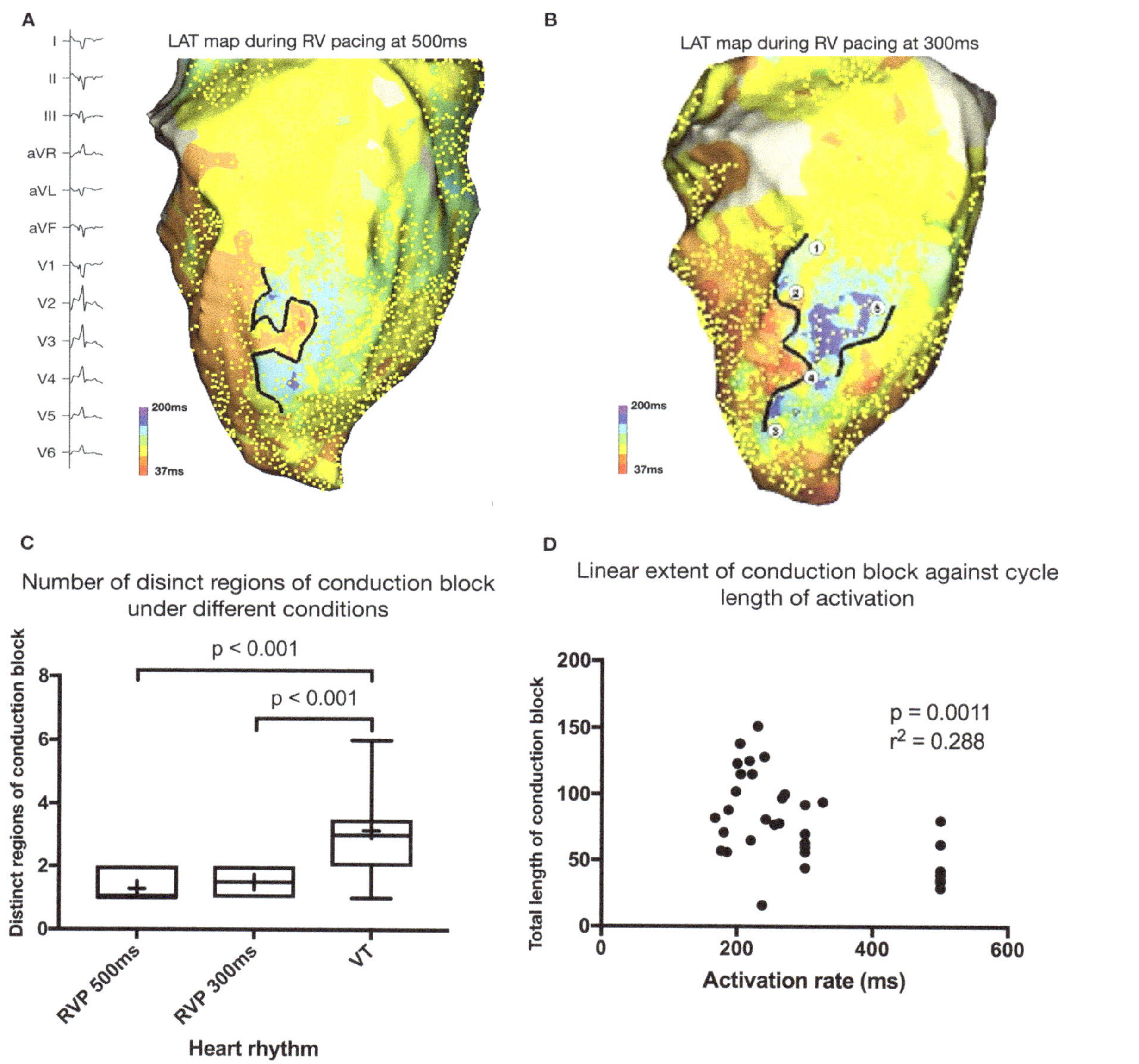

FIGURE 1 | (A) Activation map during right ventricular (RV) pacing at 500 ms. Yellow dots mark the point at which activation time was recorded. Black line represents linear conduction block during pacing at this cycle length. **(B)** Activation map during right ventricular (RV) pacing at 300 ms. **(C)** Number of distinct regions of conduction block during different heart rhythms (RV pacing at 500 ms and 300 ms and during VT). **(D)** Scatter plot of extent of linear endocardial conduction block and activation rate during pacing or VT.

Ordinal and non-parametric continuous data were compared using a Mann-Whitney U test or Kruskal-Wallis H-test as appropriate, with pairwise comparisons performed using Dunn's (1964) procedure with a Bonferroni correction for multiple comparisons where appropriate in which case adjusted p-values are presented. Two-tailed values of $p<0.05$ were considered significant. Statistical analysis was carried out in SPSS (v24, IBM Corporation, New York).

RESULTS

One post-MI pig died after CMR imaging and prior to EP study. The study protocol was completed in the remaining seven post-MI pigs and two control pigs who did not undergo CMR imaging. During this study all the VT that was induced was associated with hemodynamic compromise as defined above.

Late Gadolinium Enhanced Imaging Under Contrast Steady State

3D LGE-CMR imaging was acquired in eight animals (weight 62.6+/−3.7 kg) in the supine position under general anesthesia and CSS achieved in seven animals. In a single animal failure of the peripheral cannula interrupted the continuous Gd infusion, which prevented CSS during imaging. In the remaining seven animals 3D LGE-CMR imaging was acquired using a total Gd dose of <0.2 mmol/kg. 3D LGE-CMR was acquired in mid-diastole with a data acquisition duration of 83–104 ms, 23–42 segments, and a total imaging time of 50+/−12 min. Under conditions of CSS mean variation in $TI_{myocardium}$ was 5.2% (±3.1%, range 2.6–9.3%) and mean variation in TI_{blood} was 9.8% (±2.1%, range 6.7–13.5%). Representative imaging examples and demonstration of CSS are shown in **Figure 1**. All 3D LGE-CMR imaging is available for review online (**Supplementary Material**).

A comparison of the image quality with clinical standard 2D LGE-CMR imaging was undertaken and is included in the **Supplementary Materials.**

Induced Ventricular Tachycardia

Twenty episodes of VT-HC demonstrating a macro reentrant pattern of activation were mapped (18 complete maps, 2 incomplete) and the locations of diastolic electrograms (EGMs) assessed to be part of the reentrant circuit were identified and Labeled. A summary of the characteristics of the induced VTs is shown in **Table 1**. All mapped VTs were dependent on at least one region of conduction block that was not evident during RVP_{500}. All VTs with a complete activation map demonstrated at least two distinct regions of conduction block.

There was an increase in the extent of conduction block between RVP_{500} and VT (mean increase = 45 mm, 95% CI 27–63 mm, $p < 0.001$) and between RVP_{300} and VT (mean increase 23 mm, 95% CI 5–42 mm, $p = 0.016$), and a trend toward, an increase in conduction block between RVP_{500} and RVP_{300} (mean increase = 22 mm, 95% CI−1–45 mm, $p = 0.059$). Pearson correlation coefficient demonstrated a negative correlation between activation rate and total extent of conduction block ($r^2 = 0.288$, $p = 0.001$). These data are illustrated in **Figure 1**. Entrainment mapping was attempted in a subset of the induced VT-HC but was not successful due to failure to entrain or degeneration of the VT to ventricular fibrillation (VF).

TABLE 1 | Number of tachyarrhythmias observed and mapped per animal.

Pig	Number of episodes of non-sustained VT	Number of sustained, unmapped VTs	Number of mapped VTs	Number of episodes VF
1	67	3	0	7
2	-	-	-	-
3	27	2	4	1
4	100	3	9	4
5	22	2	2	6
6	16	3	2	10
7	88	2	2	1
8	47	3	2	8

Tissue Structure Assessment With *in-vivo* CMR at Locations With Diastolic Activation

Representative examples of diastolic EGMs recorded during VT are shown with their corresponding locations on *in-vivo* CMR in **Figure 2**. As shown in these examples, diastolic EGMs were visualized in regions with subendocardial HT (location 1), near-transmural scar (location 2) and pure HT (location 3). Tissue thinning is also seen in all locations.

A representative example of the position of a diastolic EGM, corresponding *in-vivo* imaging and episcopic auto-fluorescence cryomicrotome imaging (EACI) data is shown in **Figure 3**.

Non-enhanced tissue adjacent to regions of enhancement on *in-vivo* CMR were frequently observed in the septal area and corresponded to regions where muscle fibers traversing the RV cavity, including the moderator band, inserted into the septum. An example of this is shown in **Figure 4**, in which a corridor of preserved myocardium surrounded by dense scar forms the principal path of the diastolic isthmus of one VT, which in this case is approximately aligned with the direction of the long axis of the left ventricle.

The structural characteristics of locations at which diastolic EGMs occurred during the observed VTs were systematically examined and compared with locations at which normal EGMs were recorded. The normal EGMs were all recorded at positions with 0% scar/HT transmurality. Diastolic locations had a median scar transmurality of 33.1%, [IQR 0–77.3%, mean 37.4(±36.3) %, $p < 0.001$] and a median HT transmurality 7.6% [IQR 0–30.3%, mean 18.3(±22.9)% $p < 0.001$]. The majority (80.1%) of diastolic locations were found within areas with non-transmural scar or HT. Tissue activated in the diastolic component of VT circuits was thinner than healthy tissue (median thickness tissue with diastolic activation = 5.5 mm vs. 8.2 mm healthy tissue, $p < 0.001$) and was closer to HT (median distance from HT diastolically activated tissue 2.8 mm vs. 11.4 mm healthy tissue, $p < 0.001$). Of those diastolic locations that were in regions without scar or HT, all were within 15 mm of HT and

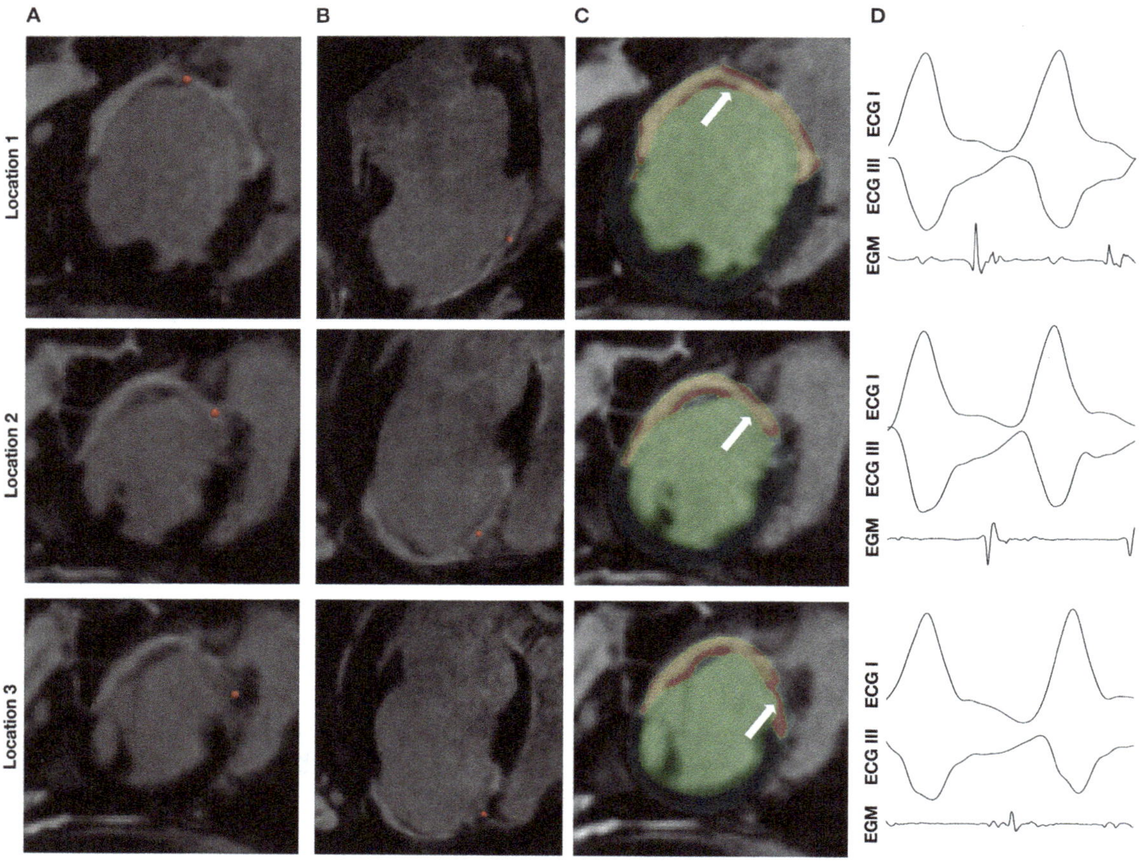

FIGURE 2 | Visualization of location of diastolic EGMs on *in-vivo* CMR. Column **(A)** and column **(B)** show short axis (SAX) and long axis (LAX) multiplanar reconstruction (MPR) of *in-vivo* CMR with the location of the corresponding diastolic EGM [column **(D)**] indicated by a red sphere. Column **(C)** shows SAX MPR of *in-vivo* CMR with segmentation of scar (yellow) and heterogeneous tissue (HT) (red) superimposed.

89% lay within 10 mm of HT. These results are illustrated in **Figure 5.**

Non-scarred Regions With Diastolic Activation During Ventricular Tachycardia

Approximately 20% of diastolic points had 0% scar/HT on *in-vivo* CMR. As noted, all regions activated during diastole during VT-HC were within 15 mm of HT. An example of EGMs recorded from a reentrant VT-HC is shown in **Figure 6**. In this example, early diastolic activation is identified within non-scarred tissue, before the wavefront continues into a region demonstrating non-transmural scar in which the remainder of the isthmus is located. On the corresponding *in-vivo* CMR and EACI data the EGMs are located adjacent to a sharp gradient in tissue thickness just outside the thinned scar region. When all locations without scar were considered, locations with diastolic activation were closer to steep gradients in tissue thickness than non-diastolic locations (diastolic locations distance = 1.2 mm (IQR 0–3.6 mm) vs. 9.7 mm (IQR 2.9–18.6 mm) for non-diastolic locations, $p < 0.001$). When diastolic locations were classified according to whether they demonstrated early, mid or late activation within the diastolic window, defined as being from the end of the QRS complex on the surface ECG, the median distance to regions of steep gradient in tissue thickness was lowest at late-diastolic sites (distance = 1.5 mm), followed by early-diastolic sites (distance = 2.8 mm) and greatest at mid-diastolic sites (distance = 3.9 mm, $p < 0.001$ for group differences and $p < 0.001$ for all pairwise comparisons).

DISCUSSION

In a chronic porcine infarct model high resolution 3D LGE-CMR acquired during contrast steady state can be used to define the structural characteristics of components of post-infarct reentrant VT circuits. Our data demonstrate that the majority of diastolic locations in this model of VT-HC are located in regions with non-transmural (<95%) scar/HT with lower tissue thickness than healthy tissue. In addition, ~20% of diastolic points during VT-HC are in non-scarred tissue that is adjacent to steep gradients in tissue thickness.

Late-Gadolinium Enhanced Imaging Under Conditions of Contrast Steady State

Establishing CSS was technically feasible and resulted in stable $TI_{myocardium}$ for prolonged periods during image acquisition. For high-resolution 3D imaging sequences used in previous

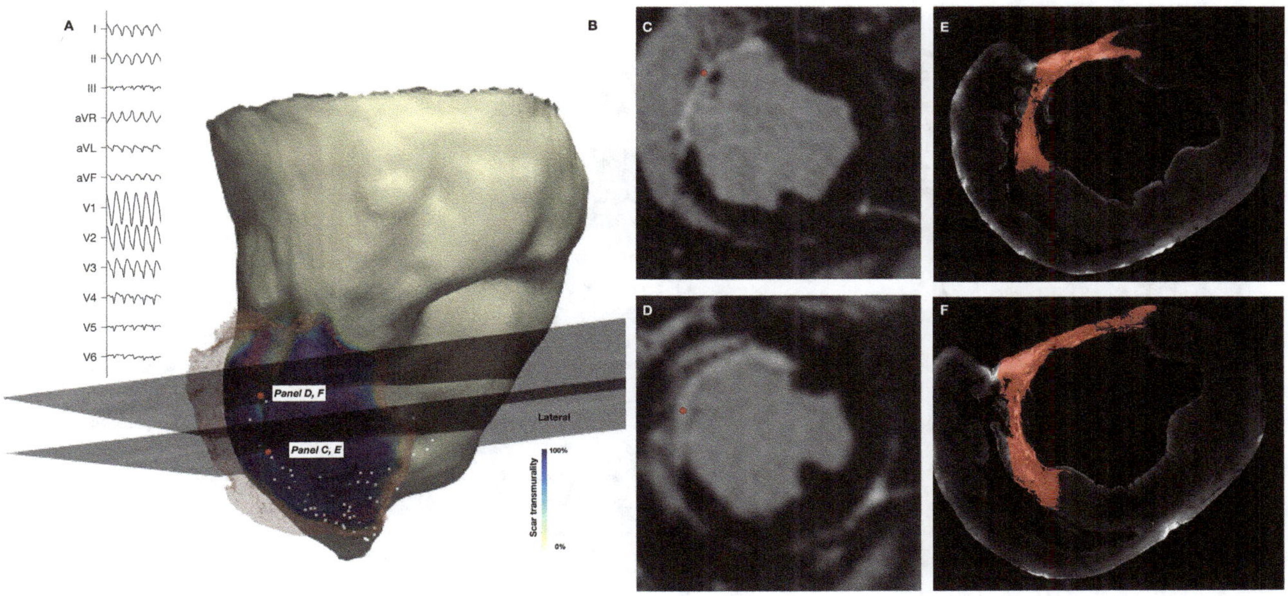

FIGURE 3 | Co-localization of diastolic locations from Electroanatomic Mapping System and *in-vivo* imaging and episcopic auto-fluorescence cryomicrotome imaging. **(A)** Surface 12-lead ECG of induced VT. **(B)** *In-vivo* CMR derived shell color coded according to scar transmurality, with translucent mesh derived from scar also shown. Location of 2 diastolic EGMs is shown (red spheres) and corresponding short axis (SAX) *in-vivo* LGE CMR slice. **(C,D)** SAX slices shown in **(B)**, with location of recorded EGM (red sphere). **(E,F)** Corresponding EACI data with segmented scar (red) superimposed.

imaging-supported VT ablation studies, $TI_{myocardium}$ drift during acquisition routinely necessitated 30–80 ms being added to the $TI_{myocardium}$ prior to the start of a 3D acquisition, which may be of up to 29 min in duration (21–23). In the present data, drift in $TI_{myocardium}$ across the course of an extended acquisition duration was always <10% and the mean was 5.2%, corresponding to an average change in $TI_{myocardium}$ of approximately 12 ms. In clinical practice, establishing CSS for 3D image acquisition even during scans of routine duration would minimize the drift in $TI_{myocardium}$ and may be helpful for optimizing image quality.

The non-standard approach to contrast delivery has not been robustly validated in this study. However, it is noted that the strategy of continuous contrast infusion, on which the protocol for the current study was based, has been validated against histological samples during extra-cellular volume mapping for the assessment of fibrosis (24). There is no consensus regarding the optimal method for thresholding LGE-CMR for scar (25), and the optimal strategy may depend on the contrast administration protocol used during imaging. The Full Width-Half Maximum technique represents a strategy with robust histological validation (26), however, clinical studies have suggested that thresholding for dense scar at 60% of the maximum SI best identifies electrophysiologically relevant left ventricular substrate. This consideration led to the current strategy being chosen for this study (17). The current study does address the unresolved issue of the optimal thresholding strategy for LGE-CMR.

The 3D LGE-CMR imaging in this study was acquired with a FA of 90° which likely resulted in reduced blood-scar contrast due to the higher T2 weighting that resulted (see **Supplementary Figure 3**). While in this study we did not feel low contrast between blood pool and scar prohibited confident identification of the blood-myocardial interface, the differentiation of endocardial scar from the blood pool could be improved in subsequent studies through using a lower flip angle. We note that this issue is encountered to some degree in all bright-blood LGE sequences and represents a motivation to the development of dark blood sequences to overcome this effect (27).

Transmurality of Scar

The calculated transmurality of scar in locations with diastolic activation reported here is lower than has been reported previously. In previous reports, mean scar transmurality at VT isthmus sites assessed using 2D 1.4 x 1.4 x 8 mm^3 LGE-CMR with scar segmented according to a Full-width at half-maximum (FWHM) threshold was 60 ± 38% (28) or using a similar 2D LGE-CMR imaging 66 ± 22%, which rose to 76 ± 16% at sites of concealed entrainment and to 70 ± 21% at termination sites (29). The use of 2D imaging, bolus contrast administration and different image analysis protocols used in previous experiments is likely to contribute to observed differences in scar transmurality. In addition, there may be mechanistic differences between the VT-HC described here and VTs studied previously, both of which included at least some hemodynamically tolerated VTs. Early reports of hemodynamically tolerated scar-mediated VT often localized the isthmus to within a thin walled LV aneurysm, which would likely be identified on CMR imaging as transmural scar (30, 31). In contrast, the re-entrant VT-HC observed in this study displayed a greater dependence on

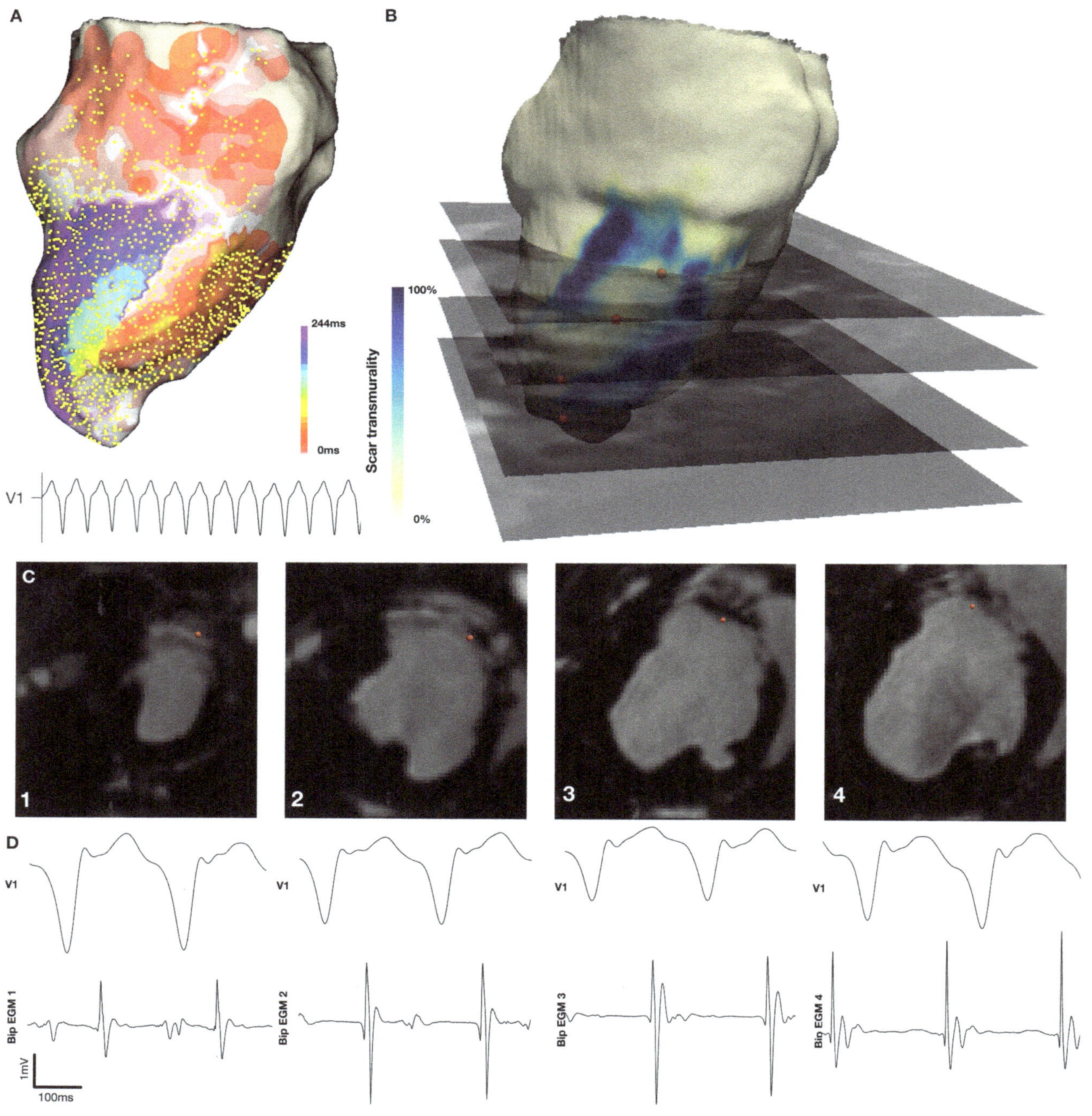

FIGURE 4 | Localization of diastolic locations on *in-vivo* CMR imaging. **(A)** Activation map demonstrating re-entrant VT with a figure 8 pattern of re-entry. **(B)** CMR derived mesh color coded according to scar transmurality with location of selected diastolic EGMs indicated by red sphere and corresponding *in-vivo* LGE CMR imaging indicated. **(C)** Diastolic EGM and corresponding location on *in-vivo* CMR at four sequential points along the diastolic isthmus of this VT.

functional rather than fixed conduction block, suggesting that the structural substrate of VT-HC may be distinct from slower and hemodynamically tolerated VTs. In addition, the use of high-resolution imaging and the measures taken to minimize artifact in this report may have contributed to an increased sensitivity for the identification of tissue with preserved viability and reduced the calculated scar transmurality at sites with diastolic activation.

Tissue Thickness

Tissue thickness has been demonstrated to be a sensitive structural marker for arrhythmogenic tissue in the post-MI

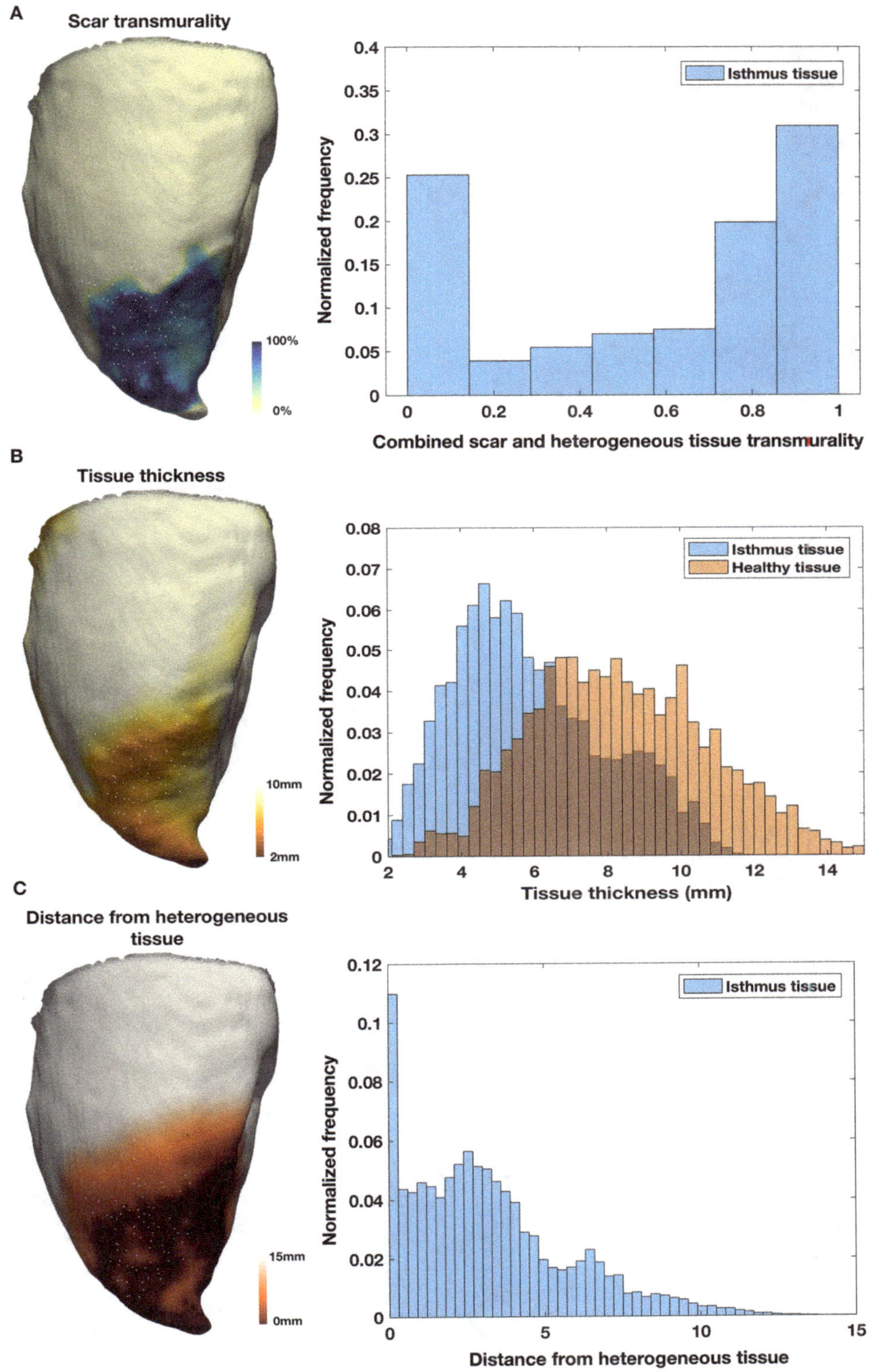

FIGURE 5 | Tissue characteristics of diastolic locations. **(A)** Example of LGE CMR derived endocardial shell color coded according tc scar transmurality and demonstrating antero-septal infarction. Histogram shows combined scar/heterogeneous tissue (HT) transmurality pooled from all locations activated during diastole in all pigs. **(B)** Example of LGE CMR derived endocardial shell color coded according to tissue thickness. Histogram shows tissue thickness pooled from all diastolic locations (blue) in all pigs compared with tissue thickness at the location of normal EGMs pooled from all pigs (red). **(C)** Example of LGE CMR derived endocardial shell color coded according to distance from HT. Histogram shows distance from HT pooled from all diastolic locations in six pigs.

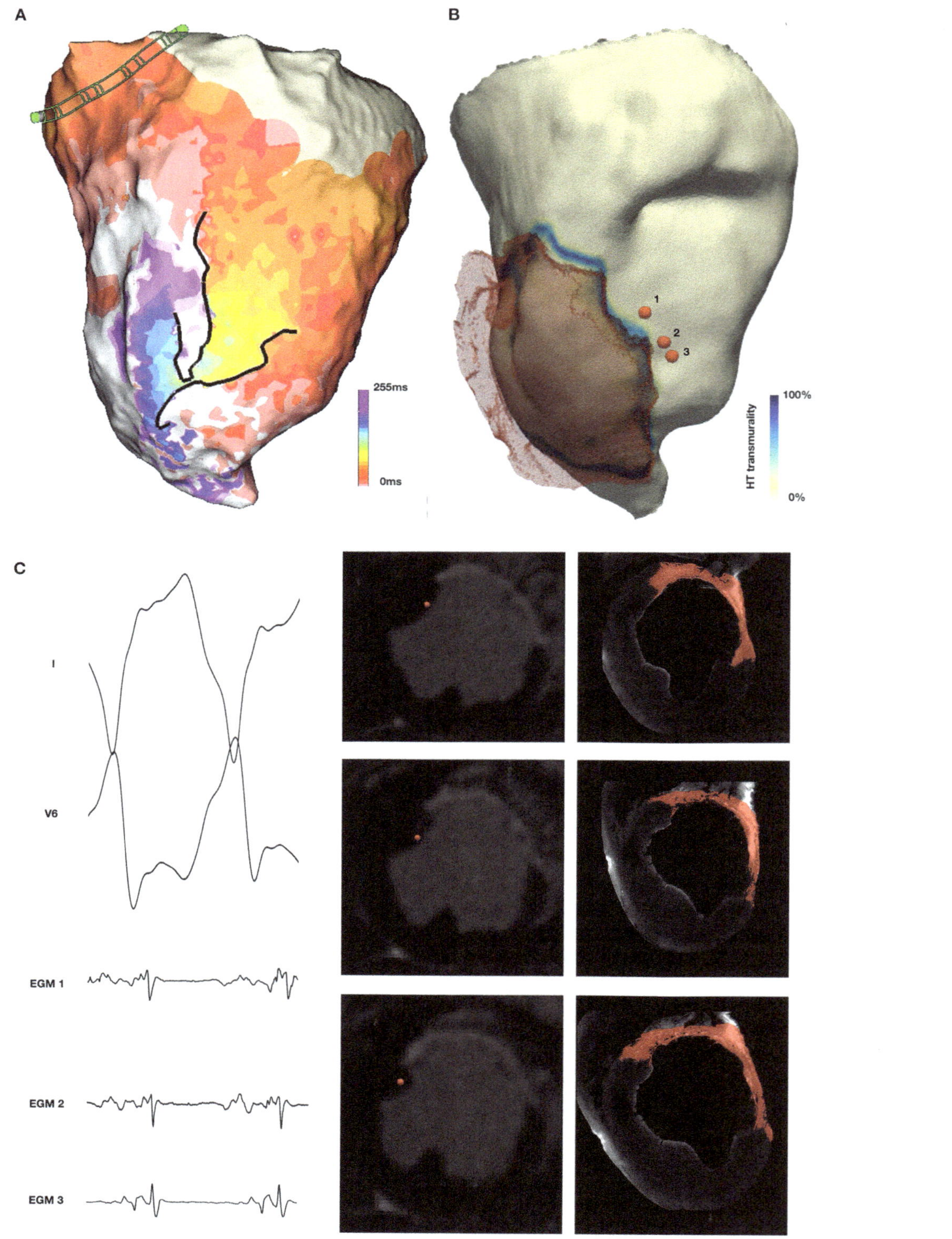

FIGURE 6 | Non-scarred tissue demonstrating diastolic activation during VT. **(A)** Activation map during VT demonstrating diastolic activation during VT (yellow to purple) with a converging pattern of activation toward a narrow channel (green) which subsequently widens prior to multiple systolic breakouts (red). **(B)** *In-vivo* CMR derived shell with translucent mesh of scar overlaid and color coded according to HT transmurality. The location of 3 early diastolic EGMs is indicated by red spheres. **(C)** Early diastolic EGM, short axis (SAX) *in-vivo* CMR and corresponding EACI imaging at locations 1, 2 and 3 demonstrating location of EGMs in tissue proximal to scar, but without enhancement in the wall at this location.

LV when assessed using coronary computed tomographic angiography (CCTA) (32). Among patients undergoing catheter ablation of drug refractory post-MI scar-related VT, 98% have been reported to demonstrate wall thinning on CCTA (32). As well as demonstrating a strong relationship between low voltage regions and local abnormal ventricular activations (LAVA), 89% of RF termination sites were located within the imaging substrate [defined as regions of wall thinning (tissue thickness < 5 mm) or severe wall thinning (tissue thickness < 2 mm)], with the majority of these located within 10 mm of the margin. The data presented here also indicate that regions of diastolic activation during VT-HC tend to be thinner than healthy tissue. However, examination of the histograms shown in Figure demonstrates that there is significant overlap between the tissue thickness assessed with diastolic activation and healthy tissue, and therefore tissue thickness alone would not adequately differentiate regions of diastolic activation during VT from healthy tissue. In the present study, the shorter VT cycle length and dependence of the VTs on functional rather than fixed anatomical conduction block, as might be expected in an aneurysm demonstrating severe wall thinning, suggests a possible explanation for why diastolic activation during VT was observed in tissue with a wider range of thicknesses than in previous reports which have used CT imaging.

Non-enhancing Tissue Activated During Diastole in VT

Approximately 20% of diastolic locations present were found in locations with no scar/HT identified on *in-vivo* imaging. This tissue was located in close proximity to HT and adjacent to steep gradients in tissue thickness. The diastolic activation of such tissue has not been previously demonstrated in the reentrant paths of hemodynamically tolerated VT. This tissue may include regions of tissue with microscopic fibrosis that occurs adjacent to scar and that is not identified by *in-vivo* LGE-CMR imaging but is likely to demonstrate distinct electrophysiological properties that promote its participation in VT-HC. Intrinsic tissue anisotropy at the scar interface, which may be enhanced in diseased ventricular tissue (33), is also likely to affect conduction behavior in this region. In canine models of scar related re-entry, it is established that the arc of functional conduction block responsible for the initiation of reentry localizes to regions of sharp gradients in tissue thickness and previous experiments have demonstrated that conduction velocity during pacing in this model is slower in regions of steep gradients in tissue thickness (34). In addition, the lowest conduction velocity (CV) in the re-entrant circuits of VTs in the same model may be found at exit sites (35). A wave of depolarization slows when transitioning from a small to a larger body of tissue due to the dispersion of the small source transmembrane current to a large number of downstream cells (source-sink mismatch) (36) and due to wavefront curvature that is a consequence of the geometric expansion of tissue encountered by a propagating wavefront. These observations suggest a mechanistic explanation for the diastolic activation of non-scarred tissue adjacent to steep gradients in tissue thickness in the reentrant path of VT-HC defined by functional conduction block, and the greatest proximity of the late diastolic component to these areas.

Unique Anatomical Characteristics of the Isthmus

In this study, tissue with scar/HT transmurality and tissue thickness across a wide range has been identified as activated during the diastolic component of the reentrant VT-HC studied. In a previous study of porcine post-MI VT-HC (10), despite high-resolution *ex-vivo* CMR (0.4 x 0.4 x 0.4 mm^3), anatomic features distinguishing HT harboring diastolic activation during VT from non-participating HT were not identified. At a histological level, structural differences exist between regions harboring a critical diastolic isthmus that distinguish this tissue from other HT (37). However, since it was impossible to identify these differences using high resolution *ex-vivo* CMR, it is extremely unlikely that such arrhythmogenic HT would be distinguishable from non-arrhythmogenic HT with CMR at current *in-vivo* resolution. The tissue in which the diastolic isthmus of VT-HC is expected to be located has been characterized in this model, however the current data does not indicate that within regions of non-transmural scar/HT, arrhythmogenic and non-arrhythmogenic substrate may be differentiated.

Limitations

Activation mapping alone was used to characterize the VT-HC circuits in this study. Entrainment mapping to confirm participation of the regions with diastolic activation was attempted but not routinely achieved and this represents a limitation of the presented data. The registration of electrophysiology and imaging data represents a major challenge when attempting to establish the structural basis for observed electrophysiological phenomena. Despite meticulous care in the registration between LGE-CMR and EAMS data, it is acknowledged that registration error has not been avoided entirely. Establishing the correct rotation around the long axis of the LV remains a significant challenge even with the use of coronary ostia and other anatomical landmarks as guidance. Change in the shape of the LV between the time of electrophysiology procedures and imaging are expected due to differences in the loading conditions, which represents an additional challenge, as do absolute limitations in the accuracy of the localization of EGM signals. The degree to which registration error affects the accuracy of results is difficult to quantify and is not accurately described by surface distance between EAMS and imaging data. There is no consensus regarding the optimal threshold to apply in order to accurately identify scar on LGE-CMR (25). The challenge of quantitatively assessing scar and fibrosis are compounded by differences in imaging parameters and contrast administration protocols, which will affect degree of hyperenhancement of tissue. The absence of standard histological data from this study due to the destructive nature of the EACI process is a further limitation of the current study and prohibits formal validation of the imaging data. Common to most large animal pre-clinical studies, this study included a relatively small number of animals, in consideration of minimizing the use of animals in experiments and cost. Despite density electrophysiological mapping data demonstrate that the imaging acquired and processing strategy reliably identified electrophysiologically relevant tissue in this model.

CONCLUSIONS

The structural characteristics of the tissue demonstrating diastolic activation during reentrant VT-HC, including non-transmural scar, mildly decreased tissue thickness and steep gradients in tissue thickness, are likely to promote functional conduction block which is demonstrated to be an important mechanism underlying the VT-HC observed in this model. The late diastolic segment of activation during VT-HC is closest to steep gradients in tissue thickness which may be a contributory factor to the maximal wavefront slowing seen in this region. The characterization of the myocardial substrate for post-MI scar mediated VT-HC could form the basis for imaging criteria to define ablation targets during future trials.

AUTHOR CONTRIBUTIONS

JW: conceived and designed study, analyzed data and prepared first draft and subsequent modifications of the manuscript. RN and SR: designed and implemented CMR protocols, assisted in acquisition of imaging and contributed to analysis of data. SK: contributed to experimental design, assisted with acquisition of electroanatomic mapping data, and contributed to analysis of data. AC: key contribution to analysis of electrophysiologic data. TA: planning and acquisition of electrophysiological data. JC, MW, and JS: electrophysiologist who acquired electro-anatomic mapping data. RK: developed computational tools for registration of imaging and electrophysiologic data. BM, CRi, SM, and LC: development of VA-ECMO protocol for hemodynamic support, delivery of hemodynamic support during electrophysiology studies. TI and JH: CMR reader. JV and MA: development of cryomicrotome imaging protocol and processing of tissue to acquire cryomicrotome imaging and approved submitted version of manuscript. SW, LO'N, RM, HC, RR, and MO'N: involved in acquisition of CMR and electrophysiological data. RM: repeat segmentation of 3d LGE CMR imaging for inter-observer reproducibility. HC, RR, and MO'N: funding holder for study. SW, LO'N, RM, HC, RR, MO'N, CT, EA, SN, and MB: planning and study design. RR and MO'N: supervisory oversight of project. CT, EA, SN, MB, HC, RR, MO'N, RM, SW, LO'N, TI, JH, BM, CRi, SM, LC, CRo, RK, JC, MW, JS, TA, AC, SK, RN and SR: substantial modifications to previous drafts of manuscript and approved submitted version of manuscript. TA, JC, MW, JS, BM, CRi, SM, LC, CRo, TI, JH, RK, SW, LO'N, RM, CT, EA, SN, MB, HC, RR, and MO'N: analysis and interpretation of data. All authors contributed to the article and approved the submitted version.

FUNDING

This work was supported by a Medical Research Council UK Clinical Research Training Fellowship (grant code MR/N001877/1) which funded JW; the Health Innovation Challenge Fund (HICF-R10-698), a parallel funding partnership between the Department of Health and the Wellcome Trust, the Wellcome Engineering and Physical Sciences Research Council (EPSRC) Centre for Medical Engineering at King's College London (WT203148/Z/16/Z); EPSRC grant (EP/R010935/1); National Institute for Health Research (NIHR) Biomedical Research Centre award to Guy's and St Thomas' National Health Service (NHS) Foundation Trust in partnership with King's College London, and by the NIHR Healthcare Technology Co-operative for Cardiovascular Disease at Guy's and St Thomas' NHS Foundation Trust. The views expressed are those of the author(s) and not necessarily those of the NHS, the NIHR or the Department of Health. The CardioHelp machine and all ECMO consumables were donated by Maquet, Getinge Group without conditions on their use. The Precision and Claris system and all EP mapping consumables were donated by Abbott without conditions on their use. This research was funded in whole, or in part, by the Wellcome Trust [Grant Number WT203148/Z/16/Z]. For the purpose of open access, the author has applied a CC BY public copyright licence to any Author Accepted manuscript version arising from this submission. This project was supported by the National Institute of General Medical Sciences of the National Institutes of Health [Grant Numbers P41 GM103545 and R24 GM136986]. SW was supported by British Heart Foundation [Grant Number FS/20/26/34952].

ACKNOWLEDGMENTS

We are grateful to the Abbott UK, France and US teams who generously loaned the Precision and Claris systems for these experiments, provided outstanding technical support and donated all the EP mapping catheters, cables and consumables, Sagar Haval, Lynn Calvert and the Maquet, Getinge Group whq generously provided a CardioHelp machine, provided technica support and donated all the ECMO consumables as well as Sophie Pernot and the staff at the Institute de Chirurgie Guidée par l'image (IHU), Strasbourg, France for their support for these experiments and the outstanding animal care they provided. We are grateful to Professor Maria Siebes for her assistance with establishing the protocol for and assistance with the processing of the cryomicrotome imaging.

REFERENCES

Mehra R, Zeiler RH, Gough WB, El-Sherif N. Reentrant ventricular arrhythmias in the late myocardial infarction period. 9 electrophysiologic- anatomic correlation of reentrant circuits. *Circulation.* (1983) 67:11- 24. doi: 10.1161/01.CIR.67.1.11

El-Sherif N, Smith RA, Evans K. Canine ventricular arrhythmias in the late myocardial infarction period. 8 epicardial mapping of reentrant circuits. *Circ Res.* (1981) 49:255–65. doi: 10.1161/01.RES.49.1.255

Qin D, Zhang Z-H, Caref EB, Boutjdir M, Jain P, El-Sherif N. Cellular and ionic basis of arrhythmias in postinfarction remodeled ventricular myocardium. *Circ Res.* (1996) 79:461–73. doi: 10.1161/01.RES.79.3.461

Stevenson WG, Friedman PL, Sager PT, Saxon LA, Kocovic D, Harada T, et al. Exploring postinfarction reentrant ventricular tachycardia with entrainment mapping. *J Am Coll Cardiol.* (1997) 29:1180–9. doi: 10.1016/S0735-1097(97)00065-X

Tung R, Mathuria N, Michowitz Y, Yu R, Buch E, Bradfield J, et al. Functional pace-mapping responses for identification of targets for catheter ablation of scar-mediated ventricular tachycardia. *Circ Arrhythmia Electrophysiol.* (2012) 5:264–72. doi: 10.1161/CIRCEP.111.967976

Jaïs P, Maury P, Khairy P, Sacher F, Nault I, Komatsu Y, et al. Elimination of local abnormal ventricular activities : a new end point for substrate modification in patients with scar-related ventricular tachycardia. *Circulation.* (2012) 125:2184–96. doi: 10.1161/CIRCULATIONAHA.111.0 43216

Al-Khatib SM, Stevenson WG, Ackerman MJ, Bryant WJ, Callans DJ, Curtis AB, et al. 2017 AHA/ACC/HRS guideline for management of patients with ventricular arrhythmias and the prevention of sudden cardiac death: a report of the American College of Cardiology/American Heart Association Task Force on Clinical Practice Guidelines and the Heart Rhythm Society. *Circulation.* (2018) 138:e272–391. doi: 10.1016/j.hrthm.2017.10.036

Dukkipati SR, Koruth JS, Choudry S, Miller MA, Whang W, Reddy VY. Catheter ablation of ventricular tachycardia in structural heart disease: indications, strategies, and outcomes—part II. *J Am Coll Cardiol.* (2017) 70:2924–41. doi: 10.1016/j.jacc.2017.10.030

Schelbert EB, Hsu LY, Anderson SA, Mohanty BD, Karim SM, Kellman P, et al. Late gadolinium-enhancement cardiac magnetic resonance identifies postinfarction myocardial fibrosis and the border zone at the near cellular level in ex vivo rat heart. *Circ Cardiovasc Imaging.* (2010) 3:743- 52. doi: 10.1161/CIRCIMAGING.108.835793

Ashikaga H, Sasano T, Dong J, Zviman MM, Evers R, Hopenfeld B, et al. Magnetic resonance-based anatomical analysis of scar-related ventricular tachycardia: implications for catheter ablation. *Circ Res.* (2007) 101:939- 47. doi: 10.1161/CIRCRESAHA.107.158980

Piers SRD, Tao Q, De Riva Silva M, Siebelink HM, Schalij MJ, Van Der Geest RJ, et al. CMR-based identification of critical isthmus sites of ischemic and nonischemic ventricular tachycardia. *JACC Cardiovasc Imaging.* (2014) 7:774–84. doi: 10.1016/j.jcmg.2014.03.013

Androulakis A, Zeppenfeld K, Paiman E, Venlet J, CA G, Schalij M, et al. Scar transmurality and composition derived from LGE MRI predicts VT. *Eur Heart J.* (2017) 38:Supplement:4088314. doi: 10.1093/eurheartj/ehx502.2017

Andreu D, Penela D, Acosta J, Fernández-Armenta J, Perea RJ, Soto- Iglesias D, et al. Cardiac magnetic resonance–aided scar dechanneling: influence on acute and long-term outcomes. *Hear Rhythm.* (2017) 14:1121- 8. doi: 10.1016/j.hrthm.2017.05.018

Sacher F, Tedrow UB, Field ME, Raymond JM, Koplan BA, Epstein LM, et al. Ventricular tachycardia ablation: evolution of patients and procedures over 8 years. *Circ Arrhythm Electrophysiol.* (2008) 1:153- 61. doi: 10.1161/CIRCEP.108.769471

Josephson ME, Anter E. Substrate mapping for ventricular tachycardia assumptions and misconceptions. *JACC Clin Electrophysiol.* (2015) 1:341- 52. doi: 10.1016/j.jacep.2015.09.001

Whitaker J, Tschabrunn CM, Jang J, Leshem E, O'Neill M, Manning WJ, et al. Cardiac MR characterization of left ventricular remodeling in a swine model of infarct followed by reperfusion. *J Magn Reson Imaging.* (2018) 48:808–17. doi: 10.1002/jmri.26005

Andreu D, Berruezo A, Ortiz-Pérez JT, Silva E, Mont L, Borràs R, et al. Integration of 3D electroanatomic maps and magnetic resonance scar characterization into the navigation system to guide ventricular tachycardia ablation. *Circ Arrhythmia Electrophysiol.* (2011) 4:674–83. doi: 10.1161/CIRCEP.111.961946

Bishop M, Rajani R, Plank G, Gaddum N, Carr-White G, Wright M, et al. Three-dimensional atrial wall thickness maps to inform catheter ablation procedures for atrial fibrillation. *Europace.* (2016) 18:376- 83. doi: 10.1093/europace/euv073

Wellens H, Brugada P, Stevenson WG. Programmed electrical stimulation of the heart in patients with life-threatening ventricular arrhythmias: what is the significance of induced arrhythmias and what is the correc stimulation protocol? *Circulation.* (1985) 72:1–8. doi: 10.1161/01.CIR.72.1.1

van Horssen P, van den Wijngaard JPHM, Brandt MJ, Hoefer IE, Spaan JAE, Siebes M. Perfusion territories subtended by penetrating coronary arteries increase in size and decrease in number toward the subendocardium. *Am J Physiol Circ Physiol.* (2013) 306:H496–504. doi: 10.1152/ajpheart.00584.2013

Fernández-Armenta J, Berruezo A, Andreu D, Camara O, Silva E, Serra L, et al. Three-dimensional architecture of scar and conducting channels based on high resolution ce-CMR: insights for ventricular tachycardia ablation. *Circ Arrhythmia Electrophysiol.* (2013) 6:528–37. doi: 10.1161/CIRCEP.113.000264

Andreu D, Ortiz-Pérez JT, Fernández-Armenta J, Guiu E, Acosta J, Prat- González S, et al. 3D delayed-enhanced magnetic resonance sequences improve conducting channel delineation prior to ventricular tachycardia ablation. *Europace.* (2015) 17:938–45. doi: 10.1093/europace/euu310

Bizino MB, Tao Q, Amersfoort J, Siebelink HJ, Bogaard PJ, Van RJ, et al. High spatial resolution free-breathing 3D late gadolinium enhancement cardiac magnetic resonance imaging in ischaemic and non-ischaemic cardiomyopathy : quantitative assessment of scar mass and image quality. *Eur Radiol.* (2018) 28:4027–35. doi: 10.1007/s00330-018-5361-y

Flett AS, Hayward MP, Ashworth MT, Hansen MS, Taylor AM, Elliott PM, et al. Equilibrium contrast cardiovascular magnetic resonance for the measurement of diffuse myocardial fibrosis: preliminary validation in humans. *Circulation.* (2010) 122:138–44. doi: 10.1161/CIRCULATIONAHA.109.930636

Schulz-Menger J, Bluemke DA, Bremerich J, Flamm SD, Fogel MA, Friedrich MG, et al. Standardized image interpretation and post-processing in cardiovascular magnetic resonance-2020 update. *J Cardiovasc Magn Reson.* (2020) 22:1–22. doi: 10.1186/s12968-020-00610-6

Amado LC, Gerber BL, Gupta SN, Rettmann DW, Szarf G, Schock R, et al. Accurate and objective infarct sizing by contrast-enhanced magnetic resonance imaging in a canine myocardial infarction model. *J Am Coll Cardiol.* (2004) 44:2383–9. doi: 10.1016/j.jacc.2004.09.020

Ginami G, Neji R, Rashid I, Chiribiri A, Ismail TF, Botnar RM, et al. 3D whole-heart phase sensitive inversion recovery CMR for simultaneous black-blood late gadolinium enhancement and bright-blood coronary CMR angiography. *J Cardiovasc Magn Reson.* (2017) 19:1–14. doi: 10.1186/s12968-017-0405-z

Desjardins B, Crawford T, Good E, Oral H, Chugh A, Pelosi F, et al. Infarct architecture and characteristics on delayed enhanced magnetic resonance imaging and electroanatomic mapping in patients with postinfarction ventricular arrhythmia. *Hear Rhythm.* (2009) 6:644–51. doi: 10.1016/j.hrthm.2009.02.018

Piers SRD, Everaerts K, Van Der Geest RJ, Hazebroek MR, Siebelink HM, Pison LAFG, et al. Myocardial scar predicts monomorphic ventricular tachycardia but not polymorphic ventricular tachycardia or ventricular fibrillation in nonischemic dilated cardiomyopathy. *Hear Rhythm.* (2015) 12:2106–14. doi: 10.1016/j.hrthm.2015.05.026

Josephson ME, Horowitz LN, Farshidi A, Spear JF, Kastor JA, Moore EN. Recurrent sustained ventricular tachycardia. 2 endocardial mapping. *Circulation.* (1978) 57:431–40. doi: 10.1161/01.CIR.57.3.440

Okumura K, Olshansky B, Henthorn RW, Epstein AE, Plumb VJ, Waldo AL. Demonstration of the presence of slow conduction during sustained ventricular tachycardia in man: use of transient entrainment of the tachycardia. *Circulation.* (1987) 75:369–78. doi: 10.1161/01.CIR.75.2.369

Yamashita S, Sacher F, Mahida S, Berte B, Lim HS, Komatsu Y, et al. Image integration to guide catheter ablation in scar-related ventricular tachycardia. *J Cardiovasc Electrophysiol.* (2016) 27:699–708. doi: 10.1111/jce.12963

Glukhov AV, Fedorov VV, Kalish PW, Ravikumar VK, Lou Q, Janks D, et al. Conduction remodeling in human end- stage nonischemic left ventricular cardiomyopathy. *Circulation.* (2012) 125:1835–47. doi: 10.1161/CIRCULATIONAHA.111.0 47274

Jang J, Whitaker J, Leshem E, Ngo L, Neisus U, Nakamori S, et al. Local conduction velocity in the presence of late gadolinium enhancement and myocardial wall thinning: a cardiac magnetic resonance study in a swine model of healed left ventricular infarction. *Circ Arrhythm Electrophysiol.* (2019) 12:e007175. doi: 10.1161/CIRCEP.119.0 07175

Anter E, Tschabrunn CM, Buxton AE, Josephson ME. High- resolution mapping of postinfarction reentrant ventricular tachycardia: electrophysiological characterization of the circuit. *Circulation.* (2016) 134:314–27. doi: 10.1161/CIRCULATIONAHA.116.021955

Fast VG, Klkber AG. Cardiac tissue geometry as a determinant of unidirectional conduction block: assessment of microscopic excitation spread by optical mapping in patterned cell cultures and in a computer model. *Cardiovasc Res.* (1995) 29:697–707.

Dhanjal TS, Lellouche N, von Ruhland CJ, Abehsira G, Edwards DH, Dubois-Randé JL, et al. Massive accumulation of myofibroblasts in the critical isthmus is associated with ventricular tachycardia inducibility in post-infarct swine heart. *JACC Clin Electrophysiol.* (2017) 3:703–14. doi: 10.1016/j.jacep.2016.11.010

Permissions

All chapters in this book were first published by Frontiers; hereby published with permission under the Creative Commons Attribution License or equivalent. Every chapter published in this book has been scrutinized by our experts. Their significance has been extensively debated. The topics covered herein carry significant findings which will fuel the growth of the discipline. They may even be implemented as practical applications or may be referred to as a beginning point for another development.

The contributors of this book come from diverse backgrounds, making this book a truly international effort. This book will bring forth new frontiers with its revolutionizing research information and detailed analysis of the nascent developments around the world.

We would like to thank all the contributing authors for lending their expertise to make the book truly unique. They have played a crucial role in the development of this book. Without their invaluable contributions this book wouldn't have been possible. They have made vital efforts to compile up to date information on the varied aspects of this subject to make this book a valuable addition to the collection of many professionals and students.

This book was conceptualized with the vision of imparting up-to-date information and advanced data in this field. To ensure the same, a matchless editorial board was set up. Every individual on the board went through rigorous rounds of assessment to prove their worth. After which they invested a large part of their time researching and compiling the most relevant data for our readers.

The editorial board has been involved in producing this book since its inception. They have spent rigorous hours researching and exploring the diverse topics which have resulted in the successful publishing of this book. They have passed on their knowledge of decades through this book. To expedite this challenging task, the publisher supported the team at every step. A small team of assistant editors was also appointed to further simplify the editing procedure and attain best results for the readers.

Apart from the editorial board, the designing team has also invested a significant amount of their time in understanding the subject and creating the most relevant covers. They scrutinized every image to scout for the most suitable representation of the subject and create an appropriate cover for the book.

The publishing team has been an ardent support to the editorial, designing and production team. Their endless efforts to recruit the best for this project, has resulted in the accomplishment of this book. They are a veteran in the field of academics and their pool of knowledge is as vast as their experience in printing. Their expertise and guidance has proved useful at every step. Their uncompromising quality standards have made this book an exceptional effort. Their encouragement from time to time has been an inspiration for everyone.

The publisher and the editorial board hope that this book will prove to be a valuable piece of knowledge for researchers, students, practitioners and scholars across the globe.

List of Contributors

Scott A. Kanner
Doctoral Program in Neurobiology and Behavior, Columbia University College of Physicians and Surgeons, New York, NY, United States

Ananya Jain
Department of Physiology and Cellular Biophysics, Columbia University College of Physicians and Surgeons, New York, NY, United States

Henry M. Colecraft
Doctoral Program in Neurobiology and Behavior, Columbia University College of Physicians and Surgeons, New York, NY, United States
Department of Physiology and Cellular Biophysics, Columbia University College of Physicians and Surgeons, New York, NY, United States
Department of Pharmacology, Columbia University College of Physicians and Surgeons, New York, NY, United States

Stefan Van Duijvenboden, Pier Lambiase and Peter Taggart
Institute of Cardiovascular Science, University College London, London, United Kingdom

Bradley Porter, Baldeep Sidhu and Justin Gould
School of Imaging Sciences and Biomedical Engineering, King's College London, London, United Kingdom

Martin J. Bishop and Reza Razavi
School of Imaging Sciences and Biomedical Engineering, King's College London, London, United Kingdom
School of Biomedical Engineering and Imaging Sciences, King's College, London, United Kingdom

David Adolfo Sampedro-Puente and Jesus Fernandez-Bes
BSICOS Group, I3A, IIS Aragón, University of Zaragoza, Zaragoza, Spain

Esther Pueyo
BSICOS Group, I3A, IIS Aragón, University of Zaragoza, Zaragoza, Spain
CIBER-BBN, Madrid, Spain

Ben Hanson
Department of Mechanical Engineering, University College London, London, United Kingdom

Christopher A. Rinaldi and Jaswinder S. Gill
Guy's and St Thomas' NHS Foundation Trust, London, United Kingdom

Tarvinder K. Taneja, Donghui Ma, Bo Y. Kim and Paul A. Welling
Department of Physiology, Maryland Center for Kidney Discovery, School of Medicine, University of Maryland, Baltimore, Baltimore, MD, United States

Gianfranco Piccirillo, Federica Moscucci, Marcella Fabietti, Ilaria Parrotta, Fabiola Mastropietri, Claudia Di Iorio, Teresa Sabatino, Davide Crapanzano, Giulia Vespignani, Marco Valerio Mariani and Nicolò Salvi
Dipartimento di Scienze Cardiovascolari, Respiratorie, Geriatriche, Anestesiologiche e Nefrologiche, Policlinico Umberto I, "La Sapienza" University of Rome, Rome, Italy

Damiano Magrì
Dipartimento di Medicina Clinica e Molecolare, S. Andrea Hospital, "Sapienza" University of Rome, Rome, Italy

Allison R. Hall, Jennifer L. Smith and Brian P. Delisle
Department of Physiology, University of Kentucky, Lexington, KY, United States

Corey L. Anderson and Craig T. January
Cellular and Molecular Arrhythmia Research Program, University of Wisconsin–Madison, Madison, WI, United States

Tooraj Mirshahi
Department of Molecular and Functional Genomics, Genomic Medicine Institute, Geisinger Clinic, Danville, PA, United States

Claude S. Elayi
Department of Cardiology, Gill Heart Institute, University of Kentucky, Lexington, KY, United States

N. Sydney Moïse and Romain Pariaut
College of Veterinary Medicine, Department of Clinical Sciences, Cornell University, Ithaca, NY, United States

Wyatt H. Flanders
Department of Physics, University of Washington, Seattle, WA, United States

Joanne J. A. van Bavel and Marcel A. G. van der Heyden
Department of Medical Physiology, Division of Heart and Lungs, University Medical Center Utrecht, Utrecht, Netherlands

Maria Teresa La Rovere
Department of Cardiology, IRCCS Istituti Clinici Scientifici Maugeri, Montescano (Pavia), Italy

Peter J. Schwartz
Center for Cardiac Arrhythmias of Genetic Origin and Laboratory of Cardiovascular Genetics, Istituto Auxologico Italiano, IRCCS, Milan, Italy

Mona M. El Refaey
Dorothy M. Davis Heart and Lung Research Institute, Wexner Medical Center, The Ohio State University, Columbus, OH, United States
Department of Physiology & Cell Biology, Wexner Medical Center, The Ohio State University, Columbus, OH, United States

Peter J. Mohler
Dorothy M. Davis Heart and Lung Research Institute, Wexner Medical Center, The Ohio State University, Columbus, OH, United States
Department of Physiology & Cell Biology, Wexner Medical Center, The Ohio State University, Columbus, OH, United States
Department of Internal Medicine, Division of Cardiovascular Medicine, College of Medicine, Wexner Medical Center, The Ohio State University, Columbus, OH, United States

David Jaap Sprenkeler, Jet D. M. Beekman, Alexandre Bossu, Albert Dunnink and Marc A. Vos
Department of Medical Physiology, Division of Heart and Lungs, University Medical Center Utrecht, Utrecht, Netherlands

Raquel G. Utrilla, Paloma Nieto-Marín, Silvia Alfayate, David Tinaquero, Marcos Matamoros, Marta Pérez-Hernández, Lorena Ondo, Juan Tamargo, Eva Delpón and Ricardo Caballero
Department of Pharmacology, School of Medicine, Instituto de Investigación Sanitaria Gregorio Marañón, Universidad Complutense, Madrid, Spain
CIBERCV, Madrid, Spain

Sandra Sacristán
CIBERCV, Madrid, Spain

Raquel de Andrés and F. Javier Díez-Guerra
Departamento de Biología Molecular and Centro de Biología Molecular "Severo Ochoa" (UAM-CSIC), Universidad Autónoma de Madrid, Madrid, Spain

Faez Al-Amodi
Institute of Cardiovascular Sciences, University College London, London, United Kingdom

Michele Orini
Institute of Cardiovascular Sciences, University College London, London, United Kingdom
The William Harvey Research Institute, Queen Mary University of London, London, United Kingdom
Department of Clinical Pharmacology, Queen Mary University of London, London, United Kingdom

Stefan Koelsch
Department of Biological and Medical Psychology, University of Bergen, Bergen, Norway

Raquel Bailón
Aragon Institute for Engineering Research, University of Zaragoza, Zaragoza, Spain
Center for Biomedical Research in the Network in Bioengineering, Biomaterials and Nanomedicine (CIBER-BBN), Madrid, Spain

Beatrice Bianchi, Lijo Cherian Ozhathil and Hugues Abriel
Swiss National Centre of Competence in Research (NCCR) TransCure, Institute of Biochemistry and Molecular Medicine, University of Bern, Bern, Switzerland

Argelia Medeiros-Domingo
Department of Cardiology, Inselspital, University Hospital Bern, Bern, Switzerland

Michael H. Gollob
Department of Medicine, Peter Munk Cardiac Centre, Toronto General Hospital, University of Toronto, Toronto, ON, Canada

Richard Ang
Centre for Cardiovascular and Metabolic Neuroscience, Neuroscience, Physiology and Pharmacology, University College London, London, United Kingdom

Nephtali Marina
Centre for Cardiovascular and Metabolic Neuroscience, Neuroscience, Physiology and Pharmacology, University College London, London, United Kingdom
Division of Medicine, University College London, London, United Kingdom

Elise Balse
Unité de Recherche sur les Maladies Cardiovasculaires, le Métabolisme et la Nutrition, Faculté de Médecine Pitié-Salpêtrière, Sorbonne Universités, UPMC Univ. Paris VI, Inserm, UMRS 1166, Université Pierre et Marie Curie, Paris, France

Hannah E. Boycott
Department of Cardiovascular Medicine, John Radcliffe Hospital, University of Oxford, Oxford, United Kingdom

Beatrice De Maria and Laura Adelaide Dalla Vecchia
IRCCS Istituti Clinici Scientifici Maugeri, Milan, Italy

Vlasta Bari and Emanuele Vaini
Department of Cardiothoracic, Vascular Anesthesia and Intensive Care, IRCCS Policlinico San Donato, Milan, Italy

Andrea Sgoifo and Luca Carnevali
Stress Physiology Laboratory, Department of Chemistry, Life Sciences and Environmental Sustainability, University of Parma, Parma, Italy
Microbiome Research Hub, University of Parma, Parma, Italy

Alberto Porta
Department of Cardiothoracic, Vascular Anesthesia and Intensive Care, IRCCS Policlinico San Donato, Milan, Italy
Department of Biomedical Sciences for Health, University of Milan, Milan, Italy

Beatrice Cairo
Department of Biomedical Sciences for Health, University of Milan, Milan, Italy

Aparecida Maria Catai and Anielle Cristhine de Medeiros Takahashi
Department of Physiotherapy, Federal University of São Carlos, São Carlos, Brazil

Vincent Portero, Simona Casini and Carol Ann Remme
Department of Experimental Cardiology, Academic Medical Center, Amsterdam, Netherlands

Ronald Wilders
Department of Medical Biology, Academic Medical Center, Amsterdam, Netherlands

Arie O. Verkerk
Department of Experimental Cardiology, Academic Medical Center, Amsterdam, Netherlands
Department of Medical Biology, Academic Medical Center, Amsterdam, Netherlands

Flavien Charpentier
L'Institut du Thorax, INSERM, CNRS, Université de Nantes, Nantes, France

Nnamdi Edokobi and Lori L. Isom
Department of Pharmacology, University of Michigan Medical School, Ann Arbor, MI, United States

Ying Fu, Shan-Shan Zhang, Shaohua Xiao, Wassim A. Basheer, Rachel Baum and Irina Epifantseva
Cedars-Sinai Medical Center, Cedars-Sinai Heart Institute, Los Angeles, CA, United States

TingTing Hong and Robin M. Shaw
Cedars-Sinai Medical Center, Cedars-Sinai Heart Institute, Los Angeles, CA, United States
Department of Medicine, University of California, Los Angeles, Los Angeles, CA, United States

Ling-cong Kong, Tian Shuang, Zheng Li, Zhi-guo Zou, Wen-long Jiang, Jun Pu and Xin-hua Wang
Department of Cardiology, Ren Ji Hospital, Shanghai Jiao Tong University School of Medicine, Shanghai, China

Shulin Wu
Department of Cardiology, Guangdong Cardiovascular Institute, Guangdong Provincial People's Hospital, Guangdong Academy of Medical Sciences, Guangzhou, China

Xiao-Gang Guo, Qi Sun, Jian-Du Yang, Hai-Yang Xie, Shu Zhang and Jian Ma
State Key Laboratory of Cardiovascular Disease, Arrhythmia Center, National Center for Cardiovascular Diseases, Fuwai Hospital, Chinese Academy of Medical Sciences and Peking Union Medical College, Beijing, China

Hui-Qiang Wei
Department of Cardiology, Guangdong Cardiovascular Institute, Guangdong Provincial People's Hospital, Guangdong Academy of Medical Sciences, Guangzhou, China
State Key Laboratory of Cardiovascular Disease, Arrhythmia Center, National Center for Cardiovascular Diseases, Fuwai Hospital, Chinese Academy of Medical Sciences and Peking Union Medical College, Beijing, China

Gong-Bu Zhou
Department of Cardiology, Peking University Third Hospital, Beijing, China

Jackson Liang
Division of Cardiovascular Medicine, Electrophysiology Service, University of Michigan Health System, Ann Arbor, MI, United States

John Whitaker, Adam Connolly, Rashed Karim, Caroline H. Roney, James Harriso, Rahul Mukherjee, Louisa O'Neill, Henry Chubb, Steven Niederer, Sébastien Roujol and Mark O'Neill
School of Biomedical Engineering and Imaging Sciences, King's College, London, United Kingdom

Radhouene Neji
School of Biomedical Engineering and Imaging Sciences, King's College, London, United Kingdom
Siemens Healthcare, Frimley, United Kingdom

Steven Kim and Thierry Aubriot
Abbott Medical, St Paul, MN, United States

Justo Juliá Calvo and John Silberbauer
Brighton and Sussex University Hospitals NHS Trust, Brighton, United Kingdom

Tevfik F. Ismail
School of Biomedical Engineering and Imaging Sciences, King's College, London, United Kingdom
Guy's and St Thomas' NHS Foundation Trust, London, United Kingdom

Brendan Murfin, Carla Richardson, Stephen Morgan, Luigi Camporota and Matthew Wright
Guy's and St Thomas' NHS Foundation Trust, London, United Kingdom

Judith de Vos and Maurice C. G. Aalders
Department of Biomedical Engineering and Physics, Amsterdam UMC, University of Amsterdam, Amsterdam, Netherlands

Steven E. Williams
School of Biomedical Engineering and Imaging Sciences, King's College, London, United Kingdom
Centre for Cardiovascular Science, University of Edinburgh, Edinburgh, United Kingdom

Cory Tschabrunn
Division of Cardiovascular Medicine, University of Pennsylvania, Philadelphia, PA, United States

Elad Anter
Cleveland Clinic, Cleveland, OH, United States

Index

www.ingramcontent.com/pod-product-compliance
Lightning Source LLC
LaVergne TN
LVHW080927210926
848485LV00004B/748